COMPANION CD-ROM RESOURCES

DORLAND'S AUDIO PRONUNCIATIONS

ANIMATIONS

Abdominal Anatomy
Anatomy of Eye
Anoxic Brain Injury
Asthma, Pathophysiology
Bowel Resection, Detorsion
Cerebral Perfusion
Cervical Nerve Examination
CPR in the Child

Esophageal Intubation
Inefficient Bag Ventilation
Meningitis
Oxygen Desaturation
Seizure in the Infant
Spinal Tap, in Child
Volvulus, Pediatric

VIDEO CLIPS

Assessment of the Newborn

Auscultation: Breath Sounds, Posterior Chest
Auscultation: Breath Sounds, Anterior Chest
Auscultation: Heart, Anterior Chest
Auscultation: Heart, Anterior Chest
Evaluation: Chest Circumference
Evaluation: Cremasteric Reflex
Evaluation: Deep Tendon Reflex
Evaluation: Galant Reflex
Evaluation: Head Circumference
Evaluation: Legs, Symmetry, and Length
Evaluation: Moro Reflex
Evaluation: Neck Rotation
Evaluation: Plantar Grasp
Evaluation: Rooting and Sucking Reflexes
Evaluation: Stepping Reflex
Evaluation: Symmetry of Gluteal Folds
Inspection and Palpation: Head and Hair
Inspection and Palpation: Genitalia (Supine Position)
Inspection: Abdomen
Inspection: Buttocks and Anus
Inspection: External Eye
Inspection: External Genitalia
Inspection: Head
Inspection: Leg Alignment
Inspection: Male Genitalia, Circumcision
Inspection: Male Genitalia, Scrotum
Inspection: Neck, Posterior
Inspection: Nose
Inspection: Rang-of-Motion, Upper Extremities
Inspection: Skin, Back
Palpation: Abdomen
Palpation: Brachial and Femoral Pulses
Palpation: Clavicle
Palpation: Femoral Pulses
Palpation: Male Breasts (Supine Position)
Palpation: Pedal Pulses
Percussion: Chest and Abdomen
Evaluation: Babinski Reflex

Pediatric Assessment

Evaluation: Motor Development
Evaluation: Palmar Grasp
Evaluation: Symmetry of Gluteal Folds
Inspection and Evaluation: Head
Inspection and Palpation: Abdomen, Umbilicus
Inspection and Palpation: Head and Neck
Inspection and Palpation: Genitalia (Supine Position)
Inspection: Ear Canal
Inspection: External Genitalia
Inspection: Eye Alignment
Inspection: Eye-Ear Alignment
Inspection: Male Genitalia
Inspection: Oropharynx, Teeth, and Tongue
Inspection: Range-of-Motion, Upper and Lower Extremities
Inspection: Tongue
Evaluation: Crawling to Standing
Evaluation: Extraocular Movement
Evaluation: Motor Development
Inspection: Ear Canal
Inspection: External Genitalia, Anus
Inspection: Female Genitalia, Anus
Inspection: Range-of-Motion, Hip
Inspection: Stance, Feet
Palpation: Abdomen
Auscultation: Breath Sounds, Anterior Chest
Auscultation: Heart, Anterior Chest
Evaluation: Balance Using Heel-to-Toe Walking
Evaluation: Balance Using Hopping
Evaluation: Balance Using Two-Foot Hopping and Heel-to-Toe Walking
Evaluation: Deep Tendon Reflex
Evaluation: Eye Fixation Using the Cover-Uncover Test
Evaluation: Fine Motor Skills
Evaluation: Finger Squeeze
Evaluation: Mouth, Cranial Nerve X
Evaluation: Muscle Strength, Neck, Shoulders, and Tongue; Cranial Nerve VII, XI, XII
Evaluation: Muscular Development
Evaluation: Pupil Responses, Direct
Inspection and Palpation: Spine for Alignment
Inspection: Ankles and Feet, Posterior
Inspection: Back
Inspection: Chest and Lungs, Posterior
Inspection: External Ear and Ear Canal
Inspection: Feet
Inspection: Female Breasts (Sitting Position)
Inspection: Leg Alignment
Inspection: Male Breasts (Sitting Position)
Inspection: Muscle Strength, Upper Extremities
Inspection: Oropharynx, Teeth, and Tongue
Palpation: Abdomen
Palpation: Chest, Anterior
Palpation: Lymph Nodes, Head and Neck
Evaluation: Six Cardinal Fields of Gaze, Cranial Nerves III, IV, and VI—Oculomotor, Trochlear, and Abducens Nerves
Inspection and Palpation: Spine for Alignment
Inspection: Fine Motor Coordination, Lower Extremities
Inspection: Fine Motor Coordination, Upper Extremities

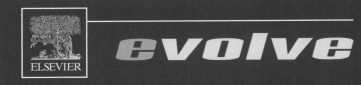

To access your Instructor Resources, visit:

http://evolve.elsevier.com/Price/pediatric/

Evolve Student Learning Resources for Price: *Pediatric Nursing, 10th ed.* offers the following features:

- **Video Assessments**
  Builds a solid foundation for nursing skills with live videos of newborn and pediatric assessments.

- **3-D Animations**
  Brings the content alive with animations of procedures, physiology, and neonatal assessments.

- **Glossary of Audio Pronunciations**
  Enhances your learning experience with an alphabetized audio pronunciation key of commonly used terms.

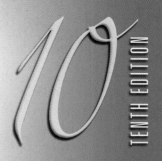

TENTH EDITION

PEDIATRIC NURSING

AN INTRODUCTORY TEXT

Debra L. Price, MSN, RN, CPNP, CNE
Assistant Professor of Nursing
Tarrant County College
Fort Worth, Texas

Julie F. Gwin, MN, RN
Associate Professor of Nursing
Tarrant County College
Fort Worth, Texas

SAUNDERS

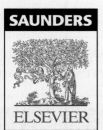

ELSEVIER

SAUNDERS
ELSEVIER

11830 Westline Industrial Drive
St. Louis, Missouri 63146

PEDIATRIC NURSING: AN INTRODUCTORY TEXT, 10TH EDITION   ISBN: 978-1-4160-4049-1
Copyright © 2008, 2005, 2001, 1997, 1992, 1987, 1981, 1976, 1970, 1965 by Saunders, an imprint of Elsevier Inc.

NCLEX®, NCLEX-RN®, and NCLEX-PN® are federally registered trademarks and service marks of the National Council of State Boards of Nursing, Inc.

Library of Congress Control Number 2007926019

ISBN: 978-1-4160-4049-1

Acquisitions Editor: Robin Levin Richman
Developmental Editor: Ryan Creed
Publishing Services Manager: Jeff Patterson
Project Manager: Anne Konopka
Design Direction: Teresa McBryan

Printed in China

Last digit is the print number: 9 8 7 6 5 4 3 2

*For my mother, **Ruth Robideau, RN.***
What an inspiration you have been in my career.
Even though you chose geriatrics and I chose pediatrics,
I cannot think of anyone whose opinion I respect more than yours.

*And to my children **Ryan** and **Christine,***
*and in-law children **Emily** and **Matthew,***
who are now a blessed addition to our family.

*And of course to my husband **Jeff***
whose dedication as a spouse is unsurpassed.

DEBRA L. PRICE

This edition is dedicated to my family.

*My husband, **John,** who supports and shares*
my interest in the field of pediatrics.

*My three boys—**Aaron, Adam,** and **Alex**—*
who continue to provide me with practical experiences
as they move through the different stages of their lives.

JULIE F. GWIN

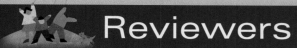
Reviewers

JANICE ANKENMANN, MSN, RN, CCRN, FNP
Instructor, Vocational Nursing
Napa Valley College
Queen of the Valley Hospital
Napa, California

MICHELE CISLO, RN, MA
Instructor, Practical Nursing
Union County College
Plainfield, New Jersey

LAURIE JO PEYRONEL, BSN, RN, MA
Instructor, Practical Nursing
Mercyhurst College Northeast
Northeast, Pennsylvania

To the Instructor

Thompson's Pediatric Nursing: An Introductory Text, **10th edition**, has been updated and revised to provide the novice pediatric nursing student with the fundamental knowledge needed to practice in a pediatric setting. We have retained many of the book's strengths—its easy-to-read, clear writing style; the organization by developmental stages; and the nursing interventions focus.

ORGANIZATION

Organized by developmental stages, this book covers pediatric nursing from infant to adolescent and also contains a separate chapter on end-of-life care for children and their families. Each chapter begins with **Objectives** and then lists **Key Terms** and their phonetic pronunciations and page reference numbers. Key Terms are in color at first mention and are defined in the **Glossary**. At the end of every chapter, **Key Points** of the chapter are briefly summarized.

A perforated **Self-Assessment** workbook at the end of this book may be used for review or as an assignment to be turned in by students. Included are matching exercises, multiple-choice questions, more Study Questions, new Community Search activities, Case Studies with Critical Thinking Questions, and Internet Activities for each chapter. Guidelines to the Case Studies are provided in the TEACH Instructor Resources.

CRITICAL CONTENT

Community-based care and care of the family are given special emphasis throughout. *Healthy People 2010 Objectives* form the basis for health promotion and are integrated into the text to provide a basis for student study.

End-of-life care is addressed in a separate chapter that includes recommendations by Last Acts, the National Task Force on Palliative Care. Topics include both psychosocial and physiological issues in providing nursing care for the terminally ill child. **Pain content** reflects current views on pediatric pain assessment and therapy. **Bioterrorism** threats and pediatric psychophysiological responses are included in Chapter 1. **Complementary and alternative therapies** are included in Chapters 1, 3, and 18. **Cultural content** is found in Chapter 1, and more coverage on cultural influences and diversity in pediatric care has been added to this edition.

NEW TO THIS EDITION

The new 10th edition has an abundance of expanded content, including **evidence-based nursing** (explained in Chapter 3), cultural influences, and more nutrition information, as well as the following new features:

- **Health Promotion** boxes (an LPN Thread) are found throughout the book, accentuating wellness and disease prevention in light of *Healthy People 2010* objectives
- **Home Care Tips** supplement the content on home care in Chapter 3: Care of the Hospitalized Child and are related to specific disorders. Since so many children now survive illness and congenital disorders well past childhood, the challenge for families and caregivers is to understand how to minister to these ongoing needs.
- **Critical Thinking Snapshots** with brief scenarios are located after Critical Thinking Questions at the end of selected Nursing Care Plans.
- New **January 2007 Recommended Childhood Immunization Schedules** (Appendix A) for children, adolescents, and catch-up growth immunizations provide the most current recommendations for pediatric immunizations.
- **The Joint Commission Lists of Dangerous Abbreviations, Acronyms, and Symbols** provide guidelines for the prevention of medication administration errors, especially serious in pediatric dosages.

LEARNING AIDS

The following learning aids are designed to guide and instruct:

- **Nursing Care Plans** with **Critical Thinking Questions** reinforce the nursing process as applied to pediatric disorders. Answers to the **Critical Thinking Questions** are provided in the TEACH Instructor Resources. Several Nursing Care Plans include **Critical Thinking Snapshots**, described above.
- **Skills** teach basic techniques used by the LPN/LVN in pediatric nursing settings.
- **Nursing Briefs** stress important content-related points.
- **Communication Alerts** identify key tips to establish successful nurse-patient-family communication.
- **Community Cues** address home care and community-based care issues.
- **Data Cues** list assessment data to cue the nurse to recognize possible pediatric disorders.

- **Internet Activities**, found in the **Self-Assessment** workbook, provide students with the opportunity to practice online research on content-related topics.
- **Online Resources** at the end of each chapter direct students to current websites related to chapter content.

ANCILLARIES
For the Instructor
Supplemental teaching aids include TEACH Instructor Resources on Evolve.

- Fully revised for the 10th edition, the **TEACH Lesson Plans** are based on the learning objectives for each chapter in the book, providing a roadmap to link and integrate all parts of the educational package.
- Open-Book Quizzes, Answers to the Self-Assessment Workbook with Guidelines for Internet Archives and Case Studies, guidelines for the Critical Thinking Questions and Snapshots in the Nursing Care Plans for Teaching English as a Second Language (ESL) students.
- **PowerPoint presentation** of text and image slides, now with annotations, has been expanded substantially from the previous edition.
- **Image Collection** includes all the illustrations and photographs from the textbook.
- **Test Bank** of approximately 500 NCLEX-PN® multiple-choice and alternate-item format questions includes the following categories: Correct Answer, Rationale, Topic, Nursing Process Step, Objective, Cognitive Level, NCLEX-PN® Category of Client Needs, and Text Page Reference.
- An online Course Management System is also provided.

For the Student
Evolve Learning Resources Website
Evolve Student Resources include WebLinks.
New to this edition of the textbook, the bind-in Companion CD-ROM includes:

- Over 90 **Video Assessments** of newborns, infants, toddlers, and children, offering a unique opportunity for students to combine visual and textbook information as they apply what they have learned.
- **3-D Animations** of neonatal procedures and physiology allow students to see procedures and difficult anatomy and physiology clearly, colorfully, and accurately portrayed for better comprehension.
- **Glossary of Audio Pronunciations** of commonly used terms includes all Key Terms and more to help students learn and apply difficult terminology.

Our knowledge and extensive experience in pediatrics have guided us in the development of this new edition. It is our hope that students will find the information clearly presented and easily understood. As reflected in our writing, we aspire to show our love of pediatrics, the children involved, their families, and the nurses who choose to pursue pediatric nursing.

DEBRA L. PRICE
JULIE F. GWIN

LPN Threads

Thompson's Pediatric Nursing: An Introductory Text, **10th edition,** shares some features and design elements with other LPN titles on the Mosby and Saunders lists. The purpose of these "LPN Threads" is to make it easier for students and instructors to incorporate multiple books into the fast-paced and demanding LPN curriculum.

The shared features in *Thompson's Pediatric Nursing,* **10th edition,** include the following:

- A **reading level evaluation** was performed on every manuscript chapter during the book's development
- Cover and internal design similarities
- Content and Special Feature threads
- Numbered lists of Objectives that begin each chapter
- Key Terms with phonetic pronunciations and page number references at the beginning of each chapter. The key terms are in color the first time they appear in the chapter. All pronunciations were reviewed by an ESL (English as a Second Language) consultant

- Critical Thinking questions and Critical Thinking Snapshots in Nursing Care Plans; answers to the Critical Thinking questions are provided in the TEACH Instructor Resources on Evolve
- Bulleted lists of Key Points at the end of each chapter
- Complete Self-Assessment Workbook in a perforated section at the back of the book. Answers are provided in the TEACH Instructor Resources on Evolve
- Complete Bibliography and Reader References list at the end of the text
- Glossary at the end of the text
- Test Bank in ExamView with the following categories of information: Topic, Step of the Nursing Process, Objective, Cognitive Level, NCLEX Category of Client Need, Correct Answer, Rationale, and Text Page Reference
- PowerPoint slide presentation in the TEACH Instructor Resources on Evolve
- Tips for teaching English as a Second Language (ESL) students in the TEACH Instructor Resources

LPN Advisory Board

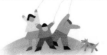

To the Student

Designed with the student in mind, ***Thompson's Pediatric Nursing: An Introductory Text, 10th Edition,*** will help you learn basic pediatric nursing care through its visually appealing and easy-to-use format. Here are some of the special features that will help you understand and apply the material.

FREE CD-ROM

The free CD-ROM packaged in your copy of *Thompson's Pediatric Nursing,* 10th edition, contains the following: **video assessments** of newborns, infants, toddlers, and children, **3-D animations** of neonatal procedures and physiology, and a **glossary of audio pronunciations** of selected terms. Using these resources as you study will help you master the material in this book. Watch for the cues throughout the text.

Chapters open with **numbered Objectives** and **Key Terms** with pronunciations. On first use within the text, each key term is highlighted in color and defined briefly. All key terms are also included in the glossary. **Audio Pronunciations** are provided on the companion CD.

Health Promotion boxes cover wellness and disease-prevention strategies.
Bioterrorism and Disaster Preparedness content is highlighted in Chapters 1 and 12.
***Healthy People 2010* Objectives** are integrated throughout the text.

Communication Alert boxes identify key tips for establishing successful nurse-patient-family communication.

Data Cues list assessment data to prompt the nurse to recognize possible pediatric disorders.

Complementary and Alternative Therapies content has been expanded in Chapters 1, 3, and 18.

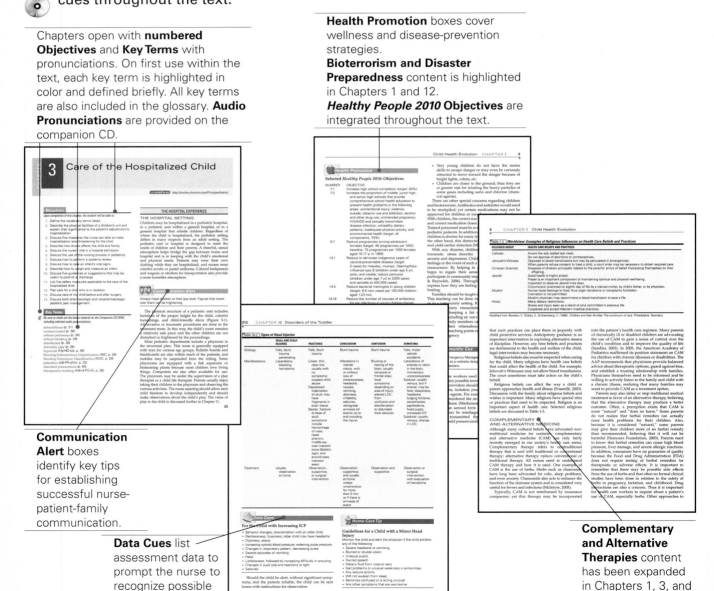

Skills provide step-by-step teaching of basic techniques used in pediatric nursing.

A Self-Assessment workbook at the back of the book includes **Matching Exercises, Multiple-choice Review Questions, Study Questions, Case Studies with Critical Thinking Questions, Internet Activities,** and more!

Nursing Care Plans reinforce nursing processes applied to pediatric disorders. **Critical Thinking Questions** are included near the end of each care plan.

Critical Thinking Snapshots with brief scenarios are provided at the end of selected Nursing Care Plans.

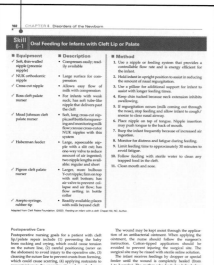

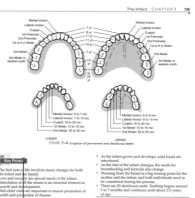

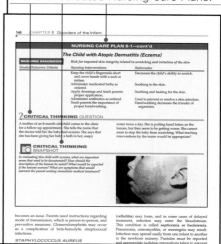

Nursing Briefs emphasize important clinical care.
Home Care Tips present guidelines for care in the home by family members and other caregivers.

Key Points, which summarize the main topics for chapter review, and **Online Resources** for further study appear at the end of each chapter.
Full-color and detailed art visually enhance the narrative.

Community Cues address home care and community-based care issues.

Acknowledgments

To Becky Law at Harris Methodist Southwest for her help with the neonate chapter. Also to Parkland Hospital burn unit and the education department for clarifying the burn information.

To Robin Richman, who never tires of my endless questions.

And finally, to Julie Gwin, my dear friend and teaching partner, with whom I so often collaborate and also share a love of pediatrics.

DEBRA L. PRICE

I would especially like to express my appreciation to all the nurses at Cook Children's Medical Center, who assist me in providing a positive learning environment for my students. And to my family, friends, and co-teachers who helped by providing support during the writing of this book.

And lastly, to Debbie Price, my friend and co-editor, who helped keep us focused during this long process.

JULIE F. GWIN

Contents

1 CHILD HEALTH EVOLUTION, 1

Evolution of Child Health, 1
Government Programs, 2
Changes in Mortality and Morbidity, 2
Health Care Today, 4
Insurance, 4
Health Promotion, 4
Emergency Preparedness, 4
Current Practice, 6
Cultural and Religious Considerations, 6
Complementary and Alternative Medicine, 8
Health Care Delivery Settings, 9
Clinics and Offices, 9
Home Care, 10
Parish Nursing, 10
Other Programs, 10

2 GROWING CHILDREN AND THEIR FAMILIES, 12

Heredity and the Developing Child, 12
Karyotype, 12
Genetic Counseling and Research, 14
Advances in Perinatology, 14
Growth and Development, 15
Clarification of Terms, 16
Characteristics of Growth and Development, 16
Growth Standards, 17
Factors That Influence Growth and Development, 18
Hereditary Traits, 18
Nationality and Race, 18
Ordinal Position, 18
Gender, 18
Environment, 18
Family, 19
Theories of Development, 19
Psychosocial Development, 19
Cognitive Development, 19
Moral Development, 20
Nursing Implications of Growth and Development, 20

3 CARE OF THE HOSPITALIZED CHILD, 23

The Hospital Experience, 23
The Hospital Setting, 23
The Child's Reaction to Hospitalization, 24
The Family's Reaction to Hospitalization, 27

The Nurse's Role, 28
Admission Process, 28
Critical Thinking and the Nursing Process, 29
Documentation, 30
Discharge Planning, 30
Data Collection, 31
Health History, 31
Systems Review, 31
Vital Signs, 31
Measurements, 34
Safety, 37
Transporting, Positioning, and Restraining the Child, 38
Medical Asepsis, 38
Preventing the Transmission of Infection, 39
Education of the Family, 41
Implications of Pediatric Surgery, 41
The Child in Pain, 41
Definition and Challenges, 41
Evaluation, 42
Intervention, 43

4 THE NEWBORN INFANT, 48

Adaptations of the Newborn Infant, 48
EXAMINATION OF THE NEWBORN INFANT, 48
Initial Exam of the Newborn Infant, 48
Airway, 48
Umbilical Cord, 49
Apgar Scoring, 50
Providing Warmth, 50
Measurements, 51
Vital Signs, 51
Characteristics of the Newborn Infant, 52
Maturity, 52
Head, 52
Nervous System, 54
Sensory System, 56
Respiratory System, 56
Circulatory System, 56
Musculoskeletal System, 57
Genitourinary System, 57
Integumentary System, 59
Gastrointestinal System, 59
Activity, 60
Reactivity, 60
Sleep, 60
Neonatal States, 61
Conditioned Responses, 61

CARE OF THE NEWBORN INFANT, 61
Identifying the Neonate, 61
Medication Administration and Screening
    Tests, 61
Nutrition, 62
    Breastfeeding Advantages, 62
    Contraindications to Breastfeeding, 63
    Technique of Breastfeeding, 63
    Possible Problems with
      Breastfeeding, 64
    Bottle Feeding, 65
    Use of Formula, 65
    Technique of Bottle Feeding, 66
Infection, 66
    Prevention of Infection, 66
    Handwashing Technique, 67
    Signs and Symptoms of Infection, 67
    Care of the Patient Unit, 67
Ongoing Care, 67
    Bathing the Baby, 67
    Clothing the Baby, 68
    Cord Care, 68
Family Relations, 68
    Getting Acquainted, 68
    Bonding/Attachment, 68
    Siblings, 68
    Spiritual Care, 69
Discharge Teaching, 69
    Home Phototherapy, 69

5   THE HIGH-RISK NEONATE, 71
The Preterm Infant, 71
    CAUSES OF PRETERM BIRTH, 72
    RISKS RELATED TO PREMATURITY, 73
    Inadequate Respiratory Function, 73
    Atelectasis, 73
    Meconium Aspiration Syndrome, 73
    Respiratory Distress Syndrome, 75
    Apnea, 75
    Sepsis, 76
    Necrotizing Enterocolitis, 76
    Hypoglycemia, 77
    Hypocalcemia, 77
    Hemorrhagic Disease, 77
    Retinopathy of Prematurity, 77
    Jaundice, 78
    SPECIAL NEEDS AND CARE OF THE PRETERM
      INFANT, 78
    Thermoregulation, 78
    Nutrition, 80
    Close Observation, 81
    Position and Skin Care, 81
    FAMILY REACTION TO THE PRETERM INFANT, 82
The Postterm Infant, 83
Infants of Mothers with Diabetes, 83
Transportation of the High-Risk
    Neonate, 83

6   DISORDERS OF THE NEWBORN, 85
Malformations Present at Birth (Congenital), 85
Immune System, 86
    Acquired Immunodeficiency Syndrome, 86
    Infections, 89
Respiratory System, 91
    Tuberculosis, 91
Cardiovascular System, 92
    Congenital Heart Disease, 92
Gastrointestinal System, 101
    Cleft Lip, 101
    Cleft Palate, 103
    Gastroschisis and Omphalocele, 104
    Esophageal Atresia and Tracheoesophageal
      Fistula Atresia, 104
Musculoskeletal System, 106
    Clubfoot, 106
    Developmental Dysplasia of the Hip, 107
Nervous System, 109
    Down Syndrome, 109
    Hydrocephalus, 110
    Myelodysplasia/Spina Bifida, 113
Perinatal Damage, 115
    Hemolytic Disease of the Newborn:
      Erythroblastosis Fetalis, 115
Intracranial Hemorrhage, 116
    Description, 116

7   THE INFANT, 119
GENERAL CHARACTERISTICS AND
    DEVELOPMENT, 119
Physical Development, Social Behavior, Care,
    and Guidance, 120
HEALTH PROMOTION AND MAINTENANCE, 120
Immunizations, 128
    Precautions/Side Effects, 129
    Importance, 131
    Concerns, 131
Nutrition Counseling of Parents, 131
    Solid Foods, 133
    Buying, Storing, and Serving Food, 133
Weaning From the Breast, 134
Teeth, 134
    Deciduous Teeth, 134
    Teething During Infancy, 134

8   DISORDERS OF THE INFANT, 136
Skin, 136
    Atopic Dermatitis (Infantile Eczema), 136
    Impetigo, 138
    Staphylococcus Aureus Infection, 140
Ears, 141
    Otitis Media, 141
Hematologic System, 144
    Iron-Deficiency Anemia, 144
    Sickle Cell Disease, 145
Respiratory System, 148

Nasopharyngitis (Common Cold), 148
Bronchiolitis, 149
Bronchopulmonary Dysplasia, 151
Lungs, 152
Cystic Fibrosis, 152
Gastrointestinal System, 156
Inguinal Hernia, 156
Umbilical Hernia, 156
Pyloric Stenosis, 156
Intussusception, 160
Hirschsprung's Disease, 162
Vomiting, 163
Fluid Imbalance, 163
Nervous System, 165
Bacterial Meningitis, 165
Genitourinary System, 167
Hydrocele, 167
Undescended Testes (Cryptorchidism), 167
Hypospadias and Epispadias, 167
Special Topics, 168
Sudden Infant Death Syndrome, 168
Failure to Thrive, 169
Child Abuse and Neglect, 170

9 THE TODDLER, 176
GENERAL CHARACTERISTICS AND
DEVELOPMENT, 176
Developmental Tasks, 176
Physical Growth, 178
Guidance and Discipline, 179
Communication, 180
Language Development, 180
Communicating with Toddlers, 180
HEALTH PROMOTION AND
MAINTENANCE, 181
Daily Care, 181
Dental Health, 181
Nutrition Counseling, 182
Toilet Independence, 183
Play, 187
Daycare, 188
Injury Prevention, 188
Epidemiological Framework, 193

10 DISORDERS OF THE TODDLER, 195
Ears, 195
Deafness, 195
Respiratory System, 197
Croup, 197
Epiglottitis, 199
Bronchitis, 199
Pneumonia, 199
Gastrointestinal System, 201
Pinworms, 201
Musculoskeletal System, 202
Fractures, 202
Dislocations, 204

Nervous System, 204
Cerebral Palsy, 204
Head Injuries, 211
Genitourinary System, 214
Wilms Tumor, 214
Special Topics, 215
Autism, 215
Poisonings, 215

11 THE PRESCHOOL CHILD, 220
GENERAL CHARACTERISTICS AND
DEVELOPMENT, 220
Theories of Development, 220
Physical, Psychosocial, and Cognitive
Development, 223
The 3-Year-Old Child, 223
The 4-Year-Old Child, 224
The 5-Year-Old Child, 225
Guiding the Preschool Child, 225
Discipline, Setting Limits, 225
Bad Language, 226
Jealousy and Sibling Rivalry, 227
Thumb Sucking, 227
Masturbation, 227
Enuresis, 228
Language and Speech Impairment, 228
HEALTH PROMOTION AND
MAINTENANCE, 229
Daily Care, 229
Preschool, 230
Play in Health and Illness, 230
Value of Play, 230
The Nurse's Role, 231
Other Aspects of Play, 233
Injury Prevention, 234

**12 DISORDERS OF THE PRESCHOOL
CHILD,** 236
Skin, 236
Burns, 236
Eyes, 240
Amblyopia, 240
Strabismus, 241
Hematologic System, 241
Leukemia, 241
Hemophilia, 245
Respiratory System, 247
Tonsillitis and Adenoiditis, 247
Gastrointestinal System, 249
Celiac Disease, 249
Musculoskeletal System, 250
Duchenne Muscular Dystrophy, 250
Nervous System, 251
Encephalitis, 251
Seizure Disorders, 252
Genitourinary System, 256
Urinary Tract Infection, 256

Acute (Poststreptococcal)
Glomerulonephritis, 257
Nephrotic Syndrome (Nephrosis), 258
Special Topics, 260
Communicable Diseases, 260
Developmental Disability, 260

13   The School-Age Child, 273
GENERAL CHARACTERISTICS AND
DEVELOPMENT, 273
Physical Growth, 273
Developmental Theories, 274
Biological and Psychosocial Development, 274
The 6-Year-Old, 274
The 7-Year-Old, 276
The 8-Year-Old, 277
The 9-Year-Old, 278
The 10-Year-Old, 278
The 11- to 12-Year-Old Period, 278
Environmental Influences, 279
School, 279
Bullying, 280
Television, 280
Video Games, 281
Peers, 282
Guidance, 282
Sex Education, 283
Latchkey Children, 284
Child Abduction, 285
Divorce, 285
Safety, 285
HEALTH PROMOTION AND
MAINTENANCE, 286
Health Examinations, 286
Daily Care, 288
Play, 288
Nutrition, 289

**14   DISORDERS OF THE SCHOOL-AGE
CHILD,** 291
Skin, 291
Pediculosis, 291
Endocrine System, 292
Diabetes Mellitus (Type 1), 292
Respiratory System, 303
Asthma, 303
Cardiovascular System, 308
Acute Rheumatic Fever, 308
Gastrointestinal System, 312
Appendicitis, 312
Musculoskeletal System, 314
Legg-Calvé-Perthes Disease (Coxa Plana), 314
Juvenile Rheumatoid Arthritis, 314
Nervous System, 318
Reye's Syndrome, 318
Brain Tumors, 318

Special Topics, 320
Overview of Emotional and Behavioral
Disorders, 320

15   THE ADOLESCENT, 324
GENERAL CHARACTERISTICS AND
DEVELOPMENT, 324
Biological Development, 325
Developmental Theories, 326
Special Needs, 328
Peer Relationships, 328
Career Plans, 328
Responsibility, 329
Emotional Needs, 329
Daydreams, 330
Heterosexual Relationships, 330
Chronic Illness/Disability, 330
HEALTH PROMOTION AND MAINTENANCE, 331
Parenting a Teenager, 331
Health Examinations, 332
Confidentiality, 332
Sexuality, 333
Homosexuality, 333
Body Piercings and Tattoos, 334
Nutrition, 334
Sports and Nutrition, 335
Personal Care, 335
Sleep, 335
Exercise, 335
Personal Hygiene, 335
Clothing, 336
Dental Care, 336
Safety, 336
Internet Solicitation, 337

**16   DISORDERS OF THE
ADOLESCENT,** 338
Skin, 338
Acne Vulgaris, 338
Hematologic System, 340
Infectious Mononucleosis, 340
Lymphatic System, 340
Hodgkin's Disease, 340
Gastrointestinal System, 342
Obesity, 342
Anorexia Nervosa, 343
Bulimia, 345
Musculoskeletal System, 345
Scoliosis, 345
Sports Injuries, 349
Genitourinary System, 352
Dysmenorrhea (Primary), 352
Sexually Transmitted Diseases, 353
Special Topics, 362
Adolescent Pregnancy, 362
Depression and Suicide, 363
Substance Abuse, 365

17 PEDIATRIC PROCEDURES, 372
  Preparation for Procedures, 372
  Basic Hygiene and Care, 373
    Bathing, 373
    Suctioning, 373
    Fever and Sponge Bathing, 373
  Collection of Specimens, 373
    Collection of Urine Specimens, 373
    Collection of Stool Specimens, 376
    Collection of Blood Specimens, 376
    Collection of Throat Cultures, 379
    Collection of Nasopharyngeal
      Cultures, 379
  Assisting with Lumbar Puncture, 379
  Administering Medications, 380
    Variations in Children, 380
    Oral Medications, 382
    Nosedrops, Eardrops, and Eyedrops, 383
    Intramuscular Injections, 384
    Subcutaneous and Intradermal
      Medications, 387
    Intravenous Medications, 387
    Rectal Medications, 388
  Principles of Fluid Balance in Children, 389
    Oral Fluids, 389
    Parenteral Fluids, 390
    Total Parenteral Nutrition, 391
  Procedures to Assist Nutrition, Digestion, and
      Elimination, 391
    Gastrostomy, 391
    Gastrostomy Button Feeding, 391
    Enema, 391
    Ostomy, 393
  Care of the Child with a Tracheostomy, 393
    Suctioning, 394
    Care of the Tracheal Stoma, 395
  Oxygen Therapy for Children, 396
    General Safety Considerations, 396
    Methods of Administration, 397

**18 END-OF-LIFE CARE FOR CHILDREN
  AND THEIR FAMILIES,** 400
  Self-Exploration, 400
  Legal and Ethical Issues Related to
      Death, 400
  Palliative Care, 401
  Child's Reaction to Death, 402
  Child's Awareness of Condition, 403
  Fears of the Child, 403
    Pain, 403
    Fear of Being Alone, 403
  Family Roles and Needs, 403
    Cultural Issues, 404
  Hospice Care, 404
  Preparing for Death, 405
  Care After Death, 406
  Family Coping, 406
  Reflection, 407

APPENDIXES

**A: Recommended Childhood and
  Adolescent Immunization
  Schedule—United States, 2007,** 408

B: NANDA Nursing Diagnoses, 410

**C: Recommendations for Preventive
  Pediatric Health Care,** 412

**D: Normal Laboratory Value for
  Children—Reference Ranges,** 415

E: Standard Precautions, 444

F: Growth Charts, 447

**G: Denver Developmental Screening
  Test—II,** 460

H: Conversion Charts, 462

**I: The Joint Commission Lists
  of Dangerous Abbreviations,
  Acronyms, and Symbols,** 463

**J: The Fourth Report on the
  Diagnosis, Evaluation, and
  Treatment of High Blood Pressure
  in Children and Adolescents,** 464

**Bibliography and Reader
References,** 468

Illustration Credits, 477

Glossary, 479

Index, 487

Self-Assessment, 497

CHAPTER 1

Child Health Evolution

Objectives

Upon completion of this chapter, the student will be able to:

1. Define or identify vocabulary terms listed
2. List historical developments that have affected the care of children
3. Contrast present-day causes of morbidity and mortality with those of the past
4. Discuss current health care trends in pediatrics and the effect they have on nursing care
5. Discuss emergency preparedness in relation to pediatrics
6. Identify the role of the pediatric nurse
7. Discuss the effects that culture, religion, and alternative medicine may have on nursing care
8. Discuss the variety of settings in which the pediatric nurse may work

Key Terms

Be sure to check out the bonus material on the Companion CD-ROM, including selected audio presentations.

anticipatory guidance (ăn-TĬS-ĭ-pa-TŌR-ē; p. 6)
bacterial agent (p. 5)
case manager (p. 10)
Children's Bureau (p. 2)
diagnosis-related groups (DRGs; p. 4)
evidence-based practice (p. 6)
Healthy People 2000: National Health Promotion and Disease Prevention Objectives (p. 4)
holistic (p. 1)
hospice (hŏs-pĭs; p. 10)
infant mortality rate (mŏr-TĂL-ĭ-tē; p. 2)
morbidity (mŏr-BĬD-ĭ-tē; p. 3)
pediatric nurse practitioner (PNP; p. 9)
pediatrics (pē-dē-ĂT-rĭks; p. 1)
toxin (p. 6)
triage (trē-ĀZH; p. 9)
viral agent (p. 6)
White House Conference on Children and Youth (p. 2)

EVOLUTION OF CHILD HEALTH

Pediatrics is the branch of medicine that deals specifically with children, their development, childhood diseases, and the treatment of such diseases. The word *pediatrics* is derived from the Greek *pais/paisos*, meaning "child," and *iatreia*, meaning "cure." The study of pediatrics began under the influence of Abraham Jacobi (1830-1919), a Prussian-born physician. Known today as the Father of Pediatrics, Jacobi paved the way for the promotion of children's health through the establishment of "milk stations," where mothers could bring sick children for treatment and learn the importance of pure milk and its proper preparation. The emergence of pediatric nursing as a specialty paralleled the establishment of pediatric departments in medical schools, the founding of children's hospitals, and the development of separate units for children in general hospitals.

In the Middle Ages, the concept of childhood did not exist. Around the age of 7 years, the child was considered to be an adult (the average life span was about 30 years.) Childhood became a separate growth stage only when large numbers of people entered the middle class and leisure time increased. Infants were surviving longer; therefore parents were more willing to become invested in them.

As a result of research into child development by such experts as Erikson and Piaget, society's view of childhood has undergone a dramatic change. Childhood has become a separate phase of life, and children's rights are protected by law and by custom. As young people have been freed from the labor of farms and factories to attend school, adolescence has also emerged as a separate entity.

The nursing care of children has evolved dramatically over the past 100 years. From its initial connection with the specialty of pediatric medicine, it has evolved into a holistic enterprise. Pediatric nursing views children as having a physical, intellectual, emotional, and spiritual nature and as having needs that differ according to developmental level. In the early part of the 20th century, the nursing of children was primarily focused on illness. Children frequently became ill and died during epidemics of communicable diseases such as measles and polio. With improved sanitation, the advent of antibiotics, and the institution of preventive measures such as immunizations and improved prenatal care, most children now survive well into adulthood. As the organic causes of death and disability have declined, pediatric nursing has become focused on improving the quality of care by providing an environment for optimal growth and development, as well as health promotion, health maintenance, and health restoration.

GOVERNMENT PROGRAMS

The government has played a key role in the evolution of child health. Lillian Wald, who founded public health nursing, and Florence Kelley, an activist who opposed child labor, were jointly responsible for the establishment of a federal Children's Bureau. In 1909, the first White House Conference on Children and Youth issued 15 recommendations, one of which called for the formation of a Children's Bureau for child welfare. Once the Children's Bureau was established in 1912, it focused on the problems of infant and maternal mortality. These investigations provided the impetus for initiatives that improved maternal and child health. The Maternity and Infancy Act provided grants to states to develop a Division of Maternal and Child Health (MCH) and influenced the creation of the American Academy of Pediatrics (AAP). The Children's Bureau was placed under the Department of Health, Education, and Welfare, which is currently known as the Department of Health and Human Services.

Studies documenting appalling working conditions for 13-year-old to 16-year-old children paved the way for a federal law that controls child labor. Before the 1930s, young adolescents worked regularly in cold, damp, and drafty sheds, standing long hours, doing wet, dirty, and sometimes unsanitary and dangerous work. School attendance was sporadic, and children were considered well educated if they finished the eighth grade. The Fair Labor Standards Act, passed in 1938, regulates working conditions for children under 18 years. More importantly, this act paved the way for the establishment of national minimum standards for child labor and provided a means for enforcement.

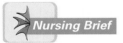

Nursing Brief

The American Academy of Pediatrics (AAP) *(http://www.aap. org)*, made up of pediatricians nationwide, and the American Nurses' Association *(http://www.ana.org)* have established positions of leadership in setting health standards for children and standards of practice for nurses caring for children and families.

In the past 30 or more years, child health care has been positively affected by several federal programs. In 1965, Medicaid and the Children and Youth Project were formed to provide care for children in low-income and inaccessible areas. Both these programs exist today, although they have been affected by budget cuts. The Special Supplemental Food Program for Women, Infants, and Children (WIC) was begun in 1966. This program serves to safeguard the health of low-income women, infants, and children up to age 5 who are at nutritional risk by providing nutritious foods to supplement diets, information on healthy eating, and referral to health care. The National School Lunch Act (1946) and Child Nutrition Act (1966) provide meals, either free or at a reduced rate, for low-income children. In 1982, the Missing Children's Act was passed, which established a clearinghouse for missing children. The Balanced Budget Act of 1997 established the State Children's Health Insurance Program (SCHIP) as Title XXI of the Social Security Act to expand insurance coverage to a large portion of uninsured children ineligible for Medicaid. Table 1-1 summarizes federal programs that affect maternal-child care.

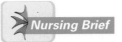

Nursing Brief

Two international organizations concerned with children are the United Nations Children's Fund *(http://www.unicef.org)* and the World Health Organization *(http://www.who.int/en/).*

The enactment of the **HIPAA** (Health Insurance Portability and Accountability Act) regulations in 1996 required strict observance of confidentiality within the hospital setting. This requirement is for the protection of the patient and is extremely important when caring for children. Adults could easily overhear and misinterpret information discussed about a child.

CHANGES IN MORTALITY AND MORBIDITY

The infant mortality rate (number of infant deaths per 1000 live births) has declined from approximately 200 in 1900 to 20 deaths in 1970 to 6.9 in 2003. Infant mortality among infants of non-Hispanic black mothers, however, is more than double that for non-Hispanic whites (U.S. Dept. of Health and Human Services, 2003).

Despite declines in infant mortality, the United States continues to rank poorly in international comparisons. Although the exact reason is unclear, countries that rank higher have national health programs. Low birth weight (LBW) has been well documented as a primary contributor to infant mortality in developed countries. Other contributing factors include African-American race, male gender, socioeconomic status, lower level of maternal education, and gestational age (longer or shorter). According to the 2002 statistics, the leading causes of infant mortality are congenital anomalies, disorders relating to short gestation and unspecified LBW, sudden infant death syndrome (SIDS), and maternal complications (see SIDS in Chapter 8).

Positive steps are being taken to help with the continual decline of infant mortality. Cigarette smoking during pregnancy has declined, and the percentage of mothers that began prenatal care within the first trimester of pregnancy has increased. The Healthy Start program *(www.hrsa.gov)* that works to expand the availability and accessibility of prenatal health

| Table 1-1 | *Summary of Federal Programs That Affect Maternal-Child Health* |

NAME	YEAR	COMMENT
Social Security	1935	Provides matching state/federal funds for maternal/child care and for children with disabilities, supports preventive health programs (immunizations, screenings)
Fair Labor Standards Act	1938	Establishes minimum working age of 16 years
Maternal–Child Health Infant Care Project	1963	Effort to decrease infant and child mortality
Children and Youth Project	1965	Targets low-income children and children in less accessible areas who need health care
Medicaid EPSDT	1965	Early and periodic screening, diagnosis, and treatment (EPSDT) for low-income children
Crippled Children's Service	1965	Services to disabled children under 21 years
WIC	1965	Supplemental food program for low-income women, infants, and children (WIC)
Head Start	1965	Assists disadvantaged preschool children, increases educational skills
National School Lunch Act and Child Nutrition Act	1966	Provides reduced or free meals to low-income families
Education for All Handicapped Children	1975	P.L. 94-142, free public education for all disabled children ages 3-21 years; provides necessary supportive services
CMHCs (Community Mental Health Centers)	1982	Effort to increase availability of mental health centers to low-income families
Missing Children's Act	1982	Nationwide clearinghouse for missing children (National Crime Information Computer)
Comprehensive Child Immunization Act	1993	Ensures that all children in the United States are protected against vaccine-preventable infectious diseases at the earliest appropriate age
Family and Medical Leave Act (FMLA)	1993	Enables eligible employees to take up to 12 weeks of unpaid leave from their jobs every year to care for newborn or newly adopted children; to care for children, parents, or spouses who have serious health conditions; or to recover from their own serious health conditions; after the leave, the law entitles employees to return to their previous jobs or to equivalent jobs with the same pay, benefits, and other conditions
State Children's Health Insurance Program (SCHIP)	1997	Provides health care coverage for children in families that earn too much to qualify for Medicaid but cannot afford private health insurance
Children's Online Privacy Protection Act	2000	Regulates the collection of personally identifiable information online from children under 13 years
Health Insurance Portability and Accountability Act (HIPAA)	2003	Developed by the Department of Health and Human Services to protect patient's medical records and other health information provided to health plans, doctors, hospitals, and other health care providers

care in more than 100 communities nationwide with higher-than-average infant mortality rates has recently received increased funding to help with the problem of infant mortality.

Childhood mortality rates have also declined. The leading cause of death in children over 1 year of age is injury from accidents; the majority of these are motor vehicle–related. Homicide remains the fourth leading cause of death in children ages 1 through 14. Homicide and suicide rank second and third, respectively, in the older adolescent age group. This reflects a continued shift in societal values and greatly affects the approach to health care for children in this age group (Box 1-1).

Childhood morbidity (illness, chronic disease, disability) is affected by general health, socioeconomic status, access to health care, and psychosocial factors. Acute illnesses, such as respiratory and gastrointestinal disorders, are common in children. At-risk children, such as those who are homeless, live in poverty, attend daycare regularly, or have decreased access

to the health care system, often have more frequent illnesses.

Because of technological advances, many premature and LBW infants who formerly would have died are surviving. Although this improvement in survival rates is encouraging, many of these infants develop chronic health problems such as bronchopulmonary dysplasia (BPD) (see Chapter 8 for further discussion on BPD).

Children with formerly fatal conditions, such as severe congenital heart disease and cystic fibrosis, are also surviving into adulthood. The AIDS epidemic has presented a spectrum of new challenges for nurses who care for infected infants and children. As incidents of childhood injury increase, the incidence rate of associated disabilities rises as well. A final important concern is the number of children and adolescents with severe emotional and behavioral problems that are caused by, or result in, school failures, violence, substance use, and risky sexual behavior.

Box 1-1 *Leading Causes of Death by Age Group in the United States*

1 TO 4 YEARS
Unintentional injuries
Congenital anomalies
Malignant neoplasms
Homicide

5 TO 14 YEARS
Unintentional injuries
Malignant neoplasms
Congenital anomalies
Homicide

15 TO 24 YEARS
Unintentional injuries
Homicide
Suicide
Malignant neoplasms

From the Centers for Disease Control and Prevention (2003). Deaths, percent of total deaths, and death rates for the 15 leading causes of death in 10-year age groups in the U.S.

HEALTH CARE TODAY

INSURANCE

One of the greatest effects on health care in the 1980s was the establishment of the Medicare system of payment for hospital stays on the basis of patient diagnosis-related groups (DRGs). This system also affected the private sector because many third-party insurance companies developed prospective payment plans of their own. These changes, along with the explosion of managed care systems in the 1990s, have led to shorter hospital stays for more acutely ill children and an increased need for earlier discharge teaching and home health care. Health maintenance organizations (HMOs) and preferred provider organizations (PPOs) are examples of managed care organizations. HMOs provide health care services for those enrolled; PPOs provide health care services to a specific group of clients at a discounted cost.

Unfortunately, access to primary care (health promotion and illness prevention) is a problem for many American families. In fact, 8.4 million children are uninsured. Significant disparity exists in the ethnic makeup of the uninsured. Specifically, 20% of all Hispanic children are uninsured, and 9% of all African-American children are uninsured, whereas only 6% of non-Hispanic white children are uninsured (Going Without: America's Uninsured Children, 2005). Many uninsured children are eligible for Medicaid or the State Children's Health Insurance Program (SCHIP) coverage. The SCHIP, enacted in 1997, provides health care coverage for children in families that earn too much to qualify for Medicaid but cannot afford private health insurance.

Aside from changes in the insurance industry, many advances have been made in medical and surgical techniques, giving rise to medical and nursing subspecialties within the area of pediatrics. For example, children with heart problems are treated by a pediatric cardiologist and cared for by pediatric cardiology nurse specialists. The complex surgery necessary for the newborn infant with a congenital defect is provided by the pediatric surgeon. Equipment to diagnose and treat illness in infants and children has become more sophisticated and specialized. Chromosomal studies and biochemical screening have made identification and family counseling more significant than ever. Acutely ill children are being cared for in special diagnostic and treatment facilities, where they receive expert attention. Many conditions that were once treated in inpatient settings are now treated in clinics, same-day surgery units, and other ambulatory settings.

Community Cue

A national program of the Robert Wood Johnson Foundation, *Covering Kids & Families,* works to connect uninsured children to low-cost and free health care coverage programs. Families can call toll-free (877-KIDS-NOW) to learn more.

HEALTH PROMOTION

Health promotion and disease prevention have become priorities. In 1990, the United States Department of Health and Human Services released a document entitled *Healthy People 2000: National Health Promotion and Disease Prevention Objectives.* This document builds on previously developed objectives to present an opportunity for Americans to take responsibility for their own health. It emphasizes equal access to health care for all segments of the population, particularly the most vulnerable. Many of these objectives apply to infants and children and are being researched and updated on an ongoing basis.

Healthy People 2010 is a follow-up to *Healthy People 2000.* Its objectives are promotion of healthy behaviors, promotion of healthy and safe communities, improvement of systems for personal and public health, and prevention and reduction of diseases and disorders.

EMERGENCY PREPAREDNESS

Emergency preparedness is essential in today's society. Recent natural disasters, along with events of terrorism and war, have increased the need for society to be prepared for emergencies, which include possible chemical, biological, or nuclear attacks. Children are especially vulnerable and are at greater risk than adults for the following reasons:

Selected *Healthy People 2010* Objectives

NUMBER	OBJECTIVE
7-1	Increase high school completion (target: 90%)
7-2	Increase the proportion of middle, junior high, and senior high schools that provide comprehensive school health education to prevent health problems in the following areas: unintentional injury; violence; suicide; tobacco use and addiction; alcohol and other drug use; unintended pregnancy; HIV/AIDS and sexually transmitted disease infection; unhealthy dietary patterns; inadequate physical activity; and environmental health (target: all components, 70%)
9-7	Reduce pregnancies among adolescent females (target: 46 pregnancies per 1000; baseline: 72 pregnancies per 1000 females aged 15-17 yr in 1995)
14-1	Reduce or eliminate indigenous cases of vaccine-preventable disease (target: 0 cases for measles, mumps, *Haemophilus influenza* type B [children under age 5 yr], polio, and rubella; reduce pertussis [children under age 7 yr] to 2000 cases and varicella to 400,000 cases)
14-4	Reduce bacterial meningitis in young children (target: 8.6 new cases per 100,000 children aged 1-23 mo)
14-18	Reduce the number of courses of antibiotics for ear infections in young children (target: 88 antibiotic courses per 100 children under 5 yr; baseline 108 antibiotic courses per 100 children under 5 yr during 1996-1997 [2-yr average])
14-22	Achieve and maintain effective vaccination coverage levels for universally recommended vaccines among young children (target: 90%)
15-20	Increase use of child restraints (target: 100%)
19-3	Reduce proportion of children and adolescents who are overweight or obese (target: 5% for children aged 6-19 yr)
19-4	Reduce growth retardation among low-income children under age 5 yr (target: 5%)

From U.S. Department of Health and Human Services (2000). *Healthy People 2010: Objectives.* Washington, D.C.: U.S. Government Printing Office. Available: *www.health.gov/healthypeople*.

- They breathe at a faster rate (inhaling more substances over a period of time).
- Their skin is thinner, and they have more skin surface in relation to total body mass (thus receiving proportionally higher doses of agents).
- They are more vulnerable to the effects of agents that produce vomiting and diarrhea (because they have less fluid reserve than adults).
- Very young children do not have the motor skills to escape danger or may even be curiously attracted to move toward the danger because of bright lights, colors, etc.

- Children are closer to the ground; thus they are at greater risk for inhaling the heavy particles of some gases including sarin and chlorine (chemical agents).

There are other special concerns regarding children and bioterrorism. Antibiotics and antidotes would need to be stockpiled; yet certain medications may not be approved for children or may have contraindications. With children, the correct size of emergency equipment and correct medication doses are extremely important. Trained personnel must be available to provide care for pediatric patients. In addition, the incubation period in children is shorter for many (e.g., biological) agents. On the other hand, this distinction could prove beneficial and yield earlier detection (Markenson, 2005).

With any disaster, children may suffer from post-traumatic stress disorder. They may demonstrate anxiety and depression. Children need to express their feelings in the event of such a disaster and be provided reassurance. By helping in some way, children can begin to regain their sense of security. They can participate in community response efforts (Markenson & Reynolds, 2006). Through play, children can also express how they are feeling and begin the process of healing.

Families should be taught emergency preparedness. This teaching can be done in the pediatrician's office or in a community setting. Knowing how to perform cardiopulmonary resuscitation, having rendezvous points, and keeping a list of emergency telephone numbers—including an out-of-state friend or relative whom all family members can contact after the event to report their whereabouts and conditions—are examples of teaching points needed to prepare families for any emergency.

Community Cue

The Federal Emergency Management Agency lists *www.fema.gov/kids* as a website designed for children to use to prepare for disasters.

Health care workers need to be vigilant, and early detection of any possible terrorism event is imperative. Health care providers should be familiar with clinical manifestations, isolation precautions, and treatments for causative agents. For example, the bacterial agent anthrax is considered the most likely candidate for a biological release (Markenson, 2005). Anthrax can be released in an aerosol form and could easily spread because it may be misdiagnosed. Although anthrax cannot be transmitted through person-to-person contact, it would present similar to influenza—but with a high fatality rate. Symptoms include fever, dyspnea, and eventually shock. Additional information on anthrax, as well as information on one of the viral

agents, smallpox, can be found in Chapter 12. The **toxin** *ricin* is a poison that can be made from processing castor beans. Symptoms of ricin inhalation poisoning include weakness, fever, cough, and pulmonary edema within 24 hours of ingestion. Death occurs 36 to 72 hours later. Treatment is supportive only; there is no cure.

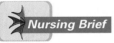

Community Cue

The Department of Health and Human Services Centers for Disease Control and Prevention (CDC) *(http://www.bt.cdc. gov/agent/agentlist.asp)* maintains an up-to-date listing of bioterrorism agents with information specific to them.

CURRENT PRACTICE

Because of the rapid changes taking place in health care today, it is the nurse's responsibility to update his or her knowledge constantly. As the role of the pediatric nurse expands, the issue of accountability becomes more important. Nurses have a responsibility to the community and to their profession. Today, involvement in community and professional organizations is not simply encouraged; it is absolutely essential for continued growth in an ever-changing society.

Nursing Brief

The Society of Pediatric Nursing is a professional organization for pediatric nurses *(www.pedsnurses.org)*.

Nurses are also expected to provide the best practice, and thereby the best outcomes, for their patients. Simply saying "Because we have always done it this way" is no longer acceptable. Health care professionals need to question current practices and find better alternatives. Through examination of research literature, nurses can analyze important evidence and improve the quality of care for their patients. This philosophy is known as **evidence-based practice**, and through its application, nurses are able to consistently apply new knowledge to practice and continually improve patient care (Windle, 2003).

The pediatric nurse may serve in a variety of roles, ranging from teaching in various settings to providing hands-on care in the hospital or clinic. Disease prevention is a focus for current health care. Health promotion and **anticipatory guidance** continue to play important roles in pediatric nursing. Caring for children in today's society requires careful assessment and early identification of children and families at risk. Working with families in a variety of settings helps to ensure the safety and needs of all children. Advocating for children and families

involves helping families to be fully informed regarding their child's care. The pediatric nurse works with other members of the health care team and with the family in providing care. Coordination and collaboration with other professionals becomes the norm. The nurse must be able to give competent, skillful care to children while maintaining a caring holistic attitude. Ethical decision making is an issue that nurses must deal with. Nurses must determine the most beneficial or least harmful action within the scope of the practice guidelines, standards, laws, and society. Incorporation of cultural and religious awareness and understanding of the family structure are also essential in providing competent nursing care. (Chapter 2 discusses the family unit.)

CULTURAL AND RELIGIOUS CONSIDERATIONS

Today, as in the past, cultural beliefs affect how a family perceives health and illness. The nurse cares for many culturally diverse patients. Each culture has its own beliefs and values. These values and beliefs are generally passed on from generation to generation. The more nurses know and understand different cultural beliefs, the easier it is to gain cooperation and trust from families. Holistic nursing includes awareness of cultural diversity and integration of this information with nursing care. It is important that one remain respectful and open-minded in discussions of cultural beliefs with the patient and family. Patient's beliefs generally cannot be changed, but the nurse should try to negotiate with the family to achieve desired goals when caring for the patient. The nurse needs to have an understanding of, and respect for, the beliefs of various cultures. When interviewing the family, it is crucial that one discuss cultural and religious preferences and determine the language that the family speaks most frequently. The nurse should discuss methods or preferences of treatment, any use of cultural and/or religious healers, and any home remedies that may have been used recently (Table 1-2).

Active listening is a key component of effective communication. Major blocks to listening are environmental distraction and premature judgment. Observe interactions with others to determine which body gestures (e.g., shaking hands or direct eye contact) are appropriate; ask when in doubt. Speak slowly and clearly to families with limited language comprehension. If possible, learn basic words and sentences of a family's language. Offer the services of an interpreter when necessary. When an interpreter is needed, be sure the interpreter knows the reason for the interview and the type of questions that are to be asked. Try to use the same interpreter each time, to provide consistency. To avoid confusion, pose questions to elicit only one answer at a time. Refrain from interrupting the family member and interpreter

Table 1-2 | *Worldview: Examples of Cultural Influences on Health Care Beliefs and Practices*

CULTURAL GROUP	HEALTH CARE BELIEFS AND PRACTICES
Mexican American	Looking at or admiring baby without touching the child can bring about *mal ojo* (evil eye). Touching the child when giving care will both prevent and treat *mal ojo*. Cold remedies are used to treat hot diseases, and hot remedies are used to treat cold diseases. Often seek *curandero*, or a folk healer, for treatment remedies and spiritual healing ceremonies. May be very modest when it comes to physical examination. Father has the dominant role; mother may influence decision making. Family values and roles need to be considered in the patient's treatment and recovery. Roman Catholicism is the predominant religion. Rely on the priest and family for prayers. Death and grief are considered "God's will."
African American	Believe illness can be from natural causes (exposure to wind, rain) or unnatural causes (witchcraft, voodoo, punishment for sin). "Granny" or "old lady" is woman in community with knowledge of herbs to treat common illnesses; many rely on folk remedies passed on from one generation to the next before seeking care from physician. "Spiritualist" will combine rituals, spiritual beliefs, and herbal medicines to cure ailments or illnesses. Some believe in the voodoo priest or priestess. Family structure is matrifocal or oriented around women.
Vietnamese American	Do not touch children on the head; the head is considered sacred, and care should be taken in touching and patting. Direct eye contact should be avoided when talking with someone who does not have equal standing in education, social standing, age, or gender. Beckoning with one's hand or finger with an upturned palm is the gesture used to beckon dogs and is considered insulting when used with people. Religions include Buddhism, Confucianism, and Taoism. Respect and harmony are the two most important values. Forces of yang (light, heat, or dryness), and yin (darkness, cold, or wetness) influence the balance and harmony of person's state of health; an imbalance causes disease. Natural elements can cause illness, such as bad food or contaminated water. Medicinal herbs and therapeutic diets can counteract the effects of natural causes. Supernatural causes of disease may be from gods, demons, or spirits. The *shaman* can restore the individual's spirit. Copper or silver bracelets, necklaces, or anklets prevent the spirit from leaving. Germs may also cause illness. Antibiotics have healing powers.
Chinese American	Forces of yang and yin influence the balance and harmony of person's state of health. Excessive eye contact may be considered impolite. May not ask questions when they do not understand. Normally, do not touch another person during conversation. Buddhist religion has the largest following. Family is based on a hierarchical structure. Chinese women are very uncomfortable when examined by male health professionals; a female nurse should be present for the examination. Colors and numbers may take on significance. The number 8 is lucky, as is the color red. The number 4 and the color white are considered unlucky. Traditional Chinese medicine is sought first before Western medicine. Acupuncture, herbal medicines, massage, etc., are used as therapies to restore yin and yang. Cultural healing practices can cause visible bruising or injury to child's skin.
Navajo	Eye contact is considered a sign of disrespect. Pointing is considered insulting. Children are taught to respect tradition and are viewed as assets. Must live in harmony with nature and supernatural forces. Medicine men and medicine women use sacred items for healing and blessing. May discuss care of a patient in the hospital with the physician. Mother retains primary responsibility for child rearing and discipline; matriarchal society.

Adapted from Giger, J., & Davidhizar, R. (2004). *Transcultural nursing* (4th ed.). St. Louis: Mosby.

while they are conversing. Avoid medical jargon whenever possible. These reminders help to bring down the communication barriers that exist when two people speak different languages.

The nurse also needs to determine whether practices and beliefs are beneficial to the child. Some practices raise concerns of abuse. An example of a cultural practice possibly considered abusive is *coining,* a Vietnamese practice that may produce welt-like lesions on the child's back when a coin, held on edge, is repeatedly rubbed lengthwise on the oiled skin

to rid the body of disease (see Figure 8-23). Another example is *burning,* a practice of some Southeast Asian groups, in which small areas of skin are burned to treat enuresis and temper tantrums (Hockenberry & Wilson, 2007). In a study done by McEvoy et al. (2005), most parents believed that disciplinary practices needed to be strict to instill in children a sense of respect for elders. Although some of these parents feared being accused of child abuse for using harsh disciplinary methods, most still found these practices important and necessary. Families need to know

RELIGIOUS GROUP	HEALTH CARE BELIEFS AND PRACTICES

Table 1-3   *Worldview: Examples of Religious Influences on Health Care Beliefs and Practices*

RELIGIOUS GROUP	HEALTH CARE BELIEFS AND PRACTICES
Catholic	Anoint the sick (called last rites).
	Do not approve of abortions or contraceptives.
Jehovah's Witness	Opposed to blood transfusions but may be persuaded in emergencies.
	When parents refuse consent to treat a child, a court order may be necessary to obtain required care.
Christian Scientist	Diseases of children principally related to the parents' errors of belief impressing themselves on their offspring.
Jewish	Good health is highly prized.
	Prayer is an important component of maintaining spiritual and physical well-being.
	Important to observe Jewish holy days.
	Circumcision practiced on eighth day of life by a trained mohel, by child's father, or by physician.
Muslim	Human body belongs to God; thus organ donations or transplants forbidden.
	Cremation is not permitted.
	Muslim physician may recommend a blood transfusion to save a life.
Hindu	Many dietary restrictions.
	Illness and injury seen as a result of sins committed in previous life.
	Cooperate and accept Western medical practices.

Modified from Bowden, V., Dickey, S., & Greenberg, C. (1998). *Children and their families: The continuum of care.* Philadelphia: Saunders.

that such practices can place them in jeopardy with child protective services. Anticipatory guidance is an important intervention in exploring alternative means of discipline. However, any time beliefs and practices are detrimental to the health and welfare of the child, legal intervention may become necessary.

Religious beliefs also must be respected when caring for the child. Many religions have health care beliefs that could affect the health of the child. For example, Jehovah's Witnesses may not allow blood transfusions. The court sometimes must take action on the child's behalf.

Religious beliefs can affect the way a child or parent approaches health and illness (Fosarelli, 2003). Discussion with the family about religious beliefs and wishes is important. Many religions have special rites or practices that need to be respected. Religion is an important aspect of health care. Selected religious beliefs are discussed in Table 1-3.

COMPLEMENTARY AND ALTERNATIVE MEDICINE

Although many cultural beliefs have advocated nontraditional medicine for centuries, complementary and alternative medicine (CAM) has only fairly recently emerged in our society's health care arena. Complementary therapy refers to nontraditional therapy that is *used with* traditional or conventional therapy; alternative therapy *replaces* conventional or traditional therapy. All nurses need to understand CAM therapy and how it is used. One example of CAM is the use of herbs. Herbs such as chamomile have long been advocated for colic, sleep problems, and even anxiety. Chamomile also acts to enhance the function of the immune system and is considered very useful for fevers and infections (McIntyre, 2005).

Typically, CAM is not reimbursed by insurance companies; yet this therapy may be incorporated into the patient's health care regimen. Many parents of chronically ill or disabled children are advocating the use of CAM to gain a sense of control over the child's condition and to improve the quality of life (Sandler, 2003). In 2005, the American Academy of Pediatrics reaffirmed its position statement on CAM for children with chronic illnesses or disabilities. The AAP recommends that physicians provide balanced advice about therapeutic options, guard against bias, and establish a trusting relationship with families. Physicians themselves need to be informed and be willing to actively listen to the family and child with a chronic illness, realizing that many families may want to provide CAM as a treatment option.

Parents may also delay or stop traditional medical treatment in favor of an alternative therapy, believing that the alternative therapy may produce a better outcome. Often, a perception exists that CAM is more "natural" and "does no harm." Some parents do not realize that herbal remedies can actually *cause* health problems for their children. Also, because it is considered "natural," some parents may give their children more of an herbal remedy than recommended, believing that it will not be harmful (Nemours Foundation, 2003). Parents need to know that herbal remedies can cause high blood pressure, liver damage, and severe allergic reactions. In addition, consumers have no guarantee of quality because the Food and Drug Administration (FDA) does not require testing of herbal remedies for therapeutic or adverse effects. It is important to remember that there may be possible side effects from the use of herbs and that often no formal clinical studies have been done in relation to the safety of herbs in pregnancy, lactation, and childhood. Drug interactions are also a concern. Thus it is important for health care workers to inquire about a patient's use of CAM, especially herbs. Other approaches to

Table 1-4	*Selected Common Herbs and Uses*
HERB	**TYPICAL USES/CONCERNS**
Black cohosh (*Actaea racemosa*)	Used for rheumatism, hot flashes, night sweats, vaginal dryness, menstrual irregularities, and premenstrual syndrome. May also induce labor. Can cause headaches and stomach discomfort.
Echinacea (*Echinacea purpurea*)	Has traditionally been used to treat or prevent colds, flu, and other infections. Believed to stimulate the immune system to fight infections. May cause allergic reactions including rashes, increased asthma, and anaphylaxis. Gastrointestinal side effects have also been reported.
Ginkgo (*Gingko biloba*)	Used to treat asthma, bronchitis, fatigue, and tinnitus (ringing in the ears). May cause headache, nausea, gastrointestinal upset, diarrhea, dizziness, or allergic skin reactions. May increase bleeding risk, so use caution with anticoagulant drugs, bleeding disorders, or scheduled surgery or dental procedures.
Kava (*Piper methysticum*)	Used as a ceremonial beverage in the South Pacific for centuries; used to help people fall asleep and fight fatigue, as well as to treat asthma and urinary tract infections. Topically has been used as a numbing agent. Today is used primarily for anxiety, insomnia, and menopausal symptoms. May cause liver damage, hepatitis, liver failure. Also can cause dystonia (abnormal muscle spasm). May interact with several drugs, including drugs used for Parkinson's disease.
St. John's wort (*Hypericum perforatum*)	Used for centuries to treat mental disorders and nerve pain. Also for use as a sedative and treatment for malaria; balm for wounds, burns, and insect bites. Possible side effects include increased sensitivity to sunlight, anxiety, dry mouth, dizziness, gastrointestinal symptoms, fatigue, headache, or sexual dysfunction. May interact with indinavir, digoxin, warfarin, birth control pills, antidepressants, cyclosporine, and irinotecan.

Data from the National Center for Complementary and Alternative Medicine (NCCAM) Fact Sheets. 2005-2006. National Institutes of Health.

CAM are discussed in Chapter 3. Table 1-4 discusses the use and risk of several common herbs.

HEALTH CARE DELIVERY SETTINGS

Although children are hospitalized when illnesses or injuries warrant (see Chapter 3), in general, they are most often cared for in a variety of other settings. These include, but are not limited to, community and school clinics, pediatrician and family practice offices, home care, children's camps, and pediatric long-term care facilities.

CLINICS AND OFFICES

Most large hospitals today have well-organized outpatient facilities and satellite or community clinics for preventive medicine and care of the child who is ill. Although substantial socioeconomic disparities are still involved in the procurement of routine preventive services, Medicaid and other similar programs have made these services available to more low-income families. Within clinics, specialty areas (particularly at children's facilities) may exist, such as cardiac clinics, orthopedic clinics, and so forth, where the student can observe and assist. In many institutions, information is distributed and education is offered on childhood immunizations, injury prevention, and parenting skills.

In many cities, groups of pediatricians practice in office settings or clinic settings removed from the hospital. Such services aid in the distribution of health services and often provide evening and weekend health coverage. In most offices or clinics, nurses constantly triage (prioritize) and respond to telephone inquiries.

The **pediatric nurse practitioner (PNP)** may care for patients in the pediatric or family practice office, give routine physical examinations at the clinic, and otherwise collaborate with the physician so that a higher quality of individual care may be attained. This nurse frequently is the primary contact person for children in the health care system. The PNP may also work in school-based clinics or health centers along with school nurses and other health care providers. School-based health centers are often an ideal location to provide primary health care for children and adolescents. (Access to quality health care for all is the number-one focus area for *Healthy People 2010*.) The role of the school nurse has expanded at the same time that school-based health centers have increased in number (Figure 1-1). Most school-based health centers provide the basics of primary health care. Health assessments, anticipatory guidance, screenings, immunizations, acute illness care, lab services, dental care, pregnancy testing, and family planning may be incorporated into these centers. Information may also be provided in regard to sexually transmitted diseases and HIV/AIDS counseling (Gustafson, 2005). School nurses provide health counseling and education and act as advocates for students with disabilities. School nurses and nurse practitioners also partner with community physicians and community organizations and may collaborate with state programs, such as SCHIP.

Another area of outpatient care is the pediatric research center, such as the one at St. Jude's Hospital in Memphis, Tennessee. St. Jude's is one of the world's premier centers for research and treatment of catastrophic diseases in children, particularly pediatric cancers, often at little or no expense to the patient. Research is also done at Shriners Hospitals, a network

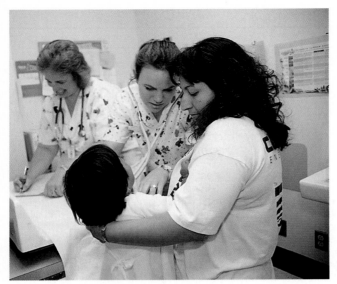

FIGURE **1-1** School-based clinics are located inside the school to provide accessible and affordable health care services to students.

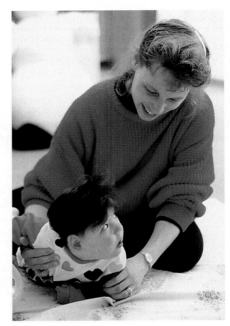

FIGURE **1-2** A home care nurse works with the child in his familiar home environment to attain his optimal level of functioning.

of pediatric specialty hospitals where children under the age of 18 receive medical care absolutely free of charge. Shriners Hospitals mainly treat patients with orthopedic conditions and burn injuries.

Elective surgery for patients with uncomplicated conditions, such as tonsillectomy or hernia repair, is also routinely done in outpatient settings. Advantages of same-day surgery include a reduction in cross infection, hospital costs, and bed use. Outpatient clinics also eliminate the need to separate the child from the family, making it less stressful for the child. In this type of setting, careful preparation and teaching must be done and assurance must be obtained that the child's home environment is adequate to meet the child's recovery needs.

As more and more medical care occurs in outpatient settings, there is an even greater reduction in the number of children who need hospitalization. It is expected that, for many children, the only exposure to medical personnel will be through brief clinic appointments. Our responsibility is to make these encounters positive for patients and families.

HOME CARE

Because hospitalizations are now briefer for most children, home care may be an acceptable alternative to a prolonged hospital stay (Figure 1-2). Technical improvements and research in specific disease entities have helped to advance the movement in home care. The result is often lower cost, increased patient satisfaction, and overall general well-being. Ongoing intravenous therapy is often maintained through home care, as is phototherapy for the newborn with jaundice. Home care, however, is not merely a matter of supplying equipment, appliances, and nursing care;

it requires assessment of the total needs of children and their families. Families need to be linked to a wide variety of network services. These services are often established by a case manager, who plays a vital role in home care arrangements. Case managers oversee a continuum of care for the patient.

For families who are facing the loss of a child, hospice is a service that offers unique help. Hospice is a program offered to children who are terminally ill, usually those with only 4 to 6 months left to live. Parents, with the help of hospice nurses and caregivers, often provide the care for their dying child at home. See Chapter 18 for more information on hospice.

PARISH NURSING

Another area of nursing that has emerged is parish nursing, a specialized practice of professional nursing that focuses on the promotion of health within the context of the values, beliefs, and practices of a faith community. Parish nursing focuses on the health care needs of all ages and provides health promotion, health maintenance, and illness prevention programs, as well as community resources and support groups. Children and adults can benefit from the services provided.

OTHER PROGRAMS

Local and national support groups for specific problems afford opportunities for families to share and support one another and to learn from others' successes and failures. Special groups and camps for children with chronic illnesses are also available. Many different types of organized camps exist in the United States. Examples include camps for children with asthma or children with cancer. Many of these camps are held in the summer months. Camp nurses perform assessments, dispense medications, provide first aid, triage health problems, and may also provide training to other staff.

Group therapy for children with stress is important in prevention of mental health problems. Children coping with depression or suicidal tendencies often need the support of group therapy. Many children also need group support if their parents are divorced, abusive, or abusing substances. Group support programs not only have the potential for improving life for the child and family but may also help reduce the high cost of medical care.

Long-term care facilities may be necessary for children with severe or profound mental retardation or for those with multiple disabilities. Placing a child in a long-term facility is a difficult decision for any family to make. A thorough assessment of the facility, with the needs of the patient kept in mind, is essential not only for the child's well-being but for the family's peace of mind as well.

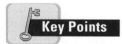
Key Points

- The Children's Bureau evolved from the first White House Conference on Children and Youth and addressed child welfare.
- Child health care has grown over the past several years as a result of federal programs and federal funding.
- The nursing care of children has evolved dramatically over the past 100 years. With this evolution, the needs of children, according to developmental level, have also evolved.
- The infant mortality rate continues to decline, although LBW is still the major contributor to infant death. An alarming increase in childhood mortality rates can be attributed to increases in homicide and suicide.

- DRGs have affected the way payment is made for hospital stays and, in combination with managed care, have led to shorter hospital stays and an increase in home health care. Insurance is lacking for many children, although programs are available to help. SCHIP has expanded insurance coverage to those ineligible for Medicaid.
- *Healthy People 2000* and *Healthy People 2010* have documented the need for Americans to take responsibility for their own health and have outlined government goals regarding health promotion and disease prevention.
- Chemical, biological, and nuclear terrorist threats are a real concern in society today. Health care workers must be aware of the special needs of children concerning these threats.
- Pediatric nurses need to be aware of cultural and religious preferences for patients and of the use of CAM such as herbs.
- Pediatric nurses care for children in a variety of settings. The care provided is directed not only at the child but at the family as well.

 Go to your companion CD-ROM for an Audio Glossary, video clips, and more.

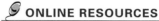 Be sure to visit the companion Evolve site at http://evolve.elsevier.com/Price/pediatric/ for WebLinks and additional online resources.

ONLINE RESOURCES

Centers for Disease Control and Prevention: http://www.cdc.gov/

Federal Emergency Management Agency: http://www.fema.gov/kids

National Center for Complementary and Alternative Medicine: http://altmed.od.nih.gov/

National Center for Health Statistics: http://www.cdc.gov/nchs/fastats/infmort.htm

The Society of Pediatric Nursing: http://www.pedsnurses.org

U.S. Department of Health and Human Services: http://www.hhs.gov/news

Growing Children and Their Families

Objectives

Upon completion of this chapter, the student will be able to:

1. Define the vocabulary words listed
2. List the stages of development from the newborn period to adolescence
3. Describe characteristics of growth and development
4. Read a growth chart
5. List six factors that influence growth and development
6. Show an understanding of the influence of the family on the developing child
7. Identify four growth and development theorists
8. Describe the predictable physical changes that take place in normal growth and development
9. Explain why nurses must have an understanding of growth and development

Key Terms

 Be sure to check out the bonus material on the Companion CD-ROM, including selected audio pronunciations.

autosome (AW-tō-sōm; p. 12)
body mass index (BMI; p. 17)
cephalocaudal development (sĕf-ă-lō-KAW-dăl; p. 16)
chromosome (KRŌ-mō-sōm; p. 12)
cognition (kŏg-NĬ-shŭn; p. 19)
development (p. 15)
growth (p. 15)
karyotype (KĂR-ē-ō-tĭp; p. 12)
Kohlberg (p. 20)
Maslow's hierarchy of needs (p. 19)
maturation (MĂCH-u-RĂ-shŭn; p. 16)
metabolic rate (MĔT-ah-BŎL-ĭk; p. 16)
multifactorial (MŬL-tĭ-făk-TŌ-rē-al; p. 15)
ossification (ŏs-ĭ-fĭ-KĀ-shŭn; p. 17)
Piaget (pē-ă-ZHĀ; p. 20)
proximodistal development (PRŎK-sĭ-MŌ-DĬS-tal; p. 16)

HEREDITY AND THE DEVELOPING CHILD

Most of us understand that something inherited is received from one's ancestors. The inheritance may be money or a desired heirloom. It is also possible to inherit physical traits and sometimes even a disorder, such as hemophilia. A person's gender and all inherited characteristics are determined at the moment of conception, when the male sperm cell unites with the female ovum. There are 23 pairs of chromosomes:

22 pairs of autosomes (chromosomes common to both genders) and one pair of sex chromosomes (XX in females and XY in males). Modern cytogenetics (*cyto,* cell; *genetic,* origin) has led to the identification of chromosomes as bearers of **genes** and of **DNA** as the key molecule of the gene. Like chromosomes, genes are paired. Although matching genes in a pair of chromosomes have the same basic function, they do not act with equal power. Some are **dominant,** others **recessive.** If a gene is dominant, its instructions are expressed. If a gene is recessive, its instructions are overpowered when it is matched with a dominant gene. If, however, a child inherits two recessive genes (one from each parent), the particular characteristics associated with this gene are expressed. When any two members of a pair of genes carry the same genetic instructions, the person carrying those genes is said to be **homozygous** for that particular trait. When the two genes in a pair carry different instructions, the person is **heterozygous** for the trait. One member of a heterozygous pair of genes is the dominant gene.

The concept of genes as dominant or recessive is important in the study of birth defects because some parents who carry defective genes can have healthy children or children who are carriers but are not affected themselves. This concept also explains how outwardly normal parents can give birth to a baby with a defect (Figure 2-1). An individual's particular set of genes is known as a **genotype.** Researchers have localized many genes to specific chromosomes, which is termed **gene mapping.** The availability of these techniques makes an accurate family health history more vital than ever.

KARYOTYPE

Geneticists are able to photograph the nuclei of human cells and enlarge them enough to see the 46 chromosomes, or karyotype. These chromosomes are cut from the picture, matched in pairs, and grouped from large to small. The result is called a **karyogram** (*karyo,* nucleus; *gram,* chart). The karyogram of a normal individual shows 22 pairs of chromosomes called **autosomes.** These chromosomes, which are alike in male and female, direct the development of the individual. An example of an autosomal defect is **Down syndrome,** also known as trisomy 21 because

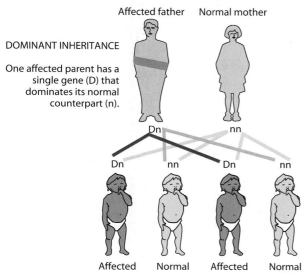

DOMINANT INHERITANCE

One affected parent has a single gene (D) that dominates its normal counterpart (n).

Affected father   Normal mother

Dn   nn

Dn   nn   Dn   nn

Affected   Normal   Affected   Normal

Each child has a 50% chance of inheriting either the D or the n from the affected parent.

A

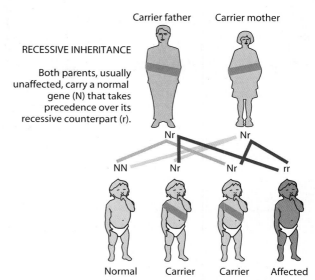

RECESSIVE INHERITANCE

Both parents, usually unaffected, carry a normal gene (N) that takes precedence over its recessive counterpart (r).

Carrier father   Carrier mother

Nr   Nr

NN   Nr   Nr   rr

Normal   Carrier   Carrier   Affected

Each child has a 25% chance of inheriting two r genes, which may cause a serious birth defect; a 25% chance of inheriting two Ns, and thus being unaffected; and a 50% chance of being a carrier, like both parents.

B

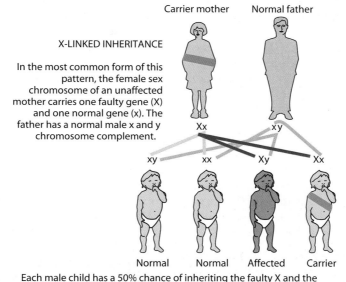

X-LINKED INHERITANCE

In the most common form of this pattern, the female sex chromosome of an unaffected mother carries one faulty gene (X) and one normal gene (x). The father has a normal male x and y chromosome complement.

Carrier mother   Normal father

Xx   xy

xy   xx   Xy   Xx

Normal   Normal   Affected   Carrier

Each male child has a 50% chance of inheriting the faulty X and the disorder, and a 50% chance of inheriting the normal x and y. Each female child has a 50% chance of inheriting the faulty X, and thus to be a carrier like the mother, and a 50% chance of not inheriting the faulty X.

C

FIGURE **2-1** Patterns of inheritance. **A,** Dominant inheritance. **B,** Recessive inheritance. **C,** X-linked inheritance.

these individuals have a third, or extra, number 21 chromosome.

The remaining pair of chromosomes are **sex chromosomes.** These differ in male and female, determining gender and secondary sexual characteristics. Defects in sex chromosomes are more prevalent than those in autosomes and account for a greater variety of abnormal conditions. The Y chromosome is small and apparently carries only the genes for masculinity. The X chromosome is much larger and carries the female genes plus many traits essential to life, such

as those that direct various aspects of metabolism, blood formation, color blindness, and defense against bacteria. When the genes that cause a specific condition are known to be carried on the sex chromosomes, the disorder is **sex-linked** (Box 2-1).

Omissions and duplications of chromosomes can occur during **meiosis** (the cell division seen only in sex cells in which the chromosomes divide in half before the cell divides in two). When either a piece of a chromosome or an entire chromosome becomes joined to another chromosome, or when broken

Box 2-1	*Examples of the Genetic Origin of Illnesses and Conditions in Children*

AUTOSOMAL ABNORMALITIES
Down syndrome (trisomy 21)
Edward syndrome (trisomy 18)
Patau syndrome (trisomy 13)
Mosaic trisomy 8 (trisomy 8)

SEX CHROMOSOME ABNORMALITIES
Klinefelter syndrome (XXY)
Double Y syndrome (XYY)
Trisomy X (XXX)
Turner syndrome (XO)

Table 2-1 *Common Malformations and Diseases Found in Children of Different Population Groups*

DISEASE	POPULATION GROUP
Cystic fibrosis	Northwestern European
Phenylketonuria	Northwestern European
Sickle cell anemia	African and Mediterranean
Tay-Sachs disease	Ashkenazi Jewish
Clubfoot	Polynesians
Cleft lip and palate	Chinese
Neural tube defects	White
Postaxial polydactyly	African
Ellis-van Creveld syndrome	Amish Mennonites
Thalassemia	Quebec, Northern New Brunswick regions
Umbilical hernias	African
Adrenogenital syndrome	Eskimo
Glucose-6-phosphate dehydrogenase (G-6-PD) deficiency	African and Chinese

segments exchange places, the abnormality is termed a **translocation.**

Mutations, or accidental errors in duplication, rearrangement, or loss of parts of the DNA genetic code, are not completely understood. Once a gene becomes abnormal, the defect is repeated whenever the chromosome on which it appears reproduces itself during normal cell division. Radiation in the form of radiographs, radium, atomic energy, and isotopes can cause mutations. Because a defect may not appear for generations, the amount of radiation to which a person can safely be exposed is difficult to determine. New gene mutations may also occur. A mutation of a gene that directs the production of an enzyme can result in a disruption of the orderly process of metabolism. These biochemical disorders are termed **inborn errors of metabolism.** Without proper direction of the enzymes, harmful chemical products accumulate in the system. If a genetic mistake affects only an unimportant link in the metabolism chain or if the body otherwise compensates, no abnormal symptoms may occur, even though a gene is defective. Some examples of inherited pathological conditions discussed in this text are cystic fibrosis, sickle cell anemia, and hemophilia.

GENETIC COUNSELING AND RESEARCH

As researchers gather more information concerning the mysteries of the gene, they are able to discover more ways to prevent and treat genetic mishaps. The role of the **genetic counselor** has broadened and taken on greater importance in recent years. Genetic counseling is the process whereby parents and families are counseled regarding the pattern of a gene's transmission and the probability of occurrence or recurrence (Table 2-1). Patterns of inheritance are known for hundreds of specific birth defects. Counselors often can suggest laboratory tests to determine whether prospective parents are carriers. A list of genetic counseling services can be obtained from the National Foundation/March of Dimes.

In specific genetic disorders in which a precise enzyme or protein is missing, it is often possible to supply the necessary factor. For example, clotting agents may be given to persons with hemophilia and pancreatic enzymes to those with cystic fibrosis. In other disorders, elimination of an offending substance can correct the problem. This is seen in phenylketonuria, in which the elimination of foods high in phenylalanine can prevent brain damage.

Medical research is on the threshold of important breakthroughs in the understanding and treatment of genetic disorders. The U.S. Human Genome Project, funded by the federal government, is locating DNA on genes. Biochemists can at this time create many of these genes in laboratories. As the genetic code is further deciphered, sending messages to the nuclei of cells and supplying the minute amount of DNA needed to correct a mistake will become possible. Gene therapy replacement is a highly experimental project that holds great potential for diseases that are the result of a defective gene, such as cystic fibrosis.

With the development of new technology, obstetric and pediatric providers are faced with questions about pediatric genetic disorders. The ethical and moral obligations for care of such disorders are a constant issue for providers. Definition of standards of care for those who receive genetic testing and counseling is crucial to this area.

ADVANCES IN PERINATOLOGY

The quality of the uterine environment is as important to the fetus as its genetic makeup. Even if the fetus is exposed to a seemingly harmless drug or minor pathogenic organism, great harm can ensue. Certain chemicals and radiation are known **teratogens.** Teratogens are chemicals, agents, or factors that cause the production of physical defects in the developing embryo. These substances are hard to pinpoint because

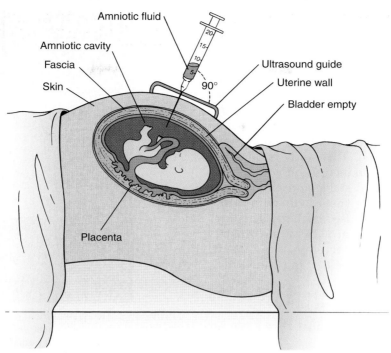

Amniotic fluid

Amniotic cavity

Fascia

Skin

90°

Ultrasound guide

Uterine wall

Bladder empty

Placenta

FIGURE **2-2** Amniocentesis. Amniotic fluid is drawn with a needle from within the amniotic sac. Cells from the fetus are in the fluid; analysis of these cells can indicate certain genetic disorders.

the defect may not be apparent for several months after delivery. Teratogens are most harmful during the first weeks after conception, before a mother is aware that she is pregnant. Many disorders are thought to be multifactorial. Cleft lip or palate, clubfoot, congenital dislocation of the hip, spina bifida, hydrocephalus, and pyloric stenosis are defects now thought to be multifactorial in origin.

Direct monitoring of a fetus and measurement of the amount of oxygen concentration in the blood of the unborn child are now possible. Both these procedures tend to be done late in pregnancy. Ultrasound sends sound beams into body tissues for determination of early pregnancy, multiple fetuses, fetal growth, location and size of the placenta, and certain malformations.

Intrauterine diagnosis has also been greatly facilitated by **amniocentesis** and **chorionic villi sampling (CVS).** Amniocentesis entails withdrawing amniotic fluid from the womb for the purpose of examining fetal cells (Figure 2-2). CVS entails withdrawing a sample from the chorionic villi space in the placenta with real-time ultrasonographic guidance. An advantage of CVS over amniocentesis is that it can be done earlier in pregnancy, usually at 9 to 12 weeks of gestation; however, CVS does pose a higher risk for miscarriage (March of Dimes, 2006). Amniocentesis depends on the production of amniotic fluid, and the earliest it can be done is at 16 weeks of gestation. Both CVS and amniocentesis can test for the same conditions, except that CVS will not screen for neural tube abnormalities (March of Dimes, 2006). The safety of these procedures is augmented with the use of ultrasonography.

Additional testing may include **percutaneous umbilical blood sampling (PUBS)** and **fetoscopy.** PUBS uses an amniocentesis technique to remove blood from the umbilical cord. This test provides information that may not be provided by other tests. Fetoscopy is a procedure by which a fiberoptic fetoscope is inserted into the uterus to identify abnormal gross abnormalities. During the procedure cells can be removed for further DNA analysis. This procedure can also provide the mechanism to perform fetal surgery, such as placement of a ventricle shunt for hydrocephalus (Cortes, 2004).

Early prenatal testing allows the detection of Rh-negative blood problems and certain types of retardation, such as that accompanying Down syndrome and Tay-Sachs disease. These prenatal tests can also enable the physician to determine the gender of the baby, which is important in sex-linked disorders.

The physician may also test the mother's blood for elevated levels of a certain fetal protein, alpha-fetoprotein (AFP). Elevated AFP levels may indicate the possibility of spina bifida (open spine) or anencephaly (absence of the brain). If elevation of AFP exists, the test may be repeated and further investigation, such as ultrasound imaging, performed.

GROWTH AND DEVELOPMENT

Growth generally refers to the processes that result in increases in size, whereas development refers to increases in complexity of form or function.

Growth is **orderly** and proceeds from the simple to the more complex. Although orderly, growth is uneven at times. Growth spurts are often followed by plateaus. The periods of most rapid growth are infancy and adolescence. The **rate** of growth varies with the individual child. Each has a timetable that revolves around established norms. Siblings within a family vary in growth and development.

Growth and development are measurable and can be observed and studied. This study is done by comparing height, weight, an increase in vocabulary, the development of physical skills, and other parameters. There are variations in growth within the systems and subsystems, because not all parts mature at the same time. Skeletal growth approximates whole body growth, whereas the brain, lymph, and reproductive tissues follow distinct and individual sequences.

CLARIFICATION OF TERMS

The stages of growth and development referred to in this chapter are as follows:

PRENATAL LIFE	CONCEPTION TO BIRTH
Newborn or neonate	Birth to 4 weeks
Infant	4 weeks to 1 year
Toddler	1 to 3 years
Preschool	3 to 6 years
School age	6 to 12 years
Adolescence	12 to 21 years

As *growth* refers to an increase in physical size, measured in inches/centimeters or pounds/kilograms, *development* refers to a progressive increase in the function of the body. The two are inseparable. **Maturation** (*maturus*, ripe) refers to the total way in which a person grows and develops, as dictated by inheritance. Although maturation is independent of environment, the timing of maturation may be affected by the environment.

CHARACTERISTICS OF GROWTH AND DEVELOPMENT

Directional Patterns

Directional patterns are fundamental to the growth of all humans. **Cephalocaudal development** proceeds from head to toe (Figure 2-3). The infant is able to raise the head before he or she can sit and gains control of the trunk before walking. The second pattern is **proximodistal development**, or inner to outer. Development proceeds from the center of the body to the periphery. These patterns occur bilaterally. Development also proceeds from the general to the specific. The infant grasps with the hands before pinching with the fingers.

Height. The newborn infant at birth has an average length of about 20 inches (50 cm). Linear growth is caused mainly by skeletal growth. Growth fluctuates throughout life until maturity is reached. Infancy

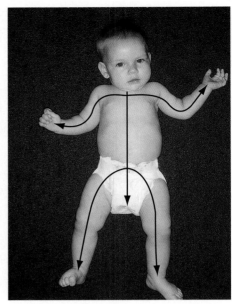

FIGURE **2-3** The development of muscular control proceeds from head to foot (cephalocaudal) and from the center of the body to its periphery (proximodistal).

and puberty are both rapid growth periods. Height is generally a family trait, although exceptions do exist. Good nutrition and general good health are instrumental in promoting linear growth. Height is measured during each well-child conference.

Weight. Weight is another good index of health. The average newborn infant weighs 7 pounds (3.25 kg). The quality of the uterine environment has a bearing on weight. Birth weight usually doubles by 5 to 6 months of age and triples by 1 year of age. After the first year, weight gain levels off to approximately 4 to 6 pounds (1.81 to 2.72 kg) per year until the pubertal growth spurt. Weight is determined at each office visit. A marked increase or decrease requires further investigation.

Body Proportions. Body proportions differ greatly in the child and adult. The head is the fastest growing portion of the body during fetal life. During infancy, the trunk grows rapidly, and during childhood, lower limb (leg) growth predominates. In adolescence, characteristic male and female proportions develop as childhood fat disappears. Alterations in proportions in the size of the head, trunk, and extremities are characteristic of certain disturbances. Routine measurements of head and chest circumferences are important indices of health. Head circumference need not be measured routinely after 3 years of age.

Metabolic Rate

The **metabolic rate** in children is higher than in adults. Infants require more calories, minerals, vitamins, and fluid in proportion to weight and height than do adults. Higher metabolic rates are accompanied by increased heat production and increased production of waste products. The body surface area of young children is far greater in relation to body weight than that of the adult. The young child loses relatively more fluid from the pulmonary and integumentary systems.

Bone Growth

Bone growth is one of the best indicators of biological age. Bone age can be determined from radiographic films. In the fetus, bones begin as connective tissue, which later is converted to cartilage. Through **ossification,** cartilage is converted to bone. The maturity and rate of bone growth vary within individuals; however, the progression remains the same. Growth of the long bones continues until **epiphyseal fusion** occurs. Bone is constantly synthesized and reabsorbed. In children, bone synthesis is greater than bone destruction. Calcium reserves are stored in the ends of the long bones.

Critical Periods

There appear to be certain periods when environmental events or stimuli have their maximal effect on the child's development. The embryo, for example, is adversely affected during times of rapid cell division. Certain viruses, drugs, and other agents are known to cause congenital anomalies during the first 3 months after conception. It is believed that sensitive periods also occur in respect to bonding, developing a sense of trust during the first year of life, learning readiness, and others. Most research in this area has been done with animals, and questions have been raised as to its application in humans.

Integration of Skills

As the child learns new skills, those skills are combined with ones already mastered. For instance, the child who is learning to walk may sit, pull herself up to a table by grasping it with her hands, balance herself, and take a cautious step. Tomorrow she may take three steps. Children connect and perfect each skill in preparation for learning a more complex one.

GROWTH STANDARDS

Growth is measured in dimensions such as height, weight, volume, and thickness of tissues. Measurement alone, without any standard of comparison, limits the interpretation of the data. Thus data have been collected and standards developed that make it possible to (1) compare the measurement for any one child with those for other children of the same age, gender, and ideally, race and (2) compare that child's present measurements with the former rate of growth and pattern of progress. The 2000 Centers for Disease Control and Prevention (CDC) growth charts are recommended for all children in the United States. These charts have been revised with samples

---

> **Box 2-2** | *BMI Calculation*
>
> **METRIC**
> BMI = (weight [kg]/height [cm] × height [cm]) × 10,000
> **ENGLISH**
> BMI = (weight [lb]/height [in] × height [in]) × 730

of children that include breastfed and formula-fed infants. The new charts include the 14 previous charts (revised), as well as two new charts that show body mass index (BMI)-for-age percentiles. These charts monitor data for infants, children, and adolescents up to age 20 years. They can also be used for low birth-weight infants. Head circumference measurements for infants and children up to age 36 months continue to reflect brain growth and size.

Body mass index has been established for use in adults for identification of overweight and obesity. BMI is calculated with height and weight measurements (Box 2-2) and can now be used to identify children as underweight, overweight, or at risk for overweight. BMI is age- and gender-specific, and a nutritional status is determined by percentiles. BMI is a tool that may indicate the need for further assessment. The importance of BMI data has been validated in studies indicating that children with BMI values of more than 95% have risk factors for cardiovascular disease (Freeman et al., 2001).

Accurate measurements are necessary in collection of data. **Length** indicates horizontal measurement; it is used before a child can stand. **Height** is measured with the child standing. Some guidelines in reading and interpreting growth charts follow:

- Children who are in good health tend to follow a *consistent* pattern of growth.
- At any age, there are wide individual differences in measured values.
- Percentile charts are customarily divided into seven percentile levels, designated by lines. These lines are generally labeled either as (1) 97th, 90th, 75th, 50th, 25th, 10th, and 3rd; or (2) 95th, 90th, 75th, 50th, 25th, 10th, and 5th.
- The median (middle), or 50th percentile, is designated with a solid black line. Percentile levels show the extent to which a child's measurements deviate from the 50th percentile, or median measurement. For instance, a child whose weight falls in the 75th percentile line is 1 percentile (1 line) *above* the median. A child whose height is at the 25th percentile is 1 percentile *below* the median.
- A BMI of more than 95% indicates a nutritional status of overweight. A BMI of more than 85% but less than 95% indicates a nutritional status of at risk for overweight. A BMI of less than 5% indicates a nutritional status of underweight.

- Deviations of two or more percentile levels from an established growth pattern necessitate further evaluation.

It is important to note that a child whose height or weight falls below the 10th percentile may be normal if the child has shown regular growth in height and weight and has a growth pattern that is comparable with that of the general population. Likewise, children whose height and weight fall in the 75th percentile may need further evaluation if this constitutes a major change from previous measurements (for example, if the child previously was in the 25th percentile). See Appendix F for examples of growth charts or visit the CDC website (*http://www.cdc.gov/growthcharts/*).

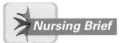
Nursing Brief

BMI is a tool that may indicate the need for further assessment.

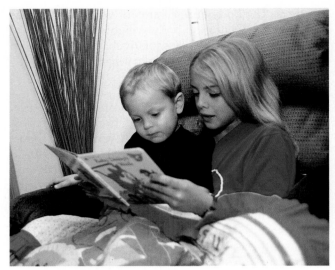
FIGURE **2-4** Siblings can play important roles in the family. Children who are secure and loved can direct their energies toward positive development.

FACTORS THAT INFLUENCE GROWTH AND DEVELOPMENT

Growth and development are influenced by many factors, such as heredity, nationality, and race, ordinal position in the family, gender, environment, and the family.

HEREDITARY TRAITS

Characteristics derived from our ancestors are determined at the time of conception by countless **genes** within each chromosome. Each gene is made up of a chemical substance called **DNA** that plays an important part in determining inherited characteristics. Examples of these inherited traits are eye color, hair color, and physical resemblances within families.

NATIONALITY AND RACE

Many ideas about physical differences between people of various nationalities and races have changed in our age of increasingly common environment and customs. For instance, persons of Japanese origin were once considered by Western standards to be short in stature. However, children of Japanese origin living in the United States are found to be comparable in height with other children in the United States.

Ethnic differences affect many areas, including speech, food preferences, family structure, religious orientation, and moral code. Ascertaining cultural beliefs and practices is important in the collection of data for nursing assessment.

ORDINAL POSITION

Whether the child is first, middle, or last in birth order in the family has a bearing on development. Younger children learn from their older brothers and sisters (Figure 2-4). The motor development of the youngest child in a family may be prolonged because this child tends to be "babied" by the others in the family. An only child tends to mature faster intellectually but, like the youngest child, is apt to be slower in motor development because much is done for her or him. Of course, the statements above are general tendencies, not absolutes, and individual variances abound.

GENDER

In general, the male infant weighs more and is longer than the female. He grows and develops at a different rate. Parents often treat boys and girls differently by providing gender-specific toys during play and by differences in expectations.

ENVIRONMENT

The physical condition of the newborn infant is influenced by the prenatal environment. The health of the mother at the time of conception and the amount and quality of her diet during pregnancy are important for proper fetal development. Infections or diseases may lead to malformations of the fetus. A healthy and strong newborn baby can adapt easily to the surroundings.

The home greatly influences the infant's physical and emotional growth and development. If a family is financially strained by an added member and the parents are unable to provide nourishing foods and suitable housing, the infant is directly affected. An uneducated mother may not know the proper methods of cooking foods to preserve nutritional value. Immunizations and other medical attention may be neglected. In addition, the baby may sense tension within the family and be affected by it.

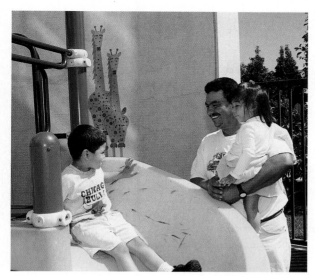

FIGURE **2-5** A single-parent family may result from divorce, death, or other events.

In contrast, when the home surroundings are secure and stable and the infant is made to feel wanted and loved, energies can be directed toward positive development. Most environments are neither completely positive nor completely negative but somewhere in between.

Intelligence, cognitive and emotional, plays an important role in social and mental development. Cognitive intellect is believed to be inherited, and emotional intellect is greatly affected by environment. These factors are related and are at times dependent on each other in the effect on growth and development. They make each person unique. If a child is ill, physically or emotionally, the developmental processes may be altered.

FAMILY

Family structure today is different from that of the past. Because of changes in women's roles in society, more women are employed. The 1990s and early 2000s have seen a great increase in both the number of women working outside the home and the number of women as the head of household. The increase in the number of single-parent families is another component of stress on the family (Figure 2-5). The traditional roles of the mother and father have changed, with many parents sharing both child care and household duties. The family is also more mobile, disrupting the family's support systems and requiring children to change schools.

As the family changes, so does the child. Children may be raised by one parent, by a relative, or in a foster home. Many children live in poverty and lack proper nutrition and health care. Currently, child care is lacking in quantity and quality, and this will be a central issue in the new millennium.

The home into which a child is born influences the child's entire life. Poverty is less detrimental to a child in a home where love and affection are present than in a home where there is discord and rejection. Each person brings to the role of parent certain attitudes about parenting based on his or her life experiences. A knowledge of growth and development can help parents set realistic goals for their children and themselves.

The effect of the family greatly affects the emotional well-being of the child. It is imperative that we, as health care providers, not only attend to families' needs, but also take advantage of their strengths and diminish their weaknesses.

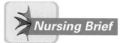

The family is an important resource for the child and the nurse.

THEORIES OF DEVELOPMENT

PSYCHOSOCIAL DEVELOPMENT

Although no one group of theories can explain all human behavior, each theory can make a useful contribution. Many experts have devoted their lives to understanding why children and families behave as they do. Some, called **systems theorists,** believe that everyone in the family (or system) is affected by everyone else in the family. This theory focuses on relations between and among the various individuals rather than on the individuals themselves. The nurse who relates to the systems theory focuses on caring for the child by caring for the whole family. The family, or system, is seen as protector, educator, resource, and health provider for the child. In turn, the child's health is seen as having an impact on each individual member of the family and on the family as a whole.

Many see human development as a composite of various theories. Maslow's hierarchy of needs is depicted in Figure 2-6, and the developmental theories of Erikson, Freud, Kohlberg, Sullivan, and Piaget are presented in Table 2-2. These theorists are discussed in later chapters where their theories relate to the specific age group discussed. Theories provide a framework for the practitioner, but it must be emphasized that humans are not a gathering of isolated parts, even though these parts may be analyzed for research purposes.

COGNITIVE DEVELOPMENT

Cognition refers to intellectual ability. Children are born with inherited potential, but this must be developed. There are a number of theories as to how learning takes place, with some disagreement as to the roles or importance of inner drives or needs and environmental stimuli. The development of logical thinking and conceptual understanding is

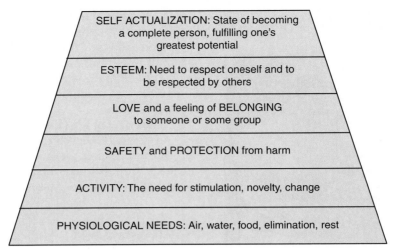

FIGURE **2-6** Maslow's hierarchy of basic needs.

a complex process. One outstanding authority on cognitive development was Jean **Piaget**, a Swiss psychologist. He proposed that intellectual maturity is attained through four orderly and distinct stages of development, all of which are interrelated. These stages are **sensorimotor** (up to 2 years), **preoperational** (2 to 7 years), **concrete operations** (7 to 11 years), and **formal operations** (11 to 16 years). The ages are approximate, and each stage builds on the preceding one.

Piaget held that intelligence consists of interaction and coping with the environment. Babies begin their interaction with reflex response. As they grow older, their use of symbolism (particularly language) increases. This gradually shifts to a here-and-now orientation (concrete operations) and finally to a fully abstract comprehension of the world (formal operations). Current theorists have identified inconsistencies in Piaget's theories; however, he remains an important pioneer in the study of intelligence.

MORAL DEVELOPMENT

Lawrence **Kohlberg** is one of the leading theorists of moral development. Kohlberg's theory is described in three levels, with two stages at each level. In the **preconventional** phase, children operate on a level of obedience to parental authority, and behavior is driven by a wish to avoid punishment. At the **conventional** level, the child is interested in pleasing others, and there is a need to maintain social order in society by maintaining law and order. At the **postconventional** level, moral principles are developed that can be used to solve complex moral and ethical dilemmas. Children pass through and reach these stages at various ages. It is believed that most children begin to develop the stages of the postconventional level only in adolescence and do not fully attain this stage until adulthood.

NURSING IMPLICATIONS OF GROWTH AND DEVELOPMENT

An understanding of growth and development and its predictable nature, including individual variation, has value in the nursing process. Such knowledge provides the basis for the nurse's anticipatory guidance to parents. For example, the nurse who knows when the infant is likely to crawl begins to expand teaching on safety precautions. The nurse also incorporates these precautions into nursing care plans in the hospital and in other health care settings.

Age-appropriate care cannot be administered when one does not have an understanding of growth and development. As the nurse explains various aspects of child care to families, the importance of individual differences is stressed. Parents tend to compare their children's development and behavior with those of other children and with information in popular magazine articles. This may relieve their anxiety or cause them to impose impossible expectations and standards. In addition, some parents have had poor role models who influenced their own experiences as children. Lack of knowledge concerning parenting can be recognized by the nurse, and suitable interventions should be used.

The nurse who understands that children are born with their own personalities can help frustrated parents cope with a newborn baby who is having difficulty settling into the new environment. During well-child visits, an assessment can determine whether an infant is merely on his or her own timetable or whether a variation from normal exists. The nurse provides anticipatory guidance to direct the parent's or caregiver's attention to upcoming events in the child's growth and development. The nurse also recognizes when to intervene to promote wellness or to prevent disease. For example, a brief visit with a caretaker may

Table 2-2   *Developmental Theories of Erikson, Freud, Kohlberg, Sullivan, and Piaget*

STAGE	ERIKSON	FREUD	KOHLBERG	SULLIVAN	PIAGET (INTELLECTUAL DEVELOPMENT)
Infancy (birth to 1 yr)	Trust/mistrust getting Tolerating frustration in small doses Recognizing mother as distinct from others and self	Orality—understanding the world by exploration with the mouth	—	Security, patterns of emotional response, organization of sensation	Sensorimotor stage (birth to 2 yr)—at birth responses are limited to reflexes; begins to relate to outside events; concerned by sensations and actions that affect directly
Toddler (1-3 yr)	Autonomy/shame and doubt Trying out own powers of speech Beginning acceptance of reality versus pleasure principle	Anality—learning to give and take	—	Mastery of space and objects	Preoperational (2-7 yr)—child is still egocentric; thinks everyone sees world as he or she does Preconceptual (2-4 yr)—forms general concepts, not yet capable of reasoning
Preschool (3-6 yr)	Initiative/guilt Questioning Exploring own body and environment Differentiation of genders	Phallic/Oedipal phase—becoming aware of self as sexual being	Preconventional or premoral morality—rules are absolute; breaking rules results in punishment (4-7 yr)	Speech and conscious need for playmates, interpersonal communication	Preceptual (4-7 yr)—capable of some reasoning, but can concentrate on only one aspect of a situation at a time
School age (6-12 yr)	Industry/inferiority Learning to win recognition by producing things Exploring, collecting Learning to relate to own gender	Latency—focusing on peer relations, learning to live in groups and to achieve	Conventional morality—rules are created for the benefit of all; adhering to rules is the right thing to do (7-11 yr)	Chumship, one-to-one relationship, self-esteem, compassion (homosexuality)	Concrete operations (7-11 yr)—reasoning is logical but limited to own experience; understands cause and effect
Adolescence (12-21 yr)	Identity/role diffusion Moving toward heterosexuality Selecting vocation Beginning separation from family Integrating personality (altruism, etc.)	Genitality	Principled morality (autonomous stage; 12 yr on)—acceptance of right or wrong on basis of own perceptions of world and personal conscience	Capacity to love, empathy, partnership (heterosexuality)	Formal operational stage (11-16 yr)—acquires ability to develop abstract concepts; oriented to problem solving

reveal that the child's immunizations are not up to date. Promotion of health can be achieved by educating the expectant mother. Other threats to health may likewise be anticipated. By knowing that specific diseases are prevalent in certain age groups, the nurse maintains a high level of awareness when interacting with these patients. This approach, based on knowledge, experience, and effective communication, helps to ensure a higher level of family care.

Finally, the nurse must understand how to provide nursing care to children of various ages so that their physical, mental, emotional, and spiritual development is enhanced according to their specific needs and comprehension.

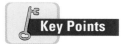

Key Points

- The genetic component of a child is based on chromosomes.
- Genetic disorders can result from mutations.
- Prenatal testing can detect some defects.
- Growth occurs in a cephalocaudal direction, which is from head to toe.
- Growth charts are used to assess a child's growth.
- BMI charts identify children who are at risk for cardiovascular disease.
- Factors influencing growth and development are heredity, nationality, race, ordinal position in the family, gender, environment, and the family.

- Maslow's hierarchy provides a framework for identifying the priority of basic human needs.
- Theorists of psychosocial development include Erikson, Freud, Kohlberg, Sullivan, and Piaget.
- Assessment of growth and development identifies the need for anticipatory guidance or nursing interventions.

Go to your Companion CD-ROM for an Audio Glossary, video clips, and more.

evolve Be sure to visit the Companion Evolve site at http://evolve.elsevier.com/Price/pediatric/ for WebLinks and additional resources.

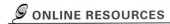

ONLINE RESOURCES

Abraham Maslow: http://www.ship.edu/~cgboeree/maslow.html

Erik Erikson: http://www.ship.edu/~cgboeree/erikson.html

Genetic disease information: http://www.cdc.gov/genomics/

Growth charts: http://www.cdc.gov/nchs/about/major/nhanes/growthcharts/clinical_charts.htm

Major personality theories: http://www.ship.edu/~cgboeree/perscontents.html

March of Dimes: http://www.marchofdimes.org

National Center for Health Statistics: http://www.cdc.gov/nchs/

New York Online Access to Health (NOAH): http://www.noah-health.org

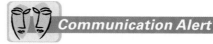 http://evolve.elsevier.com/Price/pediatric/

Objectives

Upon completion of this chapter, the student will be able to:

1. Define the vocabulary terms listed
2. Describe the physical facilities of a children's unit and explain their significance to the patient's adjustment to hospitalization
3. Discuss five measures the nurse can take to make hospitalization less threatening for the child
4. Describe how illness affects the child and family
5. Discuss the nurse's role in a hospital admission
6. Discuss the use of the nursing process in pediatrics
7. Discuss how to perform a systems review
8. Discuss how to take an infant's vital signs
9. Describe how to weigh and measure an infant
10. Discuss five guidelines or suggestions that may be useful to parents at discharge
11. List five safety measures applicable to the care of the hospitalized child
12. Plan care for a child who is in isolation
13. Discuss care of the child before and after surgery
14. Discuss both pharmacologic and nonpharmacologic pediatric pain management

Key Terms

 Be sure to check out the bonus material on the Companion CD-ROM, including selected audio pronunciations.

adventitious (p. 31)
contaminated (p. 38)
critical pathways (p. 30)
critical thinking (p. 29)
disinfected (p. 38)
dramatic play (p. 26)
hypnosis (hǐp-NŌ-sǐs; p. 46)
Nursing Interventions Classification (NIC; p. 29)
Nursing Outcomes Classification (NOC; p. 29)
palpation (pǎl-PĀ-shǔn; p. 33)
standard precautions (p. 40)
therapeutic holding (thěr-ǎ-PŪ-tǐk; p. 38)

THE HOSPITAL EXPERIENCE

THE HOSPITAL SETTING

Children may be hospitalized in a pediatric hospital, in a pediatric unit within a general hospital, or in a general hospital that admits children. Regardless of where the child is hospitalized, the pediatric setting differs in many respects from an adult setting. The pediatric unit or hospital is designed to meet the needs of children and their parents. A cheerful, casual atmosphere helps bridge the gap between home and hospital and is in keeping with the child's emotional and physical needs. Patients may wear their own clothing while they are hospitalized, and nurses wear colorful scrubs or pastel uniforms. Colored bedspreads and wagons or strollers for transportation also provide a more homelike atmosphere.

> **Communication Alert**
>
> Always meet children at their eye level. Figures that tower over them can be frightening.

The physical structure of a pediatric unit includes furniture of the proper height for the child, colorful furnishings, and child-friendly décor (Figure 3-1). All invasive or traumatic procedures are done in the treatment room. In this way, the child's room remains a relatively safe place and the other children are not disturbed or frightened by the proceedings.

Most pediatric departments include a playroom in the structural plan. This room is generally equipped with toys for various age groups. Bulletin boards and blackboards are also within reach of the patients, and mobiles may be suspended from the ceiling. Some playrooms are equipped with a fish aquarium or blossoming plants because most children love living things. Computers are also often available for use. The playroom may be under the supervision of a play therapist or a child life therapist. Parents usually enjoy taking their children to the playroom and observing the various activities. The nurse assisting should allow each child freedom to develop independently and should make observations about the child's play. The value of play to the child is discussed further in Chapter 11.

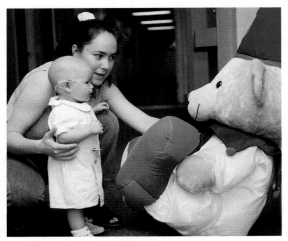

FIGURE **3-1** Children on the pediatric unit may be less anxious when the atmosphere is child-friendly.

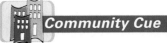
Community Cue

Child life therapists apply knowledge of theories of child development, play, stress, and coping and work with families and children to cope effectively with potentially stressful situations, both in the hospital and clinic settings (http://www.childlife.org).

Some children are not able to be taken to the playroom because of their physical condition. In such cases, the nurse should provide age-appropriate toys for the child in his or her room. If the child is in isolation, the toys generally stay in the room until the child goes home. Be sure cleaning procedures are followed once the child leaves.

Mealtimes on the children's unit may differ from those on adult units. Patients whose conditions permit may be served together around small tables. This provides a homelike setting and offers the child a social experience. If the child eats in his or her room, ensure a pleasant setting, free of odors and other noxious stimuli such as bedpans or urinals.

The daily routine in the pediatric setting also differs widely for obvious reasons. Although rigid schedules are not encouraged, children do benefit from a certain amount of routine. Meals, rest, and play are carried out at approximately the same time each day. Time for school work should also be structured. Nursing care is often delivered by consistent caregivers, promoting further security. Visiting hours on the pediatric unit are usually liberal. Parents are encouraged to stay with their child whenever possible, and most hospitals provide beds for parents.

THE CHILD'S REACTION TO HOSPITALIZATION

How a child reacts to hospitalization depends on the child's age, preparation, previous illness-related experiences, support of family and health professionals, and the child's emotional status. The major stressors of hospitalization include separation, loss of control, and bodily injury and pain (Hockenberry et al., 2005).

Infants and Toddlers

For infants and toddlers, separation anxiety is the major stressor during hospitalization. According to Hockenberry et al. (2005), three stages of separation anxiety exist: protest, despair, and denial. Unless toddlers are extremely ill, their grief and sense of abandonment are obvious. They protest loudly, watch and listen for their mother, and cry continuously until they fall asleep from sheer exhaustion.

The second stage occurs as anger turns to despair. The children look sad and lonely. They may refuse to eat. They become depressed and move about less. In the third stage—denial—children may try to deny the need for mother by appearing detached and uninterested in her visits. On the surface, children may seem to have settled in, but this is only a disguise to prevent further emotional pain. The nurse who comprehends the various separation stages sees parental visits as essential, even though the process of separation and reunion is painful. Education of the parents helps promote their continued visits and decreases feelings of inadequacy.

Toddlers also react to the loss of control they experience while hospitalized. According to Erikson, these children are involved in the task of autonomy (see Table 2-2). Activity limits, decreased opportunities for choices, and interrupted rituals contribute to a feeling of powerlessness. It is not unusual for toddlers to respond to this feeling with regression. They abandon recently acquired skills and may demand assistance with tasks that they have previously mastered. Without preparation for this, parents often find it difficult to understand the child's behavior. They need to be reminded that in this situation, this is normal behavior. Parents, however, do need to reinforce appropriate behavior, and the nurse needs to maintain a sense of sameness whenever possible.

Toddlers also are often affected by fear of injury and remember previous painful experiences. A brief explanation of the procedure followed by comfort after the procedure is often the best way to deal with this stressor.

Box 3-1 lists interventions for dealing with the stressors of hospitalization. In addition, toddlers need, within reason, to be allowed choices, which helps them to achieve control. However, questions such as, "Do you want to take your nap now?" could lead to answers such as, "I don't want to take a nap." Thus questions such as, "Do you want to take your nap now or after a story?" are better. Sometimes limits on behavior are necessary, especially if the behavior is intolerable. Parents are encouraged to support the child and use sensible limit setting if necessary.

Children should be forewarned, in keeping with their level of understanding, about any unpleasant or

Box 3-1 *Nursing Interventions for Stressors of Hospitalization*

Explain all procedures. Be honest.
Include parents in the care of the child.
Encourage the parents to stay with the child.
Maintain the routines and rituals of home.
Encourage the parents to bring familiar objects from home (stuffed animal, blanket, doll).
If the parents cannot stay with the child, encourage them to call, leave photographs, and visit when possible.
Perform all invasive procedures in the treatment room to keep the child's room a safe place for the child.
Provide for a consistent caretaker when possible.
Comfort the child after traumatic procedures if the parent is not present to care for the child.
Provide age-related diversionary activities.

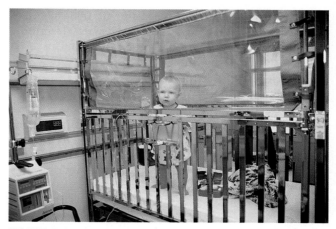

FIGURE **3-2** To facilitate autonomy, young toddlers should be allowed outside of their cribs whenever possible.

new experience that they may have to undergo while in the hospital. Be truthful about things that may hurt. This prevents a child from feeling betrayed and losing trust. Preparation and explanation should be done immediately before a procedure so that the child does not worry needlessly for an extended period of time. During the procedure, explain what is happening step by step. Immediately before something painful, tell the child that what is going to happen might hurt or be an "owie." Reassure the child that it is all right to cry or say "ouch." Allow toddlers to master the threatening experience through the use of play and fantasy.

Communication Alert

Using a stuffed animal, doll, or puppet decreases fear and helps the toddler to communicate. The nurse can use the inanimate object to assist in gaining the child's cooperation. For instance, "Let's see if your doll will take the medicine. She did! Now you try it."

Toddlers are encouraged to play with safe equipment used in their care—for instance, tongue blades and stethoscopes. Provide other toys appropriate to the developmental level, such as blocks, stacking toys, balls, and wooden puzzles. Whenever possible, toddlers should also be allowed out of the crib because confinement is frustrating for little ones who have just begun to enjoy walking (Figure 3-2). Supervised playroom activity contributes to intellectual, social, and motor development. Whenever possible, treatments should be done in the treatment room. The child's room should remain a "safe place," and the playroom should *never* be used for anything but play.

Preschoolers

Although not as obviously as the toddler, the preschooler also has separation anxiety. Preschoolers may act uncooperatively and ask frequently for their parents.

Preschoolers are significantly affected by loss of control. Not only have their schedules changed, but they are physically restricted. Children at this age are prelogical in their thinking and have difficulty distinguishing between fantasy and reality. They believe they are all-powerful and control the world around them and, in fact, may believe that their illness was caused by something they did or thought. They may feel guilty, particularly if an accident happened because of some mischief on their part, as in the case of a burn or a fall. It is important to help hospitalized preschoolers realize that hospitalization is not a punishment for something they have done wrong. Preschoolers also need choices so that they can regain some sense of control.

One of the major ways preschoolers cope with their environment is by fantasizing. Unfortunately, when in an unfamiliar environment, preschoolers' use of fantasy also contributes to their fears. Hospitalized preschoolers often have nightmares and are afraid of the dark or of unfamiliar sights and sounds. Animism, a belief that essentially gives life to inanimate objects, is a common concern of children this age (Hockenberry et al., 2005). Preschoolers often fear hospital machinery and equipment because they believe it is alive and will hurt them. This causes them to feel powerless (see Chapter 11 for further discussion).

Preschoolers fear mutilation during hospitalization and do not understand body integrity. They are afraid of bodily harm, particularly by invasive procedures and procedures that involve the genital area. Because they still have limited understanding of the inside of the body, preschool children often imagine that bodies are filled with air and will collapse when punctured or that bodies are filled with blood, which could all leak out through any artificial opening. This is why bandages (Band-Aids, for example) are so important to cover any injury, real or imagined.

Preschoolers tend to attach literal meanings to words such as *dye, draw blood, take,* or *test.* These words can have more than one meaning for the child and can be confusing. Avoid these words when describing procedures to children, and try to rephrase information in terms that are clear and understandable.

In addition to the interventions listed in Box 3-1, nurses should use their communication skills to assist the child in dealing with feelings of separation or fear. For example, the nurse might say, "Sometimes when I am in a strange place, I feel afraid." This assists the child in expressing fears. Nurses and parents should not tell a child that they will return unless they definitely intend to do so.

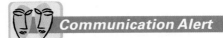
Communication Alert

Preschool children do not have a concept of time as it relates to the clock. If the child asks a question regarding time, the nurse might reply, "We will do that after cartoons" or "Mommy will come back after you eat your lunch."

The nurse must be aware of verbal and nonverbal cues from children this age. The child may withdraw or act in an aggressive manner. Parents may tell their children to "be brave" or to "act like a grown-up." This can prevent the child from verbalizing fears and discomfort.

The preschool child relieves tension through magical thinking, fantasy, and role playing. Nurses should participate readily in the child's fantasy if the fantasy is positive and appears to be helping the child achieve control. For example, if the child views the cardiac monitor as threatening because it is so loud, help the child write or draw a sign telling it to "talk softly" or "be quiet." Many children this age have imaginary friends, with whom they converse and behave as though the friends were really present in the room. Participation in this form of imagination is acceptable because displacing fears and feelings onto an imaginary friend helps a child feel more powerful.

Play is important to help the child adjust to hospitalization (Figure 3-3). Through dramatic play, children can act out situations that are part of their hospital experience. Dramatic play through the use of hospital equipment enables the child to "work through" emotions they may be dealing with. Giving a "shot" to a doll is an example of dramatic play. Puppets also help young children work through feelings. Nurses can encourage children to communicate through puppets; dolls and puppets may also be an avenue to play out situations with children.

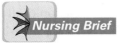
Nursing Brief

In addition to toys appropriate for the child's age group, everyday hospital supplies such as tongue depressors and bandages are often relished by the sick child.

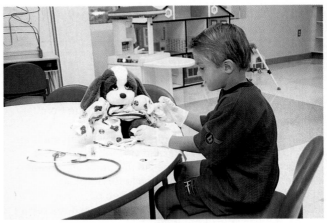
FIGURE **3-3** Play therapy is important for the hospitalized child. Note the child-sized furniture.

Preschool children may regress in their behavior when they are ill. An example would be bedwetting after the child has not had an "accident" for some time. Children may also be irritable and demanding when they are discharged. The parent should be assured that these behavior changes are temporary and the child will soon return to his or her "old self."

School-Age Children

School-age children may show some signs of parental separation anxiety, especially when they are ill. Even more so, these children miss their friends. They may fear their peers will forget them while they are away from school. On the other hand, their more sophisticated concept of time generally allows them to be patient and wait for a parent's return or a peer's visit.

School-age children are in the process of developing confidence in their abilities to control their feelings and actions. Hospitalization places them in the position of feeling out of control because it interrupts their routine and limits their independence. They may demonstrate resistive behaviors and have changes in vital signs in response to stress. Anger, boredom, frustration, and disinterest are other common manifestations of loss of control in the school-age child. These children appreciate the familiarity of objects from home and should be encouraged to bring such items to the hospital (Figure 3-4).

The school-age child fears pain and bodily harm. These children are more concerned with permanent disability or body disfigurement than are younger children. The older school-age child may also fear death.

In addition to the interventions listed in Box 3-1, school-age children can benefit from drawing and talking about drawings. This activity allows them to get in touch with their feelings because they may not have the ability or vocabulary to express their fears, worries, and concerns verbally. The use of drawings allows a child to express his or her feelings in an

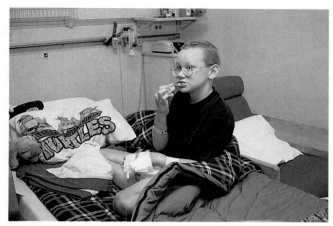

FIGURE **3-4** Familiar objects and maintenance of home routines normalize the environment and help the child cope with hospitalization.

abstract manner, and the nurse can then discuss these drawings with the child.

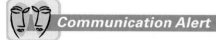

Communication Alert

Playing a board game often facilitates communication with a school-age child, who may feel uncomfortable talking to an adult. As the two participants become involved in the game, therapeutic conversation can be directed and begin to flow.

Encourage the hospitalized school-age child to be as independent as possible. Most school-age children are capable of complete self-care and can perform most daily activities independently within the modifications of their illness. Maintaining a school-age child's privacy is extremely important.

The education of the school-age child must continue throughout any illness. This gives the child a sense of continuity with the outside world, provides periods of socialization, and may reinforce weak academic areas. Some pediatric hospitals have areas designated for "school." The local school district may provide teachers to do on-site teaching. If this service is not available, family or friends may bring in school work from the child's regular teacher. This will ensure that the child does not fall behind in his or her studies. Education involves the parents, who may act as liaisons between the school and hospital. The teacher needs to be informed of the child's physical and emotional health to deal effectively with the patient. The nurse provides the children with opportunities to study undisturbed so that they are prepared for their classes. Whenever possible, diagnostic tests and treatments should be scheduled around established school routines.

Teachers should be notified if a child will be out of school for any length of time, and classmates should be encouraged to send cards, draw pictures, call, and visit if appropriate. The nurse should assist the child in displaying the cards and pictures. If possible, care should be planned around the visit of classmates and friends. Children need to maintain as much control as possible while in the hospital.

Adolescents

Adolescents may still want their parents present when they are hospitalized. They too miss their friends. However, some are hesitant to have friends visit because they are not sure how their friends will handle their illness or injury. They do not want to appear different or act differently, so compliance may be problem with a chronic disease. Even though adolescents may give the impression that they are not afraid, they actually may be terrified. They may feel that they will no longer "fit in" with their friends. Encouraging adolescents to express their fears helps alleviate these stressors and allows them to work toward maintaining or reestablishing their identity. Offer choices; this helps them maintain control and independence.

In general, fear of the unknown affects all hospitalized children. The nurse must explain in an age-appropriate manner what the child can expect, whether it pertains to unit routines or to procedures that need to be performed.

Unclear limits and expectations can best be minimized by explaining the rules and the expectations to the child. Once children understand what is expected of them, they feel less threatened and confused.

THE FAMILY'S REACTION TO HOSPITALIZATION

When a child is hospitalized, the whole family is affected. If the caregiver stays with the child in the hospital, then normal duties at home are neglected. Parents may be concerned about small children who are kept by relatives or friends. If the parents are unable to stay at the hospital, they may feel guilty about leaving the child. They may also attempt to rearrange their schedules to spend as much time as possible with the hospitalized child. Whatever the situation, the parents' needs should be identified by the nurse, and efforts should be made to decrease the anxiety the parents experience.

Parents may initially feel guilty, helpless, and anxious. They often blame themselves for the child's illness because they did not recognize early symptoms of a disease, may have delayed treatment, or were behind in preventive care. However, parents seldom are the direct cause of a child's hospital admission. Even in cases of child abuse, nothing is gained by blaming the parents. The nurse must realize that developing a trusting relationship with parents is often at the center of helping the child. This can be done only if the nurse remains objective and empathetic. The nurse should listen, acknowledge feelings, and support the family.

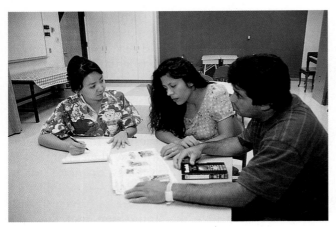

FIGURE **3-5** A variety of educational tools should be used to prepare the family and child for care.

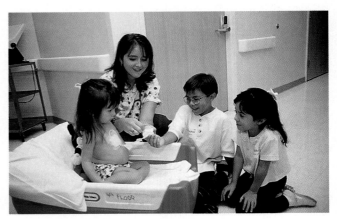

FIGURE **3-6** Siblings need to be fully informed about their sibling's care needs and condition and should be allowed to participate in care activities as much as they wish.

Parents may also fear the unknown. They may be unfamiliar with the hospital setting, procedures, treatments, and the disease itself. Explaining the rules and protocol of the hospital unit will reduce anxiety. Discussing procedures ahead of time and educating the parents on the disease process will also help to allay anxious feelings. Many children's hospitals now have educational areas designed for parents. Hospital librarians or other resource persons help parents to be *empowered* in the care of their child.

Hospitalization may cause financial problems for the family. This is especially true in the case of long-term illnesses and treatment. In addition to the obvious expense of the hospital and doctor, families often have the added costs of travel, lodging, food, and missed work. The nurse must be aware of these needs and make the appropriate referrals to social services.

As with the child, the nurse assesses the family's needs and develops interventions to meet these needs. Some of these interventions include:

- Assist parents in obtaining written and verbal information concerning the condition of the child and the treatment plan (Figure 3-5).
- Orient the family to the hospital.
- Explain all procedures.
- Refer the parents as needed to social services to assist in areas of medical expenses, food, and lodging.
- Listen to parents' concerns and clarify information.
- Involve parents in the care of the child.
- Provide for rooming-in.
- Reinforce positive parenting.
- Provide educational resources as necessary.

Siblings are also affected when a family member is hospitalized. They may experience anger, resentment, jealousy, and guilt. Suddenly attention is focused on the sick family member, and siblings may feel neglected. When routines are changed and members are separated, the needs of the siblings may not receive attention. Siblings may feel resentment. This can lead

them to feel guilty about their ill family member. The nurse can assist the parents in identifying and meeting the needs of siblings in the following ways:

- Keep siblings informed of the child's illness and progress.
- Allow siblings to visit the hospitalized child.
- Encourage siblings to provide pictures, make cards, and call.
- Allow siblings to assist with the care of the ill child if they seem comfortable doing so (Figure 3-6).

THE NURSE'S ROLE

ADMISSION PROCESS

A child must be prepared for hospitalization. If possible, the nurse should provide a tour of the pediatric unit to the parents and the child before admission. This is advisable and enables the parents to meet the people who will be caring for their child. Children and their families are often overwhelmed by the size of an institution and fear becoming lost.

Beginning as early as 6 months, the child is worried about being separated from the parents. Increased stress can lead to increased separation anxiety. After age 3 years, children may become more fearful about what is going to happen to them. Parents should try to be as matter of fact about this new experience as possible. Unless they have been hospitalized before, children can only try to imagine what will happen to them. Much detail is not provided because giving information beyond a child's understanding may create unnecessary fears. It is better to focus on the more pleasant and positive aspects—but not to the point where hospitalization seems to involve no discomforts. For example, one might mention that meals are served on a tray, that baths are taken from a basin at the bedside, and that the child will be with other children. The fact that there is a buzzer to call the nurse if necessary may add to the child's sense of security. The parents may also plan with the child what favorite toy or book to bring to the hospital. Security objects from home will help reduce anxiety in an unfamiliar setting.

In addition to explaining certain procedures, it is important to listen to patients and encourage questions. Parents should prepare children a few days, not weeks, in advance of a hospital admission. They should never lure children to the hospital under the pretense that they are actually going someplace else. In emergency situations, however, there may be little time for any preparation. In such cases, the entire medical team must try to give added emotional support to the child.

The nurse prepares the equipment for the admission procedure in advance. This saves time and frustration. Once the technical details are attended to, the nurse should concentrate on the approach to the patient and the family. The initial greeting should show warmth and friendliness. Smile and introduce yourself to the family and the child. When addressing the child, position yourself at eye level. If the child is shy, talk to the parents first. Children may need time to feel comfortable. Speak in a quiet, unhurried, and confident voice. Be prepared to meet the family's emotional needs. Many parents are stressed when their child is hospitalized.

When the child and parents are taken to the child's room, introduce them to any other children present. Parents should be seated comfortably. Explain the admission procedure carefully. Avoid discussing information in front of the child that he or she will not understand. The parents are encouraged to do as much for their child as possible, such as removing the child's clothes. Try not to appear rushed. A matter-of-fact attitude must be maintained regardless of the patient's condition. A soft voice and quiet approach are less frightening to the child. If the nurse looks anxious, it merely causes unnecessary worry for everyone. Take one step at a time. A calm nurse is more likely to reassure the family and the child than a nervous one. The nurse also should remain available to answer any questions that might arise. When a good relationship exists between parent and nurse, the child benefits from a higher level of care.

After essential admission information is documented (Figure 3-7), the nurse performs a systems review and physical examination of the child. Vital signs and measurements are obtained and recorded. Continued assessment findings are obtained and recorded throughout the hospital stay. See the Data Collection section later in this chapter for further discussion.

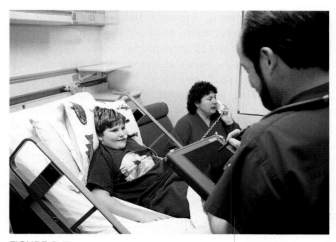

FIGURE **3-7** Documenting admission assessment findings in a computerized database organizes the information and makes it accessible to all health care providers.

CRITICAL THINKING AND THE NURSING PROCESS

Critical thinking is an expanded, systematic way of thinking. It emphasizes process, inquiry, and reasoning, as well as creativity and ingenuity, so that the nurse can draw the best conclusion regarding a situation. Critical thinking requires insight into one's ability to think and find solutions that provide the most effective nursing care. Several critical thinking exercises are used throughout this text.

Both critical thinking and the nursing process involve problem solving. The nursing process incorporates five steps: assessment, diagnosis, planning, implementation (intervention), and evaluation. In pediatrics, *both* the child and the family are the focus of the nursing process. The *care plan* is the result.

During the assessment, the data-gathering phase of the process, the nurse obtains essential information about the child's physical, social, and emotional health and about the family's adaptation to health alterations. Problems that emerge from the assessment are stated in diagnostic format. Those diagnoses approved by the North American Nursing Diagnosis Association (NANDA) are listed in Appendix B. The nurse next plans care for problems that were identified during assessment and are stated as nursing diagnoses. Priorities are set, and goals or outcomes are developed. Nursing Outcomes and goals are sometimes used interchangeably, however outcome statements are more measurable and state specific outcome criteria. In general, goal setting and outcome criteria constitute the planning phase and are the organizing structure for nursing interventions. Interventions are defined as "any treatment, based upon clinical judgment and knowledge, that a nurse performs to enhance patient/client outcomes" (Dochterman & Bulechek, 2004). The NANDA, **Nursing Outcomes Classification (NOC)**, and **Nursing Interventions Classification (NIC)** are three standardized nursing languages that were developed to facilitate communication, improve data collection and prioritizing, and assist in nursing research. Linkages between the three classifications show the connections between the patient's problem, the patient outcomes, and the nursing actions that resolve or decrease the problem. For example, if the NANDA diagnosis is *anxiety,* the NOC label might be *anxiety control,* and the NIC label might be *active listening.* The focus is on the actions necessary to reduce or eliminate a specific problem or to promote health. The evaluation phase appraises the changes experienced by the child or family in relation to achieving goals or outcomes.

Most hospitals and institutions use nursing care plans—individualized guidelines for care of the child and family. Some hospitals use preprinted, standardized care plans that are broad in nature and can be individualized to a particular patient. Care plans serve as communication tools among members of the health care team. They are a written expression of the nursing process. They state specifically what is to be done for each child and keep the focus on the child, not on the condition or the therapy. Care plans should be reviewed and updated daily. Nursing care plans appear throughout this book to illustrate the treatment of selected illnesses.

Because hospital stays, even for acutely ill children or those who have had major surgery, are becoming shorter (sometimes only 24 to 48 hours), many hospitals use written care plans and critical pathways. **Critical pathways** convert expected medical, nursing, social, and emotional outcomes for a particular problem into actions necessary to achieve the outcomes within a specified time frame. Nurses need to be especially vigilant with critical pathways to ensure that teaching and preparation for discharge are adequately provided for the child and family and that the appropriate referrals are made for follow-up care and health promotion.

DOCUMENTATION

The nurse must document initial findings when the child is admitted. Note any changes in the child's condition throughout the hospital stay. Document patient care needs and interventions done to meet those needs as well as the patient's response to the nursing care provided. Always document according to a specific time, rather than as a shift summary (Alford, 2003). Document assessment findings, significant changes of condition, and any actions based on changes of condition. Always chart with legal requirements in mind since each patient's chart is a legal document. In lawsuits it is often assumed by juries that if something was not charted, it was not done.

DISCHARGE PLANNING

Ideally, preparation for the patient's discharge begins on admission, because the goal of hospitalization is to return a more healthy and happy child to the parents. Good physical management of the patient's disease is necessary, but this is not enough. The nurse must also consider the emotional growth of the child and the education of the patient and family. This should provide a positive learning experience for all involved.

If a patient needs specific home treatment, such as hyperalimentation, colostomy care, crutches, a special diet, or insulin therapy, instructions should be given to the parents gradually throughout their child's hospitalization. These instructions should be provided in writing so that parents can refer to them as needed. If older children are to administer any treatments to themselves, they need careful explanations and supervision until both they and the parents are confident that the procedure will be carried out correctly at home. This may require home health care services.

Parents must also be prepared for behavioral problems that may arise after hospitalization. Severe stress is obvious during the patient's stay and requires in-service care and professional follow-up. In guiding the parents, the following suggestions may prove helpful:

- Recognize that after hospitalization the child may display such behaviors as clinging, regression in bowel and bladder control, aggression, fears, nightmares, and negativism.
- Allow the child to become a participating family member as soon as possible. Return former family responsibilities within the limits of the child's present abilities.
- Try not to make the child the center of attention simply because of the illness. Praise accomplishments unrelated to it.
- Be kind, firm, and consistent if the child misbehaves.
- Be truthful so that the child continues to trust you.
- Provide suitable play materials such as clay, paints, and doctor and nurse kits. Allow free play.
- Listen to the child and clear up any misconceptions about the illness.
- Do not leave the child alone for a long period or overnight until a sense of security is regained.
- Allow the child to visit hospital staff when returning for routine clinic visits.

Whenever possible, parents should be given as much notice of their child's discharge from the hospital as possible so that they can make necessary arrangements. This is particularly important if both parents work or if transportation is a problem. First, the physician writes the discharge order. Next, the approximate hour of dismissal is relayed to the parents. The intravenous (IV) or heparin lock is removed (as ordered by the physician), the child is dressed, and all personal belongings are collected. Parents are given any prescriptions written by the doctor, and discharge paperwork is completed. Most hospitals have a special discharge sheet that provides the family with written instructions regarding medications, diet, activity, and any other special precautions or procedures the child may need. The nurse prepares the discharge sheet, reviews it with the parent to determine understanding, and then has the parent sign the sheet. A copy is given to the parent, and a copy is retained on the patient's chart. Parents visit the hospital business office according to hospital procedure. According to condition, the child usually is placed in a hospital wagon, wheelchair, or stretcher and accompanies the family to the exit. The nurse assists the patient into the car as needed. State law requires that parents have car seats for infants and small children. Families without car seats may be provided with them on either a permanent or a loan basis. Charting includes time of departure and person with whom the child departs, the patient's behavior (smiling, alert, crying), method of transportation from the unit, any instructions or medications given to the patient or parents, and possibly the patient's weight and vital signs. Always check the institution's policy on dismissal.

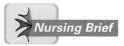
Nursing Brief

Discharge planning includes the identification and follow-up of children who may be at risk for child abuse, neglect, poverty, or a number of other conditions associated with their health problem or family lifestyle.

DATA COLLECTION

HEALTH HISTORY

Obtaining a complete health history is an important component of the assessment process. This interview process begins a relationship with the parent and child, provides useful data for the nursing process, and allows the nurse to begin to provide education and support for the family. When obtaining this information, convey an unhurried attitude, examine any cultural differences, and acknowledge any concerns the parents may have. Always clarify if unsure and summarize when necessary.

The *complete* health history (McKinney et al., 2005) includes the following:
- Statistical information (name, address, phone number, etc.)
- Client profile (eating and sleeping habits, educational level, developmental level, etc.)
- Health history (birth history, illnesses, immunizations, previous hospitalizations, allergies, etc.)
- Family history (information concerning the health status of the immediate family)
- Lifestyle and life patterns (social, psychological, physical, and cultural environment)
- Review of systems (see below)

SYSTEMS REVIEW

When examining the child, proceed in a general head-to-toe manner while collecting vital signs. In very young children, it is often helpful to examine heart, lungs, and bowel sounds first, especially if the child is quiet. Children can sit up if they prefer during the examination. Keep the child warm during the examination. Perform the least distressing aspects of the examination first. Use puppets or dolls to ease the anxiety of younger children. Allow children to handle the equipment such as the blood pressure cuff or stethoscope before the examination. Perform the most invasive procedures (such as rectal temperatures) last.

Note the facial expression and general appearance of the child. Observe posture, positioning, and body movement. Note the hygiene, any odor, drainage, discharge, or unusual skin conditions. Determine the child's nutritional status and any growth or development alterations. Observe the child's behavior. If the child is not alert and responsive, the child may be seriously ill. Inform the nurse in charge immediately if the child is lethargic or unresponsive. Always talk to the parents about how *they* think their child is doing because they know their child best. Be sure to perform a systems review on all hospitalized children at least once a shift (check the hospital policy). All hospitals have a method of recording the systems review. Be sure to document and report any unusual or abnormal findings. Table 3-1 provides a review of the body systems.

All areas of the systems review are important. It is especially important, however, to note that when auscultating the heart and lungs, the heart should have a regular rhythm. If extra sounds are detected or if the rhythm is irregular, notify the nurse in charge. The lungs should be clear to auscultation with no adventitious breath sounds. If wheezing, crackles, diminished lung sounds, or other unusual sounds are heard, report this to the nurse in charge also.

VITAL SIGNS
Pulse

When the nurse counts the pulse, the wave of blood is felt as it is forced through the artery. The pulse rate varies considerably in different children of the same age and size (Table 3-2). The normal pulse rate and respiratory rate of the newborn infant are high. Both pulse and respiratory rates gradually decrease with age until adult values are reached.

The pulse may be counted at any of the peripheral pulse points. However, an apical pulse is recommended for infants and small children. The apical pulse is heard through a stethoscope at the apex of the heart. The nurse counts the rate for 1 full minute. As previously mentioned, listen for any irregularities in rhythm. Report any irregularities to the charge nurse. Figure 3-8 shows the location of the pulses.

Respirations

The respirations of the infant and small child are counted by observing the movement of the abdominal wall because respirations are primarily abdominal at this time. The rate is counted for 1 full minute because respirations tend to be irregular during infancy. After about age 7 years, the child's respirations are measured in the same way as in the adult. Table 3-2 shows normal respiratory rates for children.

Blood Pressure

Blood pressure is defined as the pressure of the blood on the walls of the arteries. It is an index to the elasticity of the arterial walls, peripheral vascular resistance, efficiency of the heart as a pump, and blood volume. Blood pressure is lower in children than in adults. Common sites for measuring blood pressure in children are the brachial artery, radial artery, popliteal artery, and posterior tibial artery (Figure 3-9).

In the hospital setting, blood pressure is obtained on admission and at regular intervals throughout

Table 3-1 | *Review of Body Systems*

Integument	Observe for odor, color, moisture, texture, scars, bruising, lesions of the skin. Check for edema and turgor. Look at the hair for texture, quality, distribution. Inspect the nails for color, shape, and condition.
Head and neck	Observe the shape and symmetry of the head; observe the fontanel. Inspect the neck for any masses or swollen lymph nodes.
Eyes and ears	Look for symmetry. Check for any drainage. Does the child have trouble seeing or hearing?
Nose and mouth	Check for any drainage, observe the oral mucosa for color and moisture; check condition of the teeth.
Chest and lungs	Evaluate respiratory rate, rhythm, and depth. Note any retractions. Check symmetry. Listen to breath sounds with a stethoscope. Look at the color and consistency of sputum; note any cough. Note any breast development in females.
Heart	Note rate and rhythm of heartbeat with stethoscope.
Abdomen	Listen for bowel sounds in all 4 quadrants. Note peristalsis, hernias. Check the umbilicus in the newborn for drainage, odor, redness.
Genitalia and rectum	Observe for lesions, discharge, descended testes. Observe for patency of the rectum.
Back and extremities	Look for curvature of the spine. Note gait and posture and movement. Look for asymmetry of gluteal folds in an infant.

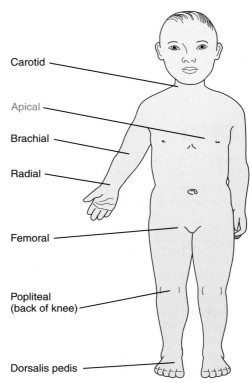

Carotid

Apical

Brachial

Radial

Femoral

Popliteal (back of knee)

Dorsalis pedis

FIGURE **3-8** Location of pulses. The apical pulse, heard through the stethoscope, needs to be counted for 1 full minute.

Table 3-2 | *Vital Signs at Various Ages*

AGE	HEART RATE (BEATS/MIN)	BLOOD PRESSURE (mm Hg)	RESPIRATORY RATE (BREATHS/MIN)
Premature	120-170*	55-75/35-45[†]	40-70[‡]
0-3 mo	100-150*	65-85/45-55	35-55
3-6 mo	90-120	70-90/50-65	30-45
6-12 mo	80-120	80-100/55-65	25-40
1-3 yr	70-110	90-105/55-70	20-30
3-6 yr	65-110	95-110/60-75	20-25
6-12 yr	60-95	100-120/60-75	14-22
12 yr	55-85	110-135/65-85	12-18

From Behrman, R. Kliegman, R., & Jenson, H. (2004). *Nelson's Textbook of Pediatrics,* (17th ed.). Philadelphia: Saunders.
*In sleep, infant heart rates may drop significantly lower, but if perfusion is maintained, no intervention is required.
[†]A blood pressure cuff should cover approximately two thirds of the arm; too small a cuff yields spuriously high pressure readings, and too large a cuff yields spuriously low pressure readings.
[‡]Many premature infants require mechanical ventilatory support, making their spontaneous respiratory rate less relevant.

the hospital stay. In the community setting, children over 3 years of age should have their blood pressure measured at the time of their physical examination. Children under 3 years of age need blood pressure evaluation if they have certain medical conditions such as congenital heart defects or renal disease (see Table 3-2 for normal blood pressure readings). It is important to remember that the child's blood pressure may be affected by time of day, age, gender, exercise, pain, medication, and emotion.

When obtaining blood pressure readings, the nurse needs to explain to the child what is about to happen. For example, the nurse might say, "This will hug your arm and feel tight for a few seconds." The child also needs to be allowed to examine the sphygmomanometer and cuff. This is followed by giving the child an age-appropriate explanation of the procedure. Afterward, the reading should be rechecked if a significant change or abnormal numbers are obtained. All readings are charted, and abnormal readings are reported to the appropriate charge nurse.

The general rule of thumb has been that the width of the cuff should cover approximately two-thirds of the upper arm, and the cuff (the inner inflatable bladder) should be long enough to encircle the extremity. See Figure 3-10 for a description of proper blood pressure cuff size. In general, systolic pressure in the lower extremities (thigh or calf) is greater than pressure in the upper extremities. In addition, a cuff that is too small causes a falsely elevated blood pressure; a cuff that is too large causes a falsely lowered blood pressure.

The most common ways to measure blood pressure are through auscultation and automated devices such as the Dinamap.

Auscultation. This is the preferred method for measuring blood pressure. Measure blood pressure as for an adult, with the pediatric stethoscope and cuff. Use the correct size. Record the systolic blood pressure at the onset of the "tapping" Korotkoff (K1) sounds. The fifth Korotkoff sound (K5), or the disappearance of Korotkoff sounds, has been established as the diastolic blood pressure (National High Blood Pressure Education Program, 2004).

Automated Devices. Devices such as the Dinamap are commonly used in pediatric settings. These can be set to measure blood pressure repeatedly and at short intervals. Remember to measure cuff size appropriately. Both systolic and diastolic pressures are recorded. An accurate reading can be obtained only if the child's arm (or leg) is held still. If the reading shows a major change from the child's baseline blood pressure, the measurement should be repeated because the machines are sensitive to movement. It is recommended that blood pressures exceeding the 90th percentile be repeated by auscultation (percentiles are listed in Appendix J).

Palpation. The nurse may occasionally obtain blood pressure readings through palpation. **Palpation** is one of the oldest methods of blood pressure measurement.

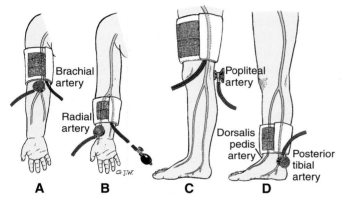

FIGURE **3-9** Common sites for measuring blood pressure in children. **A,** Upper arm. **B,** Lower arm or forearm. **C,** Thigh. **D,** Calf or ankle.

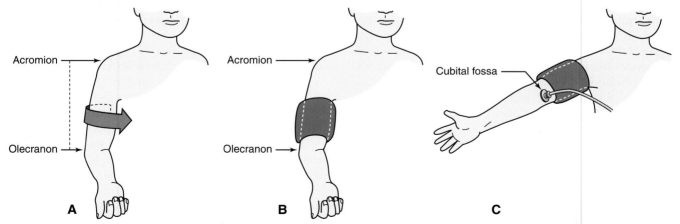

FIGURE **3-10** Determination of proper blood pressure cuff size. **A,** The cuff bladder width should be approximately 40% of the circumference of the arm measured at a point midway between the olecranon and acromion. **B,** Cuff bladder length should cover 80% to 100% of the circumference of the arm. **C,** Blood pressure should be measured with the cubital fossa at heart level. The arm should be supported. The stethoscope bell is placed over the brachial artery pulse, proximal and medial to the cubital fossa, and below the bottom edge of the cuff.

Apply the cuff and inflate above the expected pressure. Place the fingers over the brachial or radial artery. Record the systolic pressure as the point where the pulse reappears. Diastolic pressure is unobtainable. This is useful in neonates.

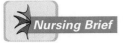

Nursing Brief

Electronic measurements are frequently used, but hypertension or hypotension that has been assessed electronically should always be verified with a manual cuff.

Temperature

Temperature measurement can be oral, axillary, rectal, or tympanic (taken from the tympanic membrane, or eardrum). Several types of thermometers are used, including electronic (digital), plastic strip, and tympanic. According to the U.S. Environmental Protection Agency (EPA), glass thermometers made of mercury should no longer be sold or used because of the risk for breakage and leakage of mercury that could create an exposure risk. Electronic thermometers can be used to obtain oral, axillary, or rectal temperatures. They are supplied with different probes, and probe covers are always used. Plastic strips are not routinely used in hospitals. The tympanic thermometer is considered a rapid, efficient, and noninvasive device for measurement of temperature. Temperatures are generally recorded in Celsius (centigrade). See Appendix H for conversions to Fahrenheit.

Rectal Temperature. A rectal temperature measurement may be preferred for the infant and for the small child who cannot hold a thermometer in the mouth without danger of biting it. Because a rectal temperature measurement may be traumatic to children, some institutions use only axillary temperatures for children who are not seriously ill. Research is ongoing in this area as measurement accuracy and temperature differences are examined. If the temperature is to be taken rectally, it should be the last vital sign obtained because it may make the child cry, which influences the pulse, respirations, and blood pressure. Table 3-3 shows normal temperature ranges.

When obtaining the rectal temperature, place the child in a comfortable position, either on the side with the knees slightly flexed or on the stomach. Infants may be in the supine position with their legs held around the ankles and then raised up. Insert the lubricated (electronic) thermometer a maximum of 1 inch into the rectum. Rectal temperatures are contraindicated in newborns because of the danger of rectal perforation and in children who have had rectal surgery or who are immunosuppressed or receiving chemotherapy.

Oral Temperature. The procedure is the same as for adults. Remember, *never* measure the temperature

Table 3-3 | *Normal Temperature Ranges for Children*

METHOD	RANGE
Oral	97.6°-99.3° F (36.4°-37.4° C)
Rectal	98.6°-100.0° F (37.0°-37.8° C)
Axillary	96.6°-98.0° F (35.8°-36.6° C)
Tympanic	98.4°-99.5° F (36.9°-37.5° C)

orally in a child who has had oral surgery or is at risk for seizures.

Axillary Temperature. The thermometer is held in the axilla with the child's arm pressed close to the body. This is a particularly good method for preschoolers who may fear invasive procedures.

Tympanic Temperature. Many hospitals use the infrared tympanic thermometer (ITT), or ear thermometer. Advantages include safety, noninvasiveness, convenience, and rapid results. Ear thermometers, however, are not as accurate, especially in younger children, specifically those less than 3 months of age. In children 3 years and younger, pull the ear down and back during this temperature measurement.

Body temperature does not remain at 98.6° F (37° C), and slight variations are considered normal. Rectal temperatures are slightly higher and axillary temperatures slightly lower than oral, but not the full degree Fahrenheit that was once thought. When temperature findings are recorded, the nurse notes the route used. If the reading is abnormal, the appropriate charge nurse should be notified. Managing fever in children is depicted in Nursing Care Plan 3-1; home care guidelines are included for parents. (Also see Skill 17-3 in Chapter 17, which describes the procedure for giving a sponge bath to manage fever.)

MEASUREMENTS
Weight

Weight must be recorded accurately on admission. Pounds are generally converted to kilograms for the pediatric patient in the hospital (see Appendix H). The weight of a patient provides a means of determining progress and also is necessary to determine the dosage of most medications. The child who has been undressed for weighing is observed for such objective symptoms as skin coloring, abrasions, bruises, rashes, swelling, or other unusual skin conditions or markings. The way in which the nurse weighs the child depends on the age.

The infant is weighed completely naked in a warm room. A fresh diaper or scale paper is placed on the scale. This prevents cross contamination—the spread of germs from one infant to another. The scale is balanced to compensate for the weight of the diaper. There are various ways of balancing scales; the nurse should request specific instruction for the particular scale used. The infant is placed gently on the scale. The nurse's nondominant hand is held slightly above the infant to ensure that the infant does not fall. The

NURSING CARE PLAN 3-1

The Child with a Fever

NURSING DIAGNOSIS *Hyperthermia, related to illness*

Goals/Outcome Criteria	Nursing Interventions	Rationale
Child's temperature between 97.4° F and 99.4° F (36.5° C and 37.4° C)	Assess temperature at least every 4 hours	Establishes baseline and shows variances
	Administer antipyretic medications (30 minutes before sponge bath) according to physician's instructions	Antipyretics lower body's "set-point" temperature
	Administer "tepid" sponge bath for fever of greater than 104° F (40° C); see sponge bath procedure	A "tepid" sponge bath lowers the body's temperature
	Assess vital signs before sponge bath	Determines a baseline for evaluation of response to treatment
	Assess vital signs 30 minutes after procedure	Determines effectiveness of procedure; expect temperature to decrease
	Cover with light clothing after procedure, prevent shivering	Shivering can increase body's temperature

NURSING DIAGNOSIS *Knowledge, deficient, related to fever*

Goals/Outcome Criteria	Nursing Interventions	Rationale
Parent understands and verbalizes the cause and treatment of fever	Determine parent's knowledge of fever	Determines how much the parent already knows and serves as an introduction to teaching
	Explain nature of fever (normal body reaction to infection); too vigorous control may mask signs of illness	Fever may actually enhance body's defense mechanisms and increase antibody activity
	Emphasize removal of excess clothing when child has a fever	Lowers body temperature
	Call physician if child looks sick and acts in a way other than normal	Parent knows child better than anyone else; degree of fever does not always reflect severity of illness
	Have parent return-demonstrate how to read a thermometer and identify normal temperature parameters	Gives parent sense of control and knowledge for home care and guidelines for calling the physician
	Explain how to administer age-appropriate/weight-appropriate dosage of antipyretic medicine for home care	Antipyretics lower the body's "set-point" temperature
	Discuss with parent tepid bath administration; remind never to use rubbing alcohol or cold water to sponge	Rubbing alcohol can be absorbed and cause too rapid heat loss; cold water can cause shivering, which in turn increases temperature

NURSING DIAGNOSIS *Knowledge, deficient, related to possible seizure (convulsion) activity*

Goals/Outcome Criteria	Interventions	Rationales
Parent understands potential for and knows how to give appropriate treatment during a convulsion	Discuss with parent potential for convulsion	Only a small number of children ever convulse with fever; however, discussion is advisable to allay anxiety
	Review management of a convulsion	Knowledge allays anxiety

NURSING DIAGNOSIS *Fluid volume, risk for deficient, related to dehydration, from increased metabolic rate*

Goals/Outcome Criteria	Interventions	Rationales
Child is hydrated, as evidenced by: • Good skin turgor • Moist mucous membranes • No weight loss	Increase fluid intake, offer "oral rehydration solutions," water, juice, Popsicles, as age-appropriate	Body's metabolic rate increases with fever; children have a higher proportion of body water; therefore more water can be lost rapidly with fever
	Monitor for dehydration at least every shift	By monitoring for evidence of dehydration, the nurse can alert the physician if changes occur

Continued

NURSING CARE PLAN 3-1—cont'd

The Child with a Fever—cont'd

NURSING DIAGNOSIS *Fluid volume, risk for deficient, related to dehydration, from increased metabolic rate*

Goals/Outcome Criteria	Interventions	Rationales
	Monitor intake and output at least once each shift	By monitoring for intake and output, the nurse can alert the physician of deviations from norm
	Weigh daily and record	Weight is a good indicator of the overall hydration status

NURSING DIAGNOSIS *Injury, risk for, related to possible seizure (convulsion) activity*

Goals/Outcome Criteria	Nursing Interventions	Rationale
Child remains free of injury, as evidenced by the absence of: • Bruising • Aspiration • Breaks in the skin	Keep side rails and/or pad up, according to hospital policy	Prevents injury from falls; prevents injury from hitting side rails
	Observe child frequently	Promotes safety by detecting subtle changes and possibly reducing complications
	Maintain suction at bedside	Keeps airway clear and prevents aspiration
	Remain with child if tub bath is given	Prevents head injury or drowning should seizure occur

❓ CRITICAL THINKING QUESTION

■ How would parents care for a child experiencing a febrile seizure at home?

nurse regulates the weights with the dominant hand. The scale should be read when the infant is lying still. If the parent is present, he or she may distract the child by waving or speaking softly. Once the exact weight is determined, the infant is removed from the scale, wrapped in a blanket, and given to the parent to soothe. Record the weight immediately. The scale paper is disposed of in the proper receptacle. An unsoiled diaper is returned with the infant. Digital pediatric scales that provide readouts in pounds and kilograms are used in many institutions. They do not require the regulation of weights. It is best to use the same scale for each measurement.

Older infants and young toddlers can be weighed in the same manner as infants but may prefer to sit up on the scale. Always protect the child from falls.

The older child is weighed in the same manner as an adult. A paper towel is placed on the scale for the patient to stand on. The patient is generally weighed in underwear or a hospital gown. The shoes are removed. If the child is unable to stand on the scale, the nurse may need to hold the child and read the combined weights. The nurse then is weighed and subtracts the weight from the combined weights to obtain the child's weight. Occasionally, a child who is wearing a cast is weighed. The nurse records this as, for example, "weight 34 pounds (15.45 kg) with cast

on right arm." Weight is recorded on the growth chart (see Appendix F).

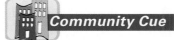
Community Cue

Temperature and weight are recorded on nearly all sick and well visits to the physician's office or clinic.

Height

The older child's height is measured at the time of weighing. Have the child stand straight (barefoot or in stocking feet) and measure with the attached marker, to the nearest 0.1 cm (0.03 inches). The infant must be measured while lying on a flat surface beside a tape measure or on a measuring board. The infant's knees should be pressed flat on the table. Place the head in the midline position; measure from the top of the head to the heel and record. Height is recorded on the growth chart (see Appendix F).

Head Circumference

Head circumference should be measured on all children less than 36 months of age and on children with neurological defects. Place a paper tape around the head from slightly above the eyebrows and pinnae of the ears to the occipital prominence of the skull.

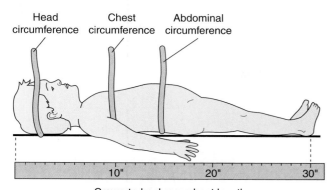

FIGURE **3-11**   Crown-to-heel recumbent measurements.

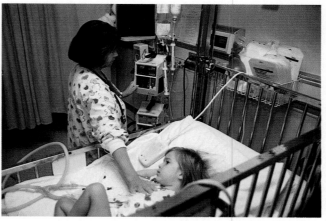

FIGURE **3-12**   Safety is always a priority. The nurse must keep at least one hand on the infant or child at all times when not properly secured.

Head circumference is recorded on the growth chart (see Appendix F). Check the institutional policy to determine whether chest or abdominal circumferences need to be measured (Figure 3-11).

SAFETY

The nurse must be especially conscious of safety measures on the children's unit. By showing concern about safety regulations, nurses not only reduce unnecessary accidents but also set a good example for the parents of children who are placed in their care. Although the physical layout of each institution cannot be altered by personnel, many simple safety measures must be carried out by the entire hospital team. The following measures apply to the children's unit.

Do

- Keep crib sides up at all times when the patient is unattended in bed. Use enclosed (bubble top) cribs for older infants and toddlers to keep them from falling or climbing out of the crib.
- Place a hand on the infant or child's back or abdomen when you turn your back to the child (Figure 3-12).
- Wash your hands before and after caring for each patient.
- Identify child by Identiband and *at least one other identifier*, such as birthday or medical record number.
- Check wheelchairs and stretchers before placing patients in them.
- Place cribs so that children cannot reach electrical outlets and appliances.
- Inspect toys for sharp edges and removable parts.
- Apply restraints correctly to prevent constriction of a part. Check institutional policy on frequency of releasing restraints and providing range of motion.
- Keep medications and solutions out of reach of the child.
- Keep the medication room locked when not in use.

- Identify the patient properly before giving medications.
- Keep lotions, tissues, disposable pads and diapers, and safety pins out of infant's reach.
- Prevent cross infection. Diapers, toys, and materials that belong in one patient's unit should not be borrowed for another patient's use. Properly disinfect any item brought out of an isolation room.
- Take proper precautions when oxygen is in use.
- Handle infants and small children carefully. Use elevators rather than stairs. Walk at the child's pace.
- Locate fire exits and extinguishers on the unit and learn how to use them properly. Become familiar with the hospital fire manual.
- Protect children from entering the treatment room, elevator, utility rooms, and stairwells.
- Use safety straps with children when they are in a highchair, swing, infant seat, stroller, and so on.
- Supervise playroom activity.
- Use electrical outlet safety plugs on the unit.
- Check hospital policy for children who are alone (for instance, policy may recommend that the door be kept open).
- Always look for small objects which can become choking hazards.

Do Not

- Do not prop nursing bottles or force-feed small children. There is a danger of choking, which may cause lung disease or sudden death.
- Do not allow ambulatory patients to use wheelchairs or stretchers as toys.
- Do not leave a child unattended in the bathtub.
- Do not leave a child unattended in a highchair, infant seat, or swing.
- Do not leave small children unattended out of their cribs in their rooms.
- Do not leave medications at the bedside.
- Do not leave a child unattended in an infant seat if it is placed on any area above the floor.

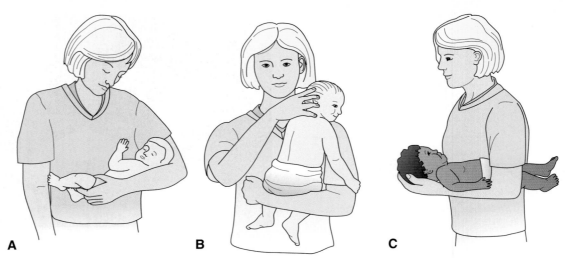

FIGURE 3-13 Three safe ways to hold a baby. **A,** The cradle position. **B,** The upright position. **C,** The football position.

- Do not leave any medication administration materials in the child's bed or infant's crib.

Many other safety measures must be carried out as each nurse becomes more familiar with the hazards of individual units. The nurse needs to continually assess the patient setting for safety issues.

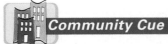

Community Cue

Be aware of safety precautions that must be taken for the child in a clinic or office setting, such as when the child is placed on the examination table.

TRANSPORTING, POSITIONING, AND RESTRAINING THE CHILD

The means by which the child is transported within the unit and to other parts of the hospital depends on age, level of consciousness, and how far the child has to travel. Older children are transported in the same way as adults. Younger children are often transported in their cribs, in a wagon or wheelchair, or on a stretcher. The side rails on a stretcher are raised during transport. Ensure that the patient's identification band is secured before leaving the unit. A notation is made about where the child is being taken and for what purpose. When a child is transferred permanently, as from the pediatric intensive care unit (PICU) to a private room, the child's new nurse should visit beforehand and meet the family.

Figure 3-13 shows three safe methods for holding a baby. Head and back support is necessary for young infants. The movements of small children are often random and uncoordinated; therefore they must be held securely. The football hold is useful when one hand needs to be free, such as for bathing the baby's head.

Restraints should rarely be used in the care of children because they restrict movement, limit autonomy, and create distress. Today's health care facilities and regu-

lating agencies clearly specify policies regarding application of restraints. When necessary, they are used to immobilize a child for diagnostic and therapeutic procedures and for safety. Documentation is required that identifies why restraints are necessary and what type of restraint is used. Restraint may be accomplished by simply holding the child or using the *least* restrictive type of physical device. Many procedures can be performed when a child is held in a secure, comfortable manner that provides close physical contact with the parent or caregiver (**therapeutic holding**). An example is when a parent securely holds the child for an injection. Restraint should be used only when other measures have failed and *never* as punishment. When restraint is necessary, it must be accompanied by increased emotional support such as rooming-in, additional attention from nurses, and suitable diversions. Always keep the patient's safety in mind when choosing the appropriate restraint. Restraints must be checked every 1 to 2 hours. To ensure that they are applied correctly, they also need to be *removed at least* every 2 hours so that they do not impair circulation, sensation, or compromise skin integrity. Table 3-4 describes some restraints for children. Figure 3-14 depicts a child in elbow restraints and a child in a jacket restraint.

MEDICAL ASEPSIS

The purpose of the medical aseptic technique is to prevent the spread of infection from one child to another or from the child to the nurse. A person (or object) is considered **contaminated** if that person has touched an infected patient or any equipment that has come in contact with the patient. People or articles that have not had any contact with the patient are considered clean.

Articles that have come in direct contact with the patient must be disinfected before they can be used by others. When something is **disinfected**, microorganisms in or on it are killed physically or

Table 3-4 *Restraints for Children*

RESTRAINT*	DESCRIPTION
Mummy	Immobilizes infant or small child for short time while procedure is performed or child is examined. Arms and legs are secured so that child cannot wiggle free. Useful for starting scalp IVs or performing nasogastric insertion.
Elbow ("no-no's")	Keeps child from reaching face or head. Covers most of arm. Must be correct size and positioned so that it does not rub against axilla or wrist. Useful for preventing touching of face, IV line, etc.
Jacket	Keeps child in bed, chair, or wheelchair. Tied in back of child and to frame of bed. Never tied to side rails.

*Check all restraints *at least* every 1 to 2 hours.

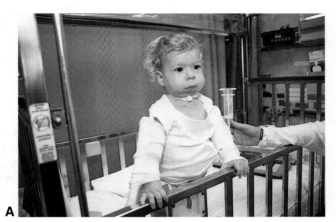
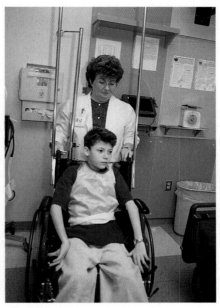

FIGURE **3-14** Two types of restraints. **A,** Elbow restraints. **B,** Jacket restraint.

chemically. The autoclave, which uses steam under pressure, is considered effective in killing most germs when the article is adequately exposed and sterilized for the proper length of time. The autoclave is used for certain nondisposable reusable items only. Items such as highchairs, IV line poles, cribs, and so forth must be properly disinfected (by chemical means) before the next patient can use them. Disinfection is done according to hospital policy, usually by the housekeeping department. Disposable items, such as needles, syringes, suction catheters, lumbar puncture trays, suture sets, nursing bottles, and oxygen tubing, are supplied to hospitals for medical asepsis purposes.

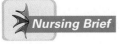

Nursing Brief

Used needles are not recapped and should be disposed of in a properly labeled, puncture-proof container. These special containers should be available in each patient room and in other areas where disposal is likely.

PREVENTING THE TRANSMISSION OF INFECTION

Children in the hospital need to be protected from nosocomial (hospital-acquired) infections. Likewise, health care workers need to be protected from infectious agents transmitted by children. Any patient who is suspected of having a contagious disease must be isolated until a definite diagnosis has been established. The Centers for Disease Control and Prevention (CDC) publish guidelines for isolation precautions that are readily available in health care institutions. These guidelines are usually located in an infection control manual. Many hospitals also have an infection control department with personnel who are specially trained to be resources in the hospital.

Pediatric hospitals and smaller children's units in general hospitals have isolation rooms or isolation set-ups. The nurse admitting the patient must take certain precautions. The purpose of the medical aseptic technique is to prevent the spread of the disease to the nurse and others. Proper handwashing cannot be overemphasized.

The patient is placed in a private room. Equipment for daily patient care is placed in the unit. This equipment includes a thermometer, stethoscope, bath equipment, etc. Such equipment remains there until the patient is discharged, and then it is treated by terminal disinfection. Disposable equipment is discarded in the proper receptacle. Linen is changed daily. Having on hand an ample supply of gowns, masks, and gloves also saves time and energy. A clean area is prepared according to hospital procedure. Remember that the floor is always considered contaminated. Anything that touches the floor must be properly cleaned or discarded (in or out of isolation). Toys must be washable. They may be borrowed from the playroom but must be disinfected before they can be returned. Because there is no satisfactory method of disinfecting books, reading should be limited to magazines or materials that are not highly prized by the owner. In the case of highly communicable diseases, reading material is discarded during the terminal disinfection of the unit.

When blood pressure is taken, a disposable blood pressure cuff is used. Built-in wall units reduce the danger of contamination. If a Dinamap is used, it must be disinfected after use and before taking it into another patient room. When a flashlight, otoscope, or ophthalmoscope is used, it is protected by a technique paper. Any equipment that comes in direct contact with the patient must be disinfected. All the specimens that leave the room are placed in a clean outer container according to hospital procedure. The hot water and detergents used in hospital dishwashers are sufficient to decontaminate dishes, glasses, cups, and eating utensils, so no special precautions are needed.

Throughout this book, emphasis is placed on the role of the nurse in preparing a safe environment for the child and parents. Of all the dangers in surroundings, none is more serious than disease-bearing organisms. Nurses must understand the importance of protecting themselves and others. This is accomplished with standard precautions. Standard precautions are followed because a history and physical examination cannot identify all patients infected with HIV or other blood-borne pathogens. Therefore body fluid precautions are taken with *all* patients. In addition to standard precautions, transmission-based precautions are designed to prevent/interrupt transmission of pathogens in the hospital. The three types of transmission-based precautions include airborne, droplet, and contact precautions (see Appendix E). Although it is vital to remember and use precautionary measures, the nurse must not forget that the patient is the primary concern. As the student's confidence increases with repetition of the details of isolation, the approach to the patient and the patient's problems is also more effective.

The following are specific techniques to be used with standard and transmission-based precautions.

Handwashing

Handwashing is the most important barrier against transmission of disease. Hands should be washed before and after contact with every patient, regardless of whether or not the nurse wore gloves during the contact. Gloves may be torn during use, and hands can become contaminated if the gloves are not properly removed. Many hospitals use gels or foams that do not require water and, dispensers are affixed either just outside or just inside the patient's door. Using these on entry and exit is now a requirement of most facilities. Soap and water are still required for visible soiling.

Gloves

Gloves are worn to protect the health care worker from contact with pathogens. They must be worn when health care workers are likely to have contact with mucous membranes, nonintact skin, blood, body fluids, secretions, excretions, and contaminated items. Gloves are to be changed between patient contacts.

Masks

Masks are worn to protect the health care worker from pathogens that are shed through respiratory droplets. A mask is also worn if there is a risk of blood or body fluid being splashed or splattered. A supply of disposable masks is kept outside the patient's room. A fresh one should be donned each time the health care worker enters the room. A mask is used once and discarded. It should *never* be allowed to hang around the neck and then be placed back over the face. It should cover the nose and mouth and should be changed at least once every hour. Do not touch a mask once it is in place. Remove it after removing the gown when leaving the unit, and do not touch the part that comes in contact with the face. Discard the mask in the room.

Gowns

When giving direct care to the child in isolation, the health care worker wears a gown to protect clothing from contamination. A gown is also worn to protect skin when procedures and patient care activities are likely to generate splashes or sprays of blood or body fluids. Without a gown, bacteria and other disease-causing organisms could be carried on the uniform, endangering the health of other patients. Sweaters should not be worn in isolation units. On the children's unit, the nurse must be particularly conscientious because small children need to be held for feedings and comforting. The nurse's relationship with the child is very direct. Caregivers wear disposable paper gowns that are used only once and then discarded. When the gown is put on, it is tied in the back. To remove, first untie the waist strings and the neckband, remove gloves if worn, and then discard. Remember to wash your hands. Use technique papers to open the door. Be sure to discard these papers in the patient's room and to close the door. The health care worker's shoes

Patient/Family Teaching Tips for the Child in Isolation

Wash hands on entering and exiting.
Gowns, masks, and even gloves may be required while in the patient's room.
Articles brought to the patient must be washable or disposable.
Always remove gowns, masks, and gloves before leaving the patient's room.
Do not take articles from the room.

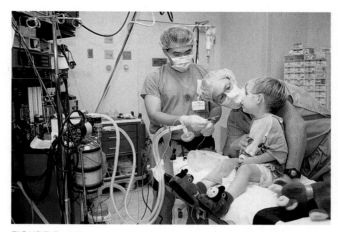

FIGURE **3-15** A parent's presence in the preoperative area can help reduce the child's separation anxiety. However, the child must be prepared for the parent wearing operating room garb.

are always a source of contamination, so hands need to be thoroughly washed if they come into contact with shoes. Contaminated linen and trash are disposed of according to hospital procedure.

Protective Eyewear

Goggles or face shields are worn if there is a risk of blood or body fluid being splashed or splattered. They are for one-time use and are disposed of with the trash.

EDUCATION OF THE FAMILY

Visitors are usually restricted to members of the immediate family. Check the hospital's policy on sibling visits. Isolation information is posted near the patient's door. Box 3-2 lists patient and family teaching tips when the child is in isolation.

Education of family members is an ongoing process. Points that need to be emphasized include the importance of immunizing children, the proper care of food (particularly perishables), the proper cooking of meats, the need for cleanliness in food preparation, and the importance of handwashing. Review with the family the primary ways in which infectious diseases are spread. Other modes of transmission, such as crowded living conditions, insects and rodents, and sandbox hazards, may also be topics to explore.

IMPLICATIONS OF PEDIATRIC SURGERY

The pediatric surgical patient needs to be shown the part of the body that requires surgery. The nurse can sketch a body outline and draw a circle around the operative site. The nurse should give simple information about the system that will be affected and stress that this is the only area of the body that will be involved. It may also be helpful to use anatomically correct dolls. The nurse must be careful if any procedure involves the genital area, especially if the patient is a preschool boy. Preschool boys are very afraid of castration. Therefore, when possible, the male child should be allowed to look at his penis after the procedure to reassure himself that it has been fixed and not cut off.

Children need to know what to expect on the day of surgery. Whenever possible, the child should attend a preoperative class. Children are particularly fearful of surgery and need both physical and psychological preparation. The child should be able to easily understand explanations and information. In addition, listening to the child is especially valuable for clarifying misunderstandings. Ask the child to point to the operative site on a body outline and then ask, "Can you show me what they are going to fix?" After explaining anesthesia, allow the child to play with the mask (Figure 3-15). Both children and adults need reassurance that they will not awaken during surgery. Be careful of expressions such as being "put to sleep" because a child may associate this with the death of a pet. It is important to always be truthful because this establishes trust. In addition, a study by Wollin et al. (2004) suggested that when there was less waiting time involved, with lots of toys, books, and posters to distract children, there was less anxiety among children waiting for surgery. Finally, nursing interventions after surgery are aimed at helping the child master a threatening situation and at minimizing physical and psychological complications. (See the index for specific operations.)

Tables 3-5 and 3-6 summarize preparation for surgery and postoperative care, comparing the child's needs with those of the adult.

THE CHILD IN PAIN

DEFINITION AND CHALLENGES

Pain in children has long been researched. Historically, children have not always been medicated properly for pain control. There is still a concern that pain in children is often undermedicated. Numerous myths, as well as deficient knowledge, contribute to the lack

Table 3-5 | *Preparation of the Child for Surgery*

PROCEDURE	ADULT	CHILD	MODIFICATION
Consent	Yes	Yes	Parent or legal guardian
Blood work	Yes	Yes	Age-appropriate restraint
Urinalysis	Yes	Yes	Age-appropriate collection (U-bag)
			Assist school child
			Age-appropriate instructions
Evaluation for respiratory infection, nutritional status	Yes	Yes	Use more objective observations in infants and toddlers because of limited verbal skills
Allergies	Yes	Yes	Indicate clearly on chart and patient wrist band
NPO	Yes	Yes	Increase fluids before NPO
			Length of time may vary with age and type of surgery (6-12 hr)
			Remove goodies from bedside stand
			No gum
			Supervise hungry ambulatory patients carefully
Vital signs	Yes	Yes	Approach child carefully, explain, demonstrate
Void before surgery	Yes	Preferred	Not always possible in infants and toddlers
Bath	Yes	Yes	Hospital gown; may wear underwear or pajama bottoms depending on age, type of surgery
Identification	Yes	Yes	Identiband
Teeth	Yes	Yes	Check for loose teeth, orthodontic appliance
Skin preparation	Yes	Possible	May be done in operating room
Nails	Yes	Yes	Trim, remove nail polish
Glasses or contact lenses	Yes	Yes	Have children and adolescents remove glasses and contact lenses
Enemas	Possible	Possible	Not routine
Transportation	Yes	Yes	Crib or stretcher
			Parents may accompany to OR door
Emotional preparation	Yes	Yes	Preoperative tour
			Group and individual puppet play
			Body drawings of parts involved
			Play selected by child as mode of expression
			Support parents during surgery
Sedation	Yes	Yes	Usually 20 min before surgery
Record all pertinent data	Yes	Yes	Essentially same, with pediatric modifications as indicated by preceding

NPO, Nothing by mouth.

of effective management (AAP Policy Statement, 2001). Unfamiliarity with use of sedative and analgesic agents in children and fears of oversedation, respiratory depression, and addiction contribute to undermedicating (Zempsky et al., 2004). In recent years, this problem has become a growing concern of health care providers. It is now known that children of all ages experience pain and are entitled to appropriate pain management. Pain is an individual, subjective experience, and health care providers need to identify and treat pain adequately. The American Pain Society (APS) describes pain assessment as the "fifth vital sign." In collaboration with the American Academy of Pediatrics (AAP), the APS has written a policy statement on pain management in children *(http://www.aap.org/policy/9933.html)* to ensure that all children receive adequate treatment of pain (AAP, 2001).

EVALUATION

When evaluating pain in children, always ask them about past pain experiences and known coping mechanisms. Also ask the parents about the child's past pain experiences. Be sure to identify words the child uses for pain, reaction to pain, and management of pain.

In addition, when evaluating the child, include precipitating factors, location, onset, duration, quality, intensity, and characteristics of the pain. Always observe nonverbal cues as well. For accurate assessment of pain, several pain scales have been developed. Depending on the developmental stage, children use different strategies to deal with pain. Pain is assessed using self-report if the child is old enough. Similar to adults, most older school-age children and adolescents are able to report pain on a scale of 1 to 10. A pictorial tool often used for preschool and young school-age children is the Wong-Baker FACES Pain Rating Scale (Figure 3-16). With this tool, the child looks at several pictures of faces ranging from happy to sad and then chooses whichever face reflects his or her pain (Hockenberry et al., 2005). A second pictorial pain assessment tool is the Oucher Scale for 3-year-old to 7-year-old children. It consists of six photographs of a white child's face representing levels ranging from "no hurt" to "biggest hurt you could ever have" and includes a vertical scale with numbers from 0 to 100.

Table 3-6 | *Summary of Postoperative Care of the Child*

PROCEDURE	ADULT	CHILD	MODIFICATION
Return from recovery room	Yes	Yes	Notify parents (parents may be allowed in recovery room) Smaller patients generally in crib Age-appropriate safety precautions
Note general condition, alertness	Yes	Yes	Infant and toddler cannot verbalize fear or pain
Vital signs	Yes	Yes	Every 15-30 min until stable Blood pressure reading sometimes omitted for infant
Evaluation for shock	Yes	Yes	Essentially same
Assessment of operative site for bleeding, dressing intactness	Yes	Yes	Essentially same Elevate casted extremities Circle drainage
Restraints	Possible	Probable	May be necessary to protect IV line Remove periodically for range of motion per hospital policy
Connect dependent drainage (urinary catheter), Levin tubes, oxygen	Yes	Yes	Prepare child for sight and noises of equipment, draw pictures to clarify purpose
Position patient	Yes	Yes	Abdomen or side unless contraindicated (no pillow)
IVs	Yes	Yes	Infusion pump for pediatric patients Monitor rate meticulously because infants and small children respond quickly to fluid shifts Measure and record intake and output
Assess elimination	Yes	Yes	Bowel and bladder
Relief of pain	Yes	Yes	Hold, comfort small children unless contraindicated Be sensitive to behavioral changes such as increase in irritability, crying, regression, nail biting, passivity, withdrawal Administer pain relievers as ordered Involve parents in care Provide transitional object such as blanket, favorite toy, pacifier Be aware of transcultural considerations that provide familiarity and comfort
NPO	Yes	Yes	Until fully awake Babies are started on clear fluids by bottle unless contraindicated Avoid brown or red liquids, which may be confused with old or fresh blood Monitor bowel sounds
Consider diet	Yes	Yes	Advance from clear to full liquids to soft to regular diet
Observe for complications	Yes	Yes	Turn, cough, deep-breathe, dangle feet, ambulate early; less of a problem in children; splint operative site (with small pillow) when child coughs

NPO, Nothing by mouth.

There are scales for African-American and Hispanic children also.

For infants and very young children, behavior is observed to assess pain. The FLACC (Face, Legs, Activity, Cry, and Consolability) scale is one tool that can be used for this young age group (Table 3-7). FLACC measures each of the five identified categories on a scale of 0 to 2, resulting in a total score between 0 and 10. The higher the total score, the more pain the child is experiencing (Merkel et al., 2002).

INTERVENTION

Nursing Care Plan 3-2 provides examples of nursing diagnoses related to pain in children.

Management of pain in children includes pharmacological interventions. Physicians will order pain medications for children depending on the intensity of the pain. Oral administration is generally used for mild to moderate pain. When the child needs immediate pain relief for more intense pain, intravenous administration is indicated. For moderate to severe pain expected to persist, continuous dosing or around-the-clock dosing at fixed intervals is recommended. Dosage is always adjusted, depending on patient response. When giving opioids or nonopioids, be sure the dosages are appropriate for the child's weight and age. (See Chapter 17 for dosage calculations.) Pediatric drug reference books are readily available in hospitals that care for children. Safe dosage guidelines should *always* be followed.

Nonopioid analgesics are often used to control children's pain. They are most effective for mild-to-moderate pain and have antipyretic effects as well. They do not produce dependence or tolerance. Examples of nonopioid analgesics are acetaminophen and ibuprofen.

Opioids are used to manage most forms of moderate to severe acute and chronic pain. They can be administered by most routes; generally, they are given

TRANSLATIONS OF WONG-BAKER FACES PAIN RATING SCALE*

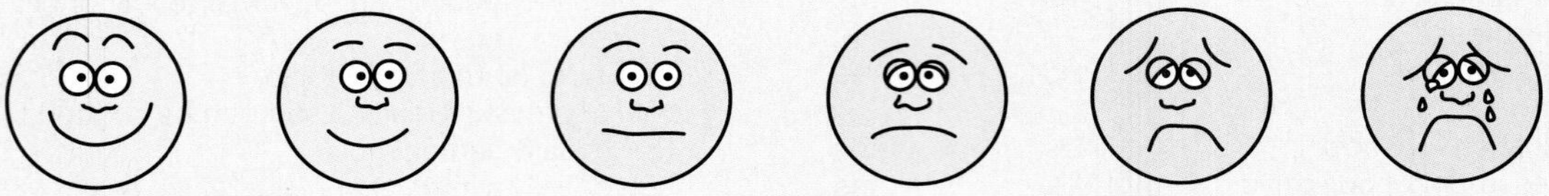

0–5 coding	0	1	2	3	4	5
0–10 coding	0	2	4	6	8	10
ENGLISH	No hurt	Hurts little bit	Hurts little more	Hurts even more	Hurts whole lot	Hurts worst
SPANISH	No duele	Duele un poco	Duele un poco más	Duele mucho	Duele mucho más	Duele el máximo
FRENCH	Pas mal	Un petit peu mal	Un peu plus mal	Encore plus mal	Très mal	Très très mal
ITALIAN	Non fa male	Fa male un poco	Fa male un po di piu	Fa male ancora di piu	Fa molto male	Fa maggiormente male
PORTUGUESE	Não doi	Doi um pouco	Doi um pouco mais	Doi muito	Doi muito mais	Doi o máximo
BOSNIAN	Ne boli	Boli samo malo	Boli malo više	Boli još više	Boli puno	Boli najviše
VIETNAMESE	Không dau	Hồi dau	Dau hỏn chút	Dau nhiêu hỏn	Dau thât nhiêu	Dau qúa dô
CHINESE†	無痛	微痛	較痛	更痛	很痛	劇痛
GREEK	Δεν Πσναï	Πσναï Λιγο	Πσναï Λιγο Πιο Πολν	Πσναï Πολν	Πσναï Πιο Πολν	Πσναï Παρα Πολν
ROMANIAN	No doare	Doare puţin	Doare un pic mai mult	Doare şi mai mult	Doare foarte tare	Doare cel mai mult

FIGURE **3-16** Brief Word Instructions (Above)

Point to each face using the words to describe the pain intensity. Ask person to choose face that best describes own pain and record the appropriate number. NOTE: Rating scale can be used with people 3 years and older.

Original instructions:

Explain to the person that each face is for a person who feels happy because he has no pain (hurt) or sad because he has some or a lot of pain. **Face 0** is very happy because he doesn't hurt at all. **Face 1** hurts just a little bit. **Face 2** hurts a little more. **Face 3** hurts even more. **Face 4** hurts a whole lot. **Face 5** hurts as much as you can imagine, although you don't have to be crying to feel this bad. Ask the person to choose the face that best describes how he or she is feeling. Rating scale is recommended for persons age 3 years and older.

NOTE: In a study of 148 children ages 4 to 5 years, there were no differences in pain scores when children used the original or brief word instructions. (In Wong D, Baker C: *Reference manual for the Wong-Baker FACES Pain Rating Scale*, Duarte, Calif, 1998, City of Hope Mayday Pain Resource Center; also available on website: http://evolve.elsevier.com/Wong/essentials/).

orally or intravenously. Although opioid analgesics can cause psychological and physical dependence, it is important not to withhold pain medication when this type of pain control is necessary. Tolerance or physical dependence may develop if opioids are used over a long period of time. Reducing doses over several days will help prevent withdrawal symptoms. Side effects of opioids may include respiratory depression, sedation, mental confusion, constipation, pruritus, nausea, and/or vomiting. Children often sleep after receiving an analgesic, but this does not mean they are pain free. Always evaluate the opioid's effect on pain and monitor vital signs after administering any analgesic. Examples of opioids commonly given orally in pediatrics are codeine and oxycodone; morphine is often given by the IV route. In pediatrics, the use of

Table 3-7 *FLACC Scale*

CATEGORY	SCORE		
	0	1	2
Face	No particular expression or smile	Occasional grimace or frown, withdrawn, disinterested	Frequent to constant frown, clenched jaw, quivering chin
Legs	Normal position or relaxed	Uneasy, restless, tense	Kicking or legs drawn up
Activity	Lying quietly, normal position, moves easily	Squirming, shifting back and forth, tense	Arched, rigid, or jerking
Cry	No cry (awake or asleep)	Moans or whimpers, occasional complaint	Crying steadily, screams or sobs, frequent complaints
Consolability	Content, relaxed	Reassured by occasional touching, hugging, or talking to; distractible	Difficult to console or comfort

From Merkel, S.I., Voepel-Lewis, T., Shayevitz, J.R., & Malviya, S. (1997). The FLACC: A behavioral scale for scoring postoperative pain in young children. *Pediatr Nurs,* 23(3), 293-297. Used with permission. © The Regents of the University of Michigan and the University of Michigan Health System. Can be reproduced for clinical and research use.

NURSING CARE PLAN 3-2

The Child in Pain

NURSING DIAGNOSIS *Pain, acute, related to surgery, injury, etc.*

Goals/Outcome Criteria	Interventions	Rationales
Patient demonstrates decrease in pain, as evidenced by: • Vocalizing decreased pain • Nonverbal signs (relaxed body position, decreased crying) • Vital signs within normal limits	Assess and record subjective and objective signs of pain	Documentation serves as a baseline and ongoing evaluation
	Use an assessment tool to measure pain	Provides for consistency in assessment
	Use nonpharmacologic techniques of pain control as needed	May be less painful; child has control
	Use pharmacologic methods to control pain as needed	Keeping pain under control helps child move more easily, preventing complications of immobilization
	Include the parents in the care	Parents' presence may reduce fear and anxiety, therefore reducing the amount of pain experienced
	Medicate before painful procedures	Helps child cope with painful procedures
	Monitor vital signs at least every 4 hours	Changes can indicate a change in level of pain

NURSING DIAGNOSIS *Anxiety related to anticipation of pain*

Goals/Outcome Criteria	Interventions	Rationales
Child shows a decrease in anxiety by: • Verbalizing decreased anxiety • Decreased crying • Interacting with staff • Participating in activities	Assign a consistent caregiver	Can make child more at ease
	Involve parents in care of child	Reduces anxiety
	Explain all procedures to child	Knowing what to expect helps reduce anxiety
	Follow home rituals when possible	Routines make child less anxious
	Allow the older child some control	Control helps child cope with situation
	Reassure preschool children that they are not to blame for illness and are not being punished	Are "magical thinkers" and believe they can cause illness

? CRITICAL THINKING QUESTION

■ How does the nurse identify and treat pain in an infant versus pain in a school-age child?

meperidine (Demerol) is controversial and therefore uncommon.

Pain medication may also be administered rectally, by intramuscular (IM) injection, transdermally, or topically. The subcutaneous and intranasal routes are also mentioned in the literature but are seldom used. The rectal route is occasionally used. Acetaminophen suppositories, for example, may be ordered rectally if the child has been vomiting or has difficulty swallowing. Children generally fear needles; therefore the IM route is rarely used. The transdermal route (patch) is generally reserved for chronic pain control. Topical application is often aimed at eliminating or reducing pain from most procedures involving skin puncture (intramuscular injection or intravenous insertion). EMLA (eutectic mixture of local anesthetics) cream is one example. It must be applied as a "dollop" over the site and covered by an occlusive dressing 1 hour or more before the procedure to be effective. Vapocoolant sprays may also used immediately before injections. In addition, the intradermal route is often used for local (skin) anesthesia such as lidocaine (Xylocaine). Finally, oral sucrose is often used when an infant is undergoing a painful procedure. It seems to be more effective when given in combination with a pacifier (Zempsky et al., 2004).

Patient-controlled analgesia (PCA) has also been used successfully with children. Typically, children are old enough to understand PCA when they are school-age and older. This programmable infusion pump is used to self-administer medication boluses at preset dose and time intervals, generally via the IV route. There is a lockout interval between doses so that the patient cannot inadvertently self-deliver too much medication. Morphine is often the drug of choice to use with the PCA pump. The epidural/intrathecal route has been used successfully when short-term or long-term analgesia is needed. The direct effect of the analgesia (in the epidural space of the spinal column) produces few and rare side effects.

Pain management may also include nonpharmacologic interventions, which may be used in conjunction with pharmacologic interventions or by themselves. Such interventions are often referred to as *complementary or alternative medicine (CAM)*, and it is important to evaluate the success of these methods as well. For instance, music therapy (Figure 3-17) may be used to promote guided imagery or relaxation. (See Chapter 18 for a discussion of guided imagery, relaxation, biofeedback, and distraction.) Hypnosis is another complementary form of pain management. In this altered state of consciousness, suggestions can lead to changes in behavior or, in the case of pain, altered physical sensations (The National Pain Foundation, 2006). The *TENS* (transcutaneous electric nerve stimulation) *unit* has also proven helpful in pain management and uses electric stimulation to relieve pain. *Acupuncture* is based on a theory that energy, or

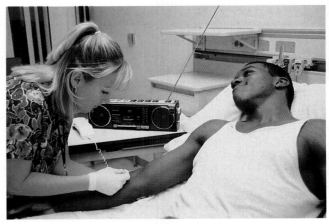

FIGURE **3-17** The adolescent listens to soothing music to promote relaxation and coping during stressful procedures.

chi, flows through the body along channels (meridians) that are connected by acupuncture points. Pain occurs when the flow of energy is obstructed. With insertion of fine needles at specific (acupuncture) points along the meridians involved, health can be restored because the flow of energy is no longer obstructed and balance is achieved. With children, the obvious concern is the fear of needles. However, in a study done by Kemper et al. (2000), pediatric patients with pain (chronic, severe) found acupuncture treatment pleasant and helpful.

Chiropractors see pediatric patients as well as adult patients. Chiropractors use a holistic approach to treating all patients. They treat patients whose health problems are associated with the body's muscular, nervous, and skeletal systems, specifically the spine. Two other forms of manual healing include massage therapy and healing touch (practitioners place their hands on or near the patient's body to direct energy). Many hospitals now include a massage therapist on site. However, insurance companies generally do not pay for massage. (See Box 18-2 for a list of other complementary methods.)

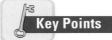

Key Points

- The pediatric hospital unit is designed to create a cheerful, casual atmosphere to help meet the needs of children.
- All children react differently to hospitalization. Parents and health care providers need to minimize the stressors of hospitalization as much as possible.
- Critical thinking and the nursing process are methods of problem solving that guide the care of the hospitalized child.
- Discharge planning begins on admission, and teaching is done throughout the child's hospitalization, not just when the child is about to leave the hospital.
- Accurate measurement of vital signs is crucial to perform a thorough and accurate evaluation of the child.

- Following safety measures is of the utmost importance when caring for children in any health care setting.
- Restraints are only used when absolutely necessary and according to institution policy.
- Medical asepsis guidelines must be strictly followed to prevent the spread of infection.
- Fears of a child who is about to undergo surgery need to be alleviated before surgery.
- A thorough evaluation of a child with pain and appropriate pharmacologic or nonpharmacologic interventions are essential for the child's well-being.

 Go to your Companion CD-ROM for an Audio Glossary, video clips, and more.

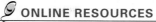 Be sure to visit the companion Evolve site at http://evolve.elsevier.com/Price/pediatric/ for WebLinks and additional online resources.

ONLINE RESOURCES

AAP (American Academy of Pediatrics), APS (American Pain Society) policy statement on pain: http://www.aap.org/policy/9933.html

Centers for Disease Control and Prevention: http://www.cdc.gov

Children's Health: http://www.kidshealth.org

The Newborn Infant

evolve http://evolve.elsevier.com/Price/pediatric/

Objectives

Upon completion of this chapter, the student will be able to:

1. Define the vocabulary terms listed
2. Discuss the importance of airway maintenance in the neonate
3. Identify the range of average measurements in the newborn infant
4. Discuss normal vital signs of the newborn
5. Describe the importance of thermoregulation
6. Briefly describe three normal reflexes of the neonate (including approximate age of disappearance) and the tests for their appearance
7. With a systems approach, summarize the pertinent nursing interventions in the care of the neonate (e.g., "circulatory system: check color and warmth, explain principles to parents")
8. Discuss safety issues such as identification and newborn screenings
9. Describe precautions to prevent infection while caring for a newborn
10. List four signs of infection in the neonate
11. Compare and contrast breastfeeding and formula feeding
12. Summarize the principles involved in teaching a new mother how to breastfeed her newborn, bathe her newborn, and provide cord care
13. Discuss behaviors that would indicate that bonding is taking place between the infant and the mother
14. Describe discharge teaching needs of the parents

Key Terms

Be sure to check out the bonus material on the Companion CD-ROM, including selected audio pronunciations.

acrocyanosis (ăk-rō-sī-ă-NŌ-sĭs; p. 52)
anuria (ă-NŪ-rē-ă; p. 57)
Apgar score (p. 50)
auditory brainstem response (p. 56)
caput succedaneum (KĂP-ĕt sŭk-sĕ-DĀ-nē-ĕm; p. 52)
cephalhematoma (sĕf-ăl-hē-mă-TŌ-mă; p. 52)
circumcision (sĭr-kŭm-sĭzh-ŭn; p. 57)
cold stress (p. 50)
cradle cap (p. 53)
fontanel (fŏn-tă-NĔL; p. 53)
hypospadias (hī-pō-SPĀ-dē-ăs; p. 57)
icterus neonatorum (ĭk-tĕr-ŭs nē-ō-nā-TŌR-ŭm; p. 59)
molding (p. 52)

Moro reflex (p. 54)
neonatal intensive care unit (NICU; p. 49)
nonshivering thermogenesis (THER-mō-JĔN-ĕ-sĭs; p. 50)
rooting reflex (p. 54)
thermoregulation (THER-mō-rĕg-ū-LĀ-shŭn; p. 51)

ADAPTATIONS OF THE NEWBORN INFANT

When a baby is born, an orderly process of adaptation from fetal life to extrauterine life takes place. All the body systems undergo some change. Respirations are stimulated by chemical changes within the blood and by chilling. Sensory and physical stimuli also appear to play a role in respiratory function. Gentle physical contact is used to provide stimulation to begin breathing. Cold, pain, touch, movement, and light are other stimuli that affect the stimulation of respirations. With the first breath, which initiates the opening of the alveoli, the newborn enters the world of air exchange and begins an independent existence. In addition, this process begins cardiopulmonary interdependence. Fetal circulation is depicted in Figure 4-1. The ability of the neonate to metabolize food is hampered by immaturity of the digestive system, particularly by deficiencies in enzymes from the pancreas and the liver. Although the kidneys are developed structurally, their ability to concentrate urine and maintain fluid balance is limited. This is because of a decreased rate of glomerular flow and limited renal tubular reabsorption. Most neurological functions are also primitive (see the individual body systems discussed subsequently in this chapter).

EXAMINATION OF THE NEWBORN INFANT

INITIAL EXAM OF THE NEWBORN INFANT

AIRWAY

Regardless of the site of delivery (home, birthing room, taxicab), clearing the neonate's airway is an immediate concern. A rubber bulb syringe or a special trap connected to suction may be used. This produces very low suction, which protects the delicate tissues while removing secretions. Spontaneous breathing should begin within a

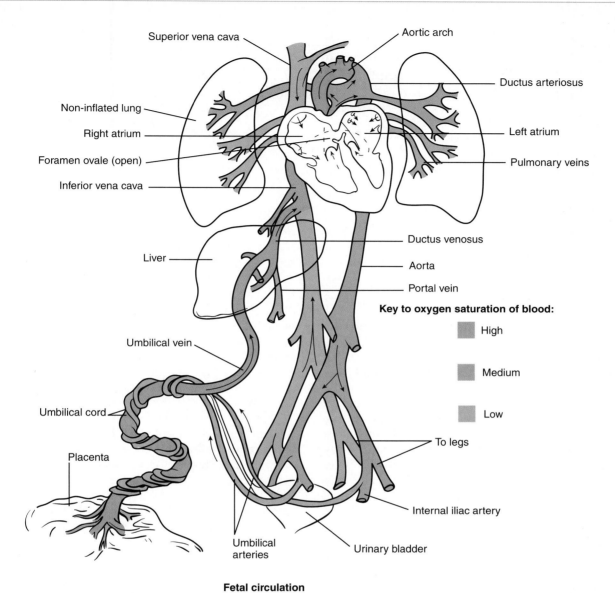

Superior vena cava

Aortic arch

Ductus arteriosus

Non-inflated lung

Right atrium

Left atrium

Foramen ovale (open)

Pulmonary veins

Inferior vena cava

Liver

Ductus venosus

Aorta

Portal vein

Key to oxygen saturation of blood:

High

Medium

Low

Umbilical vein

Umbilical cord

To legs

Placenta

Internal iliac artery

Umbilical
arteries

Urinary bladder

Fetal circulation

FIGURE **4-1** Diagram of fetal circulation showing the placenta, umbilical vein, and umbilical arteries. The fetal bypasses are also shown. These are the ductus venosus, ductus arteriosus, and foramen ovale.

few seconds. If there are no complications, the newborn is placed on a warming table where care can be given and the newborn's general condition can be observed. The newborn is dried gently with a soft cloth to remove excess blood from the face, scalp, and body. This also provides stimulation. Mothers who are alert are given their child to hold and inspect.

If spontaneous breathing does not occur, resuscitative measures are taken. The need for resuscitation often can be anticipated from the history of the mother's pregnancy, abnormal progression of labor, the size of the neonate, and the difficulty of delivery. Well-trained personnel and properly functioning equipment are imperative. Periodic review of techniques is also necessary. Resuscitation methods are directed toward clearing the airway, inflating the lungs, and maintaining circulation. The administration of appropriate drugs,

such as naloxone hydrochloride (Narcan), atropine, sodium bicarbonate, epinephrine, dextrose, or calcium gluconate, may also be warranted. Procedures range from the simple to the more complex. Measures such as tactile stimulation (rubbing the neonate's back), assisted ventilation with bag and mask or endotracheal tube, and external cardiac massage may be necessary. The infant is then transferred to the nursery in a prewarmed transport isolette. Assisted ventilation via a mechanical respirator may be necessary in the neonatal intensive care unit (NICU).

UMBILICAL CORD

The umbilical cord, which is attached to the placenta at birth, is cut by the attending physician. Before the clamp is applied, the cord is inspected to determine that two arteries and one vein are present. A single

Table 4-1 | *Apgar Scoring System*

The Apgar scoring system provides a quick and accurate way of evaluating a baby's physical status right at birth, regardless of any combination of weaknesses or debilities. The physician or nurse observes the five signs and records the score for each. Each sign is evaluated according to the degree to which it is present: 0 (poor), 1 (fair), or 2 (good). The five scores are then added together. Apgar scores range from 0 to 10. A score of 10 means the baby is in the best possible condition. A score of 9 or 8 indicates good condition; 7, 6, 5, or 4 indicates fair condition. A score of 3, 2, 1, or 0 indicates poor condition and the need for prompt diagnosis and treatment of specific disorders.

SIGN	0	1	2	SCORE
Heart rate: strong and steady?	Not detectable	Slow (less than 100)	Above 100	—
Respiratory effort: breathing frequently and regularly?	Absent	Slow, irregular	Good; crying	—
Muscle tone: kicking feet and making fists?	Flaccid	Some flexion of extremities	Active motion	—
Reflex irritability; lusty cry elicited if catheter is pushed up one nostril or soles of feet are prodded?	No response	Grimace	Cry; cough or sneeze	—
Color: pink all over, or hands and feet bluish?	Blue, pale	Body pink, extremities bluish	Completely pink or absence of cyanosis	—
			TOTAL	—

umbilical artery is often indicative of genitourinary anomalies. The findings are recorded.

Cord blood may be collected at the request of the parents. This is the blood that remains in the umbilical cord and placenta following birth. Cord blood is stored at a blood bank. This blood serves as an abundant source for stem cells, which are genetically distinctive to the baby. These cells contribute to the development of all tissues, organs, and systems in the body. They can transform into other types of cells in the body and create new growth and development. They may be used one day to help treat problems such as heart disease, cancers, and stroke. Cost can be a factor, however, and if parents do not wish to bank their baby's cord blood, it can be donated.

The cord stump may be painted with a substance to help dry the cord and prevent infection. This dye may cause a temporary purplish discoloration. Parents should not try to rub this off. The cord stump gradually shrinks, discolors, and finally falls off. This process usually takes 10 to 14 days. The cord should be off by 2 weeks. Until the umbilical wound is completely healed, the blood vessels of the cord and their extension into the abdomen are potential portals of entry for disease organisms. Redness, odor, or discharge from this area should be reported to the physician. The nurse observes the cord for bleeding, particularly during the first 24 hours.

APGAR SCORING

A system for recording the condition of the neonate and the need for resuscitation was devised by Dr. Virginia Apgar and is currently used in many delivery rooms. The first assessment is made 1 minute after delivery. This generally produces the lowest score. A second evaluation is made after 5 minutes. Table 4-1 shows how to determine the Apgar score. An infant with a score of 8 to 10 is in good condition and needs only routine suction and observation. Infants with a

score of 4 to 7 require various forms of intervention and close observation. An infant with a score of 0 to 3 needs resuscitation and care in the NICU. Apgar scores, however, are not the sole indicator used to evaluate the long-term prognosis of a child.

PROVIDING WARMTH

One of the most critical needs of the infant is control of body temperature. This is especially true if the infant is at high risk (Chapter 5 discusses the high-risk neonate). The neonate is at risk for heat loss immediately on delivery. The newborn does not have the ability to produce or conserve heat that an older infant does. A newborn cannot shiver to generate heat. Through a process called nonshivering thermogenesis, brown fat is metabolized to increase metabolic rate and to generate heat. Brown fat is a fat store located in the axillae, between the scapulae, in the mediastinum, around the liver, and down the spine. If not corrected, cold stress can actually cause metabolic and physiologic problems in the neonate such as hypoglycemia (low blood sugar) and hypoxia (low oxygenation).

Radiant warmers are available in most delivery rooms. The newborn is thoroughly dried (especially the hair) to eliminate evaporative heat loss and placed uncovered under radiant heat. If the newborn is placed on the mother's chest, skin-to-skin contact should be maintained. A cap for the newborn prevents heat loss (Figure 4-2). The nurse remains with the mother and the newborn to ensure their safety, to monitor progress, and to ensure that the newborn stays warm. Table 4-2 discusses types of heat loss.

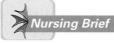
Nursing Brief

Be aware of the total surface area—the smaller the infant, the greater the surface area in proportion to weight. Be aware—the smaller the infant, the greater the heat loss potential.

MEASUREMENTS

The newborn is weighed and measured immediately after birth. The length of the average neonate is 19 to 21.5 in (48.25 to 54.5 cm). The weight varies from 6 to 9 lb (2700 to 4000 g). Girls generally weigh a little less than boys. In the first 3 to 5 days after birth, the newborn loses about 7% to 10% of the birth weight. This is from the loss of excess extracellular fluid and meconium and from limited food intake, especially in breastfed infants. The total weight loss for the newborn should not exceed 10%; this amount of weight loss is reflective of dehydration. By the 10th day of life, birth weight should be regained. Weight loss is expected, and parents should not be alarmed by it. For a more accurate assessment of weight, neonates are weighed naked on the same scale at the same time each day.

Head circumference is generally between 33 and 35 cm (13 to 15 in). This measurement may be somewhat less because of the molding process during a vaginal delivery (Figure 4-3). Within 2 to 3 days, it is usually the normal size. Chest circumference is 30.5 to 33 cm (12 to 13 in). Head circumference is generally about 2 to 3 cm (1 in) greater than the chest circumference.

VITAL SIGNS
Temperature

The most accurate way to determine body temperature is to measure it with a thermometer. The initial temperature of the neonate is generally taken via the axillary route. It is not usually taken rectally because this method could cause perforation of the mucosa. Tympanic thermometers are not as accurate in a newborn. Daily routine temperatures are taken in the axilla. Review the procedure for evaluation of vital signs in Chapter 17.

The neonate has an immature heat-regulating system. Thermoregulation (regulation of heat) requires close monitoring. The newborn's temperature falls immediately after birth to about 96° F (35.5° C). Within a few hours, it climbs slowly to a range of 98° F to 99° F (36.6° C to 37.2° C). The body temperature is influenced by the temperature of the room and the number of

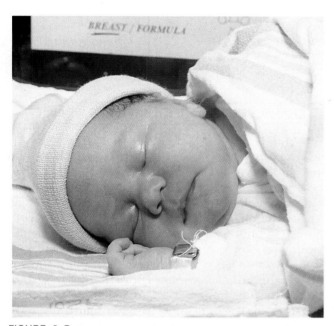

FIGURE **4-2** It is important that the newborn stay warm because heat is easily lost. Note the hat and the identification bracelet.

Table 4-2 | **Heat Loss in the Neonate**

TYPE OF HEAT LOSS	MECHANISM	CONDITIONS CONTRIBUTING TO HEAT LOSS	NURSING INTERVENTIONS
Evaporation	Heat lost by evaporation of moisture from the skin and with body fluids from mucous membranes	Increased skin permeability, increased respirations, and insensible water loss (25% of heat loss)	Dry quickly after birth/keep infant warm and dry (including head) Change wet diapers/clothing Bathe only after infant's temperature is stable Monitor/support infants experiencing rapid respirations
Conduction	Heat lost to surfaces with direct contact with them	Cool temperature of objects the infant comes into direct contact with	Warm equipment having direct contact with the infant Warm hands before touching the infant Use paper on scale to weigh; use blankets on other surfaces
Convection	Heat lost by air moving over the skin	Drafts and cool air (air conditioning)	Avoid exposure to drafts/cool air Ensure oxygen is warmed and humidified whenever used Transport in prewarmed isolette
Radiation	Transfer of heat to cooler, solid objects in the environment not in contact with the infant	Cool environment of hospital unit including walls and windows	Keep infant's bed away from outside walls and windows Keep infant clothed with hat; wrap warmly Use temperature probe in isolette to monitor the infant's temperature

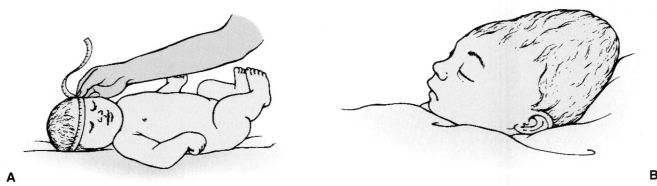

A **B**

FIGURE **4-3 A,** The circumference of the head is measured with the frontal occipital circumference (FOC). **B,** Molding of the head occurs as the bones of the fetal head overlap at the suture lines to conform to the mother's pelvis.

blankets covering the newborn. The temperature of the nursery, or the mother's room in the case of rooming-in, should be 68° F to 75° F. The humidity should be 45% to 55%. The air in the room also needs to be fresh, but there should be no drafts.

Another sign of the neonate's system immaturity is acrocyanosis (*acro,* extremity; *cyanosis,* blue color) or peripheral blueness of the hands and feet and sometimes of the lips. The hands and feet are also cooler than other parts of the body. The neonate has difficulty adapting to changes in temperature. Because heat perception is poor, the newborn must be monitored closely whenever an external heat source, such as a radiant warmer, is used. The newborn should also be wrapped in a blanket when leaving the nursery.

Heart Rate and Blood Pressure

An apical heart rate should be auscultated for 1 full minute (discussed in Chapter 3). The pulse rate is between 120 and 160 beats per minute. This rate may increase if the infant is crying and decrease if the infant is sleeping. As a general rule, however, if the pulse is above 160 or drops below 120, it should be reported. Blood pressure is low, and use of the correctly sized cuff is important. The average blood pressure at birth is 80/46 mm Hg.

Respirations

Respirations may be irregular and should be counted for 1 full minute. Normal respirations are 40 to 60 breaths per minute and then drop to 30 to 50 breaths per minute after the first 24 hours. They are typically shallow and unlabored.

After the newborn's temperature and vital signs have become stable, the newborn is bathed and dressed in a diaper and a shirt. The newborn is wrapped in blankets and placed in a bassinet. If there are concerns about possible choking during the first few hours after birth, hospital personnel can place the infants on their sides, propped up against the side of the bassinet for stability. However, the infants should be placed on their backs as soon as possible (AAP Policy Statement, 2005).

CHARACTERISTICS OF THE NEWBORN INFANT

MATURITY

Several differences are seen between a premature and a full-term infant. Muscle tone is decreased in the infant who is not full-term. The position that the infant maintains can also indicate low gestational age. When in a prone position, the full-term infant lies with the pelvis high and the knees drawn up under the abdomen. The premature infant that is placed in a prone position lies with the pelvis low and the knees at the side of the abdomen, with the hips flexed. In the supine position, the infant of 28 to 32 weeks' gestational age lies in a frog-like position with the lower limbs extended and the hips abducted. The full-term infant in a supine position lies with the limbs strongly flexed. Differences also exist in the hand movement of the infant across the chest to the opposite side of the neck. The reach of an infant of 28 weeks' gestation can extend well past the acromion, whereas the hand of the full-term infant does not go beyond that point. If the hand is put behind the neck to the opposite side, the same difference between the ages is noted. This is called the **scarf sign** (Figure 4-4). The premature infant is further discussed in Chapter 5.

HEAD

The newborn infant's head is proportionately large in comparison with the rest of the body because the brain grows rapidly before birth. The head may be out of shape from molding, which occurs as the fetal head conforms to the size and shape of the mother's pelvis. Another condition that can alter the shape of the newborn's head is caput succedaneum, which is edema of the newborn's scalp resulting from pressure against the cervix. This condition usually clears within 24 to 48 hours. Occasionally, a **hematoma** (*hemato,* blood; *oma,* tumor) protrudes from beneath the scalp. The cephalhematoma takes longer to subside, but it usually clears by the time the infant is 2 to 4 weeks of age (Figure 4-5).

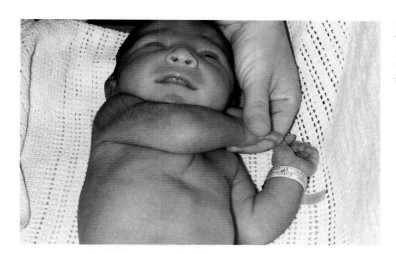

FIGURE **4-4** Examining the newborn baby for maturity. The full-term neonate's elbow resists attempts to be brought farther than the midline of the chest. Little or no resistance is seen in the preterm infant. This is called the scarf sign.

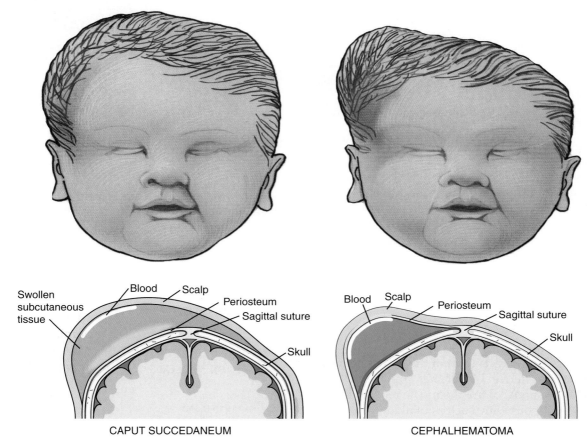

FIGURE **4-5** Caput succedaneum *(left)* and cephalhematoma *(right)* are common birth injuries.

Some neonates have a large amount of hair that eventually is replaced by new hair. The infant's hair should be washed when the newborn is bathed and then can be brushed into place. Some infants develop cradle cap (seborrheic dermatitis), characterized by yellow, oily, crust-like scales on the scalp and forehead. Using baby oil to soften the scales, massaging with a soft baby brush, and then shampooing the area with a mild shampoo will help eliminate cradle cap.

Fontanels are junctures at the cranial bones that can be felt as soft spots on the cranium of the young infant. Two can be palpated on the neonate's head. The fontanels may be smaller immediately after birth than several days later because of molding. The anterior fontanel is diamond-shaped and located at the junction of the two parietal and the two frontal bones. It usually closes by 12 to 18 months of age (Figure 4-6). The posterior fontanel is triangular and located between the occipital and the parietal bones. It is much smaller than the anterior fontanel and has usually ossified by the end of the second month. The pulsating of the anterior fontanel may be seen by the nurse. These areas

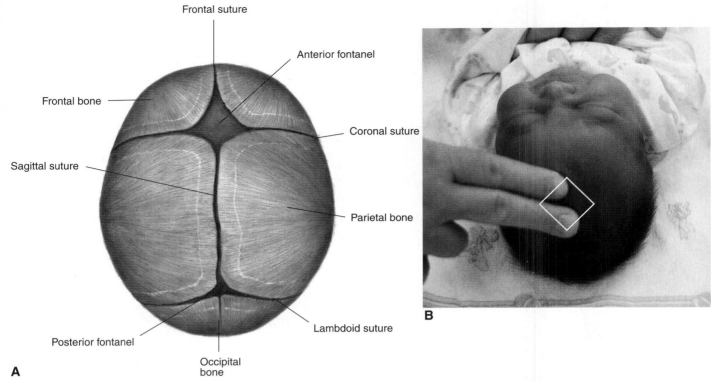

FIGURE **4-6** **A,** Location of sutures and fontanels. **B,** Palpating anterior fontanel.

are covered by a tough membrane, and there is little chance of their being injured with ordinary care.

The features of the newborn's face are small. The mouth and lips are well developed because they are necessary to obtain food. The neonate can both taste and smell. In fact, the mother's scent appears to stimulate the neonate to smell breast milk and to search for the nipple.

NERVOUS SYSTEM
Reflexes

The nervous system directs most of the body's activity. The neonate can move his or her arms and legs vigorously but cannot control them. The reflexes that a full-term baby is born with, such as blinking, sneezing, gagging, rooting, sucking, and grasping (Figure 4-7 and Table 4-3), help keep the child alive. The rooting reflex causes the infant to turn the head in the direction of anything that touches the cheek, such as in anticipation of food. The nurse should remember this when helping a mother breastfeed her infant. If the breast touches the infant's cheek, the newborn turns toward it to find the nipple. The infant can also cry, swallow, and lift the head slightly when lying on the stomach. If the crib is jarred, the newborn extends the extremities and then draws the legs up and folds the arms across the chest in an embrace position. The hands open, but the fingers often remain curved. This is normal and is called the Moro reflex (Figure 4-8). Its absence may indicate abnormalities of the nervous system.

Table 4-3	_Neurological Signs Present at Birth in the Newborn_	
REFLEX	**OCCURRENCE**
PROTECTIVE REFLEXES	
Blink	
Gag	
Cough	
FEEDING REFLEXES	
Root	
Suck	
Swallow	
MUSCLE TONE REFLEXES	**AGE OF DISAPPEARANCE**
Moro	1-3 mo
Tonic neck	5-6 mo
Palmer grasp (hand)	~4 mo
Planter grasp (foot)	4-6 mo
Babinski	Variable—not diagnostic until after 2 yr of age
REFLEXES OF VISION	**AGE OF APPEARANCE**
Horizontal following	4-6 wk
Vertical following	2-3 mo
Blinking to a threat	6-7 mo

The **tonic neck reflex** is a postural reflex that is sometimes assumed by babies while asleep (Figure 4-9). The head is turned to one side, with the arm and leg extended on the same side, whereas the opposite arm and leg are flexed in a "fencing" position. This reflex disappears around the 20th week of life. Prancing movements of

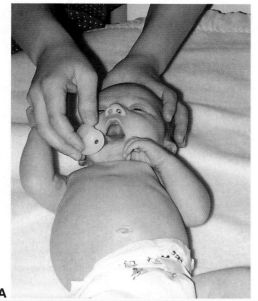

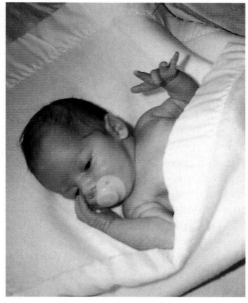

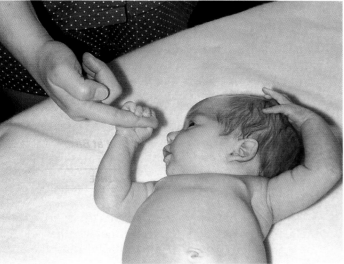

FIGURE **4-7** **A,** Rooting reflex. The infant opens the mouth and turns the head toward the pacifier stimulating the cheek. **B,** Sucking reflex. Vigorous sucking movements are initiated when an object is placed in the infant's mouth. **C,** Grasp reflex (palm). Transverse stimulation of the midpalm leads to a grasp by the infant.

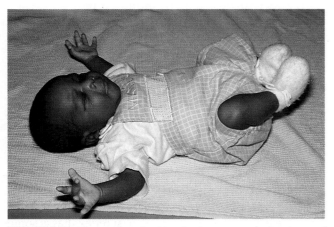

FIGURE **4-8** Moro reflex. Sudden jarring causes extension and abduction of the extremities and spreading of the fingers.

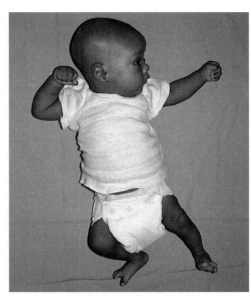

FIGURE **4-9** Spontaneous tonic neck reflex.

the legs, seen when a newborn is held upright on the examining table, are termed the **dancing reflex.**

SENSORY SYSTEM
Vision

Although vision is the most poorly developed sense at birth, the neonate can see sizes, shapes, colors, and patterns and is able to fixate points of contrast. The infant shows preference for observing a human face and follows moving objects. Visual stimulation thus becomes an important ingredient in caring for the baby. Auditory toys and contrasted colors attract the neonate. Sensory overload, of course, should be avoided.

Most newborn infants appear cross-eyed because their eye muscle coordination is not fully developed. At first the eyes appear to be blue or gray; however, the permanent coloring becomes fixed between the third and sixth month.

Hearing

Hearing in newborns is thought to be keener than was once believed. Increased response to vocal stimulation, particularly higher-pitched female voices, can be documented. The ears and nose need no special attention, except for cleansing. This can be done during the bath with a soft cloth. Cotton-tipped applicator sticks are dangerous to use. They may cause injury if inserted too far or if the newborn moves suddenly.

Undetected hearing loss can cause a child to develop problems in speech, language, and cognitive development and can also lead to development of behavioral problems. Hearing loss is a common birth defect, occurring in up to 3 per 1000 newborn infants, and needs to be identified as soon as possible. In the past, parental observation and assessment by health care providers have not been reliable in identifying hearing loss in the first year of life. In 2000, the Joint Committee on Infant Hearing (JCIH) recommended universal screening of hearing loss before hospital discharge. This screening is endorsed by the American Academy of Pediatrics (AAP). The auditory brainstem response (ABR) screening test detects hearing loss. The detection of hearing loss and early interventions aid the child in achieving academic and social success because they allow for the development of thinking and visual or spoken language skills.

RESPIRATORY SYSTEM

Before birth, a baby is completely dependent on the mother for all vital functions. The fetus needs oxygen and nourishment to grow. These are supplied through the bloodstream of the pregnant woman by way of the placenta and the umbilical cord. The fetus is relieved of the waste products of metabolism through the same route. The lungs are not inflated and are almost completely inactive. The circulatory system is adapted only to life within the uterus. Little blood flows through the pulmonary artery because of natural

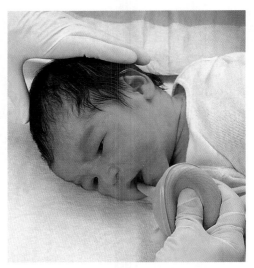

FIGURE **4-10** Suctioning with a bulb syringe may be necessary to remove secretions from the infant's mouth or nose.

openings within the heart (foramen ovale) and vessels that close at or shortly after birth. When the umbilical cord is clamped and cut, the lungs take on the function of breathing in oxygen and removing carbon dioxide. The first breath taken helps expand the collapsed lungs. The physician assists the first respiration by holding the infant's head down and removing mucus from the passages to the lungs. The newborn's cry should be strong and healthy. The most critical period for the neonate is the first hour of life, when the drastic change from life within the uterus to life outside the uterus takes place.

The nurse refers to the patient's chart to review the Apgar score and to determine whether or not there were any particular difficulties during the birth process. The orders left by the doctor are reviewed. The nurse must observe the newborn *very closely.* Respiratory distress may be indicated by the rate and character of respirations, color (watch for cyanosis), and general behavior. *Sternal retractions* should be reported immediately. Mucus may be seen draining from the nose or mouth. Gentle suctioning with a bulb syringe may also be indicated. The bulb is depressed and the tip is inserted into the mouth or nose (Figure 4-10). The depression is slowly released, creating the necessary suction. When this procedure is done orally, the tip is inserted into the side of the mouth to avoid stimulating the gag reflex (see Chapter 17 for this procedure). Suction the mouth before the nose, if both are necessary. Instruct parents in the use of the bulb syringe and keep one beside the infant during the early weeks.

CIRCULATORY SYSTEM

The mother's blood has brought essential oxygen to each cell of the fetus during life in the uterus. This supply is cut off when the umbilical cord is severed after

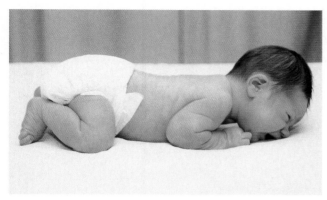

FIGURE **4-11** The newborn is barely able to lift his or her head while lying prone.

birth. From this moment on, the newborn infant has not only a systemic circulation but also a pulmonary circulation.

The circulation of the fetus differs from that of the newborn in that most of the blood bypasses the lungs (see Figure 4-1). Some of the blood goes from the right atrium to the left atrium of the heart through an opening, the foramen ovale, in the septum. Some of the blood goes from the pulmonary artery to the thoracic aorta by way of the **ductus arteriosus** (see Figure 4-1).

Murmurs are generated by turbulence of blood flow through the heart. They are classified as systolic, diastolic, or continuous. They are graded from 1 to 6 based on increasing loudness. Murmurs may be thought of as functional (innocent) or organic (from improper heart formation). Functional murmurs are caused by the sound of blood passing through a normal heart. Organic murmurs result from blood passing through abnormal openings or normal openings that have not yet closed. Most heart murmurs in the newborn period have been found to be functional, tend to come and go (transient), and tend not to be serious. However, murmurs should be reported to the physician and the newborn should be checked periodically to rule out other possibilities.

MUSCULOSKELETAL SYSTEM
Movements, Eye Coordination, Tremors

The bones of the newborn infant are soft because they are made up chiefly of cartilage, with only a small amount of calcium. The skeleton is flexible. The joints are elastic to accommodate passage through the birth canal. Because the bones of the child are easily molded by pressure, the position must be changed frequently. If the baby lies constantly in one position, the bones of the head can become flattened.

Movements of the neonate are random and uncoordinated. The newborn lacks the muscular control to hold the head up (Figure 4-11). The development of muscular control proceeds from head to foot and from the center of the body to the periphery (discussed in Chapter 2). The baby, therefore, holds up the head

before sitting erect. In fact, the head and neck muscles are the first ones under control. The legs are small and short and may appear bowed. There should be no limitation of movement. Fingers clenched in a fist should be separated and observed.

Freedom of movement is observed as the baby stretches, sucks, and makes faces. The whole body moves vigorously when the newborn cries. Tremors of the lips and extremities during crying are normal. Constant tremors during sleep, which are accompanied by eye movements and are not related to any particular stimuli, may be pathological. The morning assessment provides an excellent opportunity for the nurse to inspect and evaluate the newborn's condition. When handled, the infant should not feel limp. General body proportions are noted. Bathing is also an excellent way to provide the neonate with stimulation.

GENITOURINARY SYSTEM

The kidneys function normally at birth but are not fully developed. The glomeruli are small. Renal blood flow is only about one third of that in an adult. The ability to handle a water load is reduced, as is the excretion of drugs. The renal tubules are short and have a limited capacity for reabsorbing important substances such as glucose, amino acids, phosphate, and bicarbonate. There is a decrease in the ability to concentrate urine and to cope with fluid imbalances. The infant should void within the first 24 to 48 hours after birth. The newborn may void in the delivery room, and it may not be observed. The nurse must keep an accurate record of the frequency of urination. Anuria (absence of voiding), changes in color, and any unusual findings should be brought to the attention of the physician. The newborn is not sent home unless voiding is observed.

Male Genitalia

The genitals are undeveloped at birth. The testes of the male child descend into the scrotum before birth. Occasionally, they remain in the abdomen or inguinal canal. This condition is called *cryptorchidism* (undescended testes). The prognosis is good with proper surgical treatment.

The penis is covered by a sleeve of skin called the foreskin or prepuce. After the foreskin separates from the glans, it can be pulled back away from the glans toward the abdomen. This is called foreskin retraction. This should never be forced because it can harm the penis and cause pain, bleeding, and tears in the skin. Most boys are able to retract their foreskins by age 5 years. Parents should be taught to wash all the male infant's body parts and not to forcibly retract the foreskin. Erection of the penis is common and has no significance.

Circumcision is the surgical removal of the foreskin. The procedure has been subject to much controversy. Among the risks are infection and hemorrhage. Infants with congenital anomalies of the penis, such as hypospadias (the opening of the urethra on the

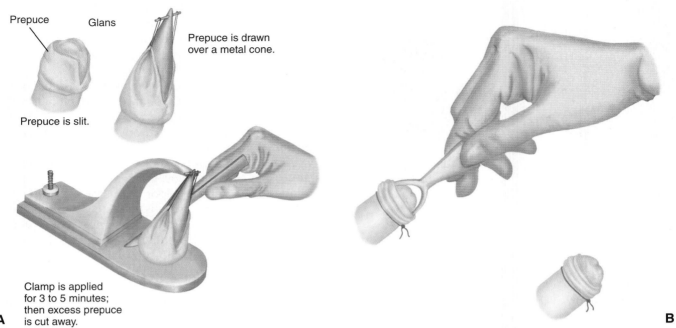

Prepuce

Glans

Prepuce is drawn over a metal cone.

Prepuce is slit.

Clamp is applied for 3 to 5 minutes; then excess prepuce is cut away.

A

B

FIGURE **4-12** **A,** Circumcision with the Gomco (Yellen) clamp. The physician pulls the prepuce over a cone-shaped device that rests against the glans. A clamp is placed around the cone and prepuce and is tightened to provide enough pressure to crush the blood vessels. This prevents bleeding when the prepuce is removed after 3 to 5 minutes. **B,** Circumcision with the Plastibell. The physician places the Plastibell, a plastic ring, over the glans, draws the prepuce over it, and ties a suture around the prepuce and Plastibell. This prevents bleeding when the excess prepuce is removed. The handle is removed, leaving only the ring in place over the glans. The Plastibell falls off in 5 to 8 days.

undersurface of the penis), should not be circumcised because the skin may be needed for surgery. Studies show that the risk for penile cancer and urinary tract infections are reduced in circumcised men compared with those who are uncircumcised; however, the incidence of such illness is so low that circumcision cannot be justified for prophylaxis (Hirji et al., 2005). A discussion of the pros and cons of this procedure should be included as part of prenatal and postpartum education. The parents' knowledge and understanding of the procedure of circumcision is necessary because a surgical consent form must be signed before this procedure can be performed.

When circumcision is desired, it is performed after 12 hours of age. This period of time allows the newborn to adjust from the stress of birth and for bonding to begin. The newborn is restrained on a circumcision board. The foreskin is freed with a probe, an incision is made the length of the foreskin, and a Hollister Plastibell, Mogen clamp, or Gomco clamp is used to control blood loss. Excess foreskin is removed with a scalpel or a scissor (Figure 4-12). After surgery, it is important for the nurse to observe for bleeding, irritation, and voiding.

When a Plastibell is used, a string is tied over a fitted plastic ring beneath the foreskin. As the area heals, the plastic rim drops off in 5 to 8 days after the circumcision. Parents are instructed not to remove the plastic ring prematurely. No special dressing is required, and the newborn may be bathed and diapered as usual. A dark brown or black ring encircling the plastic rim is natural. This will disappear when the rim drops off. Instruct parents to consult their physician if there are any questions, there is increased swelling, the ring has not fallen off within 8 days, or the ring has slipped onto the shaft of the penis.

When a Mogen or Gomco clamp is used, a dressing of Vaseline (or another petroleum jelly) is applied to the end of the penis to protect it from sticking to the diaper. Vaseline or a Vaseline dressing will be used until healing is complete, which takes approximately 7 to 10 days.

Community Cue

The Jewish religious custom of circumcision, comparable to baptism in the Christian faith, is performed on the eighth day after birth if the baby's condition permits. The baby receives his Hebrew name at this time.

Female Genitalia

The female genitals may be slightly swollen. Blood-tinged mucus may be discharged from the vagina 3 to 5 days after birth. This is from withdrawal of hormones transmitted from the mother to the fetus. The nurse should clean the vulva from the *urethra to the anus,* with three strokes—right side, left side, and center. A clean

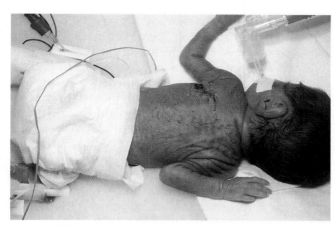

FIGURE **4-13** Lanugo in a premature neonate.

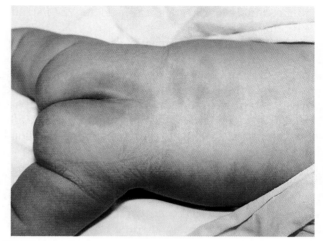

FIGURE **4-14** Mongolian spots are common in dark-skinned children. These bluish skin discolorations should not be confused with bruises.

cotton ball or clean (different) section of a washcloth is to be used for each stroke to prevent fecal matter from infecting the urinary tract. The importance of cleaning from *front to back* must be emphasized to parents.

INTEGUMENTARY SYSTEM
Skin

The skin of newborn Caucasian babies is red to dark pink in color. The skin of African-American babies is a reddish brown. Infants of Latin descent may appear to have an olive or yellowish tint to the skin. The body is usually covered with fine hair called **lanugo,** which tends to disappear during the first weeks of life. Lanugo is more evident in premature infants (Figure 4-13). **Vernix caseosa,** a cheese-like substance that covers the skin of the neonate, is made up of cells and glandular secretions and is thought to protect the skin from infection. White pinpoint pimples caused by obstruction of sebaceous glands may be seen on the nose and chin. These are called **milia** and disappear within a few weeks. **Mongolian spots,** bluish discolorations of the skin, are common in babies of African-American, Native American, or Mediterranean descent. They are usually found over the sacral and gluteal areas (Figure 4-14). They disappear spontaneously during the first years of life. Be careful not to confuse Mongolian spots with bruises that can occur from child abuse. Pallor or generalized cyanosis is not normal and should be reported.

Some hospitals still identify newborn babies with footprints, although many hospitals now have more advanced identification techniques. This method may still be used because the skin is so constructed with ridges and grooves that each person has a unique pattern that never changes. Regardless of hospital policy on identification method, most parents appreciate a copy of the footprint for the baby scrapbook.

Tissue turgor refers to the condition of the skin and indicates how hydrated or dehydrated the newborn is. To test tissue turgor (elasticity), the nurse gently grasps

and releases the skin. It should spring back into place immediately. When the skin remains distorted, tissue turgor is termed *poor.*

Desquamation, or peeling of the skin, occurs during the first weeks of life. Skin on the nose, knees, elbows, and toes may break down because of friction from rubbing against the sheets. The area involved should be kept dry, and the newborn's position should be changed frequently. The buttocks also need special attention. A wet diaper should be changed immediately to prevent irritation. The buttocks should be washed and dried well. Parents should be informed that this prevents diaper rash.

Physiological jaundice, also called icterus neonatorum, is characterized by a yellow tinge to the skin. It is caused by the rapid destruction of excess red blood cells that the newborn no longer needs. This is because the atmosphere contains more oxygen than the amount present during prenatal life. Between the second and fourth day, plasma levels of bilirubin rise from a normal 1 mg/dL to an average of 5 to 6 mg/dL. Physiological jaundice becomes evident between the third and fifth day of life and lasts for about a week. This is a normal process and is not harmful to the newborn. However, genetic and ethnic factors may affect its severity, resulting in pathological hyperbilirubinemia. Evidence of jaundice is reported and charted, and the neonate is evaluated frequently to ensure safety. Jaundice is further discussed in Chapter 5.

GASTROINTESTINAL SYSTEM
Digestion

Breastfed babies may be put to breast on the delivery table to help stimulate milk production and for the psychological benefits. Bottle-fed babies usually begin their first feeding by 6 hours of age. A baby's hunger is evidenced by crying, restlessness, sucking the fist, and the rooting reflex.

The capacity of the stomach is about 15 to 30 mL at birth and increases about 15 mL each day. It reaches a capacity of 90 mL by 1 week of age.

Emptying time for the stomach is 2 to 3 hours, and peristalsis is rapid. A deficiency in pancreatic lipase limits fat absorption. The liver is immature, especially in its ability to conjugate bilirubin, regulate blood sugar, and coagulate blood.

Stools

The normal functions of the gastrointestinal tract begin after birth: food is prepared for absorption into the blood, it is absorbed, and waste products are eliminated. **Meconium,** the first stool, is a mixture of amniotic fluid and secretions of the intestinal glands. It is dark green, thick, and sticky, is passed 8 to 24 hours after birth, and continues for about 3 days. The stools gradually change during the first week. They become loose and are a greenish yellow with mucus. These are called **transitional** stools.

The stools of a breastfed baby are bright yellow, soft, and pasty. There may be three to six stools a day. With age, the number of stools decreases. The bowel movements of a bottle-fed baby are more solid than those of a breastfed baby. They vary from yellow to light brown and are generally fewer in number. There may be one to four a day at first, but gradually this decreases to one or two a day. The stools are darker when a baby is receiving iron and green when the baby is under the bilirubin lamp. Small, putty-like stools, green watery stools, and bloody stools are abnormal and should be reported. The nursery nurse keeps an accurate record of the number and character of stools each neonate has daily.

Constipation

Constipation refers to the passage of hard, dry stools. Neonates differ in regularity. Some pass a soft stool every other day. This is not constipation. The nurse explains to parents that straining in the newborn period is from undeveloped abdominal musculature. This is normal, and no treatment is necessary.

Hiccups

Hiccups appear frequently in neonates and are normal. Most disappear spontaneously. Burping the baby and offering sips of water from a bottle may help.

ACTIVITY

REACTIVITY

After delivery, the vigorous neonate exhibits a characteristic pattern of activities. These patterns are termed the **first and second periods of reactivity.** During the first period, which lasts for about 30 minutes after birth, the neonate is awake and active. The heart and respiratory rates are rapid. There is grimacing, sucking movements, and random motor activity. This is followed by a period of rest that lasts from 2 to 4 hours. At this time, the neonate is disinterested in sucking and stimulation. On awakening, there is a second period of reactivity. This second period of reactivity occurs between 2 to 6 hours of age and is when the neonate's responsiveness returns. Periods of apnea may be seen, and there is an increase in mucus. The color of the newborn infant may vary at times between mildly mottled, pink, and pale. Bowel sounds become audible, and meconium stools are passed. The second period of reactivity can either be brief or last up to several hours. After this period, the newborn becomes relatively stable.

SLEEP

The newborn sleeps approximately 15 to 20 hours a day. As the neonate matures, there is a gradual change in the quantity and quality of sleep. Differentiation between active and quiet sleep is based primarily on whether **rapid eye movement** (REM) occurs. The sleep of a newborn infant consists of approximately 50% REM sleep, as opposed to only 20% in a 5-year-old. During REM sleep, respirations are rapid and more irregular, movements of the eye are evident beneath the eyelid, and movements of the limbs and mouth may be seen. Premature infants have an even higher proportion of REM sleep than babies born at term. Investigators theorize that REM sleep may be an internal stimulus to the higher brain centers at a time when external stimulation is minimal because of only brief periods of arousal.

Positioning the infant during sleep is an important aspect of care. In 1992, the AAP recommended that infants be placed on their backs (supine) to sleep to reduce the incidence of sudden infant death syndrome (SIDS). SIDS has been reduced by more than 50% since the "Back to Sleep" campaign began (NIH, 2005). It is strongly recommended by the AAP that infants not be placed in the prone position, which is on their abdomen. The prone position has the highest incidence rate for correlation with SIDS. Although many parents fear choking in the supine position, studies have shown that this is not the case. The AAP Policy Statement (2005) also stresses the need to avoid redundant soft bedding and soft objects in the infant's sleeping environment, the hazards of adults sleeping with an infant in the same bed, the SIDS risk reduction associated with having infants sleep in the same room as adults, the importance of educating secondary caregivers, and the benefit of using a pacifier when putting the infant to sleep. Giving a pacifier at the time of sleep significantly reduces the risk for SIDS (Burke, 2006). Finally, side sleeping as a reasonable alternative to fully supine sleeping is no longer recommended.

Table 4-4 | *Behavioral States of the Newborn*

STATE	DESCRIPTION
Quiet sleep	Regular respirations
	Very few body movements
	Deep sleep
Active sleep	REM
	Respirations irregular and primarily abdominal
	Some body movements
Drowsiness	Transitional state between sleep and awake states
	Fluttering eyelids
	If eyes open, they have a glassy appearance
	Irregular respirations
	Facial grimacing
	Variable motor activity
Quiet alert	Regular respirations
	Minimal movements
	Eyes bright and shiny
	Can look at the caregiver
	Most productive state for bonding
Active awake	Increased movements
	Increased irritability
	Fussiness
Crying	Intense, rhythmic crying
	Accompanied by increased motor activity

NEONATAL STATES

Behavioral states of the newborn have been studied since 1966. In the 1980s, Dr. T. Berry Brazelton described the following six states: (1) quiet sleep, (2) active sleep, (3) drowsiness, (4) quiet alert, (5) active awake, and (6) crying. These states are a reflection of the newborn's ability to react to the environment and a reflection of the ability of the central nervous system to adjust to stimuli (Table 4-4).

CONDITIONED RESPONSES

A conditioned response or reflex is one that is learned over time. Basically, it is an unconscious response to an external stimulus. An example is the hungry baby who stops crying simply on hearing the footsteps of the mother. Emotions are particularly subject to this type of conditioning. As an infant matures, the mere sight of an object that once caused pain can precipitate fear. Learning mechanisms such as these are of particular interest to **behavior theorists,** who believe that the proper study of psychology is one that focuses only on behavior.

The **Brazelton Neonatal Behavioral Assessment Scale** has increased our understanding of the neonate's capabilities. Among other things, the scale measures the inherent neurological capacities of the neonate and responses to selected stimuli. Areas tested include alertness, response to visual and auditory stimuli, motor coordination, level of excitement, and organizational processes in response to stress. The Brazelton Neonatal Behavioral Assessment Scale is of particular value during the newborn period; it is used to describe the emerging personality of the baby and includes evaluation of infant reflexes, general activity, alertness, orientation to spoken voice, and response to visual stimuli.

CARE OF THE NEWBORN INFANT

IDENTIFYING THE NEONATE

Proper identification of the newborn is ensured by placing wristbands with preprinted, matching numbers on the newborn, the mother, and father or significant other. The mother and the newborn should have their wristbands placed before they are separated in the delivery room. The AAP recommends that two identical identification bands be placed on the infant while in the delivery room. Bracelets are usually placed on the wrist and ankle. The neonate loses weight after birth, so the bracelets must be snug. Hospitals today often take a photograph of the infant soon after birth for identification purposes. Some hospitals still use fingerprinting of the mother and footprinting of the newborn as a means of identification.

Security issues have played a major part in the care of the newborn infant. Parents must be assured that their newborn is safe and secure whenever the infant is not in their care. Nursery and postpartum nurses must follow established protocols when removing the newborn from the parents. These nurses also need to wear appropriate identification badges. Many of these are now complete with staff picture and are color-coded according to the area in which the nurse works. Parents need to be aware of these precautions. When the newborn is returned to the parents, identification bands are again checked to reestablish security. Identification is reaffirmed on admission to the nursery and before transferring the infant to any other location.

Security measures are shared and reinforced with the parents. Parents are encouraged to follow the security protocols and release their newborn to individuals according to the protocol. Stairways are secured with security codes or alarms. In some locations, an electronic device or alarm chip may be attached to the infant. These devices trigger an alarm in the event that they exit the maternity unit. In case a newborn is abducted, hospitals have an emergency code to secure elevators and exits of the building. Employees in all areas are aware of the code name for a newborn abduction and can assist in identifying and delaying the departure of any suspicious person.

MEDICATION ADMINISTRATION AND SCREENING TESTS

Vitamin K (AquaMephyton) is administered immediately after birth to promote blood clotting and prevent hemorrhage in the neonate. A mild vitamin

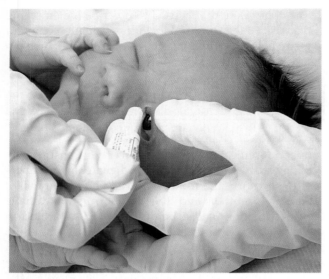

FIGURE **4-15** A ribbon of ointment is administered into each conjunctival sac to prevent chlamydial ophthalmia and gonococcal ophthalmia.

K deficiency is not unusual in newborns and is common in preterm infants. The neonate's intestinal flora is sterile at birth, and as a result, the newborn is unable to synthesize vitamin K. A normal intestinal flora is established after birth. Vitamin K is administered intramuscularly into the lateral aspect of the thigh.

All infants should receive the first dose of hepatitis B vaccine soon after birth and before hospital discharge. The hepatitis B vaccine is administered intramuscularly into the lateral aspect of the thigh. This immunization is the first in the *series* of three hepatitis B injections that the infant receives. Hepatitis B is further discussed in Chapter 7.

A 0.5% erythromycin ointment is instilled in the neonate's eyes to prevent chlamydial ophthalmia and gonococcal ophthalmia (Figure 4-15). A 1% tetracycline solution is also effective against these conditions. The ointment needs to be administered within 1 hour after birth. Mild inflammation may occur, and any discharge from the eyes should be reported.

Blood work such as a hematocrit determination and a glucose recording may be indicated if the newborn is having difficulty adjusting to the environment. Hypoglycemia (low blood sugar) is discussed in Chapter 5. Screening tests for metabolic conditions that, if left untreated, could lead to conditions such as mental retardation are done after birth. PKU and hypothyroidism screenings are required in every state. Forty-nine states require galactosemia screenings, and selected states screen for hemoglobinopathies (Kenner & Moran, 2005).

- **Phenylketonuria (PKU):** A genetic metabolic disorder that can result in mental retardation if left untreated. No signs and symptoms are usually present at birth. Treatment consists of a low-phenylalanine diet; foods high in protein are also avoided.
- **Hypothyroidism:** A condition in which the thyroid gland does not produce sufficient thyroid hormone; can result in mental retardation, growth delay, lack of activity, feeding problems, and abnormal facial appearance if untreated. Signs and symptoms may include skin mottling, a large fontanel, a large tongue, hypotonia, slow reflexes, and a distended abdomen; may be asymptomatic (McKinney et al., 2005). Treatment consists of lifelong thyroid hormone replacement (levothyroxine).
- **Galactosemia:** Condition in which infants cannot properly digest milk or sugar; can result in mental retardation, cataracts, liver disease, or even death if untreated. Signs and symptoms include intrauterine growth retardation and hypoglycemia; vomiting and diarrhea occur after feedings. Treatment is a lifelong lactose-restricted diet.
- **Hemoglobinopathies:** Conditions such as sickle cell anemia, which can result in serious complications or infections if untreated. Sickle cell anemia is discussed in Chapter 8.

Others screenings may be required, based on individual state regulations. Specimens are obtained before 72 hours of age and preferably after 24 hours of protein feeding (Rhead & Irons, 2004). With the current trend toward early discharge of mothers and newborns, it is imperative that parents understand the importance of possible follow-up screening and keep the scheduled laboratory appointment.

 Community Cue

Pediatrix Screening (*http://www.pediatrix.com*) provides a newborn screening service that can detect more than 50 disorders in newborns. Screening must be ordered by the physician and is paid for by the family.

NUTRITION

BREASTFEEDING ADVANTAGES

The nurse can play an important role in teaching, supporting, and encouraging the nursing mother. Breast milk provides immunological, nutritional, and psychosocial advantages. Compared with cow's milk, breast milk contains more iron, sugar, vitamins A and C, and niacin. Breast milk has less protein and calcium than cow's milk, but the amounts present are better utilized by the baby. Breast milk is more digestible because its fat globules are smaller, and it is free from bacteria. It provides the baby with greater

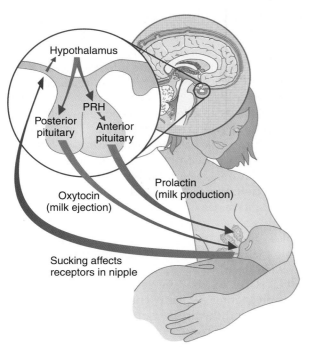

FIGURE **4-16** Milk release during breastfeeding.

immunity to certain childhood diseases. Breastfed babies are less prone to intestinal upsets. In brief, the quality of the mother's milk is suited to the needs of the baby.

Practical factors in favor of breast milk include the fact that it saves time and money. It is also delivered to the newborn in the proper quantity; the more frequently a woman nurses, the more breast milk produced (Figure 4-16). Breast milk provides the newborn with the most recommended nutrition, and it aids the mother physically. As the baby nurses, the mother's uterus contracts, thus hastening its return to a normal size and shape. Furthermore, mothers receive emotional satisfaction, and bonds of attachment are enhanced during feeding.

Breast milk can be stored in the refrigerator for up to 24 hours (some sources say 48 hours) and in the freezer for up to 3 months. Frozen breast milk should be thawed under warm running water and not in the microwave. Thawed breast milk should never be refrozen.

In order to prevent rickets, 200 international units of oral vitamin D daily are recommended for breastfed infants, beginning during the first 2 months of life and continuing until daily consumption of vitamin D–fortified formula or milk is 500 mL (Gartner & Greer, 2003).

Although the nurse must keep in mind that breastfeeding is highly recommended, the individual choice of the mother should be respected. Ensuring that the baby receives the best nutrition available is always the ultimate goal.

CONTRAINDICATIONS TO BREASTFEEDING

Nursing is contraindicated in infants with galactosemia; in mothers with active tuberculosis, herpes simplex lesions on a breast, active drug abuse (street drugs); and in mothers who are receiving chemotherapy or radioactive therapy (AAP Policy Statement, 2005). Mothers who are HIV-positive should not breastfeed, even if they are in relatively good health because the virus can be passed through breast milk. Certainly, the mother who has a personal preference not to breastfeed should not be forced to do so.

Occasionally, elevated levels of bilirubin occur in the breastfed infant. This is known as *true breast milk jaundice.* Breastfeeding may be interrupted for 1 to 2 days and formula given to the infant, phototherapy may be initiated, or both may be done. With the decrease in bilirubin and the resumption of breastfeeding, bilirubin levels do not increase significantly (Behrman et al., 2004).

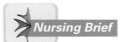
Nursing Brief

If a pacifier is used, instruct parents to obtain the type that is of one-piece construction to prevent choking. It should not be tied around the neonate's neck. Be sure breastfeeding is well established to avoid nipple confusion.

TECHNIQUE OF BREASTFEEDING

In the establishment of lactation, the mother's milk goes through three stages: colostrum, transitional milk, and mature milk. Colostrum secretion is watery and yellowish, begins early in pregnancy, increases, and may last for several days after delivery. Transitional milk replaces colostrum after 2 to 4 days and lasts until about 2 weeks postpartum, when mature breast milk is present. The neonate is generally put to breast immediately or shortly after delivery. Current research supports this practice because it appears to increase early maternal-infant attachment, increase milk production, and decrease the chances of engorgement. The sucking of the neonate stimulates the production of milk. The let-down reflex, by which the milk is squeezed into the large ducts and nipples, is stimulated by the infant's sucking or sometimes even by the baby's crying. The mother feels a vague tingling sensation in her breasts when this occurs. If she is tense or tired, this feeling can be inhibited. The crying infant does not usually stimulate the let-down reflex until the mother has been conditioned to the infant's crying. Supplemental nursery feedings are to be avoided in favor of more frequent nursing. If the mother has a good fluid intake, an ample diet with extra milk, an adequate vitamin intake, and moderate rest and exercise, most difficulties are eliminated. Factors to be emphasized are depicted in the Home Care Tip box.

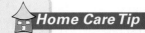

Home Care Tip

Summary of Breastfeeding Instructions for the Mother

INFORMATION	RATIONALE
1. Wash hands before proceeding; wash nipples with warm water, no soap.	Prevents infection of the newborn and breast.
2. Position options: • Comfortably seated in chair with back and arm support (baby in football position). • Side-lying with pillow beneath head, arm above head. • Mother needs to experiment initially to find most comfortable positions for her. • Entire body of infant turned to mother's breast.	Alternating positions facilitates breast emptying and prevents sore nipples.
3. Stroke baby's cheek with nipple.	Uses rooting reflex; baby will turn toward nipple.
4. Baby's mouth should cover entire or large amount of areola.	Compresses ducts, lessens tension on nipples.
5. Initially, both breasts are used; the first side for about 10 minutes; on the other, breastfeed for unlimited time (at least another 10 minutes).	Allows for let-down on the first breast.
6. After the milk supply has come in (by day 8 at the latest), the baby can nurse as long as he or she wants on the first breast (up to 20 minutes) and then the second breast, if the baby is interested. Alternate breasts at the start of each feeding (Schmitt, 2005).	Allows baby to get the high-fat, calorie-rich hind milk. Nursing at second breast increases milk production.
7. Retract breast tissue from baby's nose during sucking.	Baby releases nipple if unable to breathe.
8. Break suction by placing finger in corner of baby's mouth.	Removing baby in this way prevents irritation to nipples.
9. The neonate is nursed shortly after birth and approximately every 2-3 hours thereafter.	Initial feedings provide colostrum; establishing a pattern helps baby develop own schedule.
10. Burp baby after each breast and after feeding.	Rids stomach of air bubbles, reduces regurgitation.

POSSIBLE PROBLEMS WITH BREASTFEEDING

Although many women nurse successfully with few problems, some concerns include the neonate who does not eat well, sore and cracked nipples, and breast engorgement. Some babies do not seem to nurse vigorously and fall asleep after 5 minutes only to wake again when they are put in their crib. The mother can first try shifting the baby to the other breast. Babies can obtain a major portion of what is in the breast after 5 minutes of nursing. With further sucking, a second let-down occurs, which supplies the newborn with milk that is higher in fat.

There are several remedies for sore and cracked nipples. It is important to instruct mothers to be certain that the baby takes a large amount of the areola into the mouth when sucking. To accomplish this, the mother slides all the fingers under the breast to lift and support it for the baby. The thumb is placed above the areola, and the breast is moved so that the nipple lightly tickles the baby's lower lip. The baby is brought to the breast, *not* the breast to the baby. Time limits on each breast are no longer thought to prevent nipple soreness. Positioning of the newborn is more effective in decreasing nipple soreness than is limiting the time at the breast. When breaking suction before removing the infant from the breast, the mother should insert a finger into the infant's mouth beside the nipple. Frequent nursing provides continued stimulation of the breast and relieves fullness. After breastfeeding is established, the mother should continue feeding on the first side as long as the infant nurses vigorously, then burp the baby, and then continue on the other breast.

The nipples and areola should be washed with water and then allowed to dry thoroughly. Airing the nipples and applying a small amount of expressed breast milk to the areola has been found to be successful in the treatment of cracked or sore nipples. Ointments have become controversial in breast care because they can cause irritation, contamination, and allergic reactions. It is also important to keep breast pads dry to decrease contamination.

Breast engorgement occurs mainly in the first week of nursing. The breasts become swollen, firm, and tender, and there is less nipple protrusion. Prevention consists of emptying at least one breast at each feeding. The nurse also instructs the mother to purchase a well-fitting nursing bra and to wear it 24 hours a day. Treatment consists of breast massage during feedings, which aids in the release of oxytocin, which causes the let-down reflex. Also, frequent feedings (every 2 to 3 hours) are helpful in emptying the breasts at each feeding. It may be necessary to soften the areola region first by hand expression of milk if the nipple is too hard to get into the baby's mouth. Warm, moist compresses or a warm shower before feeding may also provide relief. Ice packs may be applied between feedings.

BOTTLE FEEDING

Newborn babies whose parents choose to bottle feed are given formula. Modern research has made such feedings safe and nutritionally adequate. The composition of formulas is designed to closely resemble breast milk.

Studies have indicated that babies tolerate cool or room-temperature formula equally as well as formula that has been heated slightly. If room-temperature formula is used, there is no chance of burns from overheated bottles; also, time and energy are conserved. Bottles should not be warmed in the microwave, because these ovens heat unevenly. Formula tends to get too hot in the center and gives a false reading to a person feeling only the outside of the bottle. Also, microwave heating continues for a period after the bottle has been removed from the unit, thus warming the formula further. Burning of the newborn's mucosa and mouth has resulted. Bottles are best heated under warm running water.

The mother or nurse needs to be relaxed and comfortable when feeding the neonate (Figure 4-17). The newborn's head and back are supported in the crook of the arm. The baby should be warm and dry. Propping the bottle on a pad deprives the baby of the pleasure of being held and loved. It is also dangerous because the baby may choke if the flow of milk is too rapid. A baby's natural tendency to push the tongue out when the nipple is placed in the mouth (the tongue retrusion reflex) should not be taken as an indication that the infant is not hungry.

USE OF FORMULA

Most formulas used today in hospitals and homes are commercially prepared. Formulas may be purchased with or without iron, according to the physician's preference and the neonate's needs. Vitamins have been added. Modified formulas are used in feeding preterm infants because of their need for a variation in the whey/casein and calcium/phosphorus ratios.

Always wash hands before handling formula. In homes with dishwashers, the high temperature of the water used in the dishwasher is excellent for cleaning the bottles. Ideally, nipples of bottles should be washed and rinsed by hand because they can be damaged by the high temperature in the dishwasher.

Basically, prepared formulas come in four forms: (1) ready to use in cans (use as-is without dilution); (2) in concentrated form (which must be diluted with an equal amount of water); and (3) in powdered form (1 scoop of powdered formula for every 2 ounces of water).

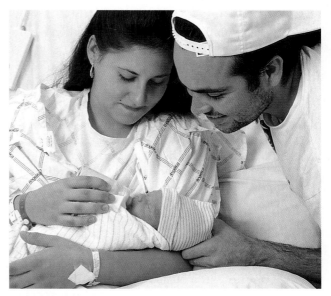

FIGURE **4-17** The mother (or father) should hold the infant close during feeding. Hold the bottle so that the baby receives formula and not air.

When using powdered formula or concentrated liquid, it is important that the nurse determine the mother's understanding of the proportions by reviewing the product directions with her. Some products sold in the United States are packaged with directions in several languages. Tap water may be mixed with powder if the water is from an uncontaminated source. If unsure, the water should be boiled rapidly for 5 minutes and cooled.

Expense governs the choice of formula for many families. In general, the more convenient, the higher the cost. Some nursing bottles use sterilized thin plastic nursing containers that come in rolls. These are inserted into the holder and filled according to the manufacturer's directions.

Leftover formula should not be rewarmed for future feedings because bacteria thrive at room temperature. This can be averted by filling the bottle with the approximate amount the baby generally drinks. Persons who need to sterilize formulas because of travel or personal circumstances are taught the aseptic or terminal heat methods. These are well outlined in government pamphlets and baby books. The services of the public health nurse are invaluable in many instances. Cultural considerations that have a bearing on practices such as feeding a newborn baby can be evaluated at this time.

Regardless of the method used, all bottles, nipples, and other utensils must be thoroughly cleaned. Bottles and nipples are scrubbed with a bottle brush in hot, soapy water and rinsed well in hot, clear water. Water is squeezed through nipple holes during washing and rinsing. Bottles are placed upside down on a rack to drain.

TECHNIQUE OF BOTTLE FEEDING

The following points should be observed when feeding the baby by bottle:

1. Change the infant's diaper if needed.
2. Wash hands.
3. Hold the baby unless doing so is contraindicated. If a baby cannot be removed from the crib, sit by the infant and elevate the head and shoulders.
4. Use of a burp cloth (clean diaper, bib, or towel) under the baby's chin is helpful.
5. Observe the kind and amount of formula in the bottle.
6. Let a few drops of formula fall on the inner aspect of your wrist to test (only necessary if it was warmed).
   a. Temperature: It should be warm but not hot.
   b. Size of nipple hole: Formula should drop but not flow in a steady stream. If the holes are too small, the weak neonate tires and fails to finish the feeding. If they are too large, the baby may choke or miss the satisfaction received from sucking.
7. Do not contaminate the nipple.
8. Hold the bottle so that the nipple is full of formula. This prevents the baby from swallowing air.
9. Burp the baby halfway through the feeding and at the end of the feeding with one of the following methods:
   a. Place a diaper or small towel over your shoulder to protect your gown. Place the baby firmly against your shoulder and gently pat its back.
   b. Place the baby in a sitting position. Put a towel beneath its chin. Support its chest and head with one hand. Gently rub its back with the other.
10. The feeding should take 15 to 20 minutes. A newborn will probably take 2 to 3 ounces of formula every 3 to 4 hours for the first few weeks, progressing to 4 ounces every 4 hours by the end of the first month. Do not hurry the baby or force the infant to eat too much.
11. Leave the baby clean and dry. Place the baby who is *awake* on the right side to promote digestion (Figure 4-18). Remember, however, that babies should *sleep on their backs*.
12. Chart the amount of formula offered, the amount taken and retained, any regurgitation or vomiting, how the formula was taken, and whether or not the baby appeared satisfied after the feeding. (Note that regurgitation is an overflow of milk that occurs shortly after feeding, whereas vomiting means bringing up a more substantial amount of partially digested milk.)

For discharge teaching, remind the parents that the baby who is fed when hungry ("demand feedings")

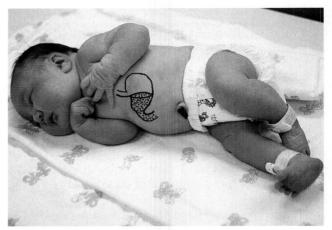

FIGURE **4-18** Right-side-lying position after feeding while awake. Supine positioning is recommended during sleep.

soon adopts a flexible schedule. Prompt fulfillment of the baby's needs assures the infant that the world is a good place to live.

INFECTION

Infections that are relatively harmless to an adult may be fatal to the newborn infant. Symptoms are often subtle in the early stages, the recognition of which can be crucial (Table 4-5). Portals of entry are the respiratory tract, the gastrointestinal tract, the genitourinary tract, and breaks in the skin. The portals of exit are the same as those just mentioned, and the organisms are in the excretions from the various systems: sneezes, sputum, vomitus, feces, saliva, urine, and discharges from the skin and mucous membranes. Nursery standards are developed and enforced by various professional agencies such as the AAP, hospital accreditation boards, and local health agencies. Provisions governing space, control of temperature and humidity, lighting, and safety from fire and other hazards are considered. Each newborn infant has her or his own bassinet/crib, bath equipment, and linen supply. Any communal equipment is sterilized after each use.

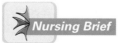

Nursing Brief

Advise parents to limit the neonate's exposure to crowds during the early weeks of life.

PREVENTION OF INFECTION

Nursery personnel wear scrub uniforms while in the nursery and put cover gowns on if they leave the nursery. Nails are kept short and clean. Artificial nails should not be permitted because they may harbor bacteria. Students should investigate the policy of the institution in which they are practicing. A nurse

Table 4-5	*Clinical Manifestations of Neonatal Sepsis*
SYSTEM	**SIGNS AND SYMPTOMS**
Integumentary	Temperature instability (may be increased, decreased, or both)
	"Does not look well"
	Rash
Cardiovascular	Tachycardia
	Decreased perfusion, capillary refill
	Hypotension
	Cyanosis, pallor, or mottling
Gastrointestinal	Feeds poorly
	Abdominal distention
	Vomiting
	Diarrhea
Respiratory	Nasal flaring, retractions, grunting
	Tachypnea
	Cyanosis
	Apnea
Central nervous	Lethargy
	Irritability
	Hypotonia
	Seizures (late sign)
Hematopoietic	Jaundice (late sign)
	Hepatomegaly, splenomegaly (late signs)
	Petechiae, purpura (late signs)
	Anemia (late sign)

who has a fever, skin infection, or gastrointestinal disease should not work in the nursery. Because many hospitals have open visiting, all visitors should be cautioned not to come if they are sick.

HANDWASHING TECHNIQUE

The most effective procedure used in the prevention of infections is **proper handwashing.** The nurse must conscientiously wash and rinse the hands and forearms before and after caring for each newborn or handling equipment. Handwashing before care protects the newborn, and handwashing after care protects the nurse. Although most organisms are transmitted by direct contact, some are capable of remaining alive for a time outside the body and may be transferred indirectly by articles. Personnel entering the newborn nursery initially scrub their hands with an antiseptic. Afterward, they wash their hands with soap under running water. Parents and relatives should be taught the importance of this simple but highly effective procedure.

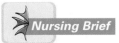
Nursing Brief

When washing hands, make sure the water flows from the least to the most contaminated area (keep hands lowered). Use friction and rub well between the fingers and around the nails. Wash hands, wrists, and forearms. Wash for a minimum of 10-15 seconds. If there is no foot pedal, turn the faucet off with a clean paper towel.

SIGNS AND SYMPTOMS OF INFECTION

The following signs and symptoms of infection in newborns and infants should not only be recognized and reported to the charge nurse but taught to parents as well:

- Temperature above 100° F (37.8° C) or below 97° F (36° C)
- Refusal to take nourishment
- Rashes or skin lesions
- Loose, watery stools
- Discharge from eyes, nose, or umbilicus
- Vomiting
- Lethargy or irritability
- Others, as indicated in Table 4-5

The ill newborn is isolated from other newborns. If warranted, the baby will be placed in the neonatal intensive care unit (NICU) with specific isolation guidelines.

CARE OF THE PATIENT UNIT

A baby in the newborn nursery is usually placed in a small, transparent bassinet equipped with a bath tray that can be pulled out. Drawers below the bassinet hold the newborn's linens and supplies. Supplies in the newborn's crib are to be used only for that newborn. With this, the rate of cross contamination can be reduced. The head of the newborn's crib should be considered the clean area. This is where the bulb suction should be placed. The bottom of the crib is less clean, so that is where soiled diapers should be placed until they can be removed from the crib. When making a crib, the nurse places the baby at the bottom and tucks the clean sheet in at the top of the mattress and then puts the baby at the top of the crib and tucks the sheet in at the bottom.

The newborn infant in the hospital may wear a hospital shirt and diaper and should be wrapped in at least one blanket, or may wear clothes from home. Remind parents to wash new baby clothing before it is worn (see Clothing the Baby). Be sure the baby remains warm enough. *Remember that babies are transported in their bassinet; they are never carried. Anyone carrying an infant in a hallway should be questioned.*

ONGOING CARE

BATHING THE BABY

The bath is an excellent time to observe the naked newborn infant. Always bathe the baby in a warm area. Bath water should be approximately 38° C (100° F). Special attention must be given to areas of the skin that come in contact with each other because chafing may occur. These areas are on the neck, behind the ears, in the axillae, and in the groin. They should be dried well to prevent evaporative heat loss. Because powder can be irritating to the respiratory tract, it is not used in the hospital and parents are discouraged from using it at home. Lotions and the type of soap used vary with each institution. The procedure for bathing the newborn infant is described in Chapter 17.

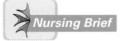

Nursing Brief

Emphasize flexibility in the timing of the bath. Stress the need to gather all materials beforehand to avoid leaving the neonate unattended or chilled. The nurse attempts to help parents relax by emphasizing that there is nothing difficult about bathing a baby.

CLOTHING THE BABY

Parents should be taught that babies should be dressed as other family members are dressed. They do not need an extra blanket or extra clothing unless they are in a cool environment. New parents should prewash all of the baby's clothes, linens, and washable accessories in a mild detergent before they are used. Clothes should be easy to put on and take off. Safety should always be kept in mind.

CORD CARE
New Patient Teaching
- The cord clamp is removed once the end of the cord is dry and crisp, usually about 24 hours after birth.
- Parents need to check for redness, odor, swelling, or any drainage (report any of these to the physician).
- The base of the cord may be wiped with alcohol 2 to 3 times a day, although this is no longer a necessity as once believed.
- The diaper should be folded below the cord to keep it dry and free from urine contamination.
- Until the cord falls off, parents should only sponge-bathe their baby.

The cord will fall off in about 10 to 14 days.

FAMILY RELATIONS

GETTING ACQUAINTED

The nurse can play an important role in helping the family make the transition to parenthood. If the parents have attended parenting classes, they know more of what to expect as they begin their new roles. Regardless, having the nurse spend time with the new family is invaluable. The nurse calls the baby by name, encourages holding the baby *en face,* discusses particular behavior patterns, and points out unique characteristics that help enhance the bonding process (Figure 4-19). This is especially important if the baby differs from the parents' perceived "fantasy child" in

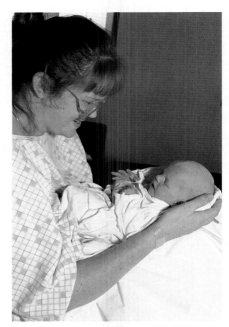

FIGURE **4-19** The mother demonstrates the *en face* position as she becomes acquainted with her newborn. She positions her infant so that their faces are aligned, aiding the eye contact that is important in the bonding process.

terms of gender, physical attributes, or health. Nursing assessment includes the observation of specific parenting behavior, such as the amount of affection shown to the baby, the level or lack of interest in the child, and the amount of time spent interacting with the baby. In addition, the nurse should look for the amount of stimulation and the amount of physical and eye-to-eye contact that occurs between the parents and the child. The extent to which the parents encourage the involvement of siblings and grandparents is also noteworthy in assessing the attachment process. This information provides a basis for nursing intervention that may serve to foster positive family relationships.

BONDING/ATTACHMENT

Although the terms **bonding** or **attachment** are sometimes used interchangeably, they actually have different meanings. Bonding is thought to occur soon after birth, and attachment occurs gradually during the first year of the infant's life. Maternal attachment behaviors include gazing at, kissing, touching, and holding the infant *en face*, along with talking to the infant in a higher-pitched voice than normal. The father is included in the bonding process, as are other family members. The nurse can point out various behaviors of the neonate, encourage eye contact, and provide periods of privacy for the couple.

SIBLINGS

Brothers and sisters—siblings—are less likely to regard a new baby as an intruder or a rival if they are made to feel that the baby is theirs as well as their parents'. If the other children feel wanted, accepted, and cherished, their jealousy of the newborn baby will be minimized.

Classes to help siblings prepare for a new baby are held in some hospitals. Questions are answered and a tour of appropriate areas given. These classes help the staff become acquainted with the rest of the family before delivery and enable them to directly involve the siblings. Two common questions from toddlers are "Why doesn't the baby have any hair?" and "When are you going to take the baby back to the hospital, Mommy?"

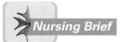
Nursing Brief

On returning home from the hospital, if siblings are waiting, it is helpful for the father to arrive carrying the baby. This leaves the mother's arms free for hugs before introductions are made.

SPIRITUAL CARE

If the condition of a neonate is poor, parents who are Christians may wish to have the baby baptized. The minister or priest should be notified. Parents of other religious affiliations may have special requests or rituals as well. Occasionally, parents attach small pins or medals to the baby's blankets or clothing. The nurse must be extremely careful not to lose these because they are probably of great sentimental and/or religious value to the parents, particularly if the baby dies.

DISCHARGE TEACHING

Since the hospital stay is short, there is a lot of importance placed on discharge teaching beginning at admission. Before discharge, follow-up appointments for visits with the pediatrician and the obstetrician are made. Families who are cared for by physicians and nurses in hospital clinics and public health clinics should be informed of the location of these facilities, and appointments should be made before discharge. The case manager may be involved in the planning and implementation of this care. This ensures that the infant receives care in well-baby clinics in the areas of anticipatory guidance, immunizations, growth and development, physical assessment, nutrition, and emotional health.

New Patient Teaching for Discharge
- Feeding, bathing, skin care, cord care, elimination
- Recognizing illness
- How to take the baby's temperature
- How to contact the baby's doctor
- Safety issues, including proper use of car seat

- Follow-up medical care (well-child care, immunizations)
- Support groups offered by hospitals for new parents or outside groups such as La Leche League or infant support groups

Involve the newborn's parents as much as possible in the daily care. This allows them to have some degree of comfort in the infant's care before being dismissed from the hospital.

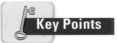
Community Cue

Newborns leaving the hospital should be placed in an approved car seat. The seat should be placed in the back seat of the car, facing the rear. Most communities have programs to assist parents in obtaining an approved car seat for their newborn before discharge.

HOME PHOTOTHERAPY

Because most women and newborn infants are discharged home by 48 hours after birth, there has been an increase in home phototherapy. Physiological jaundice, which occurs 2 to 3 days after birth, may not be evident at discharge. If the bilirubin level rises to the level that phototherapy is needed, home phototherapy is an option to keep the infant and mother in their own environment.

Referral for home phototherapy is based on the infant's health, weight, and bilirubin levels and the ability of the family to comply with the home program. The equipment is usually provided by an outside vendor. A nurse assists the family in the discharge teaching, set-up, and care throughout the treatment. The family keeps records concerning the baby's temperature, feedings, appearance of the eyes (color, drainage, lesions), number of wet diapers, and number and description of stools. Close follow-up with the physician and at least daily bilirubin levels are done to monitor the infant's condition.

Key Points

- Establishment of respirations begins the newborn's adaptation to extrauterine life.
- The Apgar score, which is done at 1 and 5 minutes after birth, is a quick assessment of the newborn's response to extrauterine life.
- Heat loss is a major consideration in caring for the newborn in the delivery area.
- Reflexes present at birth include protective reflexes, feeding reflexes, and reflexes involving muscle tone.
- The newborn is born with the ability of all the senses to function. These are vision, hearing, tasting, smelling, and feeling.
- Issues of concern for the newborn are respiration, circulatory changes, thermoregulation, and feeding.

- The quiet alert state is most conducive for bonding.
- Placing babies to bed on their backs has reduced the incidence of SIDS.
- Newborns need to be properly identified before leaving the delivery room or being separated from their mothers.
- Vitamin K and erythromycin eye ointment are medications given to the newborn shortly after birth.
- Breast milk provides nutrition and immunoglobulins, which provide immunological protection.
- Proper positioning of the newborn at the breast does more to diminish nipple soreness than does limiting the time at the breast.
- Newborns can receive proper nutrition if they are bottle-fed.
- Handwashing is the most effective method to decrease the spread of infections.
- Discharge teaching is important for all families of newborns, but it is especially important for first-time parents.
- When discharged from the hospital, the newborn needs to be placed in an approved car seat. The car seat must continue to be used at all times when the newborn is transported in a vehicle.

 Go to your Companion CD-ROM for an Audio Glossary, video clips, and more.

evolve Be sure to visit the companion Evolve site at http://evolve. elsevier.com/Price/pediatric for WebLinks and additional online resources.

ONLINE RESOURCES

Joint Committee on Infant Hearing (JCIH): http://www.jcih.org

La Leche League for breastfeeding mothers: http://www.lalecheleague.org

Newborn Screenings: http://www.pediatrix.com

5 The High-Risk Neonate

Objectives

Upon completion of this chapter, the student will be able to:

1. Define the vocabulary terms listed
2. Differentiate between the low–birth weight, the very low–birth weight, and the extremely low–birth weight neonate
3. List three causes of preterm birth
4. Describe the possible complications of a high-risk birth
5. State the nursing care needed for each complication
6. Contrast the techniques of feeding the preterm and the full-term neonate
7. Discuss two ways to help facilitate the maternal-infant bonding process for a preterm neonate
8. List three characteristics of the postterm baby

Key Terms

Be sure to check out the bonus material on the Companion CD-ROM, including selected audio pronunciations.

atelectasis (ă-tĕ-LĔK-tă-sĭs; p. 73)
grunting (p. 73)
high-risk (p. 71)
kernicterus (kĕr-NĬK-tĕr-ŭs; p. 78)
lanugo (lă-NOO-gō; p. 73)
lecithin/sphingomyelin (L/S) ratio (LĔS-ĭ-thĭn/SFĬNG-gō-MĪ-ă-lĭn; p. 75)
macrosomia (măk-rō-SŌ-mē-ă; p. 83)
previability (prē-VĪ-ă-bĭl-Ĭ-tē; p. 73)
respiratory distress syndrome (RDS; rĕs-PĬ-ră-tō-rē, p. 75)
transport team (p. 83)

THE PRETERM INFANT

A **high-risk** infant is any infant who is at risk for sustaining medical, developmental, or psychological problems. The goal is prevention or early detection of these problems. Because of increased specialization and sophisticated monitoring techniques, many babies who would have died a few years ago are now surviving. As a result, the nurse's role has become more complex and there is a greater emphasis on subtle clinical observations. The purpose of this chapter is to acquaint the student with the high-risk infant. This allows the student to appreciate the baby's struggle for survival and understand the intense responsibility placed on those entrusted with its care.

Any neonate whose life or quality of existence is threatened is considered to be in a high-risk category and requires close professional supervision. Prematurity and low birth weight often occur together, and both of these factors are associated with increased neonatal morbidity and mortality. The less a baby weighs at birth, the greater are the risks to life during delivery and immediately thereafter.

Infants weighing less than 2500 g (5 lb, 8 oz) are classified as **low–birth weight (LBW),** and those less than 1500 g (3 lb, 5 oz) as **very low–birth weight (VLBW).** Infants weighing less than 1000 g (2 lb, 3 oz) at birth are considered **extremely low–birth weight (ELBW).** In a similar fashion, those infants weighing above the 90th percentile on intrauterine growth curves are referred to as large for gestational age (LGA). Emphasis is placed on the gestational age *and* the level of maturation (Figure 5-1). Current data also indicate that intrauterine growth rates are not the same for all babies and that individual factors must be considered.

Gestational age refers to the actual time from conception to birth that the fetus remains in the uterus. A full-term infant is born between 38 and 42 weeks after conception. Infants born at less than 38 weeks are called *preterm*, and those born at more than 42 weeks are called *postterm*. The new Ballard scoring system is used to determine gestational age. The Ballard system is an update of the Dubowitz scoring system and consists of an evaluation of physical characteristics and neuromuscular tone (see Appendix F).

Level of maturation refers to how well developed the baby is at birth and the functional ability of the organs to exist outside the uterus. The physician can determine a great deal about the maturity of the neonate through careful physical examination, observation of behavior, and family history. A baby who is born at 34 weeks' gestation, weighs 3.5 pounds at birth, has not been damaged by multifactorial birth defects, and had a good placenta may be healthier than a full-term, small-for-gestational-age baby whose placenta was insufficient for any number of reasons. The infant born at 34 weeks' gestation is also probably in better shape than a heavy but immature baby of a mother with diabetes. Each child has different, distinct needs.

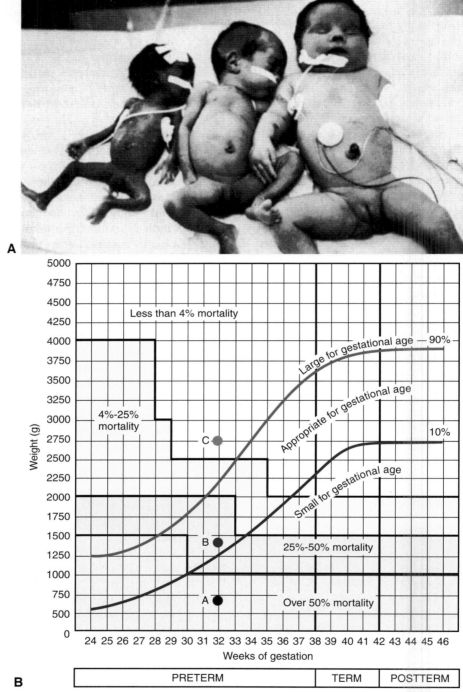

FIGURE **5-1 A,** Three babies of the same gestational age (32 weeks) weighing 600, 1400, and 2750 g, respectively. **B,** Classification of the newborn infant as indicated by relationship of weight to gestational age. The status of babies of the weights shown in **A** is plotted at 32 weeks (dots A, B, and C).

CAUSES OF PRETERM BIRTH

The causes of prematurity are numerous, but in many instances, the cause is unknown (Box 5-1). Adequate prenatal care to prevent preterm birth is extremely important. Inadequate prenatal care can result in low–birth weight infants and premature delivery. Many of these premature infants are born into families who already have socioeconomic problems. The presence of parents in special care nurseries is encouraged and commonplace. This encourages bonding and attachment. The parents may not be prepared to handle the additional strain caused by a preterm infant. Parent aides and other types of home support and assistance are vital, particularly because current studies indicate a correlation between high-risk births and child abuse and neglect.

Box 5-1 **Factors Associated with Low–Birth Weight (LBW) Infants**

- Previous LBW delivery
- Low socioeconomic status
- Low level of maternal education
- Maternal age below 16 and above 35
- Frequent pregnancies with short time between pregnancies
- Cigarette smoking
- Alcohol and/or illicit drug use
- Physical and/or psychological stress
- Maternal health issues such as malnutrition, diabetes mellitus, poor weight gain
- Pregnancy hazards such as preeclampsia (pregnancy-induced hypertension), premature rupture of the membranes, placenta previa
- Unmarried status
- African-American race

RISKS RELATED TO PREMATURITY

Premature birth deprives the neonate of the complete benefits of intrauterine life. The skin is transparent and loose. Superficial veins may be seen beneath the abdomen and scalp. There is a lack of subcutaneous fat, and fine hair called lanugo covers the forehead, shoulders, and arms. The cheese-like vernix caseosa, seen in more mature infants, is absent. The extremities appear short, and the abdomen protrudes. The nails are short. The genitals are small. If the infant is a girl, the labia majora may be open and the clitoris evident.

INADEQUATE RESPIRATORY FUNCTION

Important structural changes occur in the fetal lungs during the second half of pregnancy. The alveoli, or air sacs, enlarge, bringing them closer to the capillaries in the lungs. Failure of the alveoli to enlarge leads to many deaths, which are attributed to previability (*pre,* before; *vita,* life). In addition, the muscles that move the chest are not fully developed, the abdomen is distended and causes pressure on the diaphragm, stimulation of the respiratory center in the brain is immature, and the gag and cough reflexes are weak because of inadequate nerve supply. Surfactant (a chemical in the lungs that helps inflate alveoli) also may be deficient.

ATELECTASIS
Description

The lungs are collapsed during fetal life. Their failure to expand after birth is known as atelectasis. Although some lung expansion must take place with the first breath, full development may not occur until several days later. **Primary atelectasis,** in which the alveoli fail to expand, may occur in preterm infants, infants of mothers who are oversedated before delivery, and infants with damage to the respiratory center in the brain. **Secondary atelectasis** occurs when the lungs collapse after they have once inflated. This may be caused by viral infections, pulmonary disease, aspirated foreign material, or a mucus plug.

Signs and Symptoms

Symptoms vary with the cause and extent of the atelectasis. The infant exhibits irregular, rapid respirations. These may be accompanied by respiratory grunting and flaring of the nostrils. The skin is cyanotic and mottled. Tachycardia is generally present. Intercostal and substernal retractions may be noticeable (Figure 5-2). These symptoms cause the infant to tire and hypoxemia increases. Radiographs showing increased density, sometimes involving both lungs, confirm the diagnosis. The prognosis depends on the general condition of the baby and the cause.

Treatment

Treatment depends on the cause of the collapse. Frequent changes in position (as permitted) and oxygen therapy may be beneficial. Positioning should enhance full lung expansion and clothing should not be binding. Semi-Fowler's position may facilitate lung expansion. Oxygen must be warmed and humidified. Mechanical ventilation may be required. These babies are usually treated in the neonatal intensive care unit (NICU). Nursing care should involve close observation for changes in the respiratory status.

MECONIUM ASPIRATION SYNDROME
Description

Aspiration of stained amniotic fluid is sometimes seen in the term or postterm newborn infant. It signals that the fetus was in distress while in utero. This intrauterine stress causes relaxing of the anal sphincter and passage of meconium into the amniotic fluid. Aspiration of meconium may occur with the first breath. This results in small airway obstruction, manifested by tachypnea, hypoxia, retractions, grunting respirations, and cyanosis. Respiratory distress may be immediate or delayed, and pneumothorax may result. If the course is mild, improvement may occur within 48 hours. If the aspiration is severe, respiratory failure can occur very rapidly.

Treatment

Immediate suctioning of the nasopharynx at birth is indicated. A chest radiograph may show coarse, patchy intensities. Atelectasis sometimes occurs. Infants with respiratory distress are transferred to the NICU for close observation. These infants are treated with intravenous fluids, systemic antibiotics, exogenous (artificial) surfactant administration, and possible ventilatory support (Hockenberry & Wilson, 2007).

Grade	0	1	2

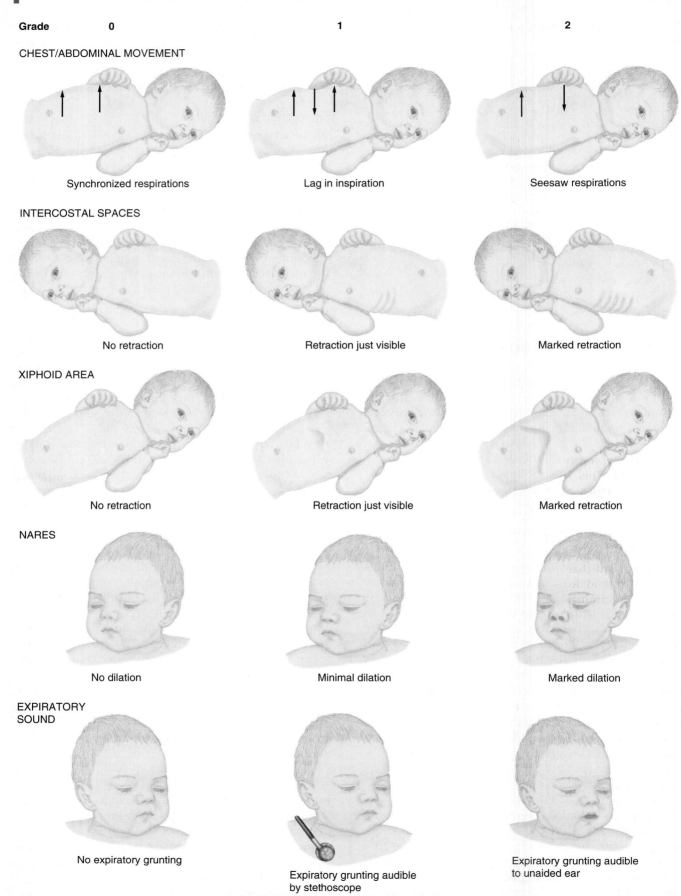

CHEST/ABDOMINAL MOVEMENT

Synchronized respirations · Lag in inspiration · Seesaw respirations

INTERCOSTAL SPACES

No retraction · Retraction just visible · Marked retraction

XIPHOID AREA

No retraction · Retraction just visible · Marked retraction

NARES

No dilation · Minimal dilation · Marked dilation

EXPIRATORY SOUND

No expiratory grunting · Expiratory grunting audible by stethoscope · Expiratory grunting audible to unaided ear

FIGURE **5-2** Indicators of respiratory distress in the neonate.

RESPIRATORY DISTRESS SYNDROME
Description

Respiratory distress syndrome (RDS), also known as *hyaline membrane disease*, is a common disorder in premature neonates. Because of the immaturity of the lungs, there is decreased gas exchange. This, together with pulmonary structural immaturity, results in absolute or functional deficiency of surfactant. Surfactant reduces the surface tension in the lung, preventing the collapse of the alveoli during expiration. Without surfactant, the alveoli must be reexpanded with each breath so as to allow adequate gas exchange to occur. As a result, the infant uses all available energy to breathe. In the absence of adequate oxygenation, there is decreased or no production of surfactant.

Signs and Symptoms

Signs of RDS may develop at birth in the premature infant. The more premature the infant and the less the infant weighs at birth, the more likely the incidence of respiratory distress. The ELBW and VLBW infants may have severe RDS at birth (Hockenberry & Wilson, 2007). Manifestations of RDS include tachypnea, nasal flaring, cyanosis, intercostal and sternal retractions, and grunting. Infants with severe RDS develop apnea and respiratory failure and need mechanical ventilation.

Treatment

The best approach to treating RDS is to prevent prematurity. This is done through prenatal care. If a problem arises and the fetus must be delivered, the treatment may involve, if there is enough time, increasing the production of surfactant. If this is not possible, the infant can be given artificial surfactant after birth.

In the event that there is time, and delivery is not necessary for at least 2 to 3 days, amniocentesis is done to determine the maturity of the fetus. A test called the lecithin/sphingomyelin (L/S) ratio can be used to detect insufficient amounts of surfactant. If insufficient amounts are found, it is possible to speed up the production of surfactant by giving the mother multiple injections of a corticosteroid such as betamethasone or dexamethasone. Administration 1 or 2 days before delivery may reduce the chance of RDS developing.

Surfactant replacement therapy is being done for the very low–birth weight infant and also for those infants who show evidence of respiratory distress during the first 24 hours of life. An exogenous synthetic form of surfactant (Exosurf) or natural form of surfactant (Survanta or Infasurf) is administered directly into the infant's endotracheal tube. This acts directly on the lungs. Surfactant may continue to be administered every 12 hours for up to four doses.

Surfactant should be administered only in the NICU, with adequate support of a neonatologist, NICU nurses, and respiratory therapists.

Surfactant has been beneficial in the treatment of RDS. In infants treated with surfactant, there has been an improvement in gas exchange, reduction in ventilatory pressures, and improved appearance of the lungs on chest radiographs. However, surfactant has not reduced the incidence of **bronchopulmonary dysplasia (BPD),** which can be a chronic lung problem. BPD is discussed in Chapter 8.

Complications of surfactant therapy include transient hypoxia and hypotension, blockage of the endotracheal tube, and pulmonary hemorrhage (Behrman et al., 2004). Research continues in areas that improve oxygenation. Currently, **liquid ventilation** and the use of **nitric oxide** are therapies that are meeting with positive outcomes in the NICU. Liquid ventilation involves the use of a **perfluorochemical** fluid for ventilation of the infant. This fluid has a low surface tension and is a solvent for oxygen and carbon dioxide. This enables gas exchange to take place through the fluid placed in the lungs. In addition, nitric oxide is a gas that causes pulmonary vasodilation and improves oxygenation. These procedures require highly skilled nursing care and are performed on infants who have not responded well to other treatments.

APNEA
Description

Apnea in the preterm infant is fairly common. Premature infants have periods of rapid respirations, followed by very slow breathing and then a period of no apparent respirations. Apnea is defined as the cessation of breathing for 20 or more seconds. This may be accompanied by bradycardia (fewer than 100 heart beats/minute) and cyanosis. Apnea in the term infant requires diagnostic evaluation. Causes may include sepsis, pneumonia, or intraventricular hemorrhage (Behrman et al., 2004).

Nursing Care

Apnea monitors, usually set at 20 seconds, help alert nurses to a cessation of respirations. This does not remove the nurse's responsibility to observe the infant for signs of respiratory distress. If the monitor alarm sounds, the nurse should *first* assess the infant for signs of distress, color, and respirations. Because of loose leads and other mechanical causes, it is not unusual for the monitor to emit false alarms. If an apneic spell has occurred, the nurse can gently rub the infant's chest or back. If stimulation fails, the nurse should suction the nose and oropharynx and reposition the infant's head by raising it to a "sniffing" position. If breathing still does not begin, the infant should be ventilated via an Ambu bag.

Infants who experience periods of apnea because of immaturity may be placed on a medication such as caffeine or theophylline to stimulate the central nervous system (CNS) (Schmidt, 2006). Stimulation of the breathing center in the CNS improves the rhythm of breathing. Nursing care includes monitoring the blood levels of these medications because toxicity can occur.

Infants known to have apneic spells often go home on monitors. Before discharge from the hospital, parents are educated about the use of home monitors. It is also imperative that the parents or the caregivers of these infants learn cardiopulmonary resuscitation (CPR) and demonstrate proficiency in CPR before discharge from the hospital.

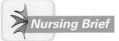

Nursing Brief

Caregivers of infants being discharged with home monitoring should have a clear understanding that the purpose of monitoring is to alert caregivers to apnea episodes and not to prevent sudden infant death syndrome (SIDS).

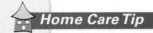

Home Care Tip

Preventing Excess Apnea
- Provide undisturbed sleep periods.
- Support the infant's head, keeping the head and neck in a straight line to avoid windpipe obstruction.
- Keep the infant's temperature stable by avoiding chilling, especially during bathing.
- Pace the infant's feeding to prevent hard and fast sucking, which can cause pauses in breathing.
- Avoid exposure to cigarette smoke (Stokowski, 2005a)

SEPSIS
Description

Sepsis or *septicemia* refers to a generalized infection in the bloodstream. All neonates are at risk for developing sepsis, but preterm infants are especially vulnerable. Newborns up to 1 month of age with an infection may have sepsis neonatorum. The infant has diminished immunity and usually there is no local inflammatory response at the site of the infection. This makes the signs and symptoms vague. Blood, urine, and cerebral spinal fluid (CSF) cultures are obtained in an attempt to determine the organism causing the infection.

Signs and Symptoms

Manifestations of sepsis are often vague, and the diagnosis is sometimes based on an infant "not looking right." All the body systems may be affected by sepsis. The classic triad of symptoms are fever, tachycardia, and vasodilation (Short, 2004). Some of the more common manifestations include hypothermia, temperature instability, changes in feeding behavior, color changes, and changes in activity. Table 4-5 shows the responses of the different systems to sepsis.

Nursing Care

Prevention of sepsis is the goal of the nurse when caring for a preterm infant. Good handwashing is imperative

before and after handling the baby or the equipment used in the infant's care. Nurses caring for infants in the NICU adhere to standard precautions when handling the infant or touching any objects in the baby's environment. The infant should be observed before handling in order to note any changes in behavior and activities. A thermoregulated environment is provided to conserve energy. Infants with sepsis are placed in an isolette to prevent the spread of infection to other neonates.

Treatment

Infants with sepsis are treated with intravenous antibiotics. Standard precautions (see Appendix E) are to be followed. These neonates are closely observed for changes in color, vital signs, neurological status, and general condition.

NECROTIZING ENTEROCOLITIS
Description

Necrotizing enterocolitis (NEC) is an acute inflammatory disease of the bowel that occurs more often in preterm and other high-risk infants. The exact cause is uncertain, but there seems to be a relationship among intestinal ischemia, bacteria in the area, and the ingestion of formula. Prematurity has been established as the major risk (Noerr, 2003). Studies have shown that there is less incidence of NEC among babies whose diet included breast milk; it is far more common among those fed formula only.

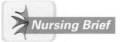

Nursing Brief

Breast milk has been shown to protect against NEC (Reber, 2004). Therefore breastfeeding or expressed breast milk should be encouraged for premature infants.

Signs and Symptoms

Early signs of NEC, such as temperature instability, apnea, and bradycardia, are difficult to differentiate from those of other diseases, especially septicemia. More specific manifestations include a distended abdomen, emesis that contains bile, blood in the stool, and diarrhea. Onset often occurs between 4 and 10 days after the initiation of feedings. Radiographic findings show a sausage-shaped dilation of the intestine. The bowel wall is described as having a *bubbly* appearance. This is from air in the submucosal surfaces of the bowel (Hockenberry & Wilson, 2007). Necrosis can occur. The bowel may require surgical resection, possibly resulting in a colostomy, ileostomy, or jejunostomy.

Nursing Care

Early recognition of the signs and symptoms of NEC aids in early treatment. Abdominal distention should be monitored by consistent abdominal circumference measurements. Temperatures should not be taken rectally because of the danger of perforation. Transmission to other infants must be prevented. Strict handwashing and other infection control measures are implemented. The infant will have a nasogastric tube for abdominal decompression, receive intravenous antibiotics, and require monitoring of laboratory values. The use of parenteral nutrition may be necessary to allow the bowel to rest. The nurse monitors vital signs and reports any abnormal findings. Orders for resuming feedings are followed closely.

HYPOGLYCEMIA
Description

The preterm infant has not remained in the uterus long enough to have sufficient supplies of fat or glycogen to mobilize glucose. Infants born to mothers with diabetes, infants small for gestational age, and infants having trouble maintaining oxygenation levels or temperature are all at risk for hypoglycemia.

Signs and Symptoms

In addition to the obvious low glucose level, determined in the plasma or blood, the nurse should watch for other manifestations of hypoglycemia. These include feeding difficulty, hunger, lethargy, apnea, irregular respiratory effort, cyanosis, a weak and high-pitched cry, jitteriness, twitching, eye rolling, and seizures.

Nursing Care

Nursing care primarily involves identifying signs and symptoms that might indicate the presence of hypoglycemia. The nurse should also control the thermal environment so that the infant does not have to expend extra energy adjusting to a cold environment. Feeding the infant also aids in preventing hypoglycemia. When feedings alone cannot maintain blood glucose concentrations at levels greater than 50 mg/dL, intravenous glucose should be started (Behrman et al., 2004).

HYPOCALCEMIA
Description

Hypocalcemia (*hypo*, below; *calcemia*, calcium in the blood) is also seen in preterm infants and sick neonates. Calcium is transported across the placenta throughout pregnancy, but particularly during the third trimester. Early birth can result in babies with lower than normal serum calcium levels. Other stressors, such as perinatal asphyxia, trauma, or diabetes in the mother, may predispose the newborn infant to hypocalcemia.

Signs, Symptoms, and Treatment

Early neonatal hypocalcemia is seen in the first 2 or 3 days of life. It usually is temporary. Symptoms include muscle cramps, tetany (muscle twitching or hand spasm), weakness, paresthesia, laryngospasm (high-pitched crowing sound), or seizure-like activity.

Late hypocalcemia usually appears about 1 week to 1 month after birth. It results when babies are fed unmodified cow's milk, which depresses the activity of the parathyroid glands. This condition, also referred to as *neonatal tetany*, is rare in developed countries, where commercial formula or human milk is used to feed the newborn. Serum calcium levels are monitored in all high-risk neonates. Normal levels range from 7.0 to 8.5 mg/dL. Hypocalcemia is treated by early feedings and calcium supplements when possible. Intravenous administration of 10% calcium gluconate may be necessary.

HEMORRHAGIC DISEASE
Description

Newborns have a deficiency of vitamin K due to the depletion of vitamin K stores. With decreased vitamin K, coagulation factors are significantly reduced, resulting in potential bleeding. The neonate's intestinal tract is sterile and, until feedings are started, unable to synthesize this vitamin.

Signs, Symptoms, and Nursing Care

Manifestations of hemorrhagic disease of the newborn usually occur on the second or third day after birth. The nurse should observe for oozing from the umbilicus or circumcision site, bloody or black stools, hematuria, bruising, and epistaxis (nosebleed). Vitamin K is given intramuscularly during the first 24 hours to all newborns to prevent this disorder.

RETINOPATHY OF PREMATURITY
Description

Retinopathy of prematurity (ROP) may result in blindness in preterm infants. This disorder was once thought to be caused by the toxic effect of oxygen on the developing blood vessels of the premature infant's retina. Other causes have since been implicated. ROP is now believed to be a complex disease of prematurity that has multiple causes such as hyperoxemia, hypoxemia, acidosis, sepsis, and shock. Infants that weigh less than 1500 g and/or have a gestational age of 28 weeks or less are to be screened for ROP. Screening should begin when the infant is 4 to 6 weeks of age or by 31 to 32 weeks after conception by an experienced ophthalmologist (Chiang & Flynn, 2006).

Treatment and Nursing Care

Prevention is the primary goal. Pediatric ophthalmologists can treat the disorder with **laser** surgery or **cryotherapy** (the therapeutic use of cold). The incidence rate may be reduced by decreasing constant bright environmental light and stimuli and by decreasing or avoiding events that cause fluctuations in blood pressure and oxygenation (Hockenberry & Wilson, 2007). Careful monitoring of arterial blood gases in infants receiving oxygen is also an important nursing measure related to prevention.

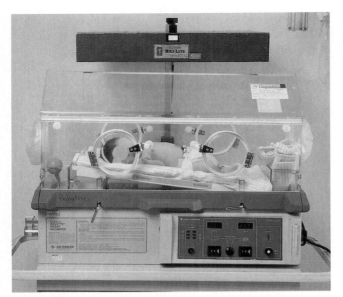

FIGURE **5-3** The infant wears eye patches when receiving phototherapy. This infant is in an incubator to maintain temperature regulation and provide protection from infection. The portholes facilitate routine infant care.

JAUNDICE
Description
The liver in the neonate is immature and, as a result, takes longer to start functioning effectively. Physiological jaundice (discussed in Chapter 4) generally occurs during the third to fifth postpartum day. In the preterm infant, the bilirubin level may be elevated for a longer time and the peak may not occur until the fifth to seventh day. It is necessary to treat physiological jaundice to prevent kernicterus or **bilirubin encephalopathy**, a syndrome of severe brain damage. Jaundice on the first day of life is *always* pathological and should not be confused with physiological jaundice.

Treatment and Nursing Care
With the prevalence of early discharges, parents should be instructed about what behaviors they should be alerted to with their new baby. They should be alert to lethargy, hypotonia, a weak suck, and color changes in skin and eyes. If the mother is breastfeeding, she should be evaluated by a lactation specialist or a professional who is experienced with breastfeeding. They should understand the importance of follow-up visits with the pediatrician. Phototherapy is the treatment for reducing or preventing rising bilirubin levels related to physiological jaundice. Phototherapy is generally initiated if the bilirubin level reaches 18 mg/dL. (It may be initiated sooner, depending on the practitioner.) The light waves used in phototherapy change the bilirubin in the skin into an excretable form (Figure 5-3). Nursing Care Plan 5-1 addresses the nursing care needed by the newborn receiving phototherapy in the hospital.

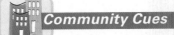
Community Cues

Fiberoptic blankets can be used in place of phototherapy lights. The baby is wrapped in the blanket, which is always kept next to the baby's skin. A receiving blanket can be wrapped over the "bili" blanket. The baby can be held for feedings and other activities. The eye patches are not necessary if only the blanket is used.

SPECIAL NEEDS AND CARE OF THE PRETERM INFANT
Care of the preterm infant is similar to that of the term infant in that the infant is assessed at birth and resuscitation is performed if indicated. Once respiratory function is established, the infant is examined for any other problems that may be present. Routine care may be delayed until the infant is stable. Stabilization of respiration and thermoregulation takes priority over all other types of care. The infant may need to be transferred from a community hospital to the NICU. This may mean immediate separation of the infant from the family unit. Obviously, issues of bonding and attachment need to be addressed in such cases.

THERMOREGULATION
One of the most critical needs of the high-risk infant is control of body temperature. The preterm infant lacks insulating fat, and because the surface area is large in proportion to the body weight, there is excessive heat loss through radiation. After birth, all high-risk infants should be dried immediately to eliminate evaporative heat loss. A radiant warmer should also be used with these infants; this decreases the heat loss and provides personnel with easy access to the infant (Figure 5-4).

The infant is placed in the isolette or radiant warmer. The infant's temperature is maintained at a constant level with a heat-sensitive probe that is taped over a nonbony prominence on either the abdomen or back. This allows the infant to become a thermostat for the radiant warmer. The infant's axillary temperature is also monitored. Overhead radiant warmers have the advantage of providing easier access to the patient while maintaining a neutral environment. The nurse should also do the following:
- Prewarm all surfaces that come in contact with the infant.
- Avoid drafts in the room.
- Use discretion in bathing the infant. Regular assessment has a much higher priority than a routine daily bath because of the danger of loss of heat through evaporation.
- Provide a plastic heat shield for very low–birth weight infants.
- Use knitted caps and booties when the infant is removed from the radiant warmer or isolette.
- Wrap the infant in a blanket if he or she is removed from the radiant warmer or isolette.

NURSING CARE PLAN 5-1

The Neonate Receiving Phototherapy

NURSING DIAGNOSIS *Nutrition, imbalanced: less than body requirements, related to newborn status and phototherapy*

Goals/Outcome Criteria	Nursing Interventions	Rationales
The infant receives adequate nutrition, as evidenced by: • Weight gain of 0.5 to 1 oz/day • Intake of 2 oz per feeding • Feeds every 3 to 4 hours if on formula • Feeds every 2 to 3 hours if breastfed • Voids at least every 4 hours • Has a stool at least every 24 hours	Weigh and assess the weight daily	Provides data to support that infant is meeting its needs
	Feed every 2 to 4 hours	Stomach of a newborn empties in 2 hours if breastfed and in 3 hours if fed formula
	Burp after each ½ oz	Allows swallowed air to be expelled, thus increasing the amount of fluid that can be taken
	Record intake	Ability to keep accurate record of intake
	Teach parents importance of feeding frequently	Sharing information increases the parents' ability to participate in care

NURSING DIAGNOSIS *Knowledge, deficient, related to the use of phototherapy*

Goals/Outcome Criteria	Nursing Interventions	Rationales
The parents show an increase in knowledge, as evidenced by: • Understanding of the process of jaundice • Knowing the benign nature of physiological jaundice • Demonstrate the ability to care for their infant • Showing positive aspects of bonding	Assess knowledge of parents	Aids the caregiver in knowing where to begin
	Give additional information in at least two different forms (e.g., verbal and written)	Use of more than one sense increases the ability to learn new information
	Encourage parent's participation in care of the infant	Allows parents to gradually increase their skills
	Reassure and praise parent's actions	Encourages learning and allows parents to see themselves as successful
	Be aware of parent's level of comfort	Allows one to give new information at the parent's level and answer questions
	Provide follow-up	Provides opportunity to answer any questions

NURSING DIAGNOSIS *Fluid volume, risk for deficient, related to increased fluid loss through skin and loose stools*

Goals/Outcome Criteria	Nursing Interventions	Rationales
The infant has adequate hydration, as evidenced by: • Good skin turgor • Moist mucous membranes • Less than 10% weight loss • Voiding at least every 4 hours	Assess infant's skin turgor and mucous membranes each shift	A quick assessment for hydration
	Weigh daily, record, and report to physician	Weight is a good indicator of the overall hydration status
	Record voiding and stools	Output of voiding is a good indicator of renal perfusion, which is an indicator of adequate hydration

NURSING DIAGNOSIS *Body temperature, risk for imbalanced, related to phototherapy*

Goals/Outcome Criteria	Nursing Interventions	Rationales
The infant has a normal temperature, as evidenced by: • Temperature between 97.6° F and 99° F axillary • Little or no acrocyanosis • Capillary refill time less than 3 seconds	Assess temperature every 4 hours	Phototherapy can increase the temperature, and if the environment is not kept warm, the temperature can decrease
	Record isolette and set temperature	Oxygen and glucose needs increase when the temperature falls outside the given parameters
	Keep skin temperature probe in place	Shows the infant's need for additional warmth; allows the infant to act as his or her own thermostat
	Dress the infant and wrap in a blanket for feedings	Decreases loss of heat from infant to environment
	Teach parents the need to maintain infant's temperature	Increases parents' understanding of importance of maintaining infant's temperature

Continued

NURSING CARE PLAN 5-1—cont'd

The Neonate Receiving Phototherapy—cont'd

NURSING DIAGNOSIS *Injury, risk for, related to high levels of bilirubin*

Goals/Outcome Criteria	Nursing Interventions	Rationales
The infant is free from neurological damage, as evidenced by: • No signs of neurological involvement (lethargy, twitching) • Bilirubin levels of less than 18 mg/dL	Assess neurological status of the infant Monitor laboratory reports concerning bilirubin levels Turn off phototherapy lights during collection of blood specimen	Aids in early recognition of any deficits Allows for prompt notification of the physician if bilirubin level increases or exceeds 18 mg/dL Phototherapy lights can alter bilirubin in specimen tubes and results can be incorrect

NURSING DIAGNOSIS *Injury, risk for, eye damage related to phototherapy*

Goals/Outcome Criteria	Nursing Interventions	Rationales
The infant is free from eye injury, as evidenced by: • No eye discharge • No redness of the eye • No corneal irritation	Apply eye patches over the infant's closed eyes while infant is under the phototherapy light Remove eye patches during feedings Assess eyes for redness, discharge, or irritation at each feeding Check the eye patches frequently to make sure they are in place	Infant's eyes should be closed to decrease the chance of irritation to the eyes and avoid corneal damage Allows eye contact and promotes parental-newborn bonding Provides earliest recognition of a problem; the earlier it is recognized, the earlier it can be treated Infants are active and patches can become displaced

NURSING DIAGNOSIS *Skin integrity, risk for impaired, related to phototherapy*

Goals/Outcome Criteria	Nursing Interventions	Rationales
The infant's skin remains intact, as evidenced by: • The skin being warm, dry, and intact in all areas • Free from any rashes, excoriation, or redness • No burns or breaks in the skin	Assess for any skin irritation at the time of each feeding Use proper phototherapy equipment (Plexiglas cover of the bulbs) Clean the diaper area gently Reposition infant every 2 hours Keep skin clean and dry and do not use powders, lotions, or oils	Phototherapy can be irritating to the thin skin of the newborn Fluorescent bulbs can break, and the Plexiglas cover protects the infant from any exposure to glass Stools are high in bilirubin, frequent, and loose; these factors can be irritating to the perineal area Increases exposure of body surface to the phototherapy lights Although the skin may become dry while the infant is receiving phototherapy, items such as oils, etc., can lead to burning of the skin

? CRITICAL THINKING QUESTIONS

■ What is the best way to manage a mother who is crying as she stands looking at her baby under the phototherapy lights and feels she is to blame for her baby turning "yellow"?

■ The mother has expressed concern about her ability to care for her new baby. How can you involve the mother in the care of the baby?

NUTRITION

Feeding of the preterm infant may be done by mouth (orally), by gavage (feeding by tube), or by parenteral methods (intravenously). Sick and very premature infants are usually given intravenous fluids. They may receive **total parenteral nutrition** (TPN) if they cannot tolerate oral or gavage feedings. TPN includes nutrients essential to meet their needs.

Parenteral feeding given intravenously through a catheter passed into the umbilical vein may be started shortly after delivery. Small amounts are given, sometimes as little as 5 mL per hour. Preterm infants younger than 32 to 34 weeks' gestation are usually fed through a nasal or gastric tube (gavage) because of their immature sucking and swallowing reflexes. As the infant matures and becomes stronger, nipple and

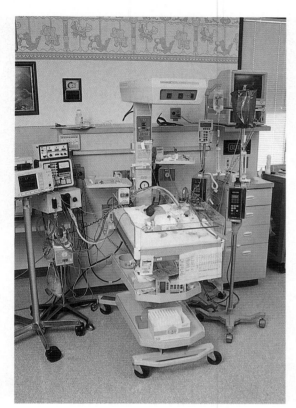

FIGURE **5-4** This infant under the radiant warmer is surrounded by equipment that can be frightening to parents. Orientation to the baby's surroundings is important for the parents.

Table 5-1	*Nursing Observations in Care of Preterm Infants*
CHARACTERISTICS	**OBSERVATIONS**
Color	Paleness, cyanosis, jaundice
Respirations	Regularity, apnea, sternal retractions, labored breathing, grunting
Pulse	Rate and regularity
Abdomen	Distention
Stools	Frequency, color, consistency
Skin	Rashes, irritations, pustules, edema, birthmarks
Cord	Discharge, odor, redness
Eyes	Discharge
Feeding	Sucking ability, vomiting or regurgitation, degree of satisfaction
Mucous membranes	Dryness of lips and mouth, signs of thrush
Voiding	Initial, frequency (1-2 mL/kg/hr is normal)
Fontanels	Sunken or bulging
General activity	Increase or decrease in movements, lethargy, twitching, frequency and quality of cry, hyperactivity

gavage feedings may be alternated. The nurse observes the infant's sucking and swallowing reflexes, weight gain, and lack of respiratory distress to determine whether nipple feeding is being tolerated. Breast milk that has been expressed and stored properly or formula may be fed to the infant when ordered. Breast milk has many advantages over commercial formula. Benefits include prevention of infection and a reduction in the rate and severity of NEC and ROP (Furman et al., 2002).

Special small and soft nipples are available for the small infant. The feeding should take no longer than 15 to 20 minutes. Feeding for longer periods uses more calories than are supplied by the feeding. The infant is fed in a semisitting position and burped gently after each half ounce. After the feeding, the infant should be placed on his or her right side with the head slightly raised. This position facilitates emptying of the stomach.

Fluid intake is recorded carefully. The nurse reports the number of voids, the color and specific gravity of the urine, and observes for signs of edema. The hydration needs of the patient are reviewed daily on the basis of intake, output, weight, blood chemistry studies, and general appearance.

CLOSE OBSERVATION

The physician examines the premature baby on a regular basis and writes specific orders concerning treatment and nursing care. The physician also relies on the assessment done by the NICU nurses and must be notified of any significant changes in the baby's condition. The experienced NICU nurse observes and charts care and treatment with great accuracy. Table 5-1 lists *general* observations to serve as a guide in premature care. Sudden changes require interventions and should be reported immediately.

POSITION AND SKIN CARE

The premature baby should not be left in one position for a long period because it is uncomfortable and may be harmful to the lungs. Positioning on the side, for example, allows drainage of secretions and prevention of aspiration. Positioning on the right side facilitates digestion (see Figure 4-18). It is always important to *gently* change the positions of preterm and high-risk infants. This is to prevent any positional deformities. Changing the baby's position also prevents pressure breakdowns on the delicate skin. The supine position requires support of the head, trunk, and extremities. Positioning aids or blankets are used to maintain positioning. The prone position may also need positioning aids to keep babies properly aligned. The prone position is used when the infant is awake. **Kangaroo care,** or skin-to-skin contact, has also been advocated for fostering intimacy and attachment between premature infants and their mothers or fathers. In this situation, the infant wears only a diaper while the parent holds the infant semiupright, against his or her skin. The parent covers the infant with his or her own clothing so as to facilitate temperature stability (Figure 5-5). Monitoring temperature remains important.

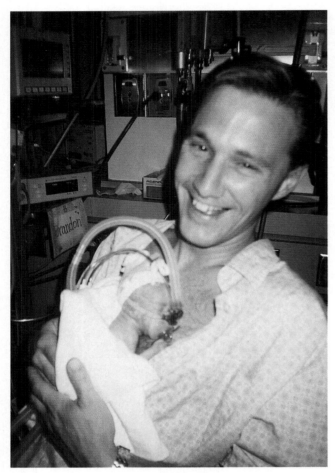

FIGURE **5-5** This father is providing kangaroo care to his preterm infant.

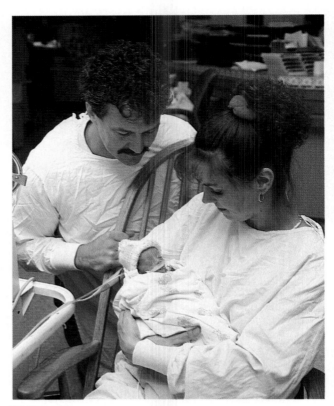

FIGURE **5-6** Parents need time to bond with their premature infant. They are taught that it is important to maintain warmth whenever the infant is removed from the radiant warmer. Note the knitted hat.

The delicate skin of the preterm infant also requires close monitoring. The skin is easily excoriated. Caution must be used with any products used on the skin; adhesives can adhere to the skin surface so well that damage can occur when these are removed. If such a breakdown should occur, the area is exposed to the air and treatment is done as prescribed by the physician (see Chapter 4 for a more extended discussion on the skin of the neonate).

FAMILY REACTION TO THE PRETERM INFANT

Parents need guidance throughout the infant's hospitalization to help prepare them for this new experience. They may be disheartened by the unattractive appearance of the premature baby. They may believe that they are to blame for the baby's condition. They may fear that the baby will die but are unable to express their feelings. They need time to look at and touch the baby and to begin to see this child as uniquely their own (Figure 5-6). This touch and immediate human contact are vital for the infant as well. The mother is usually concerned with her ability to care for such a small and helpless creature. When she feels ready, she may assist the nurse in diapering, bathing, feeding, and so on. During these times, other aspects of baby care are also stressed.

When infants need special care and are separated from their parents, there may be difficulties with bonding and attachment. Nurses need to be aware of this and help facilitate the attachment process. Whenever possible, the nurse should encourage visiting, calling, and participating in care because these are all ways of supporting the family through this crisis. Parents can help siblings accept the infant by naming the child, using the name, sharing news of progress, taking pictures of the infant, and encouraging them to send drawings and cards to the infant. Some hospitals have special areas where siblings may visit through a window.

Discharge planning should begin at the baby's birth. Parents may experience anxiety when they take their infant home. They may question their ability to care for an infant who has been receiving specialized care. They need to be confident in routine infant care and any special care the infant requires. Instructions in preventing infection should be a priority teaching goal. Follow-up visits should be scheduled and any home health care needs identified and met. The nurse should stress the importance of well-baby examinations and immunizations for this infant.

Parents need to be prepared for comments by relatives on the baby's small size and slower development. In general, the growth and development of the preterm infant should be based on the current age minus the number of weeks preterm. For example, if born at 36 weeks' gestation, a 1-month-old infant would be at a newborn achievement level. This way, no one has unrealistic expectations for the infant.

In the absence of severe birth defects and complications, the growth rate of the preterm infant nears that of the term baby by about the second year. In the presence of chronic illness, insufficient nutritional intake, or inadequate caretaking, the infant may remain below the expected growth rate.

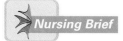

Nursing Brief

Encourage parents to talk about their feelings and fears concerning the preterm infant and how they will care for this child at home.

THE POSTTERM INFANT

The newborn baby is considered postterm if a pregnancy goes beyond 42 weeks. This is a great psychological strain on both the mother and the other members of the family, who are eagerly awaiting the birth of the baby. What causes postmaturity is not yet clear; however, it is known that the placenta does not function adequately as it ages. This could result in fetal distress, and the infant may exhibit such problems as hypoxia or meconium aspiration. Very large neonates, such as those of mothers with diabetes, are not necessarily postmature but are instead larger than normal because of rapid growth before delivery.

The mortality rate of the newborn who is delivered after 42 weeks' gestation is higher than that of a newborn delivered at term. The greatest risk for this infant is during the labor process.

The postterm infant is long and thin and looks as though he or she has lost weight. The skin is loose, especially about the thighs and buttocks. There is little downy hair (lanugo) or vernix caseosa. Loss of this cheese-like protection leaves the skin dry; it cracks and peels and is almost parchment-like in texture. The nails are long and may be stained with meconium. The baby has a good head of hair and looks alert. Many postmature babies have few adverse effects from the delay, but they still need careful observation in the nursery.

When it is determined that a pregnancy is past 40 weeks, the well-being of the mother and infant are determined by special tests. The course that is taken is determined by the results of the tests. A cesarean section is performed if there is evidence of fetal distress or a risk to the mother.

INFANTS OF MOTHERS WITH DIABETES

The successful regulation of diabetes has led to increasing numbers of women with diabetes bearing children. These infants are considered at high risk because they were exposed to high levels of maternal glucose before birth. The pancreas of the fetus responds by producing more insulin, which is an important regulator of fetal growth and metabolism. This is believed to account for the large size of these babies. Macrosomia (*macro,* large; *soma,* body) has been considered a classic symptom of babies of mothers with diabetes. Delivery may be difficult because of the infant's large size. The baby's face is large and puffy, resembling that of a child on steroids. These infants are also candidates for problems such as perinatal asphyxia, birth trauma, polycythemia, hyperbilirubinemia, hyaline membrane disease, and other complications. It is imperative that these babies be born in centers where there is expert supervision or be transferred to a regional care center shortly after birth. Nursing care includes initiating feedings early after birth, monitoring blood glucose levels closely, monitoring vital signs, and close evaluation of the infant's overall condition.

TRANSPORTATION OF THE HIGH-RISK NEONATE

Transportation of the high-risk neonate requires organization and the expertise of a special team. Successful transport depends on several factors. First, anticipating the need for the transport is vital. The infant must be stabilized before transport. Preparing and educating the parents is also extremely important. Many hospitals with a NICU have a special transport team that includes a nurse, a respiratory therapist, and sometimes a neonatologist. Baseline data, such as vital signs and blood work (blood gas and glucose levels), are obtained. The neonate is weighed if this is not contraindicated. Copies of all records are made. This includes the baby's record, the mother's prenatal history and delivery record, and pertinent admission data. A transport incubator is provided for warmth. Batteries in all equipment are kept fully charged.

The parents are shown the baby before the departure. If they are unable to hold the infant because of the infant's condition, the transport isolette is wheeled to the mother's bedside so she may observe and touch the baby. A Polaroid picture may be taken and given to the parents. On occasion, a mother is unable to see her baby because of her own unstable condition. Such situations require special empathy from nursing personnel.

Once the baby has arrived at the receiving hospital, the parents should be contacted by telephone. It is also thoughtful if the receiving hospital personnel provide feedback to the hospital personnel who initiated the transport, letting them know the results of their efforts.

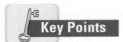
Key Points

- Gestational age refers to the time the fetus spends in the uterus from conception until birth.
- Preterm births can result from many factors, and in some cases, the cause may not be known.
- Prenatal care can decrease premature births with recognition and treatment of problems, thus delaying the process of labor.
- In the preterm infant, immaturity of all body systems, especially the respiratory system, is of concern in care and treatment.
- The immaturity of the immune system and the stress put on the immune system in high-risk conditions puts preterm newborns at risk for sepsis.
- In small preterm infants, the large surface area to body weight ratio causes an increase in the loss of body heat, creating problems related to thermoregulation.

- Nutrition issues for high-risk neonates involve their inability to meet the demands of their increased fluid and caloric requirements.
- At all times, parents and family need to be considered when caring for the high-risk neonate.

 Go to your Companion CD-ROM for an Audio Glossary, video clips, and more.

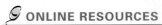 Be sure to visit the companion Evolve site at http://evolve.elsevier.com/Price/pediatric/ for WebLinks and additional online resources.

ONLINE RESOURCES

Premature Infant: http://www.premature-infant.com/

6 Disorders of the Newborn

Objectives

Upon completion of this chapter, the student will be able to:

1. Define the vocabulary terms listed
2. Describe the more common disorders of the newborn period
3. Summarize the family's needs in caring for an infant with HIV
4. Describe the nursing care of the neonate with infectious diarrhea
5. Identify the types of precautions that are necessary to prevent the spread of infection throughout the nursery
6. Discuss the important nursing care of a neonate with tuberculosis
7. Summarize the nursing goals significant to the care of the neonate with a congenital heart defect
8. Discuss modifications of these goals after heart surgery
9. Describe two feeding techniques used for the neonate with a cleft lip or cleft palate
10. Discuss the rationale for the modifications in feeding techniques
11. Summarize the needs of a neonate with tracheobronchial fistula
12. Discuss the different nursing care involved in caring for a child with a gastroschisis and omphalocele
13. Discuss the nursing measures for the neonate in a body cast
14. Differentiate between communicating and noncommunicating hydrocephalus
15. Outline the preoperative nursing care of a neonate with spina bifida cystica
16. Outline the postoperative nursing care of a neonate with spina bifida cystica
17. List three ways in which the nurse can help facilitate maternal-infant bonding when a baby is born with a birth defect

Key Terms

Be sure to check out the bonus material on the Companion CD-ROM, including selected audio pronunciations.

choroid plexus (KŌR-oid PLĚK-sŭs; p. 111)
habilitation (hă-BĬL-ĭ-TĀ-shŭn; p. 114)
hemodynamics (HĒ-mō-dĭ-NĂM-ĭks; p. 93)
hyperbilirubinemia (hī-pĕr-bĭl-ĭ-roo-bĭ-NĒ-mē-ah; p. 116)
kernicterus (kĕr-NĬK-tĕr-ŭs; p. 116)
multifactorial (MŬL-tĭ-făk-TŌ-rē-ăl; p. 113)
neural tube defects (NTD; p. 113)

shunt (p. 112)
tenesmus (tĕ-NĚZ-mŭs; p. 90)
TORCH (p. 111)
transillumination (TRĂNS-ĭ-LŪ-mĭ-NĀ-shŭn; p. 111)
tuberculosis (too-BĚR-KŪ-LŌ-sĭs; p. 91)

MALFORMATIONS PRESENT AT BIRTH (CONGENITAL)

Birth defects occur in one of every 28 births, and the effect on the infant can vary from minor to fatal. In 2003, the infant mortality rate was 6.8 deaths per 1000 live births in the United States. About two thirds of all infant deaths occur during the neonatal period, which is the first 28 days of life (March of Dimes, 2006).

A birth defect is defined as "an abnormality of structure, function, or metabolism (body chemistry) present at birth that results in physical or mental disability or death. Several thousand different birth defects have been identified. Birth defects are the leading cause of death in the first year of life" (March of Dimes, 2006). Birth defects are the cause of death in one of every five infant deaths. The March of Dimes lists three major categories of birth defects: structural/metabolic, congenital infections, and other. Because these disorders include so many conditions, it has been necessary to limit the number discussed in this chapter and to discuss others in relevant areas of the textbook (see the index for specific conditions).

In 1998, Congress passed the Birth Defects Prevention Act, which provides funding to the Centers for Disease Control and Prevention to collect and analyze data on birth defects, to support research, and to educate the public regarding birth defects. Defects present at birth often involve the skeletal system; limbs may be missing, malformed, or duplicated. Some abnormalities, such as congenital hip dysplasia (DDH), are more subtle and require alertness on the part of nurses to detect. Inborn errors of metabolism include a number of inherited diseases that affect body chemistry. There may be an absence or a deficiency of a substance necessary for cell metabolism. This is usually an enzyme. Almost any organ of the body may be damaged. Examples of inborn errors of metabolism include cystic fibrosis and phenylketonuria. In disorders of the blood, there is a reduced or missing blood component or an inability of a component to function adequately. Sickle cell anemia, thalassemia, and hemophilia fall into this group. Chromosomal abnormalities number in the hundreds. Some involve mental retardation, and some are incompatible with life. The newborn infant with Turner syndrome or Klinefelter syndrome may be retarded in physical growth and sexual development. Perinatal damage also has many causes and can be seen in a variety of forms. The most common form is premature birth. Only a few birth defects can be attributed to a single cause; most are thought to result from a combination of environment and heredity.

Some prenatal tests (ultrasound, amniocentesis, and chorionic villus sampling [CVS]) may assist in the diagnosis of certain birth defects before birth. These tests may be helpful in detecting or ruling out a possible birth defect with families that are suspected of having a history of birth defects. Medical therapies, which can be used in the prenatal period, are being developed for some defects. Prenatal surgeries also have had some success repairing congenital diaphragmatic hernias and urinary tract blockages. As medical technology improves, new interventions may have positive results for additional defects.

IMMUNE SYSTEM

ACQUIRED IMMUNODEFICIENCY SYNDROME

Description

Acquired immunodeficiency syndrome (AIDS) is caused by a retrovirus identified as the human immunodeficiency virus (HIV). This virus attacks T-helper cells that support immune functioning. T-suppressor cells that shut down the immune system are not altered by the virus. This causes an imbalance between these two cells, and the child is at great risk for infections.

The majority of the children affected contract the virus by mother-to-child transmission in utero, during birth, or through breastfeeding. With the early identification of pregnant HIV mothers and the use of antiretroviral therapy, the number of transmissions to the infant has been reduced from approximately 25% to less than 8% (Kliegman et al., 2006). Drug use and sexual transmission have been the major sources of HIV infection in the adolescent.

Because the risk for HIV transmission through blood products has diminished significantly, the main focus is preventing perinatal transmission. Pregnant women at greatest risk for carrying this disease are intravenous drug users and those with multiple sexual partners. The disease can be transferred even if the mother is asymptomatic. Many women do not know they are positive for HIV when they become pregnant and the CDC guidelines recommend that HIV screening be included in prenatal care (CDC, 2005). A portion of

| Box 6-1 | *Antiretroviral Medications* |

NUCLEOSIDE REVERSE TRANSCRIPTASE INHIBITORS
Abacavir
Didanosine (ddl)
Lamivudine (3TC)
Stavudine (d4T)
Zalcitabine (ddC)
Zidovudine (ZDV, AZT)
Zidovudine plus lamivudine

NONNUCLEOSIDE REVERSE TRANSCRIPTASE INHIBITORS
Delavirdine (DLV)
Efavirenz
Nevirapine (NVP)

PROTEASE INHIBITORS
Amprenavir
Indinavir
Nelfinavir (NFV)
Ritonavir (RTV)
Saquinavir (SQV)

children born to HIV-positive mothers remain positive. With advances in prenatal treatment with zidovudine (ZDV, also known as AZT) and the aggressive use of this treatment, the overall risk for perinatal transmission has been reduced.

Signs and Symptoms

With perinatal-acquired HIV, most infants develop symptoms by 18 to 24 months. The most common signs and symptoms in infants include failure to thrive, chronic diarrhea, repeated respiratory infections, oral candidiasis, and enlargement of the liver and spleen. Developmental delays have also been noted. Kaposi's sarcoma, which is common in adults, is rare in children. The ELISA test (enzyme-linked immunosorbent assay) can be used for children 18 months and older. PCR (polymerase chain reaction) blood test is the most commonly used test for infants. Two positive PCR tests are needed to confirm HIV. Two negative PCR tests after 1 month of age can indicate negative HIV in an exposed infant.

Treatment and Nursing Care

At present, there is no cure for AIDS. Several antiviral drugs are being used for treatment in children. Current recommended regimens include a triple combination therapy with nucleoside reverse transcriptase inhibitors, nonnucleoside reverse transcriptase inhibitors, and protease inhibitors (Box 6-1). Resistance to medications can occur, especially if the medication is not taken correctly. The child should be monitored closely. The child with AIDS has many needs, both psychological and physiological (Nursing Care Plan 6-1). All HIV-exposed infants should be given *Pneumocystis carinii* prophylaxis. Trimethoprim-sulfamethoxazole (TMP-

NURSING CARE PLAN 6-1

The Child with AIDS

NURSING DIAGNOSIS *Risk for infection related to immunosuppression*

Goals/Outcome Criteria	Interventions	Rationales
The child is free of an infection as evidenced by: • Temperature between 97.6° F and 99.6° F • No redness, drainage, or breaks in the skin • No signs of respiratory distress (coarse breath sounds, tachypnea, or restlessness)	Assess temperature	Elevation of temperature is an indication of infection.
	Assess respiratory rate and breath sounds	With immunosuppression, the child is prone to pneumonia. With an infection, oxygen needs also to be increased, and an increased respiratory rate can be seen.
	Provide the child with a safe environment	With immunosuppression, the child is susceptible to opportunistic infections such as *Candida albicans* (thrush) and *Pneumocystis carinii*.
	Promote adequate hydration	Allows for skin integrity; the skin is the first line of defense for the body. Dehydration can easily occur with an infection because of an increase in the basal metabolic rate and fluid loss through an increased respiratory rate.
	Examine the child regularly for an infection	The earlier an infection is recognized, the sooner proper treatment can be started.
	Teach parents/caregivers what signs and symptoms to report	Gives the caregivers the information needed to recognize and report an infection in its earliest possible form.

NURSING DIAGNOSIS *Imbalanced nutrition: less than body requirements related to anorexia, anemia, and thrush*

Goals/Outcome Criteria	Interventions	Rationales
The child has adequate nutrition as evidenced by: • Intake of 50% or greater of diet appropriate for age • Weight gain appropriate with growth curve • Progressive increase in growth	Frequent weights	Weight is an indicator of growth and an increase in mass.
	Record and assess intake and output	Growth depends on proper intake of both fluid and foods.
	Promote a pleasant environment when eating	A pleasant environment adds to the pleasure of eating and can influence the amount of time the child is willing to spend on eating.
	Provide favorite foods	The child tends to eat more of favorite foods.
	Teach parents/caregivers the importance of diet	Information about diet and the needs for growth influences the parent/caregiver in providing for the child.

NURSING DIAGNOSIS *Self-esteem disturbance related to disease and isolation.*

Goals/Outcome Criteria	Interventions	Rationales
The child has adequate self-esteem as evidenced by: • Expressing positive feelings about herself or himself to others • Ability to verbalize his or her fears • Ability to speak accurately about his or her disease	Assess the level of understanding the child has of the disease	It is always important to know where the individual is in regard to knowledge of the disease.
	Allow the child to verbalize his or her feelings; this can also be done through art media, such as drawings, clay, and painting	Expression of feelings makes them less explosive. The child can be helped to sort out his or her feelings once they are expressed. Unexpressed feelings can become larger and scarier than they really are.
	Promote an environment where the child is an active participant in his or her care	By being an active participant in his or her care, the child learns what is going on with the disease and can learn to separate feelings from the disease.

Continued

NURSING CARE PLAN 6-1—cont'd

The Child with AIDS—cont'd

NURSING DIAGNOSIS *Self-esteem disturbance related to disease and isolation—cont'd*

Goals/Outcome Criteria	Interventions	Rationales
	Give explanations to the child for the way care is provided and for any procedures being done	Information helps the child to know about the disease, helps to alleviate fears, and offers a sense of control over the situation.
	Allow the child to interact with others as much as possible	Interaction with others is important for proper growth and development.

NURSING DIAGNOSIS *Interrupted family processes related to the impact of the child's illness on the family*

Goals/Outcome Criteria	Interventions	Rationales
The family shows adaptive behavior as evidenced by: • Verbalization of feelings related to role function • Participation in the care of the child • Showing of mutual support and respect for other members • Utilization of appropriate external support resources	Assess this family's dynamics	The way family members interact with one another is important to determine the support that they need.
	Give opportunities for care providers to verbalize feelings	Expression is key to diminishing the power of feelings. The inability to express fears and frustrations can interfere with a positive relationship.
	Promote positive family relationships	Positive relationships need to be encouraged and supported to deal with stress of the situation. Promote the relationship, not the disease.
	Educate the family members concerning the support of each other and the disease process of the disease and what is going on aids in their support and validates their choices.	Education is a powerful tool. Family members can recognize their strength and support. Knowing the
	Alert the family members to external support resources alleviate some of the burdens and the family can use its strength to support the child.	Outside resources can be helpful to a family in stress. The resources can

? CRITICAL THINKING QUESTIONS

■ The aunt who is the caretaker of a 6-year-old with HIV asks the nurse, "When and what should I tell her about HIV?" She relates that her child has been asking her questions about why she always has to have her blood checked and why she has to take so many pills. What is the nurse's best response?

■ A 2-year-old foster child with HIV is being placed in daycare. What issues should be discussed with the family before the child begins attending the daycare?

SMZ) is the drug of choice and should be given during the first year of life. The child should be immunized against the common childhood diseases but should not receive live vaccines. Those caring for the child should observe good handwashing techniques and avoid contact with anyone who is infectious. Parents should be educated in these two areas.

Assessment for signs of infection, including vital signs, and observation of the skin and general condition of the child should be done routinely. Particular attention should be paid to the respiratory system because of the child's increased risk for infections within this system. The mouth, anal area, and skin should be assessed and care of these areas stressed.

The child should receive a high-protein, high-calorie diet. Frequent, small meals should be served. The child is on intake and output checks, and daily weights are taken.

Psychological support of the child and family is critical. The effects of isolation (and, in some cases, being ostracized) can be devastating to the developing child. Because the prognosis is poor, the nurse anticipates interventions related to the care of the child with a life-threatening disease. Many of these children come from a family already in crisis, and their support system may be weak. Family-centered interventions recommended for nurses who care for children with AIDS include (1) answering questions, (2) providing accurate information, (3) assisting the parents to move beyond guilt and blame, and (4) assisting with concrete service needs (Thurber & Berry, 1990). Many communities have support services in place that provide resources for families who are dealing with this diagnosis.

INFECTIONS
Thrush (Oral Candidiasis)

Description. Thrush is an infection of the mucous membranes of the mouth caused by the fungus *Candida.* This organism is normally present in the mother's vagina and is nonpathogenic. However, the altered conditions in the vagina produced by pregnancy may lead to the development of **monilial vaginitis.** The mucous membranes of the baby's mouth may become infected by direct contact with this infection during delivery or by contact with the mother's or nurse's contaminated hands. Cross infection of other newborn infants may then result. Breastfed infants may transfer the infection to the mother's nipples if good hygiene is not followed.

Signs and Symptoms. White patches that resemble milk curds are visible on the tongue, inner lips, gums, and oral mucosa. Initially, these are painless but do not wipe away. The patches may bleed if attempts are made to scrape them away. Because of the discomfort, anorexia may be present. The systemic symptoms are mild if the infection remains in the mouth; however, it can pass along the mucous membranes into the gastrointestinal tract, causing inflammation of the esophagus and stomach. The infant may develop a beefy red, weeping diaper rash in the genitalia area.

Treatment and Nursing Care. This infection responds well to local application of antibiotic suspensions. Nystatin, for example, may be applied with a swab. The mouth is swabbed three or four times a day, between feedings, with a sterile applicator moistened with the prescribed solution. The remainder of the dose is deposited in the infant's mouth to be swallowed, treating any other lesions of the gastrointestinal tract. With treatment, the disease is usually self-limiting in an otherwise healthy infant. Topical antifungal ointment such as nystatin may be administered to skin areas that have been affected.

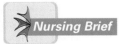
Nursing Brief

In the home, parents are taught to place nystatin or other medication slowly into each cheek pocket of the baby's mouth. Medication needs to remain in contact with "patches" as long as possible. The baby should not be fed after medication administration. Instruct parents to watch for dehydration (decrease in number of wet diapers and so on, caused by the baby's refusal to take fluids because of mouth discomfort).

Individual feeding equipment is necessary, and the equipment should be sterile. Disposable bottles or prefilled formula bottles are used. Nipples require scrupulous cleaning because they come in direct contact with the lesions. Disposable nipples and bottles are preferred. Nurses who care for neonates with thrush should direct their care toward preventing the spread of the infection and correctly applying the medication.

Prevention of this infection begins in the prenatal period. Mothers suspected of having *Candida* infection can be properly treated. Effective handwashing to prevent reinfection from the mother is necessary. This is particularly true if she is breastfeeding her infant. Nurses and other personnel must maintain a high quality of nursing care to prevent cross infection.

Infectious Diarrhea

Description. Despite improved care of the neonate, infectious diarrhea continues to be a serious problem in many areas of the world. Worldwide, the most common cause of child morbidity and mortality is diarrhea. It is responsible for 220,000 hospitalizations in the United States for children under the age of 5 (Dennehy, 2005). Diarrhea is defined as the excessive loss of water and electrolytes in stools, which usually results from disturbed solute transport in the intestine. Infectious diarrhea is highly contagious and may be fatal. It may be caused by a variety of organisms, and often the offender cannot be identified. Viral gastroenteritis is the most widespread type and is self-limiting.

Rotavirus has been found to be the major agent during the winter months. *Escherichia coli* often affects children under 2 years of age. *Shigella, Salmonella,* and *Staphylococcus* may also cause diarrhea. Diarrhea may accompany antibiotic therapy, which sometimes alters the normal flora of the intestinal tract. Food allergies, emotional strain, fatigue, and the unwise use of laxatives can precipitate this disorder in older children. Overfeeding, unbalanced diets containing excessive amounts of sweets, and spoiled foods are additional offenders in the early years.

A carefully obtained medical history yields valuable information. The age of the child is significant with regard to etiology. Travel, personal contacts, and a history of food allergy are relevant. Diarrhea may last from a few days to several weeks. **Functional diarrhea** differs from infectious diarrhea in that it is caused by an organic disease rather than an infection.

Signs and Symptoms. The symptoms of diarrhea may be mild or extremely severe. The stools are watery and are expelled with force. They may be yellowish green in color. The baby may become listless, refuse to eat, and lose weight. The temperature may be elevated, and the infant may vomit. Dehydration is evidenced by sunken eyes and fontanel and dry skin, tongue, and mucous membranes. The frequency of urination may decrease. In severe cases, the excessive loss of

Box 6-2 *Clinical Signs of Dehydration in an Infant*

MILD DEHYDRATION (5%)
Vital signs normal
Alert and thirsty
Normal turgor
Normal capillary refill time
Normal anterior fontanel
Tears present
Slight oliguria

MODERATE DEHYDRATION (6% TO 9%)
Increased heart rate and respiratory rate
Blood pressure normal or slightly decreased
Behavior: restless or irritable
Marked thirst
Turgor shows tenting
Capillary refill time is 2 to 3 seconds
Lips and mucous membranes of the mouth are dry
Anterior fontanel is sunken
Tears absent
Oliguria

SEVERE DEHYDRATION (10%)
Increased heart rate and respiratory rate
Blood pressure normal or slightly decreased
Behavior: lethargic or comatose
Turgor shows severe tenting
Capillary refill time is greater than 3 seconds
Skin is cold and clammy
Cyanosis may be present
Mucous membranes extremely dry
Anterior fontanel is severely sunken
Tears absent
Severe oliguria

bicarbonate from the gastrointestinal tract results in acidosis. The degree of dehydration and the symptoms are discussed in Box 6-2.

Treatment and Nursing Care. Constant observation of each neonate in the nursery is of utmost importance. If diarrhea is suspected, it should be reported immediately and the baby isolated. A stool specimen is sent to the laboratory for culture. The nurse must describe the stools accurately in the nurses' notes, including consistency, frequency, color, and odor; the presence or absence of blood, mucus, or pus; and the forcefulness with which the stool is expelled. In older children, cramping and tenesmus, or involuntary straining to empty the bowel, may be observed and should be recorded.

The gastrointestinal tract of the newborn infant is especially vulnerable to infection. The nurse must constantly seek to protect babies against exposure to pathogenic organisms and must adhere strictly to nursery routines. The preparation of formula requires undivided attention to prevent microorganisms from being carried to the infant through this medium. Careful feeding techniques are necessary. If a nipple becomes contaminated, a new one must be applied. Proper handwashing is essential. If clothing or blankets touch the floor, they must be relaundered before being used.

The skin of the buttocks must receive special care to prevent excoriation. Removing the diaper and exposing the area to the air may be helpful. Barrier ointments can be applied after the buttock area is cleaned and completely dried. Daily **accurate weights** are taken to help ascertain the amount of water loss. Careful observation and charting of intravenous fluids are necessary. The child is on a *strict* intake and output recording.

Diarrhea caused by bacteria and parasites may respond to drug therapy. Other cases are viral in origin, and treatment is supportive. The primary focus is on electrolyte imbalance and dehydration.

Oral glucose-electrolyte dehydration is the treatment of choice when possible. Certainly, this is effective in the infant with mild-to-moderate dehydration. Infants with moderate-to-severe dehydration may need intravenous replacement of fluids and electrolytes. Regardless of the etiology, most cases of acute diarrhea are self-limited and treatment is supportive. The cornerstone of therapy is fluid and electrolyte replacement. For most children, oral dehydration therapy is the best method of replacing fluids and electrolytes. Oral dehydration therapy is effective even when a child has severe diarrhea or vomiting. The mother who is breastfeeding should continue to breastfeed because maternal antibodies are components of breast milk.

Mild diarrhea in older children may be treated at home under a physician's direction, provided there is a suitable caregiver. Treatment is essentially the same as that for the hospitalized child, with the exception of administering intravenous fluids. Oral rehydration is obtained with recommended oral rehydration therapy (ORT). These solutions can be found in any local drug or grocery store as Pedialyte or Infalyte. They come as a liquid or as popsicles. In the past, parents have been instructed to give clear fluids. These fluids, such as flat ginger ale, carbonated soft drinks, fruit juices, tea, and popsicles, are low in electrolytes and high in glucose and should be avoided. High-sodium broths are avoided to prevent electrolyte imbalance. The BRAT diet (bananas, rice, apples, and toast) should not be used because it has low electrolytes, high carbohydrates, and little nutritional value. A diet of soft bland foods is added gradually. A regular intake is usually resumed within 2 to 3 days. Medications such as Lomotil, paregoric, and pectin, which slow intestinal mobility, are to be avoided in the treatment of children. It has been found that the intake of yogurt with live active cultures may be beneficial as part of dietary therapy for acute diarrhea because it restores the flora of the gastrointestinal tract.

In the event of an acute episode of diarrhea in a newborn nursery, newly delivered babies must not be admitted to the nursery. Separate personnel are needed to care for uninfected neonates. When the epidemic has ceased, the nursery must be thoroughly scrubbed, and all equipment must be cleaned and sterilized according to hospital procedure.

RESPIRATORY SYSTEM

TUBERCULOSIS

Tuberculosis (TB) has been around for a long time. There has been an increase in the incidence in this disease. Several factors contributing to this increase are emigration, HIV, and resistant strains. Pediatric TB directly correlates to the incidence of adult TB in the community. A child with TB is usually considered a primary infection and has been infected by contact with an infectious adult or adolescent (Robinson & El-Sadr, 2006).

Description

Tuberculosis is caused by the acid-fast bacillus, *Mycobacterium tuberculosis.* Transmission of the organism is by inhalation of an infected droplet. It begins to multiply in the lung tissue. If the primary lesion erodes into a blood vessel, dissemination of the organism can occur. When the organism spreads to other tissue, such as bone, kidney, or the brain, the condition is known as **miliary tuberculosis.**

Skin testing is the method of screening for TB. The most accurate form of skin testing is the Mantoux test, which is administered intradermally. The test should be read only by qualified medical personnel. It is recommended that children be screened at 15 months of age. If other risk factors are present, additional screenings may be needed.

Children are most vulnerable to TB when their immune system is the least mature, which is during the first 3 years of life. Another period of vulnerability is just before, during, and after puberty. The risk of becoming infected with TB increases with poverty and crowded living conditions, which can lead to poor hygiene. There is a higher incidence of TB among Native Americans, in large urban areas where poverty is a factor, and in areas where there is a large population of foreign-born individuals.

Concern about TB has increased because there has been an increase in the number of cases. Another major concern is the developing number of resistant strains. Individuals with HIV are susceptible to TB and should be screened for the exposure. Children with TB should also be tested for HIV.

Signs and Symptoms

Diagnosis is determined with tests including a positive skin test. A chest radiograph can confirm the disease. Gastric washing is done to confirm the presence of the bacillus. Infants and small children may present with a nonproductive cough and mild dyspnea. There also may be a failure to thrive. Symptoms may be variable and can include fever, anorexia, malaise, weight loss, night sweats, and mild dyspnea. As the lungs become more invaded, more respiratory symptoms may develop, such as an increase in respiratory rate, diminished breath sounds, and rales.

Treatment

Hospitalization is not necessary, except for diagnostic procedures. All hospitalized children with active TB must be in respiratory isolation. All health care workers must wear an N-95 respirator when caring for a patient with contagious TB (American Academy of Pediatrics, 2000). All other treatment can be given in a community-based environment and involves nurses in the ambulatory setting, the school, and the public health facilities.

Gastric washing is done to isolate the bacillus. Young children swallow their secretions, and the organism can be obtained from the stomach. The gastric washing is obtained in the early morning after the child has had nothing to eat during the night. A nasogastric (NG) tube is passed, and the stomach is lavaged. The gastric contents are removed and sent to the laboratory for testing.

Currently, the medication given for TB is isoniazid (INH), *given once a day,* and rifampin, *given twice a day,* for a 6-month period of time. Pyrazinamide, *given once a day,* will also be added for the first 2 months. Because of the difficulty in eradicating this organism and the importance of compliance, most experts recommend that all drug administration be directly observed (DOT) by a health care worker. A fourth drug such as streptomycin or ethambutol may be added in cases in which there are resistant strains.

Asymptomatic TB occurs when there is a positive skin test but all other diagnostic findings are negative. The child with asymptomatic TB is treated with INH for 9 months. Even if they have a negative skin test, children less than 6 years of age who have been exposed to an adult with infectious TB also receive INH therapy. These children are retested after 3 months. If the skin test is again negative, then the INH therapy can be discontinued. If the skin test is positive, the child needs a complete course of treatment.

In rare, severe cases, surgery may be needed to remove the involved tissue.

Nursing Care

Emotional support is vital for this family. The treatment of TB takes a long time. This family's life will change, and avenues of support need to be identified.

Tuberculosis is a communicable disease and therefore is reported to the public health department. A concern for some families may be their status as citizens of the United States. This concern can have an effect on the treatment of the disease because a family may not feel that they can be entirely honest with the health care team.

Parents need to know the side effects of the medication(s) given to their child. They need to understand the importance of the length of treatment. In addition, the source of infection needs to be identified so that the disease can be eradicated in the family and in other families in the community. Older children and adolescents can be involved in their own care and should assist in setting goals. Compliance increases if they are active participants.

Because stress can alter the immune system and make it less proficient, decreasing stress for these children is important. Stress may result from many factors, such as fear of bodily harm, fear of being ostracized, or fear of peer rejection, being different, or concern that they can give TB to their friends. A support group can be beneficial for these children so that they can verbalize their fears and concerns.

Proper rest and a balanced diet are important for healing. Families may need assistance in regard to a proper diet. Make sure their needs in regard to culture are addressed.

Most affected children limit their own activities. Participation in competitive sports is usually discouraged during this period of time.

CARDIOVASCULAR SYSTEM

CONGENITAL HEART DISEASE

Description

A baby born with congenital heart disease (CHD) has a defect in the structure of the heart or in one or more of the large blood vessels that lead to and from the heart. The heart or vessels have failed to develop properly during the gestational period.

The heart of the fetus is completely developed during the first 8 weeks of pregnancy. Prenatal or maternal factors associated with increased risk include alcoholism, cocaine use, rubella, exposure to *Coxsackie* virus, diabetes mellitus, ingestion of lithium salts, use of Accutane, and advanced maternal age. Genetic factors such as a history of CHD in other family members, patients with Down syndrome or other chromosomal aberrations, and patients who have other congenital defects often contribute to the incidence of CHD. Research now indicates that most congenital heart lesions are produced by a genetic-environmental interaction; that is, they are multifactorial. In other words, CHD is not one disease; there is a hereditary predisposition determined by many genes and an environmental trigger that acts to push the predisposed fetus over the threshold from normal development to abnormal development.

Heart defects are the most common birth defect and are the leading cause of birth defect-related deaths. The incidence rate of infants born with a congenital heart defect is about one per 125 to 150 deliveries (March of Dimes, 2006). Therefore the nurse must stress the need

---

Box 6-3 *Diagnostic Procedures in Congenital Heart Disease*

History
Physical examination
Chest radiography
Electrocardiography
Echocardiography
Cardiac catheterization
Laboratory studies
- Blood gases
- Hemoglobin
- Hematocrit

Box 6-4 *General Signs and Symptoms in Congenital Heart Disease*

INFANTS
Dyspnea
Difficulty feeding
Stridor or choking spells
Tachycardia
Recurrent respiratory infections
Failure to gain weight
Heart murmurs
Cyanosis
Cerebral thrombosis
Anoxic episodes

CHILDREN
Dyspnea
Decreased activity tolerance
Squatting
Tachycardia
Recurrent respiratory infections
Delayed physical development
Heart murmur and thrills
Cyanosis
Clubbing of fingers
Elevated blood pressure

---

for good prenatal care and impress on the parents the value of regular checkups at baby clinics. Many organic heart murmurs have been detected early in infancy at a periodic checkup. A careful health history is particularly useful. Other diagnostic procedures are listed in Box 6-3. The symptoms, as indicated in Box 6-4, depend on the location and type of heart defect. Some patients have mild cases and can lead a fairly normal life with medical management. Others are treated medically until the optimal time for surgery. Heart transplantation is an option in some cases.

Classification

In the past, congenital heart defects were divided into two groups: cyanotic and acyanotic. This has proved inaccurate because children with acyanotic defects may develop cyanosis and those with cyanotic disease may be pink in color. Presently, defects are classified according to the effect the defect has on the movement

Box 6-5   *Hemodynamics and Examples of Congenital Heart Disease*

INCREASED PULMONARY BLOOD FLOW
Atrial septal defect
Patent ductus arteriosus
Ventricular septal defect

OBSTRUCTIVE BLOOD FLOW
Aortic stenosis
Coarctation of the aorta
Pulmonary stenosis

DECREASED PULMONARY BLOOD FLOW
Tetralogy of Fallot
Tricuspid atresia

MIXED BLOOD FLOW
Hypoplastic left heart
Total anomalous pulmonary venous return
Transposition of the great vessels
Truncus arteriosus

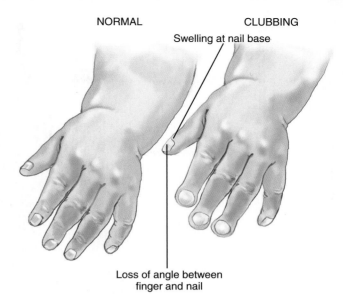

FIGURE **6-1** Clubbing in infant's fingers caused by poor oxygenation.

of circulating blood. The study of blood circulation is termed **hemodynamics** (*hemo,* blood; *dynamis,* power; Hockenberry et al., 2003). Defects can be classified as (1) defects with increased pulmonary blood flow, (2) obstructive defects, (3) defects with decreased pulmonary blood flow, and (4) mixed defects. A list of the hemodynamics and the heart defect(s) associated with each is given in Box 6-5.

Signs and Symptoms

The child with CHD may be small for age, and his or her condition may be classified as a physiological failure to thrive. This is the result of the difficulty the child has feeding and breathing at the same time. Exercise intolerance may first be identified when the infant experiences dyspnea while feeding or it may not be evident until the toddler period, when the child tends to be more active. The child may assume a **squatting position** to decrease venous return by occluding the femoral veins and thus lessen the workload of the right side of the heart. The infant can gain this same effect by lying in the knee-chest position. Clubbing of the fingers is thought to be caused by anoxia (Figure 6-1). Finally, the child tends to have frequent respiratory infections because of pulmonary vascular congestion. Some common nursing diagnoses associated with CHD are listed in Box 6-6. The normal heart is illustrated in Figure 6-2.

Defects with Increased Pulmonary Blood Flow

Patent Ductus Arteriosus. The circulation of the fetus differs from that of the neonate in that most of the fetal blood bypasses the lungs. The **ductus arteriosus** is the passageway by which the blood crosses from the pulmonary artery to the aorta and avoids the deflated lungs. This vessel closes shortly after birth; however, when it does not close, blood continues

Box 6-6   *Nursing Diagnoses Associated with Congenital Heart Disease*

Risk for infection related to reduced body defenses, debilitated state
Risk for imbalanced fluid volume related to compromised cardiac function
Imbalanced nutrition: less than body requirements related to fatigue, chronic hypoxia
Risk for activity intolerance related to imbalance of oxygen supply and demand
Delayed growth and development related to stress of chronic illness, chronic hypoxia
Interrupted family processes related to child with a long-term disease
Deficient knowledge related to chronic disease

to pass from the aorta, where the pressure is higher, into the pulmonary artery. This causes oxygenated blood to recycle through the lungs, overburdening the pulmonary circulation and making the heart pump harder. A machine-like murmur may be heard. The symptoms of this disorder may go unnoticed during infancy. However, with growth, the child experiences dyspnea, the radial pulse becomes full and bounding on exertion, and there may be growth retardation. The parents may report frequent respiratory infections.

Patent ductus arteriosus (PDA) is one of the most common cardiac anomalies (Figure 6-3). The word *patent* means open. PDA occurs twice as frequently in females as in males. In the premature infant, indomethacin may be administered to facilitate closure of the ductus. If drug treatment is not successful, surgical intervention is necessary (Murthy & Evans, 2006). Surgical repair includes ligation of the ductus through a left thoracotomy or with video-assisted thoracoscopic

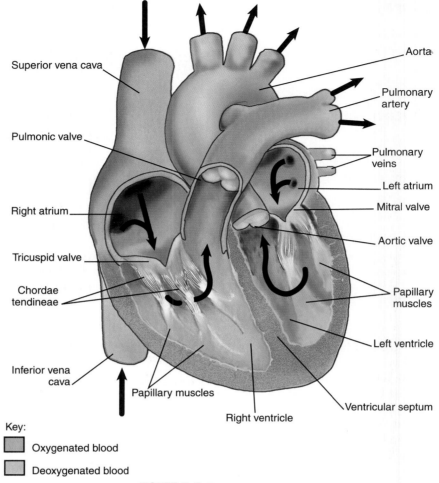

Superior vena cava

Pulmonic valve

Right atrium

Tricuspid valve

Chordae tendineae

Inferior vena cava

Papillary muscles

Right ventricle

Aorta

Pulmonary artery

Pulmonary veins

Left atrium

Mitral valve

Aortic valve

Papillary muscles

Left ventricle

Ventricular septum

Key:

Oxygenated blood

Deoxygenated blood

FIGURE **6-2** The normal heart.

(VATS). Some medical centers use occluding coils or closure devices that are placed in the patent ductus during a cardiac catheterization. If this condition is left uncorrected, the patient eventually could develop congestive heart failure (CHF) or endocarditis. The prognosis is excellent.

Atrial Ductus Arteriosus. Atrial septal defect (ASD) is one of the more common congenital heart anomalies (Figure 6-4). The incidence is higher in females than in males. There is an abnormal opening between the right and left atria. Blood that contains oxygen is forced from the left atrium to the right atrium. This type of arteriovenous shunt does not produce cyanosis unless the blood flow is reversed by heart failure. Currently, the defect can be repaired either with open heart surgery or occluding devices during cardiac catheterization. Open heart surgery requires the patient being placed on the heart-lung machine during the procedure with an extended hospital stay (Rome & Kreutzner, 2004). Occluding devices can be used with openings located in certain places along the septum and openings with a small diameter. Both procedures have good results with the occluder devices requiring shorter hospital stays.

Ventricular Septal Defect. As the name suggests, in ventricular septal defect (VSD), there is an opening between the right and left ventricles of the heart (Figure 6-5). Increased pressure within the left ventricle forces blood into the right ventricle. A loud, harsh murmur combined with a systolic tremor is characteristic of this defect. The condition can be mild or severe. The choice for repair remains surgical intervention. Use of occluding devices to close the VSD during cardiac catheterization is increasing (Rome & Kreutzner, 2004). A large percentage of small VSDs close spontaneously by 2 years of age.

Obstructive Defect

Coarctation of the Aorta. The word **coarctation** means tightening. In this condition, there is a constriction or narrowing of the aortic arch or of the descending aorta (Figure 6-6). Hemodynamic changes consist of increased pressure proximal to the defect with decreased pressure distally. The patient may not develop symptoms until later childhood. The patient has high blood pressure and bounding pulses in the upper extremities and weak pulses in the cool lower extremities. Often there are also signs of CHF. Treatment for infants and young children is surgical.

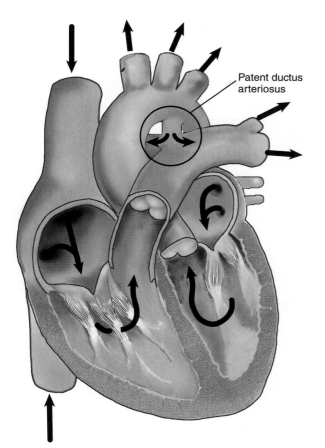

FIGURE **6-3** Patent ductus arteriosus.

Patent ductus arteriosus

During surgery, the surgeon resects the narrowed portion of the aorta and joins its ends. This joining is called an **anastomosis.** If the section removed is large, an end-to-end graft with tubes of Dacron or of similar material may be necessary. Because the graft does not grow and the aorta does, the best time for surgery is between the ages of 3 and 6 years. This is because there is a high risk for reoccurrence if the repair is done during infancy. Balloon angioplasty has also been used with some success. As with PDA, closed heart surgery is performed because the structures are located outside of the heart. The prognosis is favorable if there are no other defects.

Defect with Decreased Pulmonary Blood Flow

Tetralogy of Fallot. *Tetra* means four. In tetralogy of Fallot (Figure 6-7), there are four defects: (1) stenosis or narrowing of the pulmonary artery, which decreases the blood flow to the lungs, (2) hypertrophy of the right ventricle (enlargement of heart muscle is a result of having to work harder to pump blood through the narrow pulmonary artery), (3) dextroposition (*dextra,* right; position) of the aorta, in which the aorta is displaced to the right and receives blood from both ventricles, and (4) VSD. This is the most common of the cyanotic heart defects.

When venous blood enters the aorta, severe heart trouble is evident in the infant. Cyanosis increases with age. There is also clubbing of the fingers and toes. The

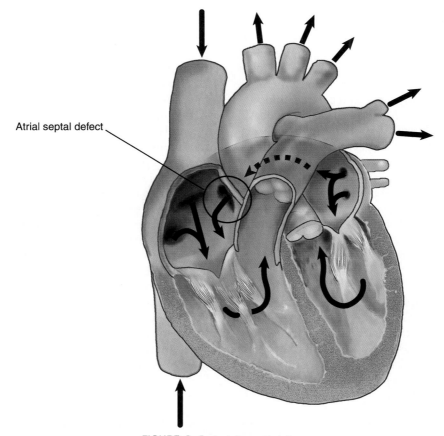

Atrial septal defect

FIGURE **6-4** Atrial septal defect.

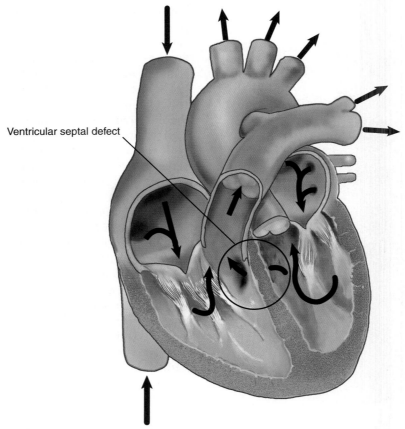

Ventricular septal defect

FIGURE **6-5** Ventricular septal defect.

child often rests in a squatting position to breathe more easily. Feeding problems, growth retardation, frequent respiratory infections, and severe dyspnea on exercise are prevalent. The red blood cells of the body increase (polycythemia [*poly,* many; *cyt,* cells; *hema,* blood]) in an effort to compensate for the lack of oxygen. All children who have cyanosis associated with their heart disease are at risk for neurological sequelae such as cerebrovascular accident. Blackouts and convulsions may also occur.

The child or infant is treated medically until surgery can be endured. A palliative surgery may be done to increase the flow of blood to the lungs. Open heart surgery is performed for the permanent correction of the defect. The optimal age for repair is 1 to 2 years of age.

Mixed Defect

Transposition of the Great Arteries. In transposition of the great arteries (TGA), the pulmonary artery leaves the left side of the ventricle and the aorta leaves the right ventricle (Figure 6-8). Because the body receives only desaturated blood, there must be other defects to maintain life (septal defects, PDA). The condition of the child depends on how much mixing of systemic and pulmonary venous blood is taking place. Infants with large septal defects or a PDA may not be as cyanotic but do develop symptoms of CHF.

No murmur is associated with TGA. If a murmur is present, it is related to the other defects. Prostaglandin E_1 (PGE_1), which keeps the ductus arteriosus open, and a balloon atrial septostomy may be used as palliative measures. Corrective surgery is usually performed within the first 2 weeks of life. The mortality rate depends on the severity of the defect, the maturity of the infant, the type of procedure performed, and any other complicating factors.

Hypoplastic Left Heart Syndrome. With hypoplastic left heart syndrome (HLHS), the left side of the heart is underdeveloped (Figure 6-9). There is hypoplasia of the aorta and left ventricle and mitral valve involvement. Therefore the systemic circulation is provided by the right side of the heart. It is necessary for the ductus arteriosus and the foramen ovale to remain patent to provide oxygenated blood to the body. Prostaglandin E_1 (PGE_1) is administered to maintain a PDA. Without interventions the infant survives only a few months. Options for treatment include surgical treatment, which is done with a several-staged approach, and heart transplants. Mortality rates are high. Although transplants have been successful, there are issues of donor availability, organ rejection, infection, and immunosuppression (Zeigler, 2003).

Congestive Heart Failure. An infant with a severe heart defect may develop congestive heart failure (CHF). CHF is not a disease in itself but rather symptoms

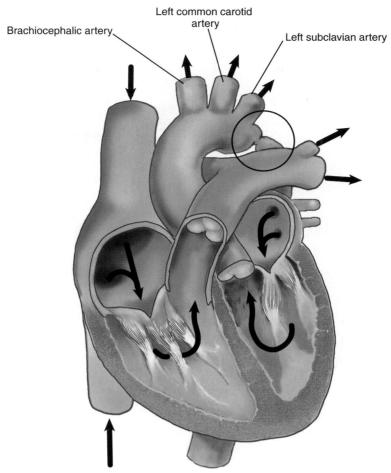

Brachiocephalic artery

Left common carotid artery

Left subclavian artery

FIGURE **6-6** Coarctation of the aorta

caused by an underlying heart defect. The nurse must constantly be on the alert for signs and symptoms of this condition. Some of these symptoms are cyanosis, pallor, rapid respiration, rapid pulse, feeding difficulties, fatigue, failure to gain weight, edema, and frequent respiratory infections.

Cyanosis. When observing the baby's color, the nurse notes whether the cyanosis is general or localized. If it is localized, the exact location is recorded in the nurse's notes (e.g., hands, feet, lips, or around the mouth). Is the cyanosis deep or light? Is it constant or transient? Sometimes a baby's color improves when crying and sometimes it gets worse. This observation is significant. If overt cyanosis is not apparent in the black infant, observe the mucous membranes of the mouth, the palms of the hands, and the bottoms of the feet. As a result of chronic pooling of the blood in the capillaries of the extremities, clubbing of the fingers and toes may also be evident. The infant may be very pale or may have a mottled appearance.

Patients with Tetralogy of Fallot often have hyper-cyanotic spells called "tet" spells. They are a result of the body's inability to provide adequate oxygenation. The infant becomes acutely cyanotic. The spells may be precipitated by events that increase the demand for oxygenation, such as crying, feeding, or defecation. Prompt nursing actions should include calming the infant, placing the infant in a knee-chest position, and providing supplemental oxygen.

Rapid Respirations. Respirations over 60 per minute in a newborn infant who is at rest indicates distress. The amount of dyspnea does vary, and in more acute cases, it is accompanied by flaring of the nostrils, mouth breathing, and sternal retractions. The baby has more trouble breathing when flat in bed than when being held upright. Signs of air hunger are irritability, restlessness, and a weak and hoarse cry.

Rapid Pulse. This is **tachycardia.** A pulse rate of over 150 beats per minute is important. It occurs because the heart pumps harder, trying to get sufficient oxygen to all parts of the body.

Feeding Difficulties. When the nurse tries to feed these patients, they tire easily. The infant may refuse to suck after a few ounces. When placed in the crib, the infant may cry and appear hungry. The infant may also choke and gag during feedings; the pleasure of sucking is spoiled by the inability to breathe.

Poor Weight Gain. The infant may fail to gain weight. A sudden increase in weight, however, may indicate the beginning of heart failure.

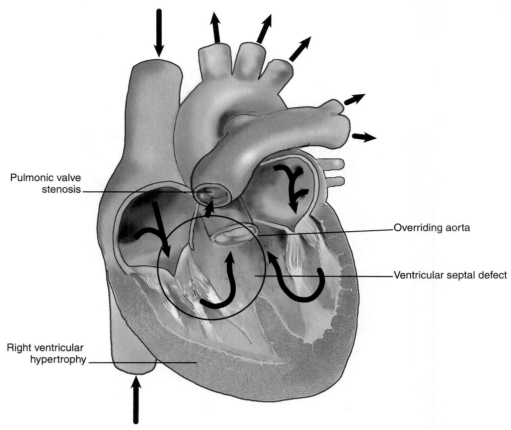

Pulmonic valve stenosis

Overriding aorta

Ventricular septal defect

Right ventricular hypertrophy

FIGURE **6-7** Tetralogy of Fallot showing the four defects: (1) pulmonary stenosis, (2) VSD, (3) dextroposition of the aorta, and (4) right ventricular hypertrophy.

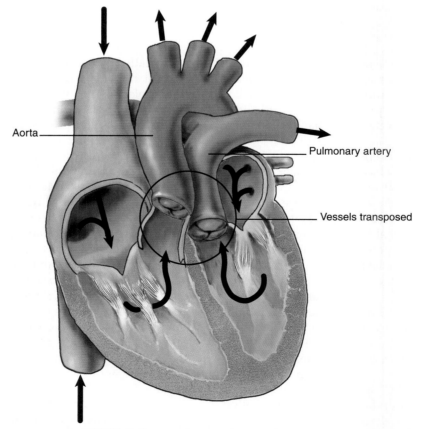

Aorta

Pulmonary artery

Vessels transposed

FIGURE **6-8** Transposition of the great arteries.

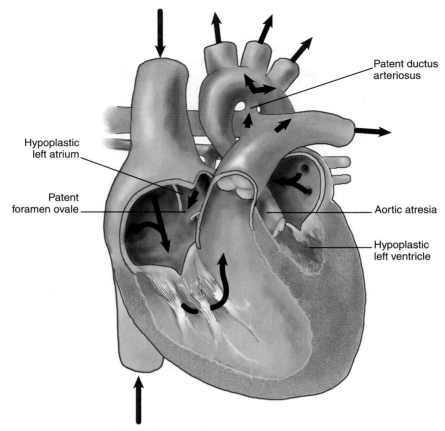

Hypoplastic
left atrium

Patent
foramen ovale

Patent ductus
arteriosus

Aortic atresia

Hypoplastic
left ventricle

FIGURE **6-9** Hypoplastic left heart syndrome.

Edema. The nurse should observe for puffiness about the eyes and, occasionally, in the legs, feet, and abdomen. Urine output should be monitored because it may decrease with CHF.

Exercise Intolerance. The infant may sleep excessively and fall asleep during feedings. As the patients grow, they may not be as active as other children and may have delayed motor development. Older children may also fatigue easily and be intolerant of exercise.

Treatment and Nursing Care

Nursing goals in the care of the newborn infant can be adapted for all children with heart defects. These are (1) to reduce the work of the heart, (2) to improve respiration, (3) to maintain proper nutrition, (4) to prevent infection, (5) to reduce the anxiety of the patient, and (6) to support and instruct the parents.

The nurse must organize care so that the baby is not unnecessarily disturbed. The patient needs a great deal of energy. A complete bath and linen change are luxuries that an infant with a serious heart defect cannot afford. The infant should be fed early if crying and late if asleep. The physician orders the position in which the infant should be placed. In some cases, the knee-chest position facilitates breathing; in other cases, elevating the head may be helpful (Fowler's position). Older babies may be placed in infant seats.

Small frequent feedings are scheduled. The physician may use a higher-calorie formula to maintain adequate intake. The infant is fed in an upright position and burped frequently. The nipple should be soft and the hole large enough for easy sucking. Older children generally tolerate a special diet of no added salt with a restriction on high-sodium foods. In some cases, nasogastric (NG) tube feedings are advantageous because they are less tiring for the patient. Oxygen is administered to relieve dyspnea. As breathing becomes easier, the baby begins to relax. A soft voice with gentle care soothes the patient. Whenever possible, the infant is held and loved during feedings.

In pediatric patients, digoxin (Lanoxin) is the most commonly prescribed oral digitalis preparation. Lanoxin is preferred because of its rapid action and shorter half-life. The action of the agent is to slow and strengthen the heartbeat. The nurse counts the patient's pulse for 1 full minute before administering the medication. A resting apical pulse is most accurate. Because the normal pulse ranges vary at different ages, the physician usually indicates at what pulse rate the drug is to be withheld. If this information is not available, it should be obtained from the physician as soon as possible to prevent confusion and a possible error. When the drug is withheld, the physician must be notified. A common guideline is to withhold the medication if an infant's pulse is below 90 to 110 beats per minute and below 70 beats per minute in older children. However, the nurse should also be aware of significant drops from the child's previous reading. Tachycardia and irregularities in the rhythm of the pulse are significant and should be reported. Symptoms of toxic effect include nausea, vomiting, anorexia, irregularity in rate and rhythm of the pulse, and a sudden change in pulse.

If the baby is discharged while still receiving medication, the parents are taught how to take the pulse and what signs to be alert for when administering the drug.

Diuretics such as furosemide (Lasix) or chloro-thiazide (Diuril) are useful in reducing edema. Careful monitoring of serum electrolyte levels can identify electrolyte imbalance, particularly potassium depletion. The nurse should teach the parents of older patients to recognize foods high in potassium, such as bananas, oranges, milk, potatoes, and prune juice. Diapers are weighed to determine urine output. Daily weights of the baby also help the physician determine the effectiveness of the diuresis.

Complications other than cardiac decompensation (heart failure) may arise before or after surgery. With the increase in numbers of red blood cells circulating within the body (polycythemia), the blood becomes sluggish and prone to clots. When this is accompanied by dehydration, the threat of cerebral thrombosis may become a reality.

An accurate record of intake and output is essential. Signs of dehydration, such as thirst, fever, poor skin turgor, apathy, sunken eyes or fontanel, dry skin, dry tongue, dry mucous membranes, and a decrease in urination, should be brought to the immediate attention of the nurse in charge. Pneumonia can occur rapidly. Fever, irritability, and an increase in respiratory distress may indicate this condition. The patient's position is changed regularly to help prevent this setback.

Chest tubes may be used after surgery to remove secretions and air from the pleural cavity and to allow reexpansion of the lungs. These are attached to underwater seal drainage bottles or a commercially manufactured disposable system such as Pleur-Evac. Units for infants and older children are available. This system must be *airtight* to prevent collapse of the lung. Drainage bottles are always kept below the level of the chest to prevent backflow of secretions. This is especially important during transportation. Two rubber-shod Kelly clamps are available at all times for emergency clamping of tubes. These are applied to the tubes as close as possible to the child's chest if a break in the system occurs. A petrolatum-covered gauze dressing also needs to be available for immediate application over the insertion site when the tubes are removed. This provides an airtight seal over the site.

The nurse working in a cardiac unit should be alert for emergencies such as cardiac and respiratory arrest and should be competent in cardiopulmonary resuscitation techniques and the necessary modifications required for pediatric patients.

The parents of the child need support and understanding over a long period of time. A mother's fears and dependencies come to the surface when she gives birth to a baby with a defect. Because the heart is the body's most vital organ, this type of diagnosis causes a great deal of apprehension and anxiety. The physician has to reassure the parents without minimizing the danger involved. If the condition permits, the infant is sent home under medical supervision until the preferred age for surgery. Every effort must be made by the family to provide a normal environment that is within the infant's limits. It is easy for parents to become overpermissive because they do not wish the child to become unnecessarily excited. The child senses this and soon gains control of the home. This is difficult for everyone but is especially exhausting and confining for the mother. Limit setting, such as 5 minutes of chair time, if done with consistency, is beneficial.

The patterns formed during infancy can build the framework of a healthy personality for the patient. The child with a heart condition who is well integrated into family life has a definite advantage over the child who is made to think he or she is an invalid. Routine naps and early bedtime provide adequate rest for most patients. As these patients grow, they usually set their own limits on the amount of activity they can handle. Substitutions can be made for strenuous activities, such as bicycle riding, and for rigorous competitive games. The child receives the usual childhood immunizations. Prompt treatment of infections is important. A suitable diet with adequate fluids is necessary and iron-rich foods encouraged. Dental care should also be regular. All-day attendance in school may be too tiring for the child, so special provisions in this area may be necessary. The child additionally needs careful evaluation before any type of minor surgery, such as a tonsillectomy, is performed.

Some children need hospitalization occasionally for various tests or problems. Simple explanations must be given to patients regarding this condition. They should be allowed to handle and to see hospital equipment before its use whenever feasible. Cardiac surgery is generally performed at a regional medical center where the necessary costly equipment is available. The American Heart Association has established standards and recommendations for centers that care for children with congenital heart defects. Whenever possible, a continuum of nursing care by an experienced registered nurse who follows the patient throughout hospitalization is desirable for both the physical and the psychological welfare of the patient. The physician may also refer the parents

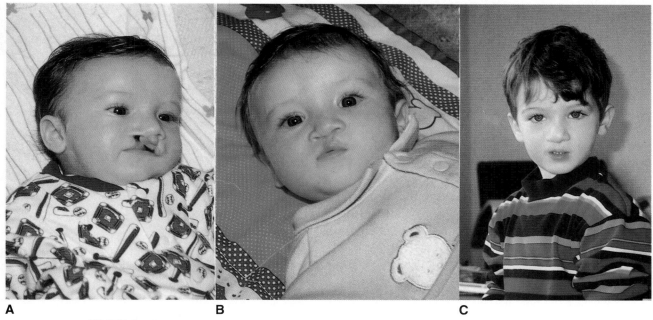

FIGURE **6-10** Child with cleft lip and palate at birth **(A)**, immediately after lip repair **(B)**, and at 3 years of age **(C)**.

of the infant to a social worker who assists them in seeking needed services and financial assistance. The financial burden on the parents for years of medical and surgical necessities is phenomenal. All avenues for financial aid should be explored by qualified personnel.

GASTROINTESTINAL SYSTEM

CLEFT LIP
Description

A cleft lip is characterized by a fissure or opening in the upper lip and is a result of the failure of the embryonic structures of the face to unite. In many cases the condition seems to be caused by hereditary predisposition, coupled with a minor deviation in the intrauterine environment. This disorder appears more frequently in boys than in girls and may occur on one or both sides of the lip. The extent of the defect may vary from slight to severe. Sometimes it is accompanied by a **cleft palate,** a fissure in the midline of the roof of the mouth. Cleft lip and palate are common congenital anomalies, occurring in about 1 in approximately 700 births.

Treatment and Nursing Care

The initial treatment is surgical repair. The cleft lip is repaired first because it interferes with the infant's ability to eat. The baby cannot create a vacuum in the mouth and is unable to suck. Surgery not only improves the infant's sucking, it also greatly improves the appearance. Currently, it is performed any time after birth if the infant's general health is good and

there is no infection. Most infants are repaired around 10 weeks of age (Figure 6-10)

Before surgery, a complete physical examination is given and blood tests are ordered. Photographs may also be taken. Any signs of infection, such as a cold, should be reported to the head nurse. The doctor may order restraints to prevent the patient from scratching the lip and to allow the patient to become accustomed to the restraints because they will be necessary after surgery. An Asepto syringe with a rubber tip or a Haberman feeder is used to feed the baby before and after surgery because the sucking motion must be avoided to decrease tension on the suture line. Sometimes a soft, cross-cut nipple can be used before surgery.

Feeding Method for Neonates with Cleft Lip, Cleft Palate, or Both. Babies with cleft lip and/or cleft palate can be fed by bottle or by breast. Use of special nipples will assist meeting the baby's sucking need and promote muscle development for speech. Breastfeeding is possible for these babies but may require the assistance of a lactation specialist. Skill 6-1 describes a feeding method that may be used for babies with both cleft lip and cleft palate. After the infant has established a feeding routine, the infant should be able to complete the feeding in 18 to 30 minutes. An infant who requires a longer feeding period could be working too hard and expending too many calories. This would not promote growth, which is a goal for these infants. It is important for the nurse and the caregiver to remain flexible and patient in feeding these infants. It may require trying several different systems and techniques before the best one is found (Figure 6-11).

Skill 6-1 Oral Feeding for Infants with Cleft Lip or Palate

■ Equipment	■ Description	■ Method
✓ Soft, thin-walled nipple (preemie nipple)	• Compresses easily; readily available	1. Use a nipple or feeding system that provides a controllable flow rate and is energy efficient for the infant.
✓ NUK orthodontic nipple	• Large surface for compression	2. Hold infant in upright position to assist in reducing the amount of nasal regurgitation.
✓ Cross-cut nipple	• Allows easy flow of milk with compression	3. Use a pillow for additional support for infant to assist with longer feeding times.
✓ Ross cleft palate nurser	• For infants with weak suck; has soft tube-like nipple that delivers past the cleft	4. Keep chin tucked because neck extension inhibits swallowing.
✓ Mead Johnson cleft palate nurser	• Soft, long cross-cut nipple; soft bottle for squeezing and monitoring milk flow; can use cross-cut or NUK nipples with this system	5. If regurgitation occurs (milk coming out through the nose), stop feeding and allow infant to cough/sneeze to clear nasal airway.
✓ Haberman feeder	• Large, squeezable nipple with a slit cut; has one-way valve to reduce amount of air ingested; two nipple lengths available: regular and short	6. Place nipple on top of tongue. Nipple insertion may push tongue to the back of mouth.
		7. Burp the infant frequently because of increased air ingestion.
		8. Monitor for distress and fatigue during feeding.
		9. Limit feeding time to approximately 30 minutes to avoid fatigue.
✓ Pigeon cleft palate nurser	• Larger, more bulbous Y-cut nipple; firm on top with soft bottom; has air valve to prevent collapse and air flow; has flow setting in bottle collar	10. Follow feeding with sterile water to clean any trapped food in the cleft.
		11. Clean mouth and nose.
✓ Asepto syringe, rubber tip	• Readily available; places with milk beyond cleft	

Adapted from Cleft Palate Foundation. (2002). *Feeding an infant with a cleft.* Chapel Hill, NC: Author.

Postoperative Care

Postoperative nursing goals for a patient with cleft lip/palate repair include (1) preventing the baby from sucking and crying, which could cause tension on the suture line, (2) careful positioning (*never* on the abdomen) to avoid injury to the operative site, (3) cleaning the suture line to prevent crusts from forming, which could cause scarring, (4) applying restraints to prevent injury to the operative site and use of a **Logan bow** (to reduce tension on the suture line), and (5) cuddling and other forms of affection to provide for the infant's emotional needs. This last is of particular importance because the baby is unable to obtain the usual satisfactions from sucking.

The wound may be kept moist through the application of an antibacterial ointment. When applying the ointment, the nurse should follow the surgeon's instruction. Cotton-tipped applicators should be avoided to prevent injuring the surgical site. The surgical site may be rinsed with sterile saline solution.

The infant receives feedings by dropper or special feeder until the wound is completely healed (from 1 to 2 weeks). The mother who feeds her baby before surgery and is allowed to assist with feedings during hospitalization should have minimal difficulty after discharge. The immediate improvement as a result of surgery is encouraging to the parents, particularly if the child must have further surgery for cleft palate repair.

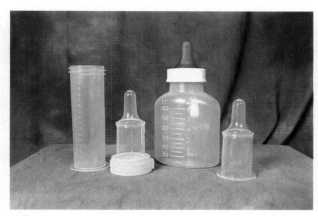

FIGURE **6-11**   Devices used to feed an infant with cleft lip and palate. *Right to left,* Haberman feeder and Mead Johnson Nurser.

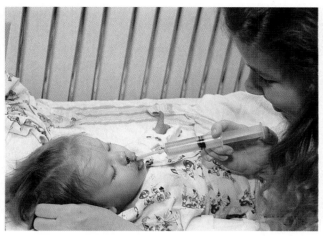

FIGURE **6-12**   After a cleft lip repair, a syringe with a rubber tip is used for feeding to prevent trauma to the incision.

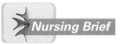
Nursing Brief

Mothers of babies with cleft lip or palate can breastfeed the infant. It requires patience and time on the part of the mother, infant, and nurse.

CLEFT PALATE
Description
A cleft palate is more serious than a cleft lip. It forms a passageway between the nasopharynx and the nose, which not only complicates feeding but easily leads to infections of the respiratory tract and middle ear and is generally responsible for speech difficulties later in life. Unlike cleft lip, cleft palate is more common in girls than in boys.

Treatment
The best time for surgery is subject to controversy, although some surgeons prefer if possible to operate before 18 months of age, so that speech patterns are not affected. With the advances in surgical techniques, many centers are electing to repair the cleft palate in the neonatal period (Merritt, 2005). To facilitate communication, a dental speech appliance may be used if surgery has been deferred or has been contraindicated because of extensive malformation. This appliance must be changed periodically as the child grows.

The management of the child with a cleft lip and palate requires expert teamwork over a long period of time. The emotional problems that sometimes occur with this condition may require more extensive attention than the repair itself. A child born with a facial deformity encounters many problems. It is difficult to be unattractive when society places such importance on good looks. A mother's first reaction to a disfigured newborn infant may be one of shock, hurt, disappointment, and guilt. Some parents may regard the deformity as a result of their inadequacies. They may desire to hide the child from relatives and friends. Feedings are difficult and are not relaxed in the initial period. As the child grows, irregular tooth eruptions, drooling, delayed speech, and intermittent hospitalizations and frequent clinic appointments can be frustrating. The developing child senses the feelings of the parents and acquires either a positive or a negative attitude about himself or herself accordingly. The patient and the family need understanding, a concrete basis for hope, and practical advice.

In large cities, special cleft palate clinics are available where several specialists can work together in convenient consultation. The parents should be informed of the resources available in the state in which they live. Financial assistance is usually indicated because of the length of treatment required.

Postoperative Management and Nursing Care
Nutrition. Fluids are best taken by a cup, although an Asepto syringe with a rubber tip (gravity feeder) may be used (Figure 6-12). The nurse should find out the preference of the plastic surgeon before feeding the child. Hot foods and liquids should be avoided to prevent injury to the surgical site. All objects should be kept out of the mouth. This includes straws, tongue blades, spoons, forks, and pacifiers. A wide-bodied spoon may be used if the food is fed from the side of the spoon and does not come in contact with the roof of the mouth. The diet progresses from a clear to a full liquid diet. The child may go home on a soft diet (nothing harder than mashed potatoes).

Oral Hygiene. The mouth is kept clean at all times. Feedings should be followed by a little water. The doctor may prescribe a mild antiseptic mouthwash.

Restraints. Elbow restraints are generally sufficient. They should be removed under supervision one at a time periodically to prevent constriction of circulation and to allow normal movement. In the home they may

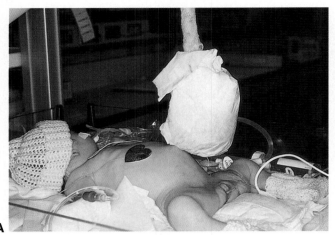

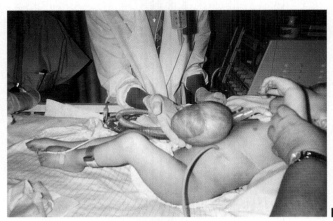

A

B

FIGURE **6-13** **A,** If an omphalocele or gastroschisis is too large to repair immediately, a Silastic silo is placed over the exposed viscera and the intestines are gradually reduced into the abdominal cavity over a period of days. **B,** A child with an omphalocele whose condition was too unstable to permit surgical reduction. The sac covering the intestines has toughened over time.

be made out of rolled cardboard tied with a string. It is important to prevent the child from placing fingers or objects in the mouth. Teach the child to keep the tongue away from the sore part of the mouth.

Speech. Speak slowly and distinctly to the patient and encourage the child to pronounce words correctly. Children who have had extensive repairs or have associated deafness need the help of a speech therapist. Others simply require a minimum of help from their parents.

Diversion. The goal is for the child to cry as little as possible. Play should be quiet, particularly in the immediate postoperative period. Read to the child or help the child color.

Complications. Otitis media and dental problems may accompany this condition. The parent must be instructed to take the child to the physician at the first signs of earache. Visits to the dentist should be regular.

GASTROSCHISIS AND OMPHALOCELE
Description

These two defects allow abdominal contents to herniate outside the abdominal cavity. The gastroschisis usually occurs to the right of the umbilical cord. It is usually a small defect and involves only the bowel. It does not have a sac covering the defect. An omphalocele is a herniation of the gut into the umbilical cord. It is generally a large defect involving the bowel, liver, spleen, bladder, uterus, or ovaries. It is contained in a translucent sac with amniotic fluid. If the defect can be identified with ultrasound, a cesarean section is usually indicated.

Treatment and Nursing Care

After delivery, care is given to prevent rupture of the sac with the omphalocele. Any exposed viscera is covered with warm saline-soaked gauze covered with plastic dressing to prevent radiant heat loss. The infant requires monitoring of respirations, temperature, and hydration status. Surgical repair is necessary for both defects. Small defects may be repaired by replacing the exposed viscera back into the abdominal cavity. For large defects, the surgical repair may require a staged repair. A Silastic silo or tube-like material is sutured around the defect. The abdominal contents are within the silo and are slowly pushed into the abdominal cavity (Figure 6-13). This procedure may take 7 to 10 days, which allows for the abdominal cavity to expand to accommodate the bowel.

During the reduction period, the infant is at risk for infection, hypothermia, dehydration and shock, and decreased lower extremity circulation. When the bowel is completely reduced into the abdominal cavity, the infant returns for complete closure. Postoperative care requires pain control. Nursing priorities include monitoring respiratory and circulatory status and bowel function. Total parenteral nutrition (TPN) provides nutritional needs until bowel function has returned. Feeding is introduced slowly as tolerance is monitored. With the improvement of parenteral nutrition and neonatal care survival rates can be as high as 90% (Cowles & Stolar, 2006)

ESOPHAGEAL ATRESIA AND TRACHEOESOPHAGEAL FISTULA ATRESIA
Description

Esophageal atresia (EA) is a congenital defect in which the esophagus fails to connect to the stomach. It ends in a blind pouch. Most cases are associated with tracheoesophageal fistula (TEF), which is characterized by an abnormal connection or fistula between the esophagus and the trachea (Figure 6-14). There may be a maternal history of polyhydramnios (excess of amniotic fluid in pregnancy).

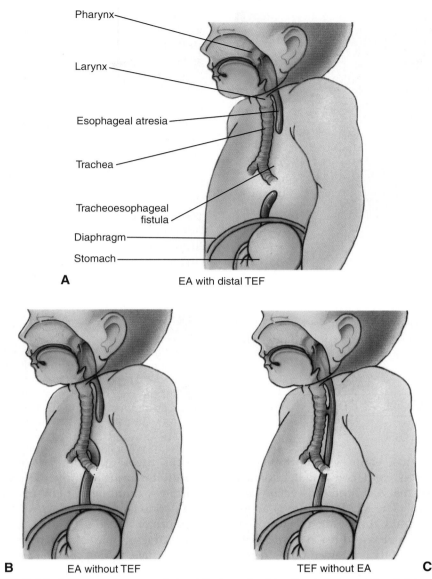

Pharynx

Larynx

Esophageal atresia

Trachea

Tracheoesophageal fistula

Diaphragm

Stomach

A   EA with distal TEF

B   EA without TEF

TEF without EA   **C**

FIGURE **6-14** **A,** The esophagus ends in a blind pouch with a fistula between the distal esophagus and trachea. **B,** EA without fistula. **C,** TEF without EA.

Treatment and Nursing Care

At birth, the infant is seen with excessive oral secretions through coughing, choking, and cyanosis. These symptoms may worsen when feeding is attempted. Respiratory distress can present when the excessive secretions are aspirated or when the secretions pass into the trachea through a fistula. If an EA is not present, diagnosis may be more difficult. Diagnosis is determined by attempting to pass a small-bore NG tube into the esophagus. If passage is not possible, radiograph is used to diagnosis the defect.

A low-suction catheter is placed in the blind pouch to control secretions. The infant is maintained in an upright position to reduce the risk for aspiration. Priority nursing interventions include monitoring respiratory status, maintaining NPO (nothing by mouth) status, and administering oxygen. Antibiotics are given

for possible infection related to aspiration pneumonia. A gastrostomy tube or button is placed to provide nutrition and gastric decompression.

Surgical intervention is necessary. It involves reattaching the ends of the esophagus and ligation of the fistula. If the distance between the two ends of the esophagus is too far, surgery to connect these may be delayed. The esophagus may need to be lengthened before the ends can be attached.

Postoperative care involves care of a chest tube, a gastrostomy tube, and an NG/orogastric tube connected to low suction. As with any postoperative patient, the nurse needs to monitor respiratory status, hydration status, thermoregulation, pain, and infection and assist in providing bonding between parent and infant. As the infant progresses toward discharge, parents need education regarding home care and

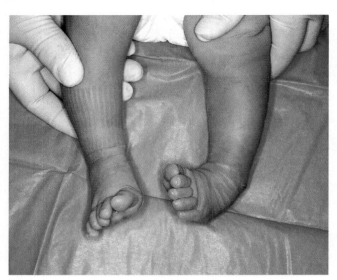

FIGURE **6-15** The child with clubfoot has a flexed ankle, a turned heel, and an adducted forefoot.

feedings. This may be more relevant for infants who require further surgical interventions.

MUSCULOSKELETAL SYSTEM

CLUBFOOT
Description

Clubfoot, one of the most common deformities of the skeletal system, is a rigid congenital anomaly characterized by a foot that has been twisted inward or outward (Figure 6-15). The incidence rate is about 1 in 730 births. Many mild forms are the result of improper position in the uterus and resolve with little or no treatment if the extremity is allowed unrestricted activity. In contrast, true clubfoot does not respond to exercise. Many believe that this is because of an abnormal degree of compression and molding of the infant's feet in the uterus. Several types are recognized. Talipes (*talus,* heel; *pes,* foot) equinovarus (*equinus,* extension; *varus,* bent inward) is seen in 95% of cases. The feet are turned inward and the child walks on the toes and the outer borders of the feet. The condition generally affects both feet. Boys are affected twice as often as girls.

Treatment and Nursing Care

The treatment of clubfoot should be started as early as possible; otherwise, the bones and muscles continue to develop abnormally. During infancy, conservative treatment consisting of manipulation and casting to hold the foot in the right position is carried out. Manipulation and casting are repeated every few days for the first 1 to 2 weeks and then at 1- to 2-week intervals. This is done to allow for the rapid growth during this period. If manipulation does not work, surgery is performed. Surgery involves releasing tight

tendons and repositioning and pinning the foot bones. The goal is to complete the treatment by 1 year of age so that the child can use normal shoes when he or she starts walking.

Cast Care. Most casts are made of synthetic materials (fiberglass, polyurethane, or a combination). Synthetic casts dry quickly (in less than 30 minutes) and are lighter, which allows for greater mobility. However, they are not as strong as plaster and are more expensive.

The gauze containing the material for a plaster cast is placed in warm water before being applied over stockinette and cotton batting. It takes approximately 24 to 48 hours for the cast to dry. The cast should be left uncovered until it dries. The cast dries from the inside out. The child should be turned every 2 hours. When lifting the cast, the nurse should use the palms, not the fingers, to prevent indentations that could press on the underlying skin and cause damage.

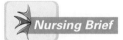

> **Nursing Brief**
>
> Important in the long-term care of orthopedic patients is educating parents about orthopedic devices, cast care, exercise and hygiene, and treatment goals. The nurse explains the importance of frequent clinic visits, reinforces physician information, and clarifies directions as necessary.

The toes are left exposed for observation. **The nurse checks them for signs of poor circulation, which would be indicated by pallor, cyanosis, swelling, coldness, numbness, pain, or burning.** If the child's circulation is impaired, the cast may be slit to relieve the pressure or it may need to be removed and reapplied. The nurse should also report irritation of the skin around the edges of the cast and lack of movement of the toes. Adhesive petals may be placed around the edges of the cast to prevent skin irritation.

It is difficult to keep a child's cast free of food particles, which cause skin irritation. The patient needs careful supervision during mealtime so that he or she does not place bits of food under the edges of the cast. Powder and oil should not be used after the bath because they may cause irritation.

If surgery on tendons and bones has been performed, the nurse must also observe the cast for evidence of bleeding. If a discolored area appears on the cast, it is circled and the time is recorded. Further bleeding can then be estimated. If bleeding is noted, the patient's vital signs are also checked and compared with preoperative readings.

Emotional Support. The nurse is an important figure in the care of the long-term patient. Nurses should review the normal growth and development of children in the patient's age range to anticipate some of the problems and to educate caretakers in parenting.

In general, children from birth to 4 years of age suffer the most from being separated from their

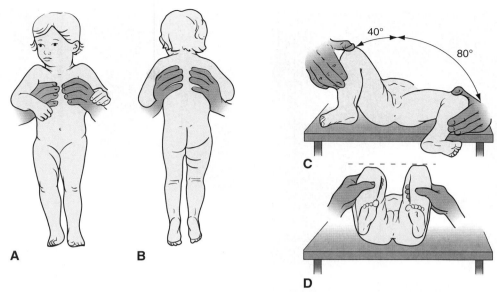

FIGURE **6-16** Three classic signs of DDH. **A** and **B,** unequal skin folds; **C,** limitation of abduction; and **D,** unequal knee height.

parents. They cry loudly when their parents leave and need the nurse to console them. They may be slow in developing certain motor abilities and in many cases regress to earlier behavior. This is particularly true of bowel and bladder control. The nurse should not shame a child if an "accident" occurs.

The parents can give helpful information about their child. Be a good listener. Parents should be encouraged to participate in the care of their hospitalized child, because it brings them emotional relief and reassures the child.

The financial burdens of hospitalization, surgery, and continued medical supervision pose a real problem. If the nurse suspects that the parents need financial help, a social service referral should be made.

DEVELOPMENTAL DYSPLASIA OF THE HIP
Description
Developmental dysplasia of the hip (DDH) is a common orthopedic deformity. The incidence is about 10 in 1000 live births. The term **hip dysplasia** is a broad description applied to various degrees of deformity that may involve subluxation or dislocation and may be either partial or complete. The head of the femur is partly or completely displaced from a shallow hip socket (acetabulum). Both hereditary and environmental factors appear to be involved in the cause. Hip malformation, joint laxity, breech position, and race may all contribute. DDH is seven times more common in girls than in boys. Newborn infants seldom have complete dislocation. When the baby begins to walk, the pressure exerted on the hip can cause a complete dislocation. Accordingly, early detection and treatment are of particular importance in this condition.

Signs and Symptoms
Subluxation of the hip is commonly discovered at the time of the newborn examination. Ongoing screening for DDH should be done during routine health examinations of the baby during the first 6 months of life. One of the most reliable signs is a limitation of abduction of the leg on the affected side. When the infant is placed on the back with knees and hips flexed, the physician can press the femur related to the normal hip back until it almost touches the examining table. On the affected side, however, this can be accomplished only partially. Also the knee on the side of the dislocation is lower and the skin folds of the thigh are deeper and are often asymmetrical. When the infant is prone, one hip is higher than the other (Figure 6-16). In some infants younger than 4 weeks, the physician can actually feel and hear the femoral head slip into the acetabulum under gentle pressure. This is called Ortolani's sign or Ortolani's click and is considered diagnostic. If the child has begun walking and has had no treatment, a characteristic limp is displayed. Bilateral dislocation may occur; however, unilateral dislocation is more common. Radiographs and ultrasound scans confirm the diagnosis.

Treatment
Treatment is begun as soon as the dislocation is detected. The physician attempts to form a normal joint by keeping the head of the femur within the hip socket. This constant pressure enlarges and deepens the acetabulum, thus correcting the dislocation. The bones of small children are fairly pliable because they contain more cartilage than bones of adults.

Treatment of the hip dysplasia depends on the age of the child. In the neonate, abduction of the hips is maintained with the use of the Pavlik harness

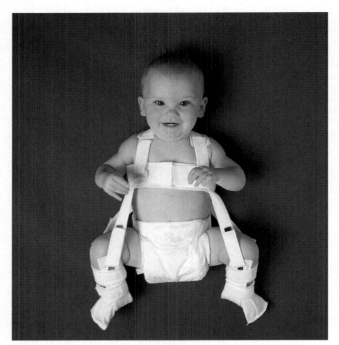

FIGURE **6-17** The Wheaton™ Pavlik Harness is used to maintain the hips in a position of flexion and abduction.

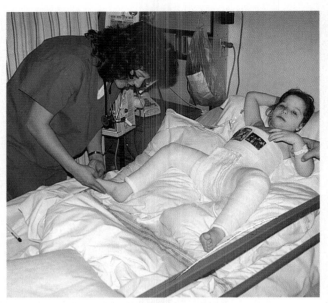

FIGURE **6-18** A spica cast after hip surgery.

(Figure 6-17). The harness is worn full time for 2 months, then with a decrease in wearing time. The Pavlik harness allows the infant to move the legs. If the dislocation is severe or has not been detected until the child has begun to walk, it may be necessary to use traction. This pulls the head of the femur down to the correct position opposite the acetabulum. After the traction has stretched the muscles enough to allow the hip to be placed in the acetabulum, the dislocation is reduced with general anesthesia and a spica cast is applied to hold the abduction. This type of cast is shown in Figure 6-18. The length of time that the patient remains in the cast varies according to progress, growth, and the condition of the cast; however, it is usually from 5 to 9 months. During this time, the cast may be changed about every 6 weeks. Sometimes surgery is necessary. In this case, open reduction of the dislocation or repair of the shelf of the hip bone is done. A cast is applied after surgery to keep the femur in the correct position.

Nursing Care

In the nursery, the nurse carefully observes each infant during the morning bath to detect signs of a dislocated hip. When the baby is prone, the nurse observes the buttocks for variation in size. The legs of the infant should be equal in length. The infant should be kicking both legs, not just one. There should be no difference in the depth of the skin folds of the baby's upper thighs. In the well-baby clinic, the nurse notes the posture and gait of older children and records observations.

Infants who progress well with the Pavlik harness remain at home. The parent and baby visit the physician regularly. They need instruction regarding skin care while the infant wears the harness. A T-shirt and long socks can protect the infant's skin from rubbing. The parents need assurance that they may hold the baby and sit him or her in a chair. They should also be encouraged to ask questions of the clinic nurse and doctor.

The child who is admitted to the hospital with a diagnosis of DDH should be given as much personal attention as possible. The first admission will set the pattern for future hospitalizations; therefore it is important that the child make a satisfactory adjustment. The nurse should become familiar with the child's daily schedule, and every effort should be made to provide patients who are hospitalized for many weeks with a homelike environment.

The type of cast that is used is called a **body spica cast.** It encircles the waist and extends to the ankles or toes. General cast care should be reviewed at this point (see the Cast Care section under Clubfoot in this chapter). Skill 6-2 describes how to turn and position a child in a body cast. Other aspects pertinent to this particular type of cast are discussed in the following paragraphs.

Firm, plastic-covered pillows are placed beneath the curvatures of the cast for support. Older children may benefit from an overhead bar and trapeze. The room should be adequately ventilated. A fracture bedpan should be available in the bedside table.

The head of the patient's bed should be slightly elevated so that urine or feces drains away from the body of the cast. Do not elevate the head or shoulders of a child in a body cast with pillows because this thrusts the patient's lower chest against the cast and can cause discomfort or respiratory difficulty. To prevent soiling of the cast from urine and feces, plastic wrap or wide

Skill 6-2 | Turning and Positioning a Child in a Body Cast

■ Method

1. Use two people to turn a child in a body cast.
2. Lift the child and place in the prone position.
3. Do not use crossbars between the legs as handles.
4. With the patient in the prone position, place a pillow under the chest and under each leg to prevent pressure on the toes.
5. With a bedpan, support the upper back and legs with pillows so that body alignment is maintained.

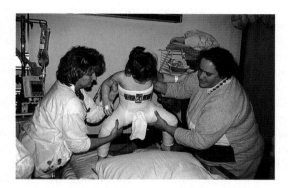

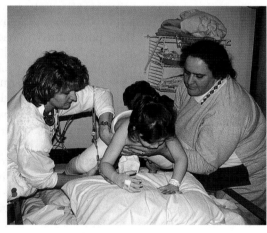

cloth tape can be tucked around the edges of the cast at the openings between the legs. A disposable diaper can be tucked under the edges around the buttocks for the same purpose. As these coverings become soiled, they must be changed immediately. Frequent changing of position is important; bed patients need to be turned often. Infants may be held in a parent's lap after the cast has dried. A ride on a stretcher or a wagon to the playroom or around the hospital provides a change of position and a change of scene.

Itching is a particular problem with a patient in a body cast. If at all possible, before the cast is applied, a strip of gauze should be placed beneath the stockinette that protects the skin from the cast. The gauze strip comes out at the opened area. It can be gently moved back and forth beneath the cast to provide relief from itching. When the strip becomes soiled, a clean one is tied to one end of the soiled gauze and pulled through the cast and the soiled portion is removed. Other methods that might cause injury to the skin beneath the cast are discouraged because any break in the skin under a cast is difficult to heal. Use of a fan facing toward the opening of the cast may relieve the discomfort. Avoid giving children small objects that could be inserted inside the cast.

The child with a long-term disability such as this needs help in meeting the everyday needs of life. The child is growing and developing rapidly. Therefore frequent adjustments in home and clinic care are necessary. Dressing and clothing are a problem. The child also cannot use regular furniture or much of the play equipment enjoyed by other children. Transportation is also difficult. Children in spica casts can be transported from their rooms by placing them in a wagon that has been built up with pillows. They can also be elevated with pillows when eating. Refer parents to home health care because most of these children need a pediatric orthopedic wheelchair to be mobile.

NERVOUS SYSTEM

DOWN SYNDROME

Description

Down syndrome is one of the most common genetic birth defects. The incidence of Down syndrome is approximately 1 in 800 live births; it is higher in children born of mothers 35 years old or older. However, sometimes a baby with Down syndrome is the first child of a young mother. Depending on the cause, her following children may be normal. There are three known causes of Down syndrome, all of which involve abnormalities of the chromosomes. In the most common type, **trisomy 21 syndrome,** the total chromosome count is 47 instead of the normal 46. This accounts for 95% of cases. It is a result of **nondisjunction,** or failure of a chromosome to follow the normal separation process into daughter cells. The earlier in the embryo's development this occurs, the greater the number of cells affected. With translocation which occurs with 3% to 4% of cases, a piece of chromosome in pair 21 breaks off and attaches itself to another chromosome. Parents should have genetic counseling as translocation is usually hereditary. Mosaicism occurs in 1% to 3% of cases and results in the body cell having either normal or abnormal chromosomes. Mosaicism and trisomy 21 are not hereditary

Signs and Symptoms

The signs of this condition, which are apparent at birth, are close-set and upward-slanting eyes, small

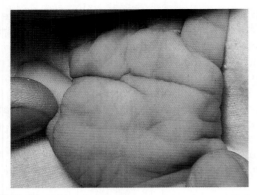

FIGURE **6-19** Bridged palmar crease, seen in some infants with Down syndrome.

head, round face, flat nose, mouth breathing, and a protruding tongue that interferes with sucking. The hands of the baby are short and thick, and the little finger is curved. In addition, there is a deep, straight line across the palm, called the **simian crease** (Figure 6-19). There is also a wide space between the first and second toes. Undeveloped muscles (hypotonia) and loose joints enable the child to assume unusual positions. Physical growth and development may be slower than normal (Table 6-1 and Home Care Tip box). Most children are mildly to moderately retarded. Because of recent advances in medicine, education, and available resources, these children have been able to progress farther than previously possible. Congenital heart deformities may be associated with this condition. It is important to remember that no one child exhibits all the possible physical characteristics of Down syndrome.

Home Care Tip

Self-Help Skills

SKILL	CHILDREN WITH DOWN SYNDROME		NORMAL CHILDREN	
	AVERAGE (MO)	RANGE (MO)	AVERAGE (MO)	RANGE (MO)
EATING				
Finger feeding	12	8-28	8	6-16
Using spoon/fork	20	12-40	13	8-20
TOILET TRAINING				
Bladder	48	20-95	32	18-60
Bowel	42	28-90	29	16-48
DRESSING				
Undressing	40	29-72	32	22-42
Putting clothes on	58	38-98	47	34-58

From Levine, M.D., Carey W.B., & Crocker, A.C. (1999). *Developmental-behavioral pediatrics* (3rd ed.). Philadelphia: Saunders, with permission.

Children with Down syndrome are very lovable. However, they are restless and somewhat more difficult to train than normal youngsters. Their resistance to infection is poor, but their life span has increased with the widespread use of antibiotics. The incidence rate of acute leukemia is higher in these children than in the normal population. They are also at risk for development of respiratory infections and otitis media. Children with Down syndrome are also prone to speech and hearing problems.

Nursing Care

Nurses need to be aware of their own feelings before they can give effective support to the child with a disability and the parents. They must have patience and understanding. The children are encouraged to help themselves within their ability, even though it may take more time. This is especially true when they are ill and hospitalized. Early infant stimulation enables children with Down syndrome to reach milestones as rapidly as possible.

With increased stimulation, love and encouragement from the family, and the utilization of community resources, the child's potential for progress has increased. The child with Down syndrome no longer needs to be institutionalized.

With an increase in funding, more and more programs and community facilities suited to the short-term and long-term needs of children with Down syndrome are becoming available. Some community facilities are group homes, foster homes, and boarding homes. The nurse should become familiar with services located in and near the community. Sometimes parents cannot accept the fact that their baby is different and are ashamed to tell anyone of the baby's condition. The parents need to grieve over the loss of the normal child they do not have. This should not be interpreted as a lack of love for the child they do have. It takes exceptional strength to accept this diagnosis. Empathy from the nurse is of particular importance. Allowing parents to become involved in care and planning for the infant from the start facilitates bonding. The staff's warm concern and care cannot be overemphasized. Pampering the baby by putting a little curl in the hair, for example, shows that others care even though this baby is different. Parents watch for evidence of rejection of their child; they are sensitive to such things as placement in the nursery.

Several organizations provide support to the child with Down syndrome, among them the National Down Syndrome Congress, the National Association for Retarded Citizens, and the National Association for Down Syndrome.

HYDROCEPHALUS
Description

Hydrocephalus (*hydro*, water; *cephalo*, head) is a condition characterized by an increase in cerebrospinal fluid (CSF) in the ventricles of the brain, which causes an increase in the size of the head and pressure changes in the brain. It occurs as a result of an imbalance between

Table 6-1 | *Developmental Milestones*

MILESTONE	CHILDREN WITH DOWN SYNDROME		NORMAL CHILDREN	
	AVERAGE (MO)	RANGE (MO)	AVERAGE (MO)	RANGE (MO)
Smiling	2	1½-3	1	½-3
Rolling over	6	2-12	5	2-10
Sitting	9	6-18	7	5-9
Crawling	11	7-21	8	6-11
Creeping	13	8-25	10	7-13
Standing	10	10-32	11	8-16
Walking	20	2-45	13	8-18
Talking, words	14	9-30	10	6-14
Talking, sentences	24	18-46	21	14-32

From Levine, M.D., Carey, W.B., & Crocker, A.C. (1999). *Developmental-behavioral pediatrics* (3rd ed.). Philadelphia: Saunders, with permission.

production and absorption of CSF. Hydrocephalus may be congenital or acquired. It may occur in conjunction with a meningomyelocele or as a sequela of infections, including congenital TORCH infections (TORCH stands for **t**oxoplasmosis, **o**ther, **r**ubella, **c**ytomegalovirus, and **h**erpes simplex), encephalitis, or meningitis, or because of perinatal hemorrhage. The symptoms depend on the site of obstruction and the age at which it develops. Although there are many causes of hydrocephalus, all result in either an impairment of CSF absorption within the subarachnoid space (communicating hydrocephalus) or an obstruction of CSF flow within the ventricles (noncommunicating hydrocephalus). Hydrocephalus may proceed slowly or rapidly. Two forms of hydrocephalus are the Arnold-Chiari malformation and the Dandy-Walker syndrome. Because hydrocephalus can cause progressive cerebral damage, early recognition and treatment are important.

It should be recalled that the brain and spinal cord are surrounded by fluid, membranes, and bone. The three membranes, called **meninges,** are the dura mater, the arachnoid, and the pia mater. The arachnoid mater, also known as the middle membrane, resembles a cobweb and its spaces are filled with fluid. CSF is also found in spaces of the brain called **ventricles.** The primary site of formation for CSF is believed to be the choroid plexus.

Signs and Symptoms

Signs and symptoms depend on the time of onset and the severity of the imbalance. The classic sign both in congenital hydrocephalus and in hydrocephalus with onset in infancy is an increase in head size (Figure 6-20). The direction of skull expansion depends on the site of obstruction. Transillumination (*trans,* across; *illuminare,* to enlighten), or the inspection of a cavity or organ by passing a light through its walls, is a simple diagnostic procedure useful in visualizing fluid. A flashlight with a sponge rubber collar is held tightly against the infant's head in a dark room. The examiner observes for areas of increased luminosity. Another sign is a bulging anterior fontanel and separation of

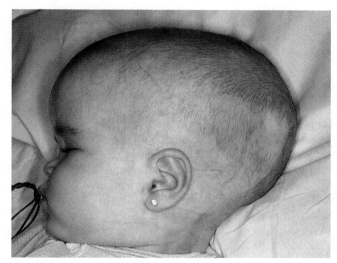

FIGURE **6-20** The head of an infant with hydrocephalus is larger than normal.

cranial sutures. The scalp is also shiny and the veins dilated. The infant appears helpless and lethargic. The body becomes thin, and the muscle tone of the extremities is often poor. In addition to the infant's shrill and high-pitched cry, irritability, vomiting, and anorexia are present. Convulsions may also occur. In severe infantile hydrocephalus, the eyes may appear deviated downward, which is known as the "setting sun" sign (Figure 6-21). Children with an onset of hydrocephalus later in childhood may have minimal enlargement of the head and display the signs and symptoms of increased intracranial pressure (ICP).

Diagnosis and Treatment

The child's head is measured daily. Echoencephalography, computed tomography (CT), or magnetic resonance imaging (MRI) is most frequently used to show the enlarged ventricles and to locate the level of obstruction. A ventricular tap or puncture may be performed in the treatment room with sterile technique. The equipment needed is the same as that for a lumbar puncture. The specimen is labeled and sent to the laboratory for analysis.

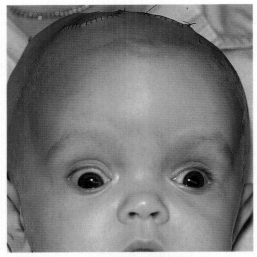

FIGURE **6-21** Marked hydrocephalus with "setting sun" sign and divergence of the eyes.

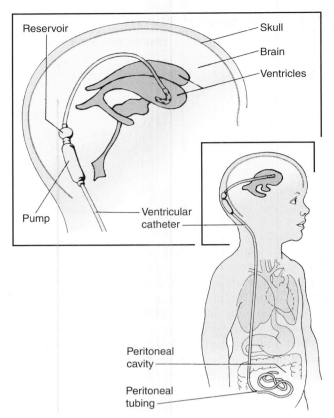

FIGURE **6-22** Placement of the VP shunt.

After careful evaluation of these and other preoperative test results, the surgeon decides whether or not to operate. The surgeon attempts to bypass or shunt the point of obstruction. A **shunt** carries the CSF to another area of the body, where it is absorbed and finally excreted. Shunting is accomplished by inserting special tubing, which is replaced at intervals during the child's growth. Two types of shunts are used: the ventriculoperitoneal (VP) shunt and the ventriculoatrial (VA) shunt. The VP shunt is the most commonly used (Figure 6-22). New shunt systems now allow for growth and have eliminated the necessity for shunt revisions. The prognosis for hydrocephalus has improved with modern drugs and surgical techniques. If the brain has not been seriously damaged before the operation, mental function can be preserved. However, motor development may occur at a slower rate, if the child cannot lift the head normally. Complications associated with shunts are usually caused by mechanical flaws (kinking or plugging of tubing) or infection. Shunt malfunction may be identified by headaches, nausea, vomiting, irritability, and lethargy. The shunt also serves as a primary spot for infection. The symptoms of shunt infections may include an unexplained fever and symptoms similar to those of shunt malfunction. If the infections persist, it may become necessary to remove the shunt.

Nursing Care

The general nursing care of an infant with hydrocephalus who has not undergone surgery presents several challenges. The child may be barely able to raise the head. Mental development is also delayed. Lack of appetite, a tendency to vomit easily, and poor resistance to infections pose additional problems.

The position of the infant must be changed frequently to prevent hypostatic pneumonia and pressure sores. Hypostatic pneumonia occurs when there is poor circulation of the blood in the lungs and when the patient remains too long in one position. It is particularly prevalent in patients who are poorly nourished, weak, or have a debilitating disease. Whenever the nurse turns the patient with hydrocephalus, the head must always be supported. To turn the patient in bed, the weight of the head should be borne in the palm of one hand and the head and body should be rotated together to prevent a strain on the neck. When the child is lifted from the crib, the head must be supported by the nurse's arm and chest. The head circumference (FOC) is measured daily. This measurement is critical, and it is necessary that the location of the measurement is marked with a marking pen on the child's head.

Pressure sores may occur if the patient's position is not changed at least every 2 hours. The tissues of the head and ears and the bony prominences have a tendency to break down. A pad of lamb's wool or a rubber sponge placed under the head may help avoid these lesions. If the skin becomes cracked, it should be given immediate attention to prevent infection. The patient must be kept dry, especially around the creases of the neck, where perspiration may collect.

In most cases, the nurse may hold the infant for feeding. The nurse sits with the arm supported because the baby's head is heavy. A calm, unhurried manner is necessary. The room should also be as quiet as possible. After the feeding, the infant is placed on the side. Do not disturb the infant once he or she is settled because the baby vomits easily. The nurse must organize daily care so that it does not interfere with meals.

Observations that need to be made include the type and the amounts of food taken, vomiting, condition of skin, motor abilities, restlessness, irritability, lethargy, and changes in vital signs. Fontanels are palpated for size and bulging. Changes in vital signs associated with increased ICP are usually a sign later in infancy. They include elevated blood pressure and a decrease in pulse and respirations. Signs of a cold or other infection should be reported to the nurse in charge immediately and recorded.

Postoperative nursing care is complex, and in addition to routine postoperative care and observations, the nurse observes the patient for signs of increased ICP and for infection at the operative site or along the shunt line. Pain issues should be included in the care of the postoperative patient.

Bacterial infection is a life-threatening complication that sometimes makes it necessary to remove the shunt. Signs of infection include poor feeding, elevated vital signs, decrease level of consciousness, vomiting, and seizure activity. The nurse should also observe for signs of inflammation at the shunt insertion site. The surgeon indicates the position desired and the activity level of the child.

If the fontanels are sunken, the infant should be kept flat because too rapid a reduction in fluid may lead to seizures or cortical bleeding. If the fontanels are bulging, the patient is usually placed in the semi-Fowler's position to assist in drainage of the ventricles through the shunt. The patient is always positioned so as to avoid pressure on the operative site. Head and chest measurements are recorded. In patients with peritoneal shunts, the abdomen should also be measured or observed to detect malabsorption of fluid. Skin care continues to remain a priority. As the patient's condition improves, parents are instructed regarding the care of the shunt.

In the presence of increased ICP, the shunt can be tested for patency by compressing the antechamber or reservoir. The physician may order the pump to be depressed a certain number of times per day to facilitate drainage.

It is important to remember that as intracerebral pressure increases, cerebral perfusion decreases or is at least compromised. A decrease in cerebral perfusion causes less oxygen to be delivered to the brain cells. Without oxygen, a cell dies, and brain cells do not replace themselves as other cells may do.

Hydrocephalus, even with a shunt, is a chronic condition, and the child needs to be followed throughout life. It is crucial to monitor this condition. It is also important that family issues and the child's own growth and development be considered.

MYELODYSPLASIA/SPINA BIFIDA

Myelodysplasia refers to a group of central nervous system (CNS) disorders characterized by abnormal development of the spinal cord and associated neural tube structures. These defects are categorized as neural tube defects (NTDs). One of these disorders is spina bifida.

Description

Spina bifida (divided spine) is a congenital embryonic NTD in which there is imperfect closure of the spinal vertebrae. There are two forms: **occulta** (hidden) and **cystica** (sac or cyst). Spina bifida occulta is a relatively minor variation of the disorder in which the opening is small and there is no associated protrusion of structures. It is often undetected and occurs most commonly at L5 and S1 levels. There may be a tuft of hair, a dimple, a lipoma, or a port-wine birthmark at the site. Generally, treatment is not necessary unless neuromuscular symptoms appear. These consist of progressive disturbances of gait, footdrop, or disturbances of bowel and bladder sphincter function.

Spina bifida cystica consists of the development of a cystic mass in the midline of the spine (Figure 6-23). **Meningocele** and **meningomyelocele** are two types of spina bifida cystica. A meningocele (*meningo,* membrane; *cele,* tumor) contains portions of the membranes and CSF. The size varies from that of a walnut to that of the head of a newborn infant.

More serious is a protrusion of the **membranes** and **spinal cord** through this opening, or a **meningomyelocele.** Although it resembles a meningocele, there may be associated paralysis of the legs and poor control of bowel and bladder functions. Hydrocephalus is common.

Although the cause of spina bifida is unknown, it is thought to be multifactorial. This would include both genetic and environmental factors. Maternal diabetes, alcohol use, hyperthermia, valproic acid use, and nutritional deficiencies may be contributing factors. The American Academy of Pediatrics recommends all women of childbearing age take a daily multivitamin that includes 0.4 mg of folic acid. For women with a previous history of an NTD birth, the recommendation is to increase the folic acid intake to 4 mg per day. The folic acid should be taken through the first trimester (American Academy of Pediatrics, 1999).

Treatment

The treatment for spina bifida is surgical closure to prevent meningeal infection. The child is observed for the development of hydrocephalus, and a shunt is placed if this occurs. Urinary retention is managed with catheterization. The prognosis for these children depends on the location of the lesion, the involvement of the spinal cord, and the presence of other anomalies. Care of the child involves a multidisciplinary approach that includes neurology, neurosurgery, urology, pediatrics, physical therapy, occupational therapy, and nursing. Depending on the extent of the defect, the child may have problems with hydrocephalus, orthopedic

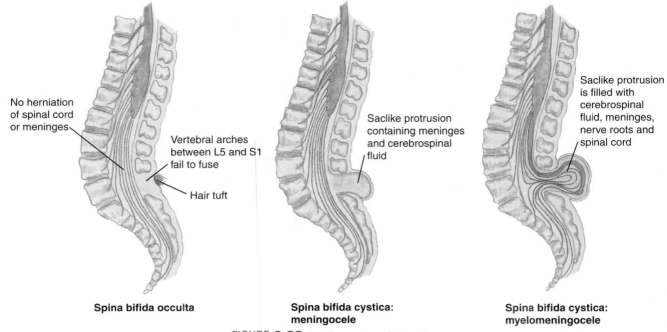

No herniation of spinal cord or meninges

Vertebral arches between L5 and S1 fail to fuse

Hair tuft

Saclike protrusion containing meninges and cerebrospinal fluid

Saclike protrusion is filled with cerebrospinal fluid, meninges, nerve roots and spinal cord

Spina bifida occulta

Spina bifida cystica: meningocele

Spina bifida cystica: myelomeningocele

FIGURE **6-23** Malformation of the spine.

defects, genitourinary abnormalities, and paralysis. Habilitation is necessary after surgery to minimize the child's disability and to put the normally functioning parts of the body to constructive use. Every effort is made to help the child develop a healthy personality so that he or she may live a happy and useful life. Eventually the child may attain some degree of fecal continence and some type of emptying of the bladder (intermittent clean catheterization). Mobility is assisted through bracing, surgery, and the use of a wheelchair.

Nursing Care

The main objectives of the extensive nursing care required include preventing infection of or injury to the sac; correct positioning to prevent pressure on the sac and deformities; good skin care, particularly if the infant is incontinent of urine and feces; adequate nutrition; tender, loving care; accurate observations and charting; education of the parents; continued medical supervision; and habilitation.

Immediate care of the sac is essentially the same whether or not the cord is involved. Upon delivery, the neonate is placed in an isolette. Moist sterile dressings of saline solution or an antibiotic solution may be ordered to prevent drying of the sac. Some method of protecting the mass is necessary if surgery is to be delayed. Pertinent nursing observations include a description of the newborn infant, the size and area of the sac, and any tears or leakage. The extremities are observed for deformities and for movement. There may be spasticity or paralysis of the limbs or they may be normal, depending on the type and location of the cyst. The head is measured to determine the possibility

of associated hydrocephalus. Fontanels are observed to provide baseline data. Lack of anal sphincter control and dribbling of urine are significant in the differential diagnosis. In general, the higher the defect is on the spine, the greater is the neurological deficit. Data are recorded along with the routine observations made for every newborn infant.

Positioning of the patient is crucial. The goal is to avoid pressure on the sac and to prevent postural deformities. When positioning patients with multiple deformities, the nurse must try to guard against aggravating existing problems. These children may also have hip dysplasia, which can be another factor in positioning the infant. The infant is usually placed prone with a pad between the legs to maintain abduction and counteract hip subluxation, and a small roll is placed under the ankles to maintain a neutral foot position. The position can be maintained with diaper rolls, blankets, or sandbags.

Postoperative nursing care involves neurological assessment and prevention of infection. The status of the fontanels and any signs of increased ICP, such as irritability or vomiting, are important. Sometimes a shunt is inserted along with the closure of the spine (see the Nursing Care section under Hydrocephalus in this chapter for a discussion of the nursing care of the patient with a shunt). Complications that can be life-threatening include meningitis, pneumonia, and urinary tract infection.

Urological monitoring is essential because many of these patients are incontinent of urine. Medication to prevent urinary tract infections is given routinely. Prolonged use of Credé's method has been replaced with clean intermittent catheterization. This is a simple procedure that ensures total emptying of the bladder. It can be performed by parents and learned by young children. It is important that this procedure be performed regularly and in a clean manner. Implanted artificial sphincters are used in some cases.

Skin care is a challenge. Diapering is generally contraindicated. Constant dribbling of feces and urine irritates the perineal area and can infect the sac or the incision. Meticulous cleanliness is necessary. Bedding must be dry and wrinkle-free. Frequent cleansing, application of a prescribed ointment or lotion, and light massage help maintain skin integrity. If range-of-motion exercises are ordered, they are performed gently. Because these children have lack of sensation below the spinal lesion, they lack the ability to be aware of skin breakdown or burns. Parents should be instructed to inspect the skin closely.

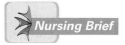
Nursing Brief

Latex allergy is common in children with spina bifida, and latex-containing toys and medical supplies should be avoided.

Feeding of the patient is facilitated by early closure of the defect. In delayed cases, gavage feedings may be used. To bottle-feed the patient, one nurse may hold the infant over the shoulder while another administers the formula. Nipple holes should be large enough to prevent exhaustion, which can occur if the infant has to work to get food. A side-lying position in or out of the crib (on the nurse's lap) is effective with some babies.

These patients need cuddling and sensory stimulation. If infants cannot be held, the nurse should soothe them by touch. Talk to them and when possible provide face-to-face (*en face* position) communication. Mobiles should be placed appropriately. Moving the incubators or cribs periodically provides diversity of view. Soft music is also soothing.

Special consideration must be given to the establishment of parent-infant relationships. This problem is complicated if the infant is transferred to a large medical center. Understanding and support need to be given to the parents. It is not unusual for them to be overwhelmed by the cyst. Most experience a sense of loss for what was to have been their "perfect baby." Steps of the grieving process may be recognized by the nurse. If the malformation is complex and incompatible with life, a decision must be made about the feasibility of surgical intervention. This is a crisis situation for the most mature of people and an area in which guidelines are not clearly defined. Information and education concerning this disorder can be obtained from the Spina Bifida Association of America.

HEMOLYTIC DISEASE OF THE NEWBORN: ERYTHROBLASTOSIS FETALIS
Description

Erythroblastosis fetalis (*erythro*, red; *blast*, a formative cell; *osis*, disease condition) is a disorder that becomes apparent late in fetal life or soon after birth. It is one of many congenital hemolytic diseases found in the neonate. There is excessive destruction of the red blood cells of the baby because of an incompatibility between the red blood cells of the mother and those of the fetus. This occurs in a sensitized Rh-negative mother who is pregnant with an Rh-positive child. Sensitization refers to the phenomenon in which the mother, during her first pregnancy or through exposure to Rh-positive blood by transfusion, has developed anti-Rh-positive antibodies, which then attack and destroy the red blood cells of the fetus. The incidence rate of erythroblastosis fetalis has greatly decreased as a result of the protective administration of Rh antibody (RhoGAM) to women at risk. In fact, incompatibility of ABO factors is now more common and certainly less severe than Rh incompatibility. The process of **maternal sensitization** to Rh-positive blood is depicted in Figure 6-24. The mother accumulates antibodies with each pregnancy; therefore the chance that complications may occur increases with each gestation. Severe reactions can cause severe anemia, hydrops, CHF, hyperbilirubinemia, brain damage, and death.

Diagnosis and Prevention

Erythroblastosis fetalis should be suspected when the mother is Rh-negative and the father is Rh-positive. During the prenatal period, an indirect Coombs test can show previous exposure to Rh-positive antigens. If there are indications that the mother is Rh-sensitized, amniocentesis can be done to detect bilirubin levels in the amniotic fluid. This procedure is not without risks and, in some cases, can sensitize the mother. Postnatally, a direct Coombs test is done on umbilical cord blood; a positive result usually indicates Rh incompatibility.

Prevention of erythroblastosis with the use of RhoGAM is now routine. An intramuscular injection can be given to the mother within 72 hours after delivery, provided she has not previously been sensitized (see Figure 6-24). RhoGAM can also be given to the pregnant woman who is Rh-negative at 28 weeks' gestation if she is not sensitized. It is additionally administered in cases of abortion or miscarriage to women who are Rh-negative. Mothers who are Rh-negative and deliver at home are candidates for RhoGAM and should not be overlooked.

Signs and Symptoms

The symptoms of erythroblastosis fetalis vary with the intensity of the disease. The infant has varying

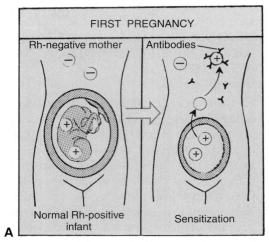
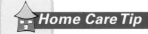
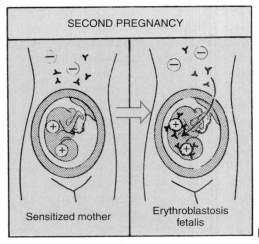

FIGURE **6-24** Development of maternal sensitization to Rh antigens. **A,** Fetal Rh-positive erythrocytes enter maternal system. Maternal anti-Rh antibodies are formed. **B,** Anti-Rh antibodies cross placental barrier and attach to fetal erythrocytes.

degrees of anemia and jaundice. The anemia is the result of hemolysis of large numbers of erythrocytes. The jaundice, termed **pathological,** differs from **physiological** jaundice in that it becomes evident within 24 hours after delivery. The infant's liver is unable to handle the massive hemolysis, and bilirubin levels rise rapidly, causing hyperbilirubinemia (*hyper,* excess; *bilis,* bile; *rubor,* red; *emia,* blood). Early jaundice should be reported immediately to the physician.

Enlargement of the liver and spleen and extensive edema may develop. The circulating blood usually contains an excess number of immature nucleated red blood cells (erythroblasts), produced in attempts by the baby's body to compensate for the destruction of its cells. As a result, the blood's ability to carry oxygen is diminished, and the blood volume is decreased. In this situation, shock or heart failure may occur. Severe jaundice may cause kernicterus, serious damage to the brain. Although this is now rare, it can leave the neonate mentally retarded and, in extreme cases, result in death.

Treatment

In the case of a fetus with severe anemia, intrauterine transfusions may be used. These transfusions may be given as often as every 2 weeks until delivery (Hockenberry & Wilson, 2007). Labor can be induced as soon as lung maturity is reached. After delivery, treatment includes a combination of phototherapy and exchange transfusion. Phototherapy may reduce the likelihood of the infant needing a transfusion or may reduce the number of transfusions needed. Treatments are instituted according to established guidelines based on laboratory findings, weight, and general condition of the infant. Nursing care of the child receiving phototherapy is discussed in the section on the high-risk infant in Chapter 5. Infants with mild-to-moderate jaundice may be treated with home phototherapy. A photoblanket or pad can be used (Figure 6-25). These

products allow for easier holding of the infant and decreased risk for eye damage (Figure 6-26). Parents should be given instructions for home care.

Home Care Tip

Home Care of Infant with Phototherapy

Instruct parents regarding fiberoptic system, including set-up and care of equipment.

Wrap unclothed infant in fiberoptic blanket from below armpits and around torso.

Protect gonads with use of diaper.

Protect infant's eyes from phototherapy light by securing fiberoptic blanket with another blanket.

Monitor infant's temperature.

Monitor infant's output for amount and description of stool. Phototherapy can cause loose green stools and cause skin breakdown.

Monitor infant's input and maintain frequent feedings to prevent dehydration and assist in the effectiveness of phototherapy.

Pick up, hold, and interact with infant during phototherapy.

Help parents understand ongoing blood tests to monitor bilirubin levels.

INTRACRANIAL HEMORRHAGE

DESCRIPTION

Intracranial hemorrhage, a common birth injury, may result from trauma or anoxia. It occurs more frequently in the preterm infant, in whom the blood vessels are fragile. Blood vessels within the skull are broken and bleeding occurs into the brain. When the diagnosis is made, the specific location of the hemorrhage should be noted: subdural or subarachnoid, epidural or intraventricular. This injury may also occur during precipitated delivery, prolonged labor, or when the

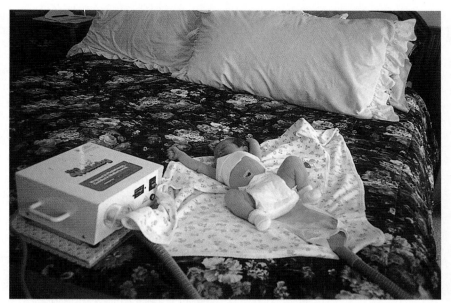

FIGURE **6-25** The fiberoptic blanket is wrapped around the infant to direct radiating light to the skin.

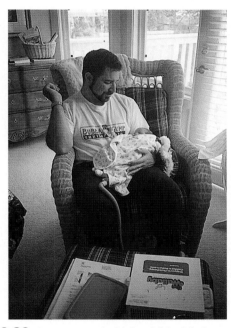

FIGURE **6-26** A parent can hold the child while he or she is receiving phototherapy via the fiberoptic blanket.

newborn's head is large in comparison with the mother's pelvis.

Signs and Symptoms

The symptoms of intracranial hemorrhage may occur suddenly or gradually. Some or all may be present, depending on the severity. They include inability to move normally, lethargy, poor sucking reflex, irregular respirations, cyanosis, twitching, forceful vomiting, a high-pitched shrill cry, and convulsions. Opisthotonic posturing may be observed. The fontanel may be tense and under pressure, rather than soft and compressible. The pupil of one eye is apt to be small and the other large. If the symptoms are mild, there is a good chance of complete recovery in most cases. Death results if there is a massive hemorrhage. The infant who survives an extensive hemorrhage may have residual defects such as mental retardation or cerebral palsy. The diagnosis is established by the history of the delivery, CT, MRI, evidence of an increase in CSF pressure, and the symptoms and course of the disease.

Treatment and Nursing Care

The newborn is placed in an isolette, which allows proper temperature control, ease in administering oxygen, and continuous observation. The baby is handled gently and as little as possible. The head is elevated. The doctor may prescribe vitamin K to control bleeding and phenobarbital if twitching or convulsions are apparent. The baby is fed carefully because the sucking reflex may be affected. The infant vomits easily. The nurse observes the baby for signs of increased ICP and convulsions. The nurse also assists the physician with such procedures as lumbar punctures and aspiration of subdural hemorrhage.

If a convulsion occurs, the nurse's observation of its character aids the physician in determining the exact location of the bleeding (see also Chapter 12). The following observations are of particular importance: Were the arms, legs, or face involved? Was the right or left side of the body involved? Was the convulsion mild or severe? How long did it last? What was the condition of the infant before and after the seizure? The nurse records observations in the nurses' notes.

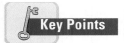

Key Points

- The March of Dimes Birth Defect Foundation classifies birth defects.
- The most common method of transmission of HIV to the pediatric population is perinatal transmission. With the prenatal use of AZT, there has been a reduction in transmitting the organism by this route.
- Rotavirus is an organism that causes diarrhea in infants and small children.
- Tuberculosis is a communicable disease and should be reported to the public health department. The public health department oversees the management and treatment of this disease.
- Congenital heart disease can lead to the development of CHF.
- Cleft lip and cleft palate cause problems with feeding the newborn.
- Tracheoesophageal fistula can be identified during feedings.
- Omphalocele has a protective covering of the internal organs, whereas gastroschisis does not.
- Clubfoot and DDH are evident at birth and need to be treated as early as possible to allow for the child's mobility as growth and development occur.
- Trisomy 21 (Down syndrome) is one of the most common forms of chromosomal abnormalities.

- Monitoring FOC is an important nursing assessment when caring for a child with hydrocephalus.
- Myelodysplasia refers to malformations of the spinal cord.
- RhoGAM has decreased the incidence rate of hemolytic disease of the newborn caused by the Rh factor, which is also known as erythroblastosis fetalis.

 Go to your companion CD-ROM for an Audio Glossary, video clips, and more.

evolve Be sure to visit the companion Evolve site at http://evolve.elsevier.com/Price/pediatric/ for WebLinks and additional online resources.

ONLINE RESOURCES

American Academy of Pediatrics: http://www.aap.org

American Cleft Palate—Craniofacial Association: http://www.cleftline.org

Centers for Disease Control and Prevention: http://www.cdc.gov

Cleft Palate Foundation: http://www.cleftline.org

Congenital Heart Defects: www.americanheart.org

March of Dimes: http://www.marchofdimes.com

Spina Bifida Association of America: http://www.sbaa.org

Upon completion of this chapter, the student will be able to:

1. Define the vocabulary terms listed
2. Discuss the nutritional needs of growing infants
3. Identify the approximate age for each of the following developments: posterior fontanel has closed, central incisors appear, birth weight has tripled, child can sit steadily alone, child shows fear of strangers
4. Describe four developmental characteristics of infants that predispose them to certain hazards; for example, "Puts everything into mouth—danger of aspiration"
5. List the immunizations given during the first year and include the approximate age for each
6. Discuss ways to educate parents about the importance of immunizations
7. Discuss precautions/contraindications of immunizations
8. Describe the physical development of infants from 1 to 12 months
9. Describe the physical and psychosocial development of infants from 1 to 12 months
10. List age-specific events and guidance appropriate for infants

Key Terms

Be sure to check out the bonus material on the Companion CD-ROM, including selected audio pronunciations.

deciduous teeth (dē-SĬD-ū-ŭs; p. 134)
encephalopathy (ĕn-sĕf-ă-LŎP-ă-thē; p. 130)
extrusion reflex (ĕk-STROO-shŭn; p. 131)
grasp reflex (p. 119)
immunization (ĭm-ū-nĭ-ZĀ-shŭn; p. 128)
parachute reflex (p. 119)
pincer grasp (p. 119)
rooting reflex (p. 131)
weaning (p. 134)

GENERAL CHARACTERISTICS AND DEVELOPMENT

The first year of life is a period of rapid growth and development. Each baby develops at an individual rate. Although growth is continuous, there are slow and rapid periods. **The most common cause for concern about a child is a sudden slowing in any aspect of development that is not typical for that age group.**

The infant is completely dependent on adults during the first months and gives little in return. Behavior is not consistent. For a baby, sucking brings comfort and relief from tensions. The nurse, understanding how important sucking is to the baby, holds the infant during feedings and allows sufficient time to suck. Infants who are warm and comfortable associate food with love. The baby who is fed intravenous fluids should be given added attention and a pacifier, which enables the infant to experience the much needed satisfaction derived from sucking. When the teeth appear, the infant learns to bite and enjoys objects that can be chewed. Gradually, the baby begins to put the fingers into the mouth. Once they can use their hands more skillfully, infants suck their fingers less often because they are able to derive pleasure from other sources.

The grasp reflex (discussed in Chapter 4) occurs when one touches the palms of the infant's hands and flexion takes place. This reflex disappears at about 3 months. **Prehension,** the ability to grasp objects between the fingers and the opposing thumb, occurs slightly later (at 5 to 6 months) and follows an orderly sequence of development. By 7 to 9 months, the parachute reflex appears. This is a protective arm extension that occurs when an infant is suddenly thrust downward when prone. By 1 year, the pincer grasp, reflecting coordination of index finger and thumb, is well established (Figure 7-1).

Love and security are vital for infants. Babies need continuous affection from their parents. Infants' needs should be met in a loving, consistent manner that enables them to trust the people with whom they interact (Figure 7-2). Parents should be assured that they will not spoil infants if they respond to their needs. Loving adults help infants to build trust and to believe that the world is a good place. This development of a **sense of trust** is key to the development of a healthy personality. A sense of trust is thought to serve as a foundation on which all subsequent tasks are based. The lack of a sense of trust can have a negative effect on the rest of a child's life because the child mistrusts people and regards the world with suspicion.

The constant care of an infant is a strain on even the most exceptional parents. If the father or mother is the full-time caregiver, he or she needs and deserves

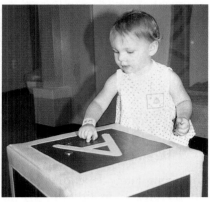

FIGURE **7-1** Pincer grasp. The 12-month-old uses the thumb and index finger to pick up small objects.

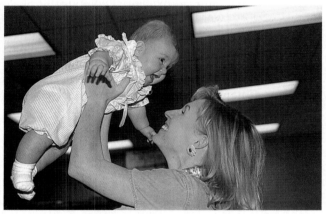

FIGURE **7-2** This 6-month-old infant responds with delight to her mother with a true social smile. Such interactive responses between parent and child promote bonding.

understanding and kind support from the spouse, the relatives at home, and the nurses in the hospital. A short break from the pressures of parenting refreshes parents, renewing their energy and allowing them to enjoy caring for the baby. A trip to the store, a walk with the baby in a stroller, or coffee with neighbors affords stimulation and provides a change of environment for the baby and for the parent. The infant who is left constantly in the crib or playpen and who is not introduced to a variety of learning experiences may become shy and withdrawn. **Sensory stimulation is essential for the development of a baby's thought processes and perceptual abilities.** Exposing babies to sights, sounds, and other stimuli helps the brain to grow. Brain growth is the most critical organic achievement of infancy.

If a mother is unable to room-in with her hospitalized infant, personnel should try to imitate her care with prompt fulfillment of the infant's physical and emotional needs. In the nursery, the baby who appears hungry should be fed first, rather than the nurse adhering to a specific routine. Wet diapers should be changed as soon as possible, and a crying child

should be soothed. The exactness of bathing or feeding the infant is not as important as the way in which it is done. Warmth and affection or the lack thereof are easily recognized by the baby.

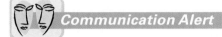

Communication Alert

The nurse can use the time spent caring for an infant to communicate with the child. While feeding, changing the diaper, and bathing, talk softly, sing, touch, and play simple games with the child.

PHYSICAL DEVELOPMENT, SOCIAL BEHAVIOR, CARE, AND GUIDANCE

Box 7-1 is a guide to infant care from the first month to the first year. Arranged with headings and in chronological order, the material has been organized so that it may be referenced easily. Although this box is a convenient reference tool, it is merely a summary of data. Some aspects of care, such as safety measures, are important throughout the entire year. The nurse should explain to parents that physical patterns cannot be separated from social patterns and that abrupt changes do not take place with each new month. Like body structures that cannot be separated from their functions, human development cannot be cleanly divided into specific areas. In addition, because no two infants are exactly alike at any given age, the following discussion is just a guide. However, individual variations do range around central norms, which serve as indicators for the evaluation of an infant or child's progress. For instance, although the time of occurrence may vary, an infant's ability to sit without support is still a marker of developmental progress.

HEALTH PROMOTION AND MAINTENANCE

The promotion of health and the prevention of disease during infancy are of the utmost importance and include all measures that improve the physical health and psychosocial adjustment of the child. The concept of periodic health appraisal is not new. In the late 1800s, "milk stations" were established in various localities throughout the United States. These stations' purpose was to reduce the number of deaths from infant diarrhea by providing safe water and milk for babies. Today, skilled health services encompass periodic health appraisal, evaluation of developmental milestones, immunizations, assessment of parent-child interactions, counseling in the developmental processes, identification of families at risk (i.e., for child abuse), health education and anticipatory guidance, referrals to various agencies, follow-up services, appropriate record keeping, and evaluation and audit by peers.

Text continued on p. 128.

Box 7-1 | *Physical Development, Social Behavior, Care, and Guidance for the First 12 Months*

ONE MONTH
Physical Development
- Gains 5 to 7 ounces weekly for the first 6 months. Has regained the weight lost after birth. Gains about 1 inch in length per month for the first 6 months. Head circumference increases by 2 cm (^{3}/4 inch) monthly for the first 3 months.
- Lifts head slightly when placed on the stomach. Pushes with toes. Turns head to the side when prone. Head wobbles. Head lag occurs when pulled from lying to sitting position.
- Obligatory nose breather (most infants).
- Clenches fists. Grasp reflexes are strong. Stares at surroundings.
- Vaginal discharge in girls and breast enlargement in boys and girls from maternal hormones received in utero are not unusual and disappear without treatment.

Social Behavior
- Makes small throaty noises.
- Cries when hungry or uncomfortable.
- Sleeps 20 of 24 hours. Awakes for 2 AM feeding.

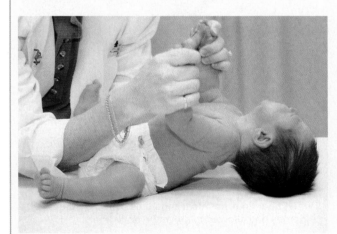

Note head lag of 1-month-old when pulled from lying position.

Care and Guidance
Sleep
- Place the infant on the back to sleep.
- The side-lying position is best used when the baby is awake and has just been fed. Place on the right side to maximize digestion.
- Use a firm, tight-fitting mattress in a crib with bars properly spaced so that the baby's head cannot be caught between them. Raise crib rails. Use no pillow.

Diet
- Give breast milk every 2 to 3 hours or iron-fortified formula every 4 hours or on demand.
- Vitamin D (400 international units/day) may be recommended in dark-skinned infants, breastfed babies, or those infants who are not regularly exposed to sunlight.
- Burp the baby well.

Immunization
- May receive second dose of **Hep B** vaccine.

Exercise
- Allow freedom from the restraints of clothing before bath.
- Provide fresh air and sunshine whenever possible.
- Sunscreen is typically not used on infants of less than 6 months of age because babies have fragile skin.
- Do not allow the baby to overheat, especially in the hot summer months.
- Provide protection from insects.
- Avoid exposure to large crowds until the immune system becomes more developed.
- Support the head and shoulders when holding the infant.
- Attend promptly to physical needs.
- Provide colorful hanging toys for sensory stimulation.

TWO MONTHS
Physical Development
- Posterior fontanel closes.
- Tears appear.
- The baby can hold the head erect in midposition.
- The baby follows moving light with the eyes.
- Grasp reflex is fading.
- The baby can hold a rattle briefly.
- Legs are active.

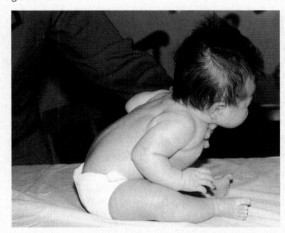

At 2 months of age, the infant needs assistance to maintain an upright position.

Social Behavior
- Smiles in response to mother's voice.
- Knows crying brings attention.
- Awakens for 2 AM feeding.

Care and Guidance
Sleep
- Develops own pattern.
- May sleep from feeding to feeding.

Continued

Box 7-1 | *Physical Development, Social Behavior, Care, and Guidance for the First 12 Months—cont'd*

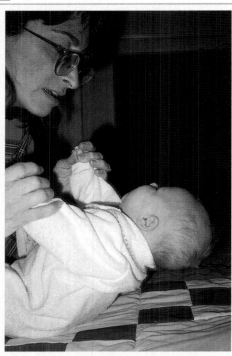

The 2-month-old shows slight head lag.

TWO MONTHS
Care and Guidance
Diet
- Feed breast milk or formula.

Exercise
- Provide a safe, flat place for baby to kick and be active. Do not leave baby alone, particularly on any raised surface. Advise parents that even the youngest of babies can roll off a changing table or bed if left unattended.
- Physical examination by the family doctor, well-baby clinic, or pediatrician.

Immunization
- See Table 7-1.

Pacifier
- If used, select for safety. Choose one-piece construction and loop handle to prevent aspiration. Introduce pacifier after breastfeeding is well established (3 weeks) to avoid nipple confusion.

Hiccups
- Are normal and subside without treatment. May offer small amounts of water.

Colic (paroxysmal abdominal pain, irritable crying)
- Usually disappears after 3 months. Place baby prone over covered hot water bottle. Use pacifier. Relieve caretaker periodically. Avoid overstimulation. Rocking, infant swing, or music box may help.
- Still completely depends on adults for physical care.
- Needs a flexible routine throughout infancy and childhood.

THREE MONTHS
Physical Development
- Primitive reflexes fading.
- Weighs 12 to 13 pounds.
- Stares at hands.
- Reaches for objects but misses them.
- Carries hand to mouth.
- Can follow an object from right to left and up and down when it is placed in front of the face.
- Supports head steady.
- Holds rattle.

Social Behavior
- Coos, babbles, chuckles.
- Cries less.
- Can wait a few minutes for attention.
- Enjoys responding to people talk.
- Takes impromptu naps.

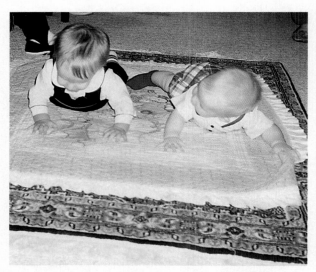

During floor time, an infant should be placed on the abdomen and allowed to move the body freely.

Care and Guidance
Sleep
- Yawns, stretches, naps in mother's arms.

Diet
- Breast milk or formula.

Exercise
- May have short play period.
- Enjoys playing with hands.
- Allow time on stomach while awake.

FOUR MONTHS
Physical Development
- Weighs about 13 to 14 pounds. Head circumference increases by 1 cm per month to age 6 months.
- Drooling indicates appearance of saliva. Can breathe when nose is obstructed.
- Lifts head and shoulders when on abdomen and looks around. Turns from back to side. Sits with support.

Box 7-1 | *Physical Development, Social Behavior, Care, and Guidance for the First 12 Months—cont'd*

Begins to reach for objects. Coordination between eye and body movements.

- Moves head, arms, and shoulders when excited. Extends legs and partly sustains the weight when held upright. Rooting, Moro, extrusion, and tonic neck reflexes are no longer present. Little head lag.

Social Behavior

- Makes consonant sounds "n," "k," "g," "p," and "b."
- Coos, chuckles, and gurgles. Laughs aloud.
- Responds to others.
- Likes an audience.
- Sleeps 8 to 10 hours at night.

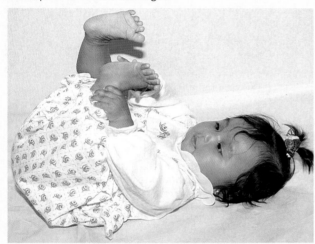

This 4-month-old infant takes pleasure in exploring her own body. She begins playing with her feet and often puts her toes in her mouth.

Care and Guidance

Sleep

- Stirs about in crib.
- Sleeps through ordinary household noises—avoid tiptoeing around.

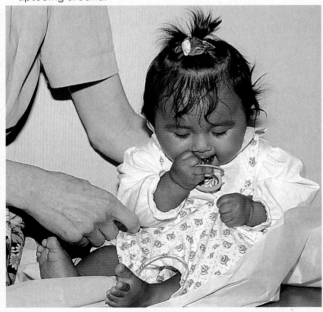

By 4 months, the infant can purposefully grasp objects with the palm of her hands.

Diet

- Feed breast milk or formula.
- May begin rice cereal.

Exercise

- Plays with hand rattles and dangling toys.
- Start acquainting the infant with a playpen where rolling safely is possible.

Immunization

- See Table 7-1.

Elimination

- May have one or two bowel movements per day.
- May skip a day.

FIVE MONTHS

Physical Development

- Sits with support.
- Holds head well.
- Grasps preferred objects.
- Puts everything into the mouth.
- Plays with toes.
- Begins showing signs of tooth eruption.

Social Behavior

- Talks to self.
- Seems to know whether persons are familiar or unfamiliar.
- Discovers parts of the body.
- Enjoys water play. Remember to never leave an infant alone in water.
- Tries to hold bottle at feeding.

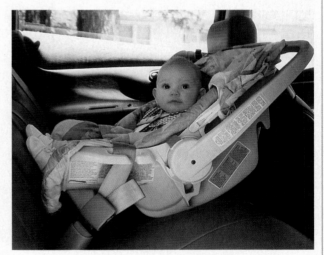

The infant rides facing the rear of the vehicle, ideally in the middle of the back seat. The infant seat is secured to the vehicle with the seat belts, and straps on the care seat adjust to accommodate the growing baby. The smaller infant needs a rolled blanket to prevent excess head movement.

Care and Guidance

Sleep

- Takes two or three naps daily in crib.

Diet

- Feed breast milk or formula.
- May have started cereal.

Continued

Box 7-1   *Physical Development, Social Behavior, Care, and Guidance for the First 12 Months—cont'd*

Exercise
- Provide space to pivot around.
- Makes jumping motions when held upright in lap.

Safety
- Check toys for loose buttons and rough edges before placing them in the playpen.
- All infants always ride in car seats. They remain rear-facing until at least 20 pounds *and* 1 year of age.

SIX MONTHS
Physical Development
- Doubles birth weight. Gains about 3 to 5 ounces per week during next 6 months.
- Grows about a half inch per month for the next 6 months. Head circumference increases $1/2$ cm ($1/4$ inch) per month for the second 6 months.
- Sits alone momentarily. Springs up and down when sitting. Hitches (moves backward when sitting).
- Turns completely over.
- Bangs table with rattle.
- Pulls self to a sitting position.
- Chewing more mature.
- Approximates lips to rim of cup.

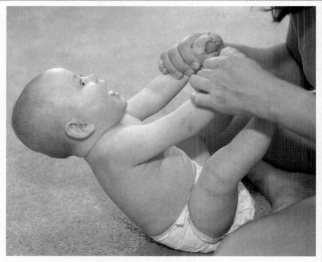

By age 6 months, no head lag is present.

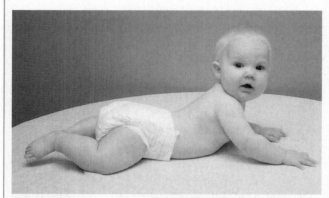

By age 6 months, the infant easily lifts the head, chest, and upper abdomen and can bear weight on the hands.

Social Behavior
- Cries loudly when interrupted from play.
- Shows increased interest in the surrounding world.
- Babbles and squeals.
- Sucks food from a spoon.
- Awakens happy.

Care and Guidance
Sleep
- Needs own room.
- Should be moved from parents' room if not previously done. Otherwise, with age, the infant may become unwilling to sleep away from them.

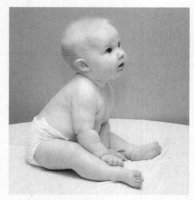

Can sit alone in tripod position, using the hands for support and stability.

Diet
- Introduce first solid foods if this has not yet been started (usually rice cereal fortified with iron).
- Iron is added for breastfed infants at 6 months with addition of cereal to the diet.

Exercise
- Grasps feet and pulls toward mouth.

Immunization
- See Table 7-1.

Safety
- Remove toxic plants from the baby's reach.
- Provide a chewable object such as a teething ring for enjoyment.

Box 7-1 | *Physical Development, Social Behavior, Care, and Guidance for the First 12 Months—cont'd*

SEVEN MONTHS

Physical Development

- Two lower teeth appear. These are the first of the deciduous teeth, the central incisors.
- Begins to crawl. Moves forward, using chest, head, and arms; legs drag.
- Can grasp objects more easily.
- Transfers objects from one hand to the other.
- Appears interested in standing.
- Holds adult's hands and bounces actively while standing.
- Struggles when being dressed.

Social Behavior

- Shifts moods easily—crying one minute, laughing the next.
- Shows fear of strangers.
- Responds to own name.
- Anticipates spoon feeding.
- Sleeps 11 to 13 hours at night.

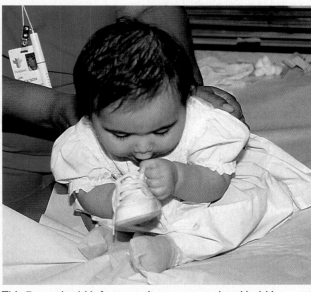

This 7-month-old infant can sit unsupported and hold her shoe. Notice how she explores it with her mouth. Parents need to learn that infants at this age put everything into their mouths. Watch for dangerous items on which the infant could easily choke.

Care and Guidance

Sleep
- Fretfulness as a result of teething may appear. This is generally evidenced by lack of appetite and wakefulness during the night. In most cases, merely soothing and offering a cup of water are sufficient.

Diet
- Add vegetables and fruits.
- Add finger foods, such as toast or zwieback.

Exercise
- Rudimentary locomotion.

EIGHT MONTHS

Physical Development

- Sits steadily alone.
- Uses index finger and thumb as pincers.
- Pokes at objects.
- Enjoys dropping articles into a cup and emptying it.

Social Behavior

- Plays pat-a-cake.
- Enjoys family life.
- Amuses himself or herself longer.
- Reserved with strangers.
- Indicates need for sleep by fussing and sucking thumb.
- Impatient, especially when food is being prepared.

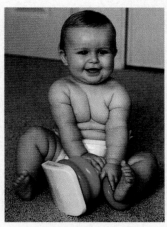

By age 8 months, the infant can sit without support and focus on play activities.

Care and Guidance

Sleep
- Takes two naps a day.

Diet
- Add vegetables and fruits.
- Continue to add new foods slowly.

Exercise
- Enjoys jump chair.
- Rides in stroller.
- Stuffed toys or those that squeak or rattle are appropriate.

Safety
- Remain with baby at all times during bath in tub.
- Protect from chewing paint from window sills or old furniture.
- Paint containing lead can be poisonous.
- Close doors to ovens, dishwashers, washing machines, dryers, and refrigerators.
- Do not leave standing water in tub, buckets, and so on.

NINE MONTHS

Physical Development

- Shows preference for the use of one hand.
- Can raise self to a sitting position.

Continued

Box 7-1 | *Physical Development, Social Behavior, Care, and Guidance for the First 12 Months—cont'd*

- Holds bottle.
- Creeps. Carries trunk of body above floor but parallel to it. More advanced than crawling.

Social Behavior
- Tries to imitate sounds (e.g., says "ba-ba" for bye-bye).
- Cries if scolded.
- Drops food from high chair at mealtime.

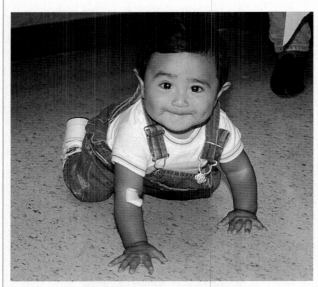

This 9-month-old infant crawls quickly, keeping his belly off the floor.

Care and Guidance
Sleep
- Has generally begun to sleep later in the morning.

Diet
- Introduce chopped and mashed foods.
- Place newspaper beneath feeding table. Use unbreakable dishes.
- Allow baby to pick up pieces of food by hand and put them into the mouth.

Exercise
- Is busy most of the day exploring surroundings. Provide sufficient room and materials for safe play.
- Help baby learn.
- See that he or she does not get into trouble.
- Distract the curious child from areas of danger. In this way, punishment is limited—avoid spankings and excessive "no's."

Safety
- Know the nationwide toll-free number for poisons (1-800-222-1222). This is operated by the American Association of Poison Control Centers through a cooperative agreement with the Centers for Disease Control and Prevention and Health Resources Services Administration.)
- Avoid tablecloths with overhangs that the baby can reach.

TEN MONTHS
Physical Development
- Pulls self to a standing position in the playpen.
- Throws toys to the floor for a parent to pick up. Cries when they are not returned.
- Walks around the furniture while holding on to it.

Social Behavior
- Knows own name.
- Plays simple games such as peek-a-boo.
- Feeds self a cookie.
- May cry out in sleep without waking.

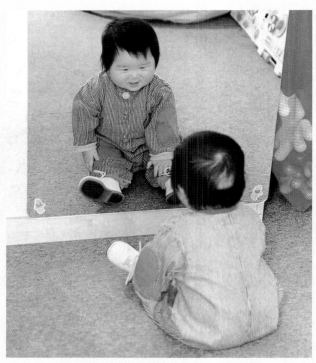

Infants this age enjoy their own image.

Care and Guidance
Sleep
- Avoid strenuous play before bedtime.
- A night-light is convenient for the parent and makes the surroundings more familiar.
- Pajamas with feet keep the baby warm because infants become uncovered easily.

Diet
- Takes juice and water from cup.
- Solid foods in general are taken well.

Exercise
- Tours around the room holding an adult's hands.
- Daytime clothing should be loose so as not to interfere with movement.

ELEVEN MONTHS
Physical Development
- Stands upright holding on to an adult's hands.

Box 7-1 | *Physical Development, Social Behavior, Care, and Guidance for the First 12 Months—cont'd*

Social Behavior
- Understands simple directions.
- Is impatient when held.
- Enjoys playing with empty dish and spoon after meals.
- Shakes head for "no."

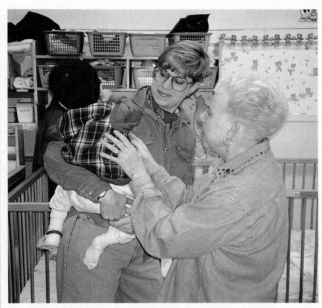

Older infants fear strangers and cling to parents.

Care and Guidance
Sleep
- Greets parents in morning with excited jargon.

Diet
- Still spills from cup.
- Enjoys blowing bubbles.

Exercise
- Plays with toys in tub.
- Enjoys gross motor activity.
- Kicks and pulls self up.

Safety
- Cover electrical outlets.
- Put household cleaners and medicines out of reach, if not previously done.
- Occasionally put baby back in sitting position in playpen; baby tends to stand until exhausted.
- Do not use baby walkers.

TWELVE MONTHS
Physical Development
- Pulse 100 to 140 beats/min. Respirations 20 to 40 breaths/min.
- Triples birth weight.
- Stands alone for short periods.

- May walk.
- Puts arm through sleeve, as an aid to being dressed.
- Six teeth (four upper and two lower).
- Drinks from a cup; eats with a spoon with supervision.
- Pincer grasp is well established.
- Handedness (the preference for the use of one hand), although not fully established, may be evidenced.

Social Behavior
- Friendly. Repeats acts that elicit a response.
- Recognizes "no-no."
- Verbalization slows owing to concentration on getting about.
- Enjoys rhythmic music.
- Shows emotions such as fear, anger, and jealousy. Reacts to these emotions from adults.
- Plays with food; removes it from mouth.

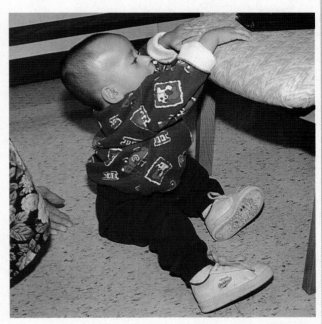

At 1 year, this infant can pull to a standing position. On a slick, hard floor, an adult should be near to catch him if he slips backward while trying to pull up.

Care and Guidance
Sleep
- May take one long nap daily.

Diet
- Gradually add egg white and fish (baked, steamed, or boiled).
- Drain oil from tuna or salmon.
- Gradually add orange juice.
- Add well-cooked table foods.
- Interest in eating dwindles.

Continued

Box 7-1 *Physical Development, Social Behavior, Care, and Guidance for the First 12 Months—cont'd*

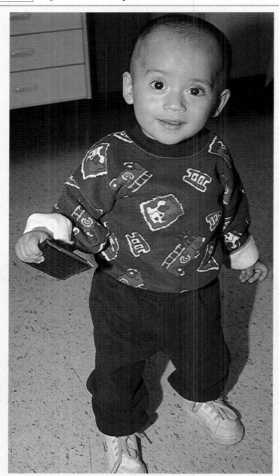

After pulling himself to a standing position, this 1-year-old can stand alone.

Exercise
- Plays in own room for an hour in the morning.
- Enjoys putting objects in a basket and then removing them.
- Places objects on head.
- Distraction is an effective way to deal with the baby's determination to do what he or she wants regardless of the outcome.

Skin test
- Tuberculin if appropriate.

Immunization
- See Table 7-1.

These services are provided in a variety of health settings. However, the kinds and quality of assistance vary. Private group practice, hospital-based clinics, and neighborhood health centers are all examples of different health settings.

Infant health care visits should be regular, and a careful health history should be obtained. Growth grids during infancy include measures of weight, length, and head circumference. The reading and recording of growth charts are described in Chapter 2. (See Appendix F for growth charts.) Several developmental screening tests may be used as well. One such test is the Denver II Developmental Screening Test (found in Appendix G). This test is used to evaluate social, fine-motor, language, and gross motor abilities from birth to 6 years. Another test, the Early Language Milestone Scale (ELM) is used from birth to 3 years to assess speech and language (PRO-ED can be contacted at 800-897-3202 or at *http://www.proedinc.com*).

The physical examination is adapted to the needs of the infant. Routine assessment of hearing and vision is an integral part of the examination. Loud noises in the newborn period should precipitate the startle or Moro reflex. Hearing is to be tested before dismissal from the hospital where the infant was born. As the infant grows, hearing can be assessed by his or her response to sounds. Vision is assessed mainly through light perception. The examiner shines a penlight into the baby's eyes and notes blinking, following to midline, and other responses. Laboratory tests are performed according to hospital policy. Screening tests for a variety of asymptomatic diseases are also important. Examples of these are the tests for phenylketonuria, galactosemia, and sickle cell anemia.

IMMUNIZATIONS

Immunizations work by having the body create antibodies to fight the weakened or inactivated germs in the vaccine. These antibodies will then know how to recognize and destroy the real disease if it poses a threat to the child. Health personnel must repeatedly stress to parents the importance of immunizations. A delay in immunizations can lead to undue risks for serious illness, with sometimes fatal complications. Measles, pertussis, and other preventable diseases continue to strike children today. Health experts warn that unless more young children are immunized, epidemics could possibly occur. Current immunization policies and recommendations have been updated in response to the changing needs of the community and the child. The nurse can emphasize to employed parents that if left unprotected, their child may become sick, resulting in a loss of valuable working hours. Immunizations prevent numerous doctor and hospital expenses. In addition, all states require immunization before a child enters school. A delay or interruption in a vaccination series does not interfere with final immunity. Restarting any series is not necessary, regardless of the length of delay. Accurate record keeping prevents confusion. **Contraindications** to routine immunizations include acute febrile conditions, some chronic diseases, a recent blood transfusion or an injection of immune serum globulin, allergy to a vaccine component, severe reaction after previous administration of an immunization, malignant disease, chemotherapy, and steroid therapy. Those individuals with an altered immune system generally do not receive live virus vaccines because multiplication of the virus could be enhanced, causing a severe vaccine-induced illness (Hockenberry & Wilson, 2007). Other stipulations are described in drug circulars. The common cold is not considered sufficient reason for delaying immunization. Any questions regarding these or other conditions should be brought to the attention of the physician or the health care provider *before* immunization.

Changes have been made in the recommendations for immunizations because of increases in outbreak of disease and the development of new vaccines. The American Academy of Pediatrics, in collaboration with the Advisory Committee on Immunization Practices of the Centers for Disease Control and Prevention and the American Academy of Family Physicians, has approved a Recommended Childhood Immunization Schedule for the United States. **The Immunization Schedule,** found in Appendix A, shows the recommendations for immunizations. The schedule is dated to ensure that health care providers are following the most recent schedule. The most up-to-date schedule can be obtained from the American Academy of Pediatrics (*http://www.aap.org*).

In the United States, by the time a child is 2 years old, he or she should be immunized against the following diseases: polio, diphtheria, tetanus, pertussis (whooping cough), hepatitis A, hepatitis B, *Haemophilus influenzae* type b, mumps, measles, rubella, varicella (chickenpox), rotavirus, and *Streptococcus pneumoniae* (pneumococcus). The influenza vaccine is now recommended for all children aged 6 to 59 months. Varicella vaccination recommendations have been updated. The first dose should be administered at age 12 to 15 months, and a newly recommended second dose should be administered at age 4 to 6 years. The new human papillomavirus (HPV) is recommended in a 3-dose schedule for females aged 11 to 12 years. (Recommended Immunization Schedules for Persons aged 0 to 18 years, United States, 2007). In February 2006, the U.S. Food and Drug Administration licensed an oral rotavirus vaccine; the three doses are to be administered at 2, 4, and 6 months of age. The meningococcal vaccine should be given to all children at the 11- or 12-year-old visit as well as to children age 2 and older with terminal complement deficiencies or functional **asplenia** or otherwise considered high risk. Table 7-1 shows the vaccines, the number of doses needed, and the recommended age when the vaccination should be administered.

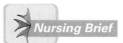

Nursing Brief

Immunizations must be stored/refrigerated correctly to ensure potency. Always check the route of administration for any vaccine because this varies.

PRECAUTIONS/SIDE EFFECTS

Precautions need to be taken when dealing with vaccines. Parents should be made aware of the possible side effects of various vaccines. These side effects are usually mild, and **the benefits of protection greatly outweigh the risks.** Other than the health care provider recommendation of the prophylactic use of acetaminophen or ibuprofen for fever or discomfort, no specific treatment is necessary. However, a persistent high fever, continued crying (longer than 3 hours), decrease in responsiveness, and/or possible seizure activity are **not** routine, and in any of these cases, the health care provider should be notified.

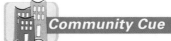

Community Cue

For vaccine information, the Immunization Action Coalition (*http://www.immunize.org*) provides extensive free provider and patient information, including translations of Vaccine Information Statements into multiple languages. In addition, suspected adverse effects of vaccinations should be reported to the Vaccine Adverse Events Reporting System (*http://www.vaers.org*) or by calling 800-822-7967.

Hepatitis B (Hep B) Vaccine. Hep B vaccine is given to the newborn before dismissal from the hospital. Some tenderness at the injection site and a mild temperature may be seen. Three doses are needed to ensure proper immunization. If the newborn's mother has a positive surface antigen for hepatitis B, the newborn will receive the hepatitis B vaccine as well as hepatitis B immune globulin (HBIG). Anaphylactic reaction to common baker's yeast is a contraindication to receiving Hep B. This vaccine is given intramuscularly.

Table 7-1 | *Immunization Doses Related to Age*

DOSE	AGE RECEIVED
HEP B	
First dose	Soon after birth; before hospital discharge
Second dose	1-2 mo
Third dose	≥24 weeks
DTAP	
First dose	2 mo
Second dose	4 mo
Third dose	6 mo
Fourth dose	15-18 mo
Fifth dose	4-6 yr
HIB	
First dose	2 mo
Second dose	4 mo
Third dose	6 mo
Fourth dose	12-15 mo
IPV	
First dose	2 mo
Second dose	4 mo
Third dose	6-18 mo
Fourth dose	4-6 yr
MMR	
First dose	12-15 mo
Second dose	4-6 yr
VARICELLA	
First dose	12-15 mo
Second dose	4-6 yr
PCV	
First dose	2 mo
Second dose	4 mo
Third dose	6 mo
Fourth dose	12-15 mo
HEPATITIS A	
First dose	12-23 mo
Second dose	6 mo after first dose
INFLUENZA	Yearly, starting at 6 mo
ROTAVIRUS	
First dose	2 mo
Second dose	4 mo
Third dose	6 mo
MENINGOCOCCAL	11-12 yr
HUMAN PAPILLOMAVIRUS (HPV)	
First dose	11-12 yr
Second dose	2 mo after first dose
Third dose	6 mo after first dose

Diphtheria-Tetanus-Pertussis Vaccine (DTP) and Diphtheria-Tetanus-Acellular Pertussis Vaccine (DTaP). DTaP contains acellular pertussis and is recommended for all doses in the series. Contraindications include encephalopathy within 7 days after administration of a previous dose of DTP/DTaP. Precautions include persistent, inconsolable crying that lasts for more than 3 hours and occurs within 48 hours of receiving a previous dose; seizures within 3 days after immunization; fever of 40.5° C (104.8° F) or above within 48 hours after the previous dose; or hypotonic-hyporesponsive episode within 48 hours of the previous dose (Hockenberry & Wilson, 2007). Possible side effects of DTaP include a mild fever and redness and swelling at the injection site. The infant/child may be fussy, and a slight decrease in appetite might be seen. These effects are temporary and should resolve in approximately 24 to 48 hours. DTaP requires excellent intramuscular injection technique to prevent complications. Pertussis vaccine is not given to children older than 7 years of age.

Haemophilus Influenzae Type B (Hib) Vaccine. The side effects from Hib vaccine are usually mild. There may be some redness at the injection site and a slight fever, which resolves itself within 2 to 3 days. Hib vaccine is administered as an intramuscular injection.

Polio Vaccine. Contraindications include anaphylactic reaction to neomycin, streptomycin, or polymyxin B. Pregnancy is a precaution with inactivated polio vaccine (IPV). In the past, the polio vaccine was given orally (OPV). Because several cases of active polio were related to the administration of OPV, the Advisory Committee for Immunization Practices of the Centers for Disease Control and Prevention, as of January 1, 2000, recommended the use of the IPV. The IPV is given as a subcutaneous or intramuscular injection. Side effects from polio vaccine are rare and consist of mild soreness at the site.

Mumps, Measles, and Rubella Vaccine (MMR). Contraindications include pregnancy, known altered immunodeficiency, or anaphylactoid reaction to neomycin, gelatin, or eggs. The MMR may be given to patients with HIV if they are not severely immune suppressed (Atkinson et al., 2002). The health care provider should be consulted regarding children who are sensitive to eggs. Measles vaccine may produce a fever and a rash, which occur about 7 to 12 days after vaccination and last only a few days. Encephalitis rarely occurs. The mumps vaccine has essentially no side effects other than an occasional mild fever. The rubella vaccine may produce a rash within a few days that may last 1 or 2 days. Joint pain and swelling can occasionally be seen about 2 weeks after vaccination. Be aware of the time delay. This is more common in older children. With the combination MMR, the side effects may include a mild fever, possibly a rash, and only occasionally mild swelling of the glands in the cheeks or the neck. MMR is administered subcutaneously.

Varicella Vaccine. This vaccine is contraindicated in immunocompromised individuals, in pregnancy, in children receiving steroids, and previous anaphylactic reaction to neomycin. However, the physician may recommend the varicella vaccine in individuals with HIV if the CD4+ T-lymphocyte count is high enough. Varicella vaccine is given at 12 to 18 months of age. Most individuals who receive the vaccine have a mild reaction. A mild vaccine-associated maculopapular or varicella rash can occur. Soreness and edema at the site and a mild fever may be the only reaction. The vaccine remains safer than the disease itself. Varicella vaccine is administered subcutaneously. NOTE: If the varicella and MMR vaccines are not given on the same day, the interval between the administrations should be at least 1 month.

Community Cue

The MMR and varicella vaccines can be safely administered to household members and caregivers of immunocompromised patients.

Pneumococcal Vaccine (PCV). This vaccine can cause fever, fussiness, or local erythema. It is given intramuscularly.

Hepatitis A Vaccine. Sensitivity to alum or phenoxyethanol is a contraindication. In some cases, local erythema (redness) may occur. Parents in high-risk areas need to have children (over the age of 2 years) immunized. This vaccine is administered with an intramuscular injection.

Influenza Vaccine. This intramuscular injection is recommended for children 6 months and older. For healthy persons aged 5 to 49 years, the live attenuated influenza vaccine (intranasal) may be used as an alternative. The influenza vaccine is contraindicated in children who have anaphylactic hypersensitivity to eggs.

Meningococcal Vaccine. The most frequent adverse reactions are pain and redness at the injection site. This intramuscular injection is contraindicated with known hypersensitivity to any component of the vaccine, including diphtheria toxoid.

Rotavirus Vaccine. This oral vaccine's precautions include altered immunocompetence, moderate to severe illness (including gastroenteritis), preexisting chronic gastrointestinal disease, and previous history of intussusception.

IMPORTANCE

Communicable diseases still pose a threat, and immunization of children is paramount. Community projects allow children to receive immunizations. Accurate records are crucial, and the parent or caregiver should keep a current immunization record for the child. Because a number of vaccines are recommended, several injections may be given at one time to an infant or child. Some vaccines protect the child from more than one disease. An example is the MMR. In addition, multiple vaccine administration during a visit does not increase the intensity or the number of side effects. Always remember to administer immunizations safely and efficiently. Children do not like "shots." The use of eutectic mixture of local anesthetics (EMLA) cream or a topical vapocoolant spray may help to decrease the pain at the injection site. See Chapter 17 for injection sites and technique.

CONCERNS

Thimerosal, a weak antibacterial agent and mercury-containing preservative used in some childhood vaccines since the 1930s, has recently been criticized because of concern over the rise of mercury toxicity in children. In 1999, the American Academy of Pediatrics, Public Health Service agencies, and vaccine manufacturers agreed that thimerosal should be reduced or eliminated in vaccines as a precautionary measure. Today, all routinely recommended pediatric vaccines manufactured in the U.S. market contain either no or only trace amounts of thimerosal (Centers for Disease Control and Prevention, 2003).

Autism is a developmental disability caused by an abnormality in the brain (see Chapter 10). Recently, an increase in the rate of autism has been seen. Although no one has an answer, some investigators believe that the MMR vaccine is associated with autism. However, multiple studies have failed to support an association between MMR vaccine and autism. In addition, the Centers for Disease Control and Prevention's National Immunization Program (2003) supports the findings that vaccines do not cause autism.

NUTRITION COUNSELING OF PARENTS

The nutrient needs of infants reflect rates of growth, energy expended in activity, basal metabolic needs, and the interaction of nutrients consumed. The baby is born with a rooting reflex, which assists in finding the nipple. The suck is rather immature because of the small mouth. There is a forward-and-backward movement of the tongue. As the infant grows, neural maturation of the cheeks and tongue enables advancement to a more mature sucking pattern that uses negative pressure to obtain milk. This occurs around the third or fourth month of age. At about this time, the extrusion reflex (protrusion), which pushes food out of the mouth to prevent intake of inappropriate food, disappears. The digestive system continues to mature. By 6 months, the digestive system is able to handle more complex nutrients and is less susceptible to food allergens. By 12 months, the stomach has expanded from 10 to 20 mL at birth to 200 mL. This increase enables the infant to consume more food at less frequent intervals. At first, most babies dislike spoon-feeding. In the beginning, they try to grasp the spoon. This gradually progresses until the child is able to scoop a little food, although the child still spills most of the contents. As the pincer grasp becomes more developed, the baby is able to pick up food with the fingers and place it in the mouth. By 2 years, the child has mastered spoon-feeding (Figure 7-3).

Parents have many concerns about feeding their infant during the first year of life. This is a time when parents are receptive to receiving nutritional education; as a result, the nurse should look for opportunities to

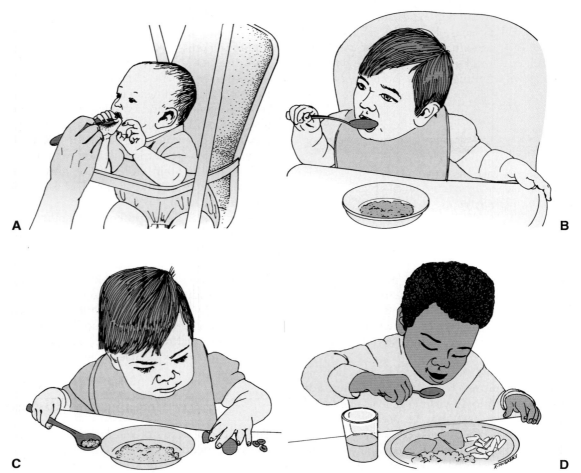

FIGURE **7-3** Development of feeding skills in infants and toddlers. **A,** At 7 months, the child shows beginning involvement with feeding and reaching for the spoon. **B,** At 9 months, the child is beginning to use the spoon independently, although there is difficulty in keeping food on it. **C,** The 9-month-old shows a refined pincer grasp to pick up food. **D,** The 2-year-old is much more skillful at self-feeding and has the ability to both rotate the wrist and elevate the elbow to keep food on the spoon.

provide sound nutritional information. It is important for the nurse to assess parental knowledge; infant development, behavior, and readiness; parent-child interactions; and cultural and ethnic practices. Nutrition care plans based on developmental levels assist parents in recognizing changes in feeding patterns. One means of assessing adequate intake is to determine whether the infant has gained 4 to 7 ounces per week for the first 6 months. Adequate hydration is evident by the infant having at least six wet diapers per day. After the feeding, the infant should fall asleep and have several hours of uninterrupted sleep. Continued monitoring of weight, height, and skinfold thickness determines whether or not the infant's diet is adequate. This can easily be done during the periodic well-baby examinations. Parents should be assured that although intake is rarely constant, varying in quantity and quality, most children do eat enough to grow normally. Forced feedings are not appropriate.

Infants need more calories, protein, minerals, and vitamins in proportion to their weight than do adults. Compared with an adult, the normal infant needs approximately three times more energy to maintain rapid growth and development. Breast milk and infant formula provide the young infant with the necessary calories (Behrman et al., 2004). Infants also have high fluid requirements. Human milk is the best food for infants of less than 6 months of age. It contains the ideal balance of nutrients in a readily digestible form (see Chapter 4). Iron-fortified infant formulas are also available. If an infant cannot tolerate milk-based formulas, soy protein–based formulas are available. These formulas are nutritionally sound and safe alternatives to cow's milk–based formulas. For the first year of life, infants should remain on human milk or iron-fortified formula. Whole cow's milk is not recommended for infants of less than 1 year of age because (1) it may create a potential for intolerance of whole milk protein; (2) an increased incidence rate of iron-deficiency anemia is associated with the intake of whole cow's milk; (3) the metabolism of whole cow's milk is difficult for the gastrointestinal tract; and (4) the high level of resulting solutes, which need to be excreted, places stress on the renal system.

SOLID FOODS

At about 4 to 6 months of age, solids are introduced. This introduction is based on the developmental readiness and the nutrient needs of the infant. Foods selected can either be commercial or home-prepared. The Home Care Tip box shows the sequence in which foods are added. Rice cereal is recommended as the first solid food because it is less allergenic than others. Three tablespoons of iron-fortified cereal mixed with breast milk or formula provide 7 mg of iron (more than half the daily requirement). Offer only small amounts at first (1 teaspoonful). Place food on the back of the infant's tongue. The consistency and amounts of solid foods are gradually increased as the infant becomes more familiar with them. *Never* mix cereal with formula in a bottle. The baby's spoon should have a long handle, and the body of the spoon should be small and shallow. Cereal is usually followed by fruits and vegetables (some parents like to introduce vegetables before fruits) and then meat. New foods should be introduced one at a time, with 4 to 7 days between each new food. This makes determination of food allergies easier if an intolerance is present.

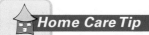

Home Care Tip

Guidelines for Introduction of Foods

1. Introduce iron-fortified baby rice cereal at about 4 to 6 months of age.
2. Add pureed vegetables and fruits, one at a time, at about 6 to 8 months (starting with vegetables may help to increase acceptance by the infant not yet exposed to the sweet taste of fruits).
3. Add pureed meats at about 6 to 8 months.
4. Add juice when the infant is old enough to drink from a cup, at about 6 months.
5. Add foods with more texture and finger foods at about 9 months (chopped meats, crackers, and so on).
6. Add allergenic foods, such as egg whites (or whole eggs), whole milk, and orange juice, after 1 year (especially important for the infant with a family history of allergies or asthma).

Modified from Peckenpaugh, N. (2003). *Nutrition essentials and diet therapy* (9th ed.). St. Louis: W.B. Saunders.

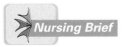

Nursing Brief

No scientific evidence supports the belief that cereal helps babies sleep through the night. Cereal should not be started before 4 to 6 months of age.

If the baby refuses a certain food, omit it temporarily. Keep mealtime pleasant. Let infants try new foods; they may like foods that the parent does not care to eat. Do not introduce new foods when the baby is ill. The amount of food consumed varies with each child.

Fruit juices are generally offered at about 6 months of age, when the infant begins to drink from a cup. An exception to this is the addition of orange juice. If family members have known allergies, orange juice is withheld until the baby is 1 year old. Other highly allergic foods that may be delayed include fish, nuts, strawberries, chocolate, and egg whites.

When the baby first begins to learn to drink from a cup, a spouted plastic cup can be helpful. Dilute the juice initially and then gradually increase the quantity to 3 to 4 ounces per day. The directions for preparing baby food at home are provided in the Home Care Tip box. Baby food can be prepared in a food grinder, blender, or food mill or by mashing the food until it is the desired texture.

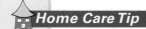

Home Care Tip

Directions for Home Preparation of Infant Foods

1. Select fresh, high-quality fruits, vegetables, or meats.
2. Be sure that all utensils, including cutting boards, grinder, knives, and the like, are thoroughly cleaned.
3. Wash hands before preparing the food.
4. Clean, wash, and trim the food in as little water as possible.
5. Cook the foods until tender in as little water as possible. Avoid overcooking, which may destroy heat-sensitive nutrients.
6. Do not add salt. Add sugar sparingly. Do not add honey or corn syrup to food intended for infants younger than 1 year of age. (Botulism spores have been reported in honey and corn syrup, and young infants do not have the immune capacity to resist this infection.)
7. Add enough water for the food to be easily pureed.
8. Strain or puree the food with an electric blender, a food mill, a baby food grinder, or a kitchen strainer.
9. Pour puree into an ice cube tray and freeze.
10. When the food is frozen hard, remove the cubes and store in freezer bags.
11. When ready to serve, defrost and heat in a serving container the amount of food to be consumed at a single feeding.

From Mahan, L.K., & Escott-Stump, S. (2007). *Krause's food, nutrition, and diet therapy* (12th ed.). Philadelphia: Saunders.

The infant's height and weight should progress at approximately the same rate. Variations may result from illness, malabsorption, psychological factors, overfeeding, and underfeeding. It is important to ascertain feeding procedures and practices regularly and to repeat essential information as indicated.

BUYING, STORING, AND SERVING FOOD

Baby foods stored in jars are vacuum-packed. When a jar is opened, a definite "pop" sound should be heard as the vacuum seal is broken. Also check the expiration date of the product. Dates are usually found on the caps of jars and on the sides of cereal and bakery items. Unopened jars of baby food and juices should be stored in a dry, cool place. Transfer food to a serving dish. Do not feed the infant from the jar or return leftovers to the jar because saliva may turn certain foods to liquid by digesting them in the jar. Unused portions may be stored in the refrigerator in the original jar. Special precautions should be taken to prevent burning when warming food in the microwave. When food is heated in the microwave, check its temperature because sometimes the food heats unevenly. Test all warmed foods. This can be done by tasting or by dropping a portion of a warmed liquid on the parent's inner wrist.

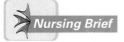

Human milk and properly prepared formula supply adequate water for the infant under normal conditions. In very hot, humid weather, the infant may need additional water.

WEANING FROM THE BREAST

Weaning is usually influenced by the mother's decision to discontinue breastfeeding or the infant's desire to breastfeed less often. Weaning is done gradually over several days or weeks. Weaning should start with daytime feedings; however, it should not be done during the first feeding of the day or the nighttime feeding. The experience should be made as pleasurable as possible for both the mother and the infant, which helps compensate for the loss of satisfaction from sucking. Weaning should not be attempted when the baby is ill. The mother can decrease her fluid consumption and the number of infant feedings and limit the time of the feeding to assist in decreasing her milk supply. Weaning from the breast is a changing point in the infant's life, and efforts should be made to make this experience as comfortable and as pleasurable as possible. Weaning is usually completed by age 1 to 2 years, although in some cultures it may continue longer.

TEETH

DECIDUOUS TEETH

The development of the 20 **deciduous teeth,** or baby teeth, begins around the fifth month of intrauterine life. The health and diet of the expectant mother affect their soundness. The 20 baby teeth erupt during the first 2½ years of life, beginning around the sixth month. It is a normal process and is generally accompanied by little or no discomfort. However, in healthy infants, there are wide individual differences in tooth eruption. A delay in teething is significant if other forms of immaturity or illness are present. The physician evaluates the process of teething during the baby's regular health checkups. The first tooth generally appears around the seventh month. The 1-year-old has about six teeth, four upper and two lower. The order in which the teeth appear is almost always the same (Figure 7-4). They are shed in about the same order in which they appear; that is, the lower central incisors first and so forth.

TEETHING DURING INFANCY

Teething refers to eruption of the crown of the tooth through the periodontal membrane. The gums may be red, swollen, and sensitive. The normal appearance of saliva and drooling at 4 months is frequently attributed to teething. However, drooling is more the result of the maturing of the salivary glands than teething. The first (deciduous) teeth act as a guide for the proper positioning of the secondary teeth. Teething does not cause infection, yet at this time, the infant's maternal antibody supply is low, making the child more prone to infection. The infant may be fussy and may wake during the night. Teething does not cause fever, nor is it responsible for respiratory tract infections, rashes, or diarrhea. Cold appears to soothe inflamed gums. A cool washcloth, a hard rubber teething ring, or a teething pretzel may bring relief. Acetaminophen or ibuprofen is useful when discomfort is clearly related to the teeth.

Good oral hygiene at this age consists of gently wiping the gums and teeth with gauze or a clean washcloth every day. Calcium, phosphorus, vitamins C and D, and fluoride help ensure healthy teeth. Bottle mouth caries is to be avoided; this can occur when an infant is regularly put to bed with a bottle of milk or sweetened juice. Sugar pools within the oral cavity, causing severe decay. It is seen most often in children between the ages of 18 months and 3 years. Eliminating the bedtime bottle or substituting water is recommended. A condition similar to nursing bottle caries is also seen in breastfed babies, particularly in infants who sleep with their mothers and nurse at will throughout the night. To prevent this, nocturnal nursing and frequent intermittent night feedings after the age of 1 year should be discouraged.

An additional cause of erosion of dental enamel is repeated exposure to gastric acids. This is now being recognized in infants with gastroesophageal reflux who are old enough to have teeth and also in teenagers with bulimia. When the effects of gastric acid are recognized early, the teeth can be protected with an acrylic sealant. In addition, parents need to be taught the tooth decaying effects of refined sugars, particularly those that are sticky and remain in the mouth for long periods of time.

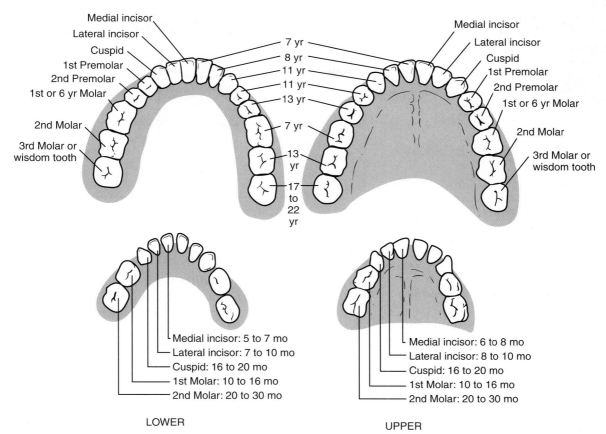

Medial incisor
Lateral incisor
Cuspid
1st Premolar
2nd Premolar
1st or 6 yr Molar

2nd Molar

3rd Molar or
wisdom tooth

7 yr
8 yr
11 yr
11 yr
13 yr

7 yr

13 yr

17 to 22 yr

Medial incisor
Lateral incisor
Cuspid
1st Premolar
2nd Premolar
1st or 6 yr Molar

2nd Molar

3rd Molar or
wisdom tooth

Medial incisor: 5 to 7 mo
Lateral incisor: 7 to 10 mo
Cuspid: 16 to 20 mo
1st Molar: 10 to 16 mo
2nd Molar: 20 to 30 mo

Medial incisor: 6 to 8 mo
Lateral incisor: 8 to 10 mo
Cuspid: 16 to 20 mo
1st Molar: 10 to 16 mo
2nd Molar: 20 to 30 mo

LOWER

UPPER

FIGURE **7-4** Eruption of permanent and deciduous teeth.

Key Points

- The first year of life involves many changes for both the infant and the family.
- Love and security are special needs of the infant.
- Stimulation of all the senses is an essential element in growth and development.
- Well-child visits are important to ensure promotion of health and prevention of disease.
- Recommended health care visits for the well infant begin soon after dismissal from the hospital, usually during the first two weeks of life and then at 1 month, 2 months, 4 months, 6 months, 9 months, and 12 months.
- Immunizations are an important aspect in the promotion of health for infants and children.
- By the age of 2 years, the child should be protected from more than 10 different communicable diseases if proper immunizations have been given.
- Considering the consequences of morbidity and mortality, the benefits of immunizations far exceed the risks.
- An adequate diet allows for proper growth and development.

- As the infant grows and develops, solid foods are introduced.
- As the diet of the infant changes, the needs for breastfeeding and formula also change.
- Weaning from the breast is a big turning point for the mother and the infant, and both individuals need to be considered during the process.
- There are 20 deciduous teeth. Teething begins around 5 to 7 months and continues until about 2½ years of age.

Go to your Companion CD-ROM for an Audio Glossary, video clips, and more.

  Be sure to visit the companion Evolve site at http://evolve.elsevier.com/Price/pediatric/ for WebLinks and additional online resources.

ONLINE RESOURCES

American Academy of Pediatrics: http://aap.org

Centers for Disease Control and Prevention: http://www.cdc.gov

Immunization Action Coalition: http://www.immunize.org

Vaccine Adverse Events Reporting System (VAERS): http://www.vaers.org

Objectives

Upon completion of this chapter, the student will be able to:

1. Define the vocabulary terms listed
2. List and discuss the more common disorders of infancy
3. Define the characteristics of the more common disorders of infancy
4. Summarize nursing care of common disorders of infancy
5. Summarize the nursing care for an infant who has infantile eczema and give the rationale for each nursing measure
6. Illustrate the anatomical difference in the ear canals of adults and children and describe the significance of this difference
7. Recommend four food sources of iron for an infant with iron-deficiency anemia
8. Explain why infants and young children are more easily dehydrated than adults
9. Define the characteristics of infants with failure to thrive
10. List four kinds of child abuse and describe the behaviors often exhibited by parent and child in each case

Key Terms

Be sure to check out the bonus material on the Companion CD-ROM, including selected audio pronunciations.

alkalosis (ĂL-kăh-LŌ-sĭs; p. 163)
anastomosis (ă-năs-tō-MŌ-sĭs; p. 161)
homeostasis (hō-mē-ō-STĀ-sĭs; p. 163)
hypotonic (hī-pō-TŎN-ĭk; p. 164)
incarcerated hernia (ĭn-KĂR-sĕr-ĀT-ĕd HĔR-nē-ăh; p. 156)
infarct (ĬN-fărkt; p. 145)
opisthotonos (ō-pĭs-THŎT-ō-nŏs; p. 165)
petechiae (pē-TĒ-kē-ē; p. 165)
respiratory syncytial virus (RSV; sĭn-SĬSH-ăl; p. 149)
syndrome of inappropriate antidiuretic hormone (SIADH; p. 165)
thrombosis (thrŏm-BŌ-sĭs; p. 145)

In infancy, children's immune systems are still developing, which can predispose them to a variety of infectious diseases. As children develop, the effect of the illnesses on this age group changes. A variety of congenital problems that present early in the child's life are also addressed in a discussion of this age group.

SKIN

ATOPIC DERMATITIS (INFANTILE ECZEMA)

Description

Atopic dermatitis is an inflammation of genetically hypersensitive skin. The pathophysiology is characterized by local vasodilation in affected areas. This progresses to **spongiosis,** or the breakdown of dermal cells and the formation of intradermal vesicles. Chronic scratching produces weeping and results in **lichenification,** or coarsening of the skin folds. The exact cause of this condition is unclear, but several factors may contribute to the condition. Factors can include a family history and/or triggers such as household aeroallergens (dust mites, cat dander, mold), environmental irritants (soaps, detergent, clothing, smoke), extreme temperatures, chemical vapors and gases, food sensitivities, and infections. Atopic dermatitis is seen less frequently in breastfed babies, and delaying introduction of solid food can decrease atopic dermatitis in the first 4 years of life. It seems to have a definite familial tendency, and emotional factors are often involved.

Development of symptoms indicate that the infant is oversensitive to certain substances called **allergens,** which enter the body via the digestive tract (food), by inhalation (dust, pollen), by direct contact (wool, soap, strong sunlight), or by injections (insect bites, vaccines). Of children who have atopic dermatitis, 50% to 60% present with symptoms in the first year of life and 80% to 85% present by 5 years of age. Overall, 10% to 20% of children are effected by the disease (Cardona et al., 2006). Many children (80%) develop the triad of atopic dermatitis, asthma, and allergic rhinitis.

Signs and Symptoms

The lesions form vesicles that weep and develop a dry crust. They are more severe on the face (Figure 8-1) but may occur on the entire body, particularly in the skin folds. Eczema is worse in winter than in the summer and has periods of temporary remission.

The infant scratches because the itching is constant and he or she becomes irritable and unable to sleep. The lesions are easily infected by bacterial or viral agents. Herpes simplex is the viral agent of particular concern.

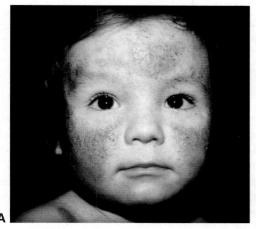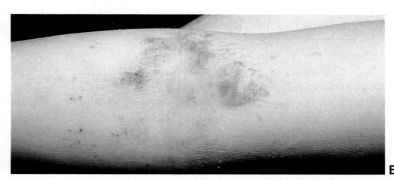

FIGURE **8-1** **A,** Infantile atopic dermatitis or eczema is shown with acute weeping lesions on the cheeks and forehead. **B,** In childhood, eczema can involve the flexor surfaces of extremities.

Infants and children with eczema should not be exposed to adults with "cold sores." Streptococcal and staphylococcal infection can also complicate the disease process. Eczema may flare up after immunization. Laboratory studies may show an increase in immunoglobulin E (IgE) and eosinophil levels.

Treatment

Treatment is aimed at maintaining the skin integrity, skin hydration, decreasing pruritus, and identification and avoidance of triggers. Treatment includes topical corticosteroids, topical immunosuppressants, and antihistamines. Corticosteroids vary from low potency to strong potency. They are used for different severities and areas of the body. Plastic wraps, snug-fitting clothes, or diapers can enhance the absorption of ointments. Topical immunosuppressants (tacrolimus or pimecrolimus) are effective on all body areas, and because they cause fewer side effects, they are appropriate for long-term usage. Antihistamines (Atarax, Benadryl) given at bedtime can help control nighttime itching and enhance sleep. Sleep deprivation is a major problem for children with atopic dermatitis. If pharmacological therapy is not effective, food allergies should be explored. Foods to which these infants may be sensitive include eggs, wheat, cow's milk, peanuts, and citrus fruits. If food allergies are identified, a restrictive diet may be required.

An emollient bath may provide a soothing effect on the infant's skin. Oatmeal and a mixture of cornstarch and baking soda are examples of substances prescribed. Tepid baths (15 to 20 minutes of soaking) and immediate application of emollient moisturizer afterward are key to skin hydration. Occlusive ointments such as Aquaphor, Eucerin, and Cetaphil are effective. Lotions are less effective and not recommended. Application of moisturizer while the skin is damp assists in hydration of the skin. Any lotions with alcohol should be avoided. A cool, wet dressing applied at night can help relieve itching and increase absorption of medication and moisturizers.

Nursing Care

The nurse plays a vital role in the treatment of patients with skin problems. During hospitalization infants with eczema are sometimes isolated for their own protection and may need additional attention. These infants are unhappy and irritable. They can tolerate the frustration of confinement more easily when their attention is diverted from their discomfort.

Children may need to be restrained if they are scratching the affected area. The kind of restraint used varies with the size and condition of the infant. Combinations of the elbow cuff, abdominal jacket, and ankle restraint are sometimes necessary. The least amount of restraint that accomplishes its purpose is the preferred choice. The restraints must be observed frequently to ensure that they are not interfering with proper circulation and removed periodically to allow for movement. Shortening fingernails and putting cotton mittens on hands and feet can be effective. The child's position must also be changed at frequent intervals to prevent pneumonia.

Medicated baths may be part of the treatment. Obtain towels and needed clothing in advance. Fill the tub and then run cold water through the faucet before turning the water off so that the handles are cool in the event that the infant grasps them. The bath should be 95° F (35° C). Place the infant in the tub for 15 to 20 minutes. Floating toys amuse the infant. **Remain with the infant at all times while the infant is in the tub.** The child should be patted or air-dried, not rubbed. Children with eczema should not be overdressed because undue warmth adds to their discomfort. One-piece soft clothing to prevent binding and irritation are recommended. Wool should be avoided.

Wet dressings are applied to reduce itching and in some cases to remove crusts. A gauze bandage is dipped into the prescribed solution (such as Burrow's solution), squeezed gently to remove excess fluid, and applied to the involved area. The bandage must cover the entire rash. Soaks are usually ordered to be done continuously, and their effectiveness depends on their being *wet*. When they are left on too long and become dried out, itching increases. This type of bandage is **not** covered with towels or rubber sheeting in an effort to protect the bed linens because the itching is relieved by the cooling effect of the medication, and covering the bandage prevents evaporation.

Wet compresses may also be applied to the face with a mask, which consists of a square piece of gauze material with openings cut out for the eyes, nose, and mouth. The mask is held in place by strings attached to the four corners. When a change of wet bandages is necessary, they are completely removed, soaked in the solution, and reapplied. Observations for the nurse to chart regarding the application of wet soaks include time of application, name of solution, strength of solution, area to which it was applied, length of time applied, general condition of the involved area (changes in the appearance or area of the rash), and comfort and tolerance of the patient during and after the procedure.

Ointments, creams, or moisturizers are used to hydrate the skin. They should be applied to damp skin after a bath. If bathing appears to worsen the skin condition, a dry bath with a nonsoap cleanser may be preferred.

The physician may prescribe an elimination diet. A basic diet consisting of only hypoallergenic foods is given to the child initially. One new food at a time is added to determine the infant's reaction. When the baby is allergic to cow's milk, a substitute such as soybean milk can be used. Vitamin supplements are needed, particularly if the infant is not consuming enough of the prescribed fruits and vegetables. The nurse charts the kind and amount of food taken at each meal and any allergic reactions that may have occurred. Plan the time so that treatments do not interfere with mealtime. Elbow restraints are removed from the toddler who is able to eat alone. The nurse assists with the patient's meals and prevents the scratching of irritated skin. Infants are held and loved during feedings because an emotional climate that discourages tension is important to the recovery of these patients.

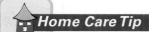

Home Care Tip

The Child with Atopic Dermatitis (Eczema)

- Use tepid water for bathing.
- Avoid irritating soaps.
- Avoid washcloths or scrubs.
- Air-dry skin and pat with soft towel.
- Apply topical corticosteroid before emollient.
- Apply emollient within 3 minutes of bath.
- Keep fingernails short and clean.
- Use cotton gloves at night.
- Use cotton sheets and pajamas.
- Moisturize skin often until skin is soft and pliable.
- Use mild laundry detergent.
- Discontinue topical corticosteroid when skin clears.

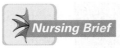

Nursing Brief

An effective moisturizer that is also inexpensive is Crisco shortening (Cardona et al., 2006)

The nurse should establish a good working relationship with the parents. Families report high stress and feelings of helplessness in caring for children with atopic dermatitis. Parents express issues with the child's sleeplessness due to itching and the child's decreased self-esteem due to their physical appearance. Parents indicate increased family financial and work problems as a result of numerous doctors' appointments. The nurse should listen to ensure that parents understand the physician's instructions and should clarify matters as needed (Nursing Care Plan 8-1).

IMPETIGO
Description
Impetigo is an infectious disease of the skin caused by staphylococci or by group A beta-hemolytic streptococci. There are two classifications: **bullous** (impetigo bullosa) and **nonbullous** (impetigo contagiosa). Both forms are generally seen in children ages 2 to 5 years. The bullous form, seen primarily in infants, is usually caused by *Staphylococcus aureus*, whereas the nonbullous type can been seen in children of all ages and is caused by either staphylococci or streptococci. Impetigo tends to spread from one area of skin to another and is quite contagious.

Signs and Symptoms
The first symptoms of a nonbullous lesion are red papules (Figure 8-2). These eventually became small vesicles or pustules surrounded by a reddened area. When the blister breaks, the surface beneath is raw and weeping and appears like a second-degree burn. The lesions may occur anywhere but are most often found on the face, neck, and extremities. A honey-colored crust forms.

Bullous lesions present as vesicles that become fluid-filled. The fluid sack can be tense or flaccid. It eventually ruptures, collapses, and leaves a base with a peeling rim (Figure 8-3). Both forms can cause itching, and the resulting scratching can spread the lesions.

Treatment and Nursing Care
The lesions may be cleaned three or four times a day with soap and water to remove crusts. This cleansing is followed by the application of topical antibiotic ointment (Bactroban). Oral antibiotics may also be given (dicloxacillin, Zithromax, or Keflex). The prognosis with proper treatment is good. Nursing care consists primarily of preventing this disease with proper **aseptic** methods. Once the diagnosis is made, preventing spread to other infants and children

NURSING CARE PLAN 8-1

The Child with Atopic Dermatitis (Eczema)

NURSING DIAGNOSIS *Imbalanced nutrition: less than body requirements related to irritability, sensitivity to certain foods, and increased metabolic needs*

Goals/Outcome Criteria	Nursing Interventions	Rationales
The child has an adequate diet, as evidenced by: • Maintenance of weight or an increase in weight • Eating at least 60% of diet for age	Assess diet according to age. Determine with history whether the child is sensitive to any specific foods. Administer hypoallergenic diet. Observe child for any food sensitivity. Administer vitamins and minerals as prescribed. Provide adequate fluids.	As the child grows, the nutritional needs change. Food sensitivity can trigger a stronger response to the condition. Hypoallergenic foods have been found to be less offensive to many people. Any food item can be a potential substance to which the body is sensitive. May be given in supplemental form to aid the body in healing and growth. Fluids are important to the child because the child's body is made up of a higher percentage of fluids than the adult's. If fluid is lost through the skin, the child can easily become dehydrated.

NURSING DIAGNOSIS *Deficient knowledge related to the nature of the disorder*

Goals/Outcome Criteria	Nursing Interventions	Rationales
The parents understand the nature of the disorder, as evidenced by: • Ability to verbalize the information given to them • Asking questions • Describing the care of and, the skin	Assess the knowledge of the parents. Instruct the parents in the care of the child's skin: • Remove clothing that might irritate the skin (e.g., wool). • Provide loose cotton clothing. • Use a mild detergent to launder clothing. • Thoroughly rinse clothing. • Bathe the child in tepid water. Expose infant to sunlight but monitor closely. Help parents identify products that contain wheat, milk, eggs, and peanuts. Advise parents to expect exacerbations and remissions.	Allows the nurse to teach the parents. These are all areas that decrease the irritation to the skin or aid in healing of the skin. Wool is an irritant to the skin. Cotton absorbs if it is loose, does not constrict. Decreases the irritation of soap in the clothing. Ensures that most of the soap is removed from the clothing. Tepid water decreases the amount of vasodilation, thus causing a decrease in stimulation to the skin and resulting in a decrease in itching. Sunlight can be healing to the skin, but because of the skin's condition, too much sunlight can cause more irritation. These foods have been found to cause allergic reactions in children. Eczema can recur. If the parents know this, treatment can be sought earlier and the intensity of the condition can be lessened.

NURSING DIAGNOSIS *Risk for impaired skin integrity related to scratching and irritation of the skin*

Goals/Outcome Criteria	Nursing Interventions	Rationales
The child is free of skin infection, as evidenced by: • Intact skin • Skin warm, dry, and pink • Skin free of discharge	Assess the skin. Describe any type of lesions. Provide elbow restraints. Hold and comfort the child as needed.	Reveals any breaks in the skin, discharge, or lesions. Allows the lesions to be monitored to see whether the condition improves or worsens. Helps the child refrain from scratching. A proper fit is important. Restraints should *never* be used in place of supervision. The child may be irritable and restless because of the condition of the skin. Holding and consoling may help the child rest.

Continued

NURSING CARE PLAN 8-1—cont'd

The Child with Atopic Dermatitis (Eczema)—cont'd

NURSING DIAGNOSIS *Risk for impaired skin integrity related to scratching and irritation of the skin—cont'd*

Goals/Outcome Criteria	Nursing Interventions	Rationales
	Keep the child's fingernails short and cover hands with a sock or mitten.	Decreases the child's ability to scratch.
	Administer medicated baths as ordered.	Soothing to the skin.
	Apply dressings and teach parents proper application.	Soothing and healing for the skin.
	Administer antibiotics as ordered.	Used to prevent or resolve a skin infection.
	Teach parents the importance of proper handwashing.	Handwashing decreases the transfer of organisms.

CRITICAL THINKING QUESTION

■ A mother of an 8-month-old child comes to the clinic for a follow-up appointment. She tells the nurse that the doctor told her the baby had eczema. She says that she has been giving her baby a bath in hot, soapy water twice a day. She is putting hand lotion on the lesions, but they seem to be getting worse. She cannot seem to stop the baby from scratching. What teaching interventions by the nurse would be appropriate?

CRITICAL THINKING SNAPSHOT

In evaluating this child with eczema, what are important areas that need to be documented? How should the description of the lesions be noted? What would be expected if the lesions worsen? What are symptoms that would warrant the parent seeking immediate medical treatment?

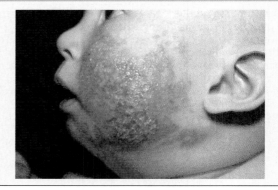

---

becomes an issue. Parents need instructions regarding mode of transmission, which is person-to-person, and preventive measures. Glomerulonephritis may occur as a complication of beta-hemolytic streptococcal infections.

STAPHYLOCOCCUS AUREUS INFECTION

Description

The bacterial genus *Staphylococcus* comprises common bacteria that are found in dust and on the skin. In normal conditions, they do not present a problem to healthy body defenses. If the number of organisms increases in infants whose general resistance is low, skin infections may occur. Neonates have fragile skin that can be traumatized with the use of electrodes or lancets. For the critically ill newborn technological advances such as indwelling catheters or hyperalimentation can provide routes for infection. An infection or abscess

(**cellulitis**) may form, and in some cases of delayed treatment, infection may enter the bloodstream. This condition is called **septicemia** or **bacteremia**. Pneumonia, osteomyelitis, or meningitis may result. Infection may spread easily from one infant to another in the newborn nursery. Pustules must be reported and appropriate isolation precautions taken to prevent further exposure.

Treatment and Nursing Care

Antibiotics effective against the particular strain are administered. Ointments may be applied locally. Some of the staphylococci have developed resistance to current drugs. Methicillin-resistant *S. aureus* (MRSA) infections have developed. When MRSA is diagnosed, vancomycin has been used. Some of these strains have become vancomycin-resistant (VRSA). There are drugs in trials that have shown promising results with both the MRSA and VRSA infections (Smith, 2005).

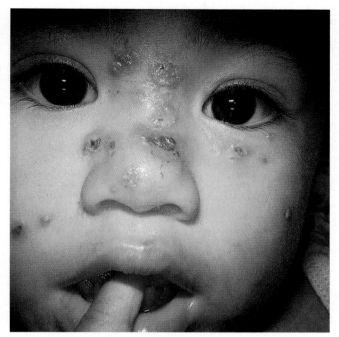

FIGURE **8-2** Lesion of impetigo contagiosa (nonbullous) on the child's face, showing the honey-colored crust.

This resistance presents difficulty in treatment and has prompted the careful use of antibiotics. Three distinctive disorders have been identified: staphylococcal scalded skin syndrome, staphylococcal scarlet fever, and toxic shock syndrome (Table 8-1; Figure 8-4).

Control of the spread of this infection is sometimes difficult because health care providers can act as carriers. The chief reservoir in the carrier for harboring this organism is the nose. To prevent staphylococcal infections, strict standards must be upheld in all facilities. The number and quality of personnel and their health status are also important factors. Washing hands before and after touching each patient and before and after handling equipment is **essential** and supported by the CDC. Medical follow-up remains important for these patients.

EARS

OTITIS MEDIA
Description

Otitis media (*ot,* ear; *itis,* inflammation of; *media,* middle) is an inflammation of the middle ear. The middle ear is a tiny cavity in the temporal bone. Its entrance is guarded by the sensitive tympanic membrane, or eardrum, which

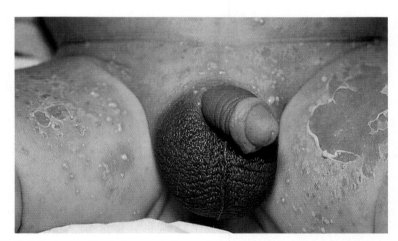

FIGURE **8-3** Infant with *Staphylococcus* diaper dermatitis has multiple small, thin-walled pustules that rupture rapidly, leaving a shallow base and superficial peeling rims.

Table 8-1 | *S. Aureus Infections*

TYPE	SIGNS AND SYMPTOMS	SKIN MANIFESTATIONS	TREATMENT
Scalded skin syndrome	Sudden onset of fever and irritability; vomiting	Generalized erythema, tender to touch, bullous lesions; skin sloughs	Antibiotics (e.g., vancomycin); fluids
Staphylococcus scarlet fever	Fever; irritability; malaise	Erythematous rash (sandpaper) in skin creases; skin cracks, weeps, and sheds	Oral antibiotics
Toxic shock syndrome	Life threatening; abrupt fever with vomiting and abdominal pain; multiorgan involvement and dysfunction; hypotension	General exanthema with macular rash; strawberry tongue; sloughing of skin	Antibiotics; fluids; cardiovascular and respiratory monitoring

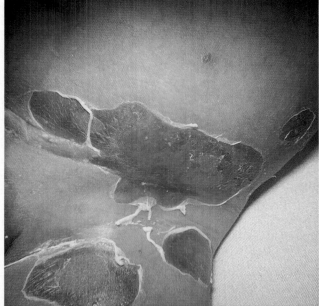

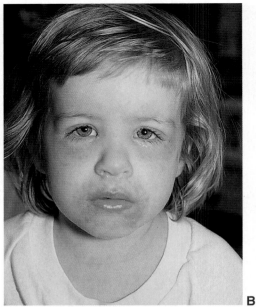

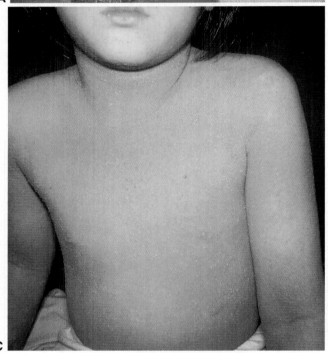

FIGURE **8-4 A,** The borders of the exfoliating skin look like rolled wet tissue paper in a child with staphylococcal scalded skin syndrome. **B,** A child with staphylococcal scarlet fever shows skin beginning to crack, fissure, and weep serous fluids. **C,** The diffuse macular skin eruption in a child with staphylococcal toxic shock syndrome.

the outside atmosphere. These protective functions are diminished when the tubes are blocked. Unequalized air within the ear creates a negative pressure that allows organisms to be swept up into the tube if it opens.

Otitis media may be the result of an upper respiratory tract infection, caused by a variety of organisms. About 40% to 50% of the infections are viral. Bacteria cause the rest of otitis media cases. Of the bacterial cases, 40% to 50% are caused by *Streptococcus pneumoniae,* which is increasingly demonstrating resistance to penicillin. Other common bacteria that cause otitis media are *Haemophilus influenzae* and *Moraxella catarrhalis.* With the use of *H. influenzae* type b vaccine (Hib) as a routine immunization, the number of cases of otitis media caused by this organism has decreased. The addition of the seven-valent *S. pneumoniae* conjugate vaccine to the immunization schedule should also decrease the incidence rate of otitis media caused by this organism (Smith, 2005). Infants are more prone to ear infections because the eustachian tube is shorter, wider, and straighter than in older children and adults. Because babies lie flat for long periods, microorganisms have easy access from the eustachian tube to the middle ear. This is thought by some investigators to be a contributing factor.

There are two types of otitis media. The acute disease is **suppurative** or **purulent otitis media (AOM).** It is most commonly caused by *S. pneumoniae* and *H. influenzae.* The second type is called **serous** or **nonsuppurative otitis media with effusion (OME).** The cause is unknown, but

transmits sound waves through the oval window to the inner ear. The inner ear contains the organs of hearing and balance. The middle ear opens into air spaces, or **sinuses,** in the mastoid process of the temporal bone. It is also connected to the throat by a channel called the **eustachian tube.** These structures—the mastoid sinuses, the middle ear, and the eustachian tube—are lined with mucous membranes. As a result, an infection of the throat can easily spread to the middle ear and mastoid. The eustachian tube also protects the middle ear from nasopharyngeal secretions and provides drainage of middle ear secretions into the nasopharynx and equalizes air pressure between the middle ear and it often occurs after an acute episode. OME is the most common cause of hearing loss and hearing impairment in children.

Signs and Symptoms

The symptoms of acute otitis media (AOM) are pain in the ear (often severe), irritability, and interference with hearing. Sucking or chewing has a tendency to increase the pain. Fever, which may run as high as 40° C (104° F), headache, and vomiting may also accompany the illness as may diarrhea. The nurse may suspect an earache in the infant who rubs the ear frequently or pulls at it. The infant may also roll the head from side to side and cry piercingly. The older child can point to the place that is tender. OME is the result of chronic otitis media. Children may be asymptomatic but may report a feeling of fullness or popping in the ears.

If an abscess forms, the eardrum may rupture as a result and pus may drain from the ear. When this happens, the pressure is relieved and the patient is more comfortable.

Complications of an ear infection include hearing loss, mastoiditis, chronic otitis media, and meningitis. These complications are rare with modern treatment. Prevention lies in the prompt treatment of respiratory infections or infected tonsils and adenoids.

Treatment and Nursing Care

The professional who examines the ears first observes their appearance and general hygiene. The lymph nodes about the ear are observed for swelling or tenderness. The patient's head is adequately stabilized to prevent injury to the ear canal from sudden, unexpected movement. Excess cerumen or wax in the ear, which may obstruct visibility, is carefully removed. The examiner ensures that no foreign bodies are lodged in the outer canal before inserting the otoscope. To straighten the canal and improve viewing, the ear is pulled **down** and **back** in infants and small children. The ear is pulled **up** and **back** in older children and adults. The physician may also perform a pneumatic otoscopic examination. The ear speculum is used to seal the ear canal, and air is expressed into the canal. The movement or lack of movement of the tympanic membrane is indicative of the degree of fluid behind the membrane. This examination has proven useful in determining the degree of the condition.

New treatment guidelines were released in 2004 by the American Academy of Pediatrics (AAP) (Box 8-1). Treatment included an observation option, pain management, and antibiotic treatment. Development of resistant strains of bacteria and misuse of antibiotics assisted in the development of new guidelines. When antibiotics are used, amoxicillin remains the drug of choice, but recurrent infections may require other antibiotics. Parents are taught to give the entire dose of the antibiotic even though the child may appear well. Parents will need to understand the new course of treatment using the guidelines and their role in the management of AOM.

Box 8-1	*Acute Otitis Media Guidelines*

- Diagnosis of AOM by history, signs and symptoms
- Assessment of pain and pain management for first 24-36 hours
- Optional treatment course of observation for 48-72 hours without antibacterial treatment; if patient fails to respond within 48-72 hours, antibacterial therapy should be started
- Treatment using antibacterial agent; high-dose amoxicillin is recommended
- Encouragement of prevention by reducing risk factors
- Insufficient evidence to recommend use of complementary and alternative medicine (AAP, 2004)

Pain control may be needed for the child with otitis media. Pain control is achieved using acetaminophen or ibuprofen. Antihistamines and decongestants are not effective and may have side effects. Eardrops (Auralgan) may be prescribed to control pain. Warm or cold compresses may be applied to the ear. The child can be placed on the affected side with the ear on top of a hot water bottle (temperature of the water 115° F, or 46° C) or on a heating pad on the low setting. Children should be placed upright to decrease pain. If the ear is draining, the outer canal can be cleaned with sterile water or hydrogen peroxide. Parents should be instructed not to use cotton swabs in the ears.

Nurses need to be aware that environmental factors have been identified that can contribute to the risk for ear infections. Daycare outside the home, parental smoking, and pacifier use has been shown to increase the risk for recurrent otitis media. Breastfeeding for at least 6 months has reduced the risk for AOM. These factors should be discussed with parents.

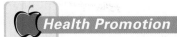

Health Promotion

Risks for Otitis Media That Need to Be Discussed with Parents

- Parental smoking
- Excessive pacifier use
- Daycare outside home

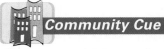

Community Cue

Parents may wish to use alternative therapies in the care of their child. Many of the herbal remedies available have not been evaluated for use in the pediatric population. These remedies are not regulated by the U.S. Food and Drug Administration (FDA) and thus may not be as labeled. Homeopathy remedies are regulated. The AAP has not made any recommendation because of insufficient evidence of effectiveness.

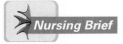

For children with recurrent AOM or chronic OME, **tympanostomy tubes** may be effective. The physician performs the procedure by completing a **myringotomy** (*myringo,* eardrum; *otomy,* incision) and inserts a tiny tube into the eardrum. These tubes require surgical placement and special care by the parents. Eventually, the tubes fall out spontaneously.

HEMATOLOGIC SYSTEM

IRON-DEFICIENCY ANEMIA
Description

The most common nutritional deficiency of children in the United States today is anemia caused by insufficient amounts of iron in the body. The incidence rate has decreased in infants as a result of the use of iron-fortified formulas and cereals. Toddlers and adolescent girls remain at risk because of rapid growth and inadequate iron intake. Anemia (*an,* without; *emia,* blood) is a condition in which there is a reduction in the amount and size of the red blood cells or in the amount of hemoglobin or both. The clinical features are related to the decrease in the oxygen-carrying capacity of the blood. Iron is needed for the manufacture of red blood cells. Iron-deficiency anemia may be caused by severe hemorrhage, the child's inability to absorb the iron received, excessive growth requirements, or an inadequate diet. Researchers have also found that whole cow's milk can precipitate gastrointestinal (GI) bleeding in some babies.

Prevention of iron-deficiency anemia begins with good prenatal care to ensure that the mother has a suitable intake of iron during pregnancy. For the first few months after birth, the newborn infant relies on iron that was stored in the system during fetal life. Iron is obtained late in the prenatal period, which has an effect on the infant's iron stores. Premature infants can deplete their iron stores by as early as 2 months of age. The normal term infant who receives unfortified formula depletes iron stores by about age 4 or 5 months. Breastfed infants rarely deplete their iron stores until after 6 months.

The highest incidence of this type of anemia occurs from months 9 to 24. During this period of rapid growth, the baby outgrows the limited iron reserve that was in the body; in addition, iron-fortified formula and infant cereals may have been eliminated from the diet. Poorly planned meals or feeding problems also contribute to this deficiency. The mother may rely too much on bottle feedings to avoid conflict at meals. Unfortunately, cow's milk contains very little iron. Instead, the amounts of solid food should be increased and the milk decreased. Boiled egg yolk, liver, green leafy vegetables; iron-fortified cereal, dried fruits (apricots, peaches, prunes, and raisins); cooked, dried beans; crushed nuts; and whole-grain bread are good sources of iron. Iron-fortified cereals eaten out of the box provide a nutritious snack.

The child's hemoglobin level is usually less than 10 g/dL. Children may have much lower hemoglobin levels before they show signs and symptoms. Typically, blood tests are done for hemoglobin, hematocrit, morphological changes in red blood cells, and iron concentration. A dietary history is also important in the diagnosis.

Signs and Symptoms

The symptoms of iron-deficiency anemia are pallor, irritability, anorexia, and a decrease in activity. Many babies are overweight because of excess consumption of milk (so-called milk babies or milkaholics). These infants may look flabby and pale. Sometimes a slight heart murmur is heard. The spleen may be enlarged. Untreated iron-deficiency anemia progresses slowly. In severe cases, the heart muscle becomes too weak to function. If this happens, heart failure follows. Screening procedures are suggested at 9 to 24 months for full-term infants and earlier, at 6 to 9 months, for low–birth weight babies.

Treatment

Iron-deficiency anemia responds well to treatment. The physician must first differentiate it from other types of anemia. Iron, usually ferrous sulfate, is given orally two or three times a day between meals. Vitamin C aids in the absorption of iron; therefore juice that is enriched with vitamin C or that naturally contains vitamin C is suggested. Read information concerning the administration of iron preparations. Some liquid preparations are taken through a straw to prevent temporary discoloration of the teeth. Recently, most available iron preparations do not have this disadvantage. Calcium interferes with the absorption of iron; therefore milk should not be given during iron supplement administration. Intramuscular iron is given in cases of malabsorption and when noncompliance with the oral route is a problem. Most children can tolerate the oral drug, and parents should be educated about the importance of compliance so the painful injections can be avoided. The injectable drug is an iron-dextran mixture (Imferon) that must be injected deep in a large muscle, with **Z-track technique** to minimize staining and irritation.

Follow-up evaluation is important. Treatment with the iron preparation is recommended for 6 to 8 weeks after the laboratory values return to normal levels. The time frame is usually about 5 months.

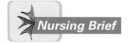

Parent Education

Parents need explicit instructions regarding the proper foods for the infant. The nurse stresses the importance of using iron-fortified formula throughout the first year of life (iron is absorbed much better from human milk than from cow's milk). Discourage the use of cow's milk before 12 months of age. The amount of milk consumed during the night and during the day is determined. Infants over 6 months of age receiving formula should not take more than 32 ounces per day. If they are receiving fresh cow's milk, the amount should be less—about 16 to 24 ounces per day. Dispel the myth that milk is a perfect food. Infants should be started on solid foods at 6 months. Review solid food intake and suggest specific iron-enriched nutrients. Consider financial, ethnic, and family preferences in discussions. The child's behavior at mealtime may also need to be addressed.

The stools of babies who are taking iron are a tarry green color. Absence of this finding may indicate poor compliance with therapy by the parents. Oral iron preparations are not to be given with milk, which interferes with absorption. These preparations also should not be given with meals. **It is important to emphasize that both dietary changes and supplemental iron therapy are necessary to eradicate iron-deficiency anemia.** Dietary changes must be lifelong to maintain good health and to prevent recurrence. Iron supplements are given until the prescription expires. Parents are encouraged to return for periodic evaluation of the child's blood status. They are also advised to remind new physicians of the condition, even though it may currently be rectified. During discussions, nurses should attempt to support parents, who usually have guilt feelings or believe they are not successful parents. It may be comforting for the nurse to reiterate that most babies are in the process of catching up on iron supplies and that the condition is not uncommon.

SICKLE CELL DISEASE
Description

Sickle cell disease (SCD) is an inherited defect in the formation of hemoglobin. It occurs mainly in populations of African descent but is also carried by some people of Arabian, Greek, Maltese, and Sicilian descent or other Mediterranean groups. Sickling caused by decreases in blood oxygen may be triggered by dehydration, infection, physical or emotional stress, or exposure to cold. Laboratory examination of the affected child's blood shows that the red blood cell has changed its shape to resemble that of a sickle blade, from which the name of the disorder is derived (Figure 8-5). These cells contain an abnormal form of hemoglobin, termed *hemoglobin* S (the sickling type). The membranes of these cells are fragile and easily destroyed. Their crescent shape makes it difficult for them to pass through the capillaries, causing a pile-up of cells in the small vessels. This clumping together may lead to a thrombosis (clot) and cause an obstruction. Infarcts, or areas of dead tissue, may result when the tissue is denied proper blood supply. These generally develop in the spleen but may also be seen in other areas of the body, such as the brain, heart, lungs, GI tract, kidneys, and bones. The patient feels pain in the affected area.

There are two types of sickle cell disorders: an **asymptomatic** (*a*, without; *symptoma*, symptom) version, referred to as **sickle cell trait,** and a much more severe form requiring intermittent hospitalization termed **sickle cell disease.** There are a variety of screening methods. Electrophoresis and high-performance liquid chromatography (HPLC) are most commonly used.

Sickle Cell Trait. This form of the disease occurs in about 10% of the African-American population in the United States. The blood of the patient contains a mixture of normal (hemoglobin A) and sickle (hemoglobin S) hemoglobins. The proportions of hemoglobin S are low because the disease is inherited from only one parent. The physician can distinguish sickle cell trait from the more severe form by studying the patient's red blood cells and hemoglobin. In sickle cell trait, the hemoglobin and red blood cell counts are normal. Although there is no need for treatment of the mild form, the patient is a carrier and genetic counseling is important. Advice might be sought from a family physician, pediatrician, or genetic specialist. The nurse encourages and supports such efforts made by the parents. The importance of regular visits to a well-child clinic or family-centered clinic is stressed.

Sickle Cell Disease. This severe form of the disease results when the child inherits the abnormal gene from each parent (Figure 8-6). **Each offspring** has one chance in four of inheriting the disease (not one of four children). The incidence rate is about 1 in 600 African Americans. The symptoms generally do not appear until the last part of the first year of life, although they may occur as early as 1 month. The first symptom may be an unusual swelling of the fingers and toes called hand-foot syndrome or **dactylitis** (Figure 8-7). Damage to the kidney's ability to concentrate urine can occur and lead to increased urination in children. Small children with SCD are difficult to toilet-train and may wet the bed for several years. When this is explained to parents as a side effect of the disease, they may be more able to accept the problem. Teenagers and adults with SCD may develop painful, slow-healing ulcers on the lower legs, particularly on the ankles.

Chronic anemia is present, which is why the disease may be referred to as sickle cell anemia. The

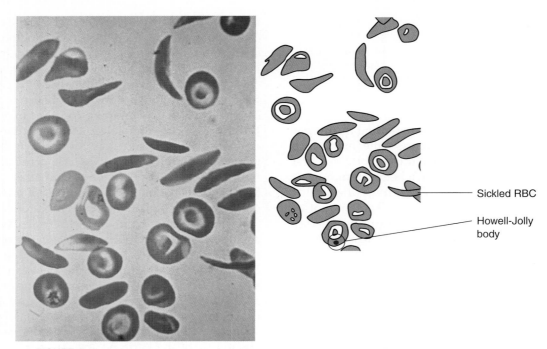

FIGURE **8-5** Peripheral blood smear from a black child with hemoglobin with SCD. Note the sickle cells.

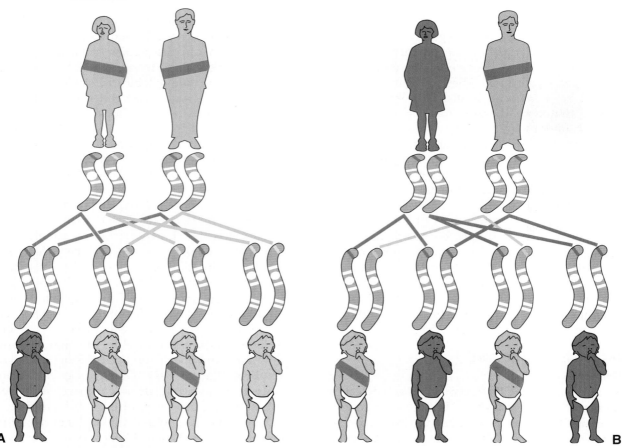

FIGURE **8-6** Genetic inheritance of SCD. **A,** When both parents are heterozygous for the hemoglobin S gene, there is a 25% probability that each child conceived will have the disease and a 50% probability that each child conceived will have the sickle cell trait. In addition, there is a 25% probability that each child conceived will have normal hemoglobin. **B,** When one parent is heterozygous and the other parent is homozygous for the hemoglobin S gene, there is a 50% probability that each child conceived will have the disease and a 50% probability that each child conceived will have the sickle cell trait.

Table 8-2 | *Summary of Types of Sickle Cell Events*

TYPE	CHARACTERISTICS	SYMPTOMS
Vasoocclusive crisis	Most common; not life threatening; obstruction of circulation; resulting in ischemia, necrosis, and infarctions	Pain, fever, dactylitis, bone and joint pain, abdominal pain, cardiovascular accident, priapism
Acute chest syndrome	Pulmonary infarcts	Chest pain, cough, fever, hypoxia, tachypnea
Dactylitis (hand-foot syndrome)	Infarction of short tubular bones, self-limiting, occurs in children 6 months to 4 years	Localized swelling of hands and feet
Acute splenic sequestration	Acute, episodic event where, for unknown reasons, blood pools in the spleen, which can result in life-threatening circulatory collapse and death; commonly preceded by acute febrile illness	Enlarged spleen, pallor, irritability, weakness, dyspnea, tachycardia, hypotension
Aplastic episodes	Diminished production of red blood cells, usually caused by viral or bacterial infection	Pallor, lethargy, faintness, anemia

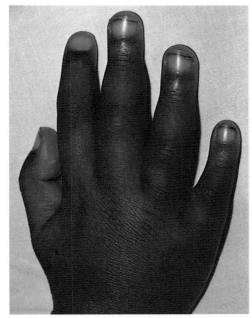

FIGURE 8-7 Hand-foot syndrome (dactylitis) in a 3-year-old child with SCD. This syndrome is primarily seen in infants and toddlers and is less frequent in the older child.

hemoglobin level ranges from 6 to 9 g/dL or lower. The child is pale, tires easily, and loses appetite. These manifestations of anemia are complicated by what is termed the **sickle cell crisis,** which can be fatal. A number of types of crises have been defined. They differ in pathology and may require somewhat different treatment (Table 8-2). Unfortunately, in some cases, the sickle cell crisis is the first evidence of the condition. For this reason, all 50 states screen all newborn infants. State screening coordinators may contact the pediatrician. Parents should be informed about the disease, the care of the child, and if necessary, a referral to a comprehensive sickle cell center (Fixler & Styles, 2002). Regularly scheduled health visits, penicillin prophylaxis, and immunizations including influenza, pneumococcal, and meningococcal vaccine should be stressed with the parents.

In a sickle cell crisis, the patient appears acutely ill with severe abdominal pain. Muscle spasms, leg pains, or painful swollen joints may be seen. Fever, vomiting, hematuria, convulsions, stiff neck, coma, or paralysis can result, depending on the organs involved. The patient may be jaundiced. Cardiac enlargement and murmurs are not uncommon. The sickle cell crises recur periodically throughout childhood; however, they tend to decrease with age. Between episodes, patients should be kept in good health. They should refrain from becoming overly tired. They also should avoid situations such as flying in an unpressurized airplane or exercising at high altitude because oxygen concentrations are already reduced in the blood. Added stress and exposure to cold may lower resistance, causing additional problems. Overheating, which can lead to dehydration, should also be avoided.

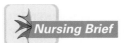

Nursing Brief

During crises, anticipate a child's need for hydration, rest, protection from infection, pain control, blood transfusions, and emotional support for life-threatening illness.

Treatment and Nursing Care

When the infant or child is hospitalized during a crisis, the treatment is supportive and symptomatic. The patient is confined to bed. Blood transfusions may be given for anemia, but they must be given conservatively to avoid iron overload. If iron overload becomes a problem, **chelation therapy** with desferrioxamine is begun. Antibiotics are given to all children with fever. Infection is the most common risk for infants with SCD, and this has prompted many practitioners to use penicillin prophylactically. Penicillin given prophylactically at 2 months of age through childhood has significantly reduced both morbidity and mortality from pneumococcal infections. Fluid intake is increased above the maintenance level for the child's age. Analgesics are given for relief of pain. Children in a severe pain crisis should receive a continuous intravenous narcotic infusion, and morphine is the drug of choice.

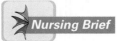
Nursing Brief

Meperidine (Demerol) is contraindicated in pain management for SCD because of the increased risk for seizures.

The nurse observes the overall appearance of the patient and assesses the developmental stage, body proportions, and the relation of height and weight to age. Facial expressions, degree of restlessness, and areas of pain are noted and recorded. Signals of dehydration are elevated temperature; a rapid, weak pulse; a sunken fontanel in infants younger than 18 months; weight loss; poor tissue turgor; dry skin, lips, and mucous membranes; and a decrease in urination. If vomiting occurs, appropriate oral hygiene is provided. The nurse observes and records infusions according to unit policy. An accurate record of intake and output is kept. Careful attention is given to the skin. Jaundice (icterus) can be detected by observing whether the skin (palms and soles) and the whites of the eyes have taken on a yellowish tinge. The patient's body position is changed gently.

Because SCD can affect muscle tone, any rigidity of the muscles should be reported. Observe eye movements, swallowing, or sucking. Note whether the child is uncomfortable when the neck is flexed to have the gown changed. Watch for twitching about the face or elsewhere.

Neurological complications such as stroke, hemiparesis, transient ischemic attack (TIA), or seizures are possible. Children should be monitored regularly. The transcranial Doppler (TCD) is effective in screening for increased blood velocity and narrowing of cerebral vessels and should be done yearly.

The prognosis is guarded. Death may result from severe anemia or secondary infection. Pregnancy may increase mortality. There is also an increased likelihood of miscarriage, premature births, and stillbirths in women with SCD. Ideally, all African-American women should be screened for the disease before pregnancy. The sickling test (Sickledex) is commonly used for screening purposes.

Surgery. The approach to splenectomy in children with SCD has been conservative. Recurrence of acute splenic sequestration becomes less likely after 5 years of age. Routine splenectomy is not recommended because the spleen generally atrophies on its own because of fibrotic changes that take place in patients with SCD. However, splenectomy is indicated in selected patients with multiple splenic events. Because

no form of prophylaxis is foolproof and because the duration of treatment is controversial, the child should continue to be carefully observed for signs of infection. Parents should be educated on how to palpate for an enlarged spleen and monitor for signs of infections (fever).

Before elective surgery, a sickle cell screening test should be performed on all African-American patients because general anesthesia places these persons at greater risk for hypoxia. With the stress of surgery and hypoxia from anesthesia, a sickle cell crisis can be precipitated.

Medication. The FDA has designated the use of hydroxyurea, an antineoplastic drug, for the palliative treatment of SCD in adults. This drug increases the production of hemoglobin F (HbF; fetal hemoglobin). HbF has a higher affinity for oxygen. Erythropoietin, which stimulates the production of red blood cells, may be used to enhance the effects of hydroxyurea. A reduction in episodes of painful vasoocclusive crisis, fewer hospitalizations, and fewer blood transfusions have been seen. Because this is an antineoplastic drug and could possibly result in mutation of genes, childbearing issues must be considered. Current studies are ongoing to determine the safety and efficacy of the use of these drugs in children as young as 2 years of age. These studies have positive results, but **hydroxyurea** use in children should be supervised by a pediatric hematologist (Fixler & Styles, 2002).

New advances with **stem cell transplantation** have produced exciting results for the child with SCD. The results are promising, with a survival rate of 90% to 95%, a cure rate of 85%, and a graft rejection rate of 10% (Fixler & Styles, 2002). Presently, only identical siblings are used for bone marrow transplantation, but other sources (cord blood) are under investigation.

RESPIRATORY SYSTEM

NASOPHARYNGITIS (COMMON COLD)
Description

A cold is the most common infection of the respiratory tract. It is caused by one or a number of viruses, principally the **rhinoviruses.** The spread from one child to another is through sneezing, coughing, and direct contact. Group A beta-hemolytic streptococci is the predominant bacterial offender. Droplets remain suspended in the air and on dust particles for short periods. The infection is transferred mainly during the initial stage. In the second phase of a cold, nasal drainage becomes thicker and purulent. Factors that contribute to the individual's susceptibility include age, state of nutrition, general health, fatigue, and emotional upsets.

As the infant becomes exposed to more children, the number of colds contracted increases. Parents may notice this particularly during the child's first few years

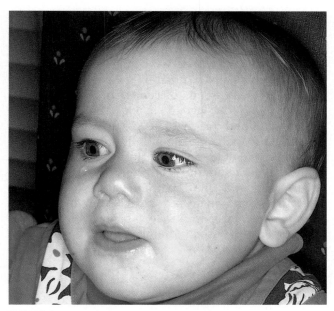

FIGURE **8-8** Common signs and symptoms of a cold include runny nose, red eyes, and fatigue.

of daycare or school because the child has had little opportunity to build up resistance. The older the child, the better he or she is able to resist infection. In temperate climates, the incidence rate of rhinoviral infection peaks in September and again in April or May.

To prevent a cold, avoid exposing children as much as possible to those with this virus. Infants less than 6 months old can acquire this infection, so they too must be protected from infected persons. Be sure to provide nourishing foods and see that the child or infant gets sufficient rest.

Signs and Symptoms

The symptoms of a cold in an infant or small child are different from those in an adult (Figure 8-8). Children's air passages are smaller and more easily obstructed. Fever as high as 104° F (40° C) is not uncommon in children less than 3 years old. Nasal discharge, irritability, sore throat, cough, and general discomfort are present, and there may be vomiting and diarrhea. The diagnosis is complicated by the fact that many infectious diseases resemble the common cold during their onset. Complications of a cold include bronchitis, pneumonitis, ear infections, and sinusitis.

Treatment and Nursing Care

There is no cure for the common cold. When a cold is suspected, treatment should be started early. The treatment is designed to relieve the symptoms. Rest, fluids, and proper diet are important. Parents are taught to watch the child for signs of dehydration. If anorexia is present, food should not be forced. The appetite gradually improves as the condition does. When high fever accompanies a cold, the physician must be consulted. Acetaminophen (Tylenol) reduces the temperature, but the correct dosage should be prescribed, particularly in patients less than 1 year old. Aqueous nose drops relieve nasal congestion. The infant needs nose drops mainly before feedings and at bedtime. When drops are instilled 10 to 15 minutes before nursing, the nasal passages are cleared and the baby can suck easily. Each child needs an individual bottle of nose drops to prevent cross infection.

Moist air soothes the inflamed nose and throat. A cold air humidifier is safe and convenient. It should be cleaned and disinfected regularly. If a great deal of moisture is indicated, as for croup, the infant may be taken to a small room, such as the bathroom, and the water faucets can be turned on to create sufficient humidity.

The older child is taught the proper way to remove nasal secretions from the nose. The mouth is opened slightly and secretions are blown gently through both nostrils at the same time. This method prevents infection from being forced into the eustachian tubes. When a large amount of nasal discharge is present, the nurse can apply petroleum jelly to the upper lip to protect it.

In the hospital, the child is isolated with proper isolation restrictions. During the initial stage of the fever, the child is kept in bed. Frequent change of position is necessary. In the home, it is difficult to keep children with a cold away from other members of the family. They must be taught to cover their mouth and nose when sneezing and to wash their hands afterward. Tissues must be properly discarded. The child should stay at home without visitors. Rest, fluids, and adequate nutrition support recovery.

BRONCHIOLITIS
Description

Bronchiolitis is an inflammation of the small airways. It occurs most often during late autumn through late spring and in children of less than 2 years of age. Bronchiolitis is usually caused by a viral infection. The most common causative organism is the respiratory syncytial virus (RSV). Children are usually exposed through other family members who have symptoms of an upper respiratory tract infection. Children who are at risk for respiratory distress have chronic lung diseases such as bronchopulmonary dysplasia (BPD) or cystic fibrosis (CF).

Inflammation of the bronchioles is associated with obstruction that is caused by edema and accumulation of mucus. There may be partial or complete obstruction. The alveoli are usually not affected. Normal gas exchange in the lung is affected. This leads to hypoxemia.

Signs and Symptoms

The infant first shows signs of a mild upper respiratory infection with rhinorrhea, sneezing, cough, and a low-grade fever. The infant's appetite may be affected.

Respiratory distress increases, and rapid breathing and wheezing develop. Bottle feeding may be difficult because of the rapid respiratory rate interfering with sucking and swallowing. As the disease progresses, nasal flaring, retractions, tachypnea (60 to 80 per minute), and cyanosis may occur. Breath sounds may be diminished if the bronchioles are severely obstructed.

Treatment

Mild cases of bronchiolitis can be managed at home. Treatment at home includes increasing the intake of fluids and increasing the humidity in the air. Also useful are antipyretics to control fever. The parents or caregiver should be instructed to bring the child back for reevaluation if any signs of increased respiratory distress occur or if the child's condition worsens.

Indications for hospitalization include a patient less than 6 months old, sleeping respiratory rates of 50 to 60 per minute or higher, hypoxemia, apnea, or the inability to tolerate oral feeding.

When the child is hospitalized, intravenous fluids are started to hydrate the child and thin the secretions. The child is placed in an atmosphere of humidified oxygen (mist tent, croupette, or nasal cannula/mask). The goal is to keep oxygen levels at 92% or better with a pulse oximeter. With severe bronchiolitis, the physician may use a bronchodilator and a corticosteroid, but these remain controversial. Antibiotics may also be used for small or severely ill infants because these infants may be susceptible to a secondary bacterial infection. Fever is controlled with antipyretics. A laboratory study of a nasopharyngeal washing should be done to determine whether the causative organism is RSV. As a precautionary measure for the safety and concern of other children, the infant is placed in contact isolation until RSV has been ruled out.

When the causative organism is RSV, no medications can effectively treat the disease. Ribavirin, antibiotics, antihistamines, and oral decongestants have been identified as being ineffective for treatment (Bradin, 2006). Medical attention has recently focused on active and passive immunizations. **RSV-immune globulin (RespiGam)** and **palivizumab (Synagis)** have been approved for use with children at high risk. Palivizumab may be preferred because of ease of administration (intramuscular); lack of interference with mumps, measles, and rubella (MMR) vaccine and varicella vaccine; and lack of complications associated with intravenous immune globulin (RespiGam). Monthly administration during RSV season (October to May) is recommended (American Academy of Pediatrics, 1998).

Nursing Care

Nursing diagnoses for the infant with bronchiolitis include the following:
- Ineffective airway clearance related to thick mucus

- Impaired gas exchange related to edema and mucus of the bronchioles
- Deficient fluid volume related to insensible fluid loss from tachypnea and decreased intake
- Anxiety related to unfamiliar environment, respiratory distress, and placement in croupette
- Deficient knowledge deficit related to disease process and treatment

The child with bronchiolitis is monitored closely for signs and symptoms of increasing respiratory distress. Breath sounds, skin color, depth and rate of respirations, and vital signs are assessed. Changes in alertness and increased anxiety can be signs of impending distress. Continuous or intermittent pulse oximetry may be used to monitor the infant's oxygen level.

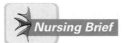
Nursing Brief

Infants with a respiratory rate of 60 breaths per minute should have nothing by mouth.

Intravenous fluids are monitored in the acutely ill child. As the child improves, oral fluids are increased and frequent small meals are offered. The child is on intake and output recording, and daily weights are taken. The fontanel and the child's skin turgor are also assessed as indicators of hydration status.

Formula-fed infants may have thickened feeding to improve swallowing dysfunction and to prevent aspiration. Breastfed infants should have more frequent feeding with shorter times. This assists in decreasing the workload of the infant and conserves energy. Nasal secretions should be removed with a bulb syringe before feedings (Allen, 2006).

The child in a mist tent should have the gown and linens changed if they become damp. Also moisture build-up should be removed from the tubing and the sides of the tent (see Chapter 17 for detailed care of the child in a mist tent). For home care, cold air humidifiers can be used but must be cleaned properly to prevent bacteria or fungal growth.

As always, parents are encouraged to stay with the child. This may be even more important because the child may already be anxious because of respiratory distress. Parents should understand the importance of the child staying in the tent. They should be included in the care and diversional activities for the child.

Preventing the spread of infection is also important. If an infant has RSV, then contact isolation is recommended. RSV is primarily spread by large droplets and fomites. RSV can survive on hands for almost an hour and on hard surfaces up to 24 hours. Nosocomial spread can be a serious nursing issue. Handwashing is extremely important in all issues of infection. All caregivers, including parents, need to know and apply measures to prevent the spread of infection.

Support of the parents is significant. Most of the infants who are in severe or critical condition are usually young infants or those who have an underlying disease. Their parents may lack confidence when it comes to the care of the infant and need to be supported and reassured in their actions. It can be frightening for them to see their infant so ill. If the infant is admitted to a critical care area, the support of the parents is crucial. Explanations should be given in terms the parents can understand. The family needs information from the physician or the nurse concerning the infant's condition, medications, treatments, and procedures. Plans for all of these issues and discharge information can aid the parents in coping with the situation. Family, friends, and clergy can be a great support for the parents.

BRONCHOPULMONARY DYSPLASIA
Description

Bronchopulmonary dysplasia (BPD) is a chronic lung disease that occurs in newborns who are premature or have pulmonary disorders that require mechanical ventilator support with high positive pressure and oxygen. The lung tissue is immature and unable to withstand tissue damage resulting from the required oxygen supplement. The resulting fibrosis and alteration in lung compliance may last from several months to years. Improvements in treatment of low–birth weight preterm infants have increased the incidence of this disorder, and continues to be the primary issue for infants less than 27 weeks (Belcastro, 2004).

Signs and Symptoms

The symptoms of BPD are directly related to the pathophysiology of the disease. Tachypnea, dyspnea, and wheezing can be a result of airway obstruction and increased airway resistance. Increased work of breathing can cause retractions and use of accessory muscles. The infants may display activity intolerance during feedings. They may be irritable and difficult to comfort. Cyanosis may develop during crying spells. Infants who needed intubation for a long period of time may have subglottic stenosis and inspiratory stridor develop. All of the symptoms can be associated with the chronic hypoxia state. The diagnosis is made on the basis of abnormal radiographic findings, signs of respiratory distress, oxygen dependency after 28 days of age, and a history of required mechanical ventilation during the first week of life.

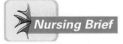

Nursing Brief

Children in severe respiratory distress should receive nothing by mouth because of the increased workload of breathing and the increased risk for aspiration.

Treatment and Nursing Care

The treatment for infants with BPD is to provide adequate oxygenation and prevent progression of the disease process. Treatment includes oxygen, drug therapy, and nutritional support. Surfactant continues to be included in the course of medical treatment (Bissenger & Carlson, 2006). Infants may continue to need oxygen after hospital discharge. These infants do not tolerate excessive or even normal amounts of fluids. They may have problems develop with accumulation of fluids in the lungs that require the use of diuretics. The use of these drugs requires the monitoring of electrolytes and edema. Oral electrolyte supplements may be given. Bronchodilators (albuterol) and steroids may promote improved lung function. These infants are at risk for respiratory infections and should be given RSV-immune globulin (RespiGam) or palivizumab (Synagis) during the RSV season.

Infants with BPD are at high risk for growth failure, and nutrition is an important issue (Thomas, 2005). They have higher metabolic needs, and providing adequate nutrition without causing overhydration can be difficult. Nursing care should be organized to provide periods of rest. Small, frequent feedings and nutritional supplements may be used. The environment should include measures to decrease stimulation.

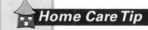

Home Care Tip

The Child with Bronchopulmonary Dysplasia

Advise parents that:
- All caregivers need CPR training.
- House and care should be smoke-free.
- Avoid contact with individuals with colds or fever.
- Avoid crowds.
- Place infant on back to sleep.
- Keep infant's room door open.

Parents may be extremely anxious caring for a child with BPD. All equipment and procedures should be explained in simple terms. Children with tracheostomies can be cared for in the home setting, and home care teaching of the equipment is needed (Figure 8-9). Extended hospitalization can interfere with the development of the normal parent-child relationship and with the normal development of the infant. Parental participation in the infant's care should be encouraged. The family's ability to cope and care for a child with a chronic illness needs to be evaluated as home discharge plans are developed. An adequate period of education may be necessary for the parents to become comfortable with the care required for their child. Families should be referred to social services to assist in providing additional support and to assist in helping the parent gain access to available community services. Parental support groups can be beneficial in providing

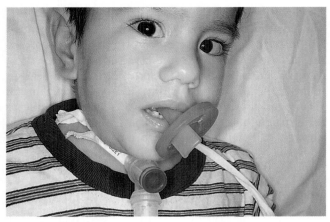

FIGURE **8-9** Humidified oxygen is provided to the child with a tracheostomy.

additional assistance with coping skills necessary for caring for a child with complex care.

LUNGS

CYSTIC FIBROSIS
Description
Cystic fibrosis (CF) is a genetic disorder that results in a multisystem disease involving the cell membrane and the electrolyte and water system of the cell. This disease affects many parts of the body but particularly the lungs and pancreas. It occurs in about 1 in 3000 live births. CF is an inherited congenital disorder. The condition is believed to be inherited as a **Mendelian recessive trait** from both parents. The parents, who are **carriers** of this disease, do not show any symptoms. When the two **genes** for the disease combine in the child at the time of conception, CF disease results. CF affects both genders equally. The survival rate of the children has increased, and many are living into adulthood. Better antibiotic control of pulmonary infection both at home and during hospitalization and increased numbers of CF centers have contributed to this success.

The gene associated with CF was identified in 1989, and it is now possible to identify healthy individuals who carry the trait. Chromosome 7 is the location of the gene responsible for CF. Sodium and chloride at the cell membrane are controlled by this gene. With a defect in the CF transmembrane regulator (CFTR) protein, secretions become thick and pasty. There are many possible mutations, which helps to explain the various degrees of involvement of the systems: respiratory and GI.

With the ability to identify the CF gene, diagnosis can be assisted with genetic analysis. Caution is noted because of the possibilities of false-positive and false-negative results. Genetic analysis can be used in conjunction with other diagnostic criteria such as the sweat test. New aggressive approaches in treatment

have resulted in increasing the life expectancy from less than 10 years to 40 years.

Signs and Symptoms
The major symptoms of CF are manifested in the respiratory tract and the GI tract. The first symptom may be seen in the newborn infant who has a **meconium ileus**. This condition is seen in approximately 10% to 20% of children who are born with CF. An overview of the manifestations of CF is shown in Figure 8-10.

Lung Involvement. Cystic fibrosis is considered the most serious lung problem in children in the United States. The air passages of the lungs become clogged with mucus. There is widespread obstruction of the bronchioles. It is hard for the patient to breathe; expiration is especially difficult. More and more air becomes trapped in the lungs (obstructive emphysema), and small areas of collapse (atelectasis) may occur. Eventually, the chest assumes a barrel shape, with increased diameter across the front and back. The right ventricle of the heart, which supplies the lungs, may become strained and enlarged. Clubbing of the fingers and toes, indicating a chronic lack of oxygen, may be present. *Staphylococcus* and *Pseudomonas* infections can easily occur in the lungs, which provide a suitable medium for these organisms to grow. This causes more thickening of the abnormal secretions, irritates and damages lung tissues, and further increases lung obstruction.

The time of onset of this disease varies. Symptoms may appear weeks, months, or years after birth. In general, the earlier the onset of the disease, the more severe the disease. Symptoms range from mild to severe. Any or all symptoms may be present in varying degrees of severity in one individual. A chronic cough develops that may produce vomiting. Dyspnea, wheezing, and cyanosis may occur. The patient is irritable and tires easily. Gradually, there is a change in physical appearance. Chest radiographs reveal widespread infection. Evidence of obstructive emphysema, atelectasis, and **fibrosis** of lung tissue may also be present. The prognosis for survival depends on the extent of lung damage. However, this is only part of the picture because CF also affects the pancreas and sweat glands.

Pancreatic Involvement. The pancreas lies behind the stomach. Some of its cells secrete **pancreatic enzymes** that drain from the pancreatic duct into the duodenum at the same area in which bile enters. Changes occurring in the pancreas are the result of obstruction by thickened secretions that block the flow of pancreatic digestive enzymes. Consequently, foodstuffs, particularly fats and proteins, are not properly used by the body.

In infants, the stools may be loose. Gradually, because of impaired digestion and food absorption, the feces of the patient become large, fatty, and foul-smelling. They are usually light in color. In spite of having a good appetite, the baby does not gain weight and may look undernourished. The abdomen becomes

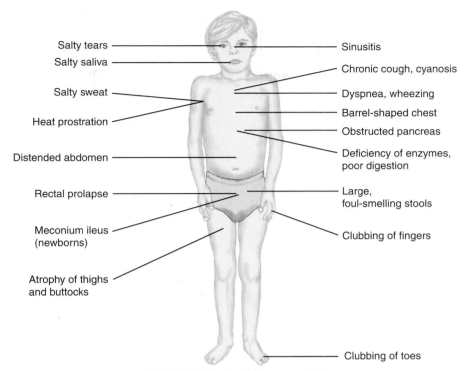

FIGURE **8-10** Manifestations of CF.

Salty tears
Salty saliva
Salty sweat
Heat prostration
Distended abdomen
Rectal prolapse
Meconium ileus (newborns)
Atrophy of thighs and buttocks

Sinusitis
Chronic cough, cyanosis
Dyspnea, wheezing
Barrel-shaped chest
Obstructed pancreas
Deficiency of enzymes, poor digestion
Large, foul-smelling stools
Clubbing of fingers
Clubbing of toes

distended, and the buttocks and thighs **atrophy** as fat disappears from the main deposit sites. Laboratory test results show a deficiency in pancreatic enzymes (trypsin, lipase, amylase).

An oral pancreatic extract such as Pancrease is given to the child with each meal and snack to replace the pancreatic enzymes the child's body cannot produce. This medication is considered specific for the disease because it aids in the digestion and absorption of food, thus improving the condition of the stools. If the child is ill and not eating, the medication is withheld.

A condition known as **meconium ileus** exists when the intestine of the newborn baby becomes obstructed with abnormally thick meconium while in utero. This is caused by the absence of pancreatic enzymes that normally digest proteins in the meconium. The abnormal, puttylike stool sticks to the walls of the intestine, causing blockage. The presenting symptoms develop within hours after birth. The absence of stools, vomiting, and abdominal distention lead one to suspect intestinal obstruction. Radiographs confirm the diagnosis. The condition is treated surgically. The death rate is high, but the prognosis is more favorable when the obstruction is detected early. Most infants who survive manifest CF. Fortunately, meconium ileus is rare because the pancreatic enzyme deficiency is seldom complete. Nevertheless, the nurse assigned to the nursery must constantly be on guard for suspicious symptoms.

Sweat Glands. The sweat, tears, and saliva of the patient with CF become abnormally salty from an increase in sodium and chloride levels. There is also an increase in the

potassium level of sweat glands. The normal amount of chloride in sweat is 1 to 60 mEq/L. Higher concentrations are considered specific for the disease. The analysis of sweat is a major aid in the diagnosis of the condition. The **sweat test,** with pilocarpine iontophoresis, is the best diagnostic study. A dilute solution of pilocarpine is applied to the arm, and a weak electrical current is used to stimulate sweating. A positive test should be repeated for confirmation. Because large amounts of salt are lost through perspiration, the patient must be observed for heat prostration. Liberal amounts of salt should be given with food, and extra fluids and salt should be provided during hot weather. Infants do not have a lot of sweat; therefore obtaining enough sweat for an accurate test may be difficult.

Complications

Cystic fibrosis is often responsible for **rectal prolapse** in infants and children. This is partly from poor muscle tone in the rectal area and excessive leanness of the buttocks of the patient.

As the disease progresses, the liver may become hard, nodular, and enlarged. There may be edema of the extremities. The retina of the eye may hemorrhage, there may be damage to the eye from swelling, and inflammation in part of the optic nerve may occur. **Cor pulmonale** (*cor,* heart; *pulmon,* lung), heart strain from improper lung function, is frequently a cause of death. **Osteoporosis** (*osteo,* bone, pore; *osis,* disease) may occur. When it is caused by CF, the bones become porous because of poor utilization of fat-soluble vitamin D, which is necessary for proper calcium metabolism.

There is a deficiency in vitamin A also because the child is unable to absorb the fats from which this vitamin is obtained.

Treatment and Nursing Care

Cystic fibrosis is a chronic condition and must be monitored and maintained daily. The family providers of care need support, as does the child. The care in a regional CF center, where all disciplines are located in one facility, can be extremely helpful because it allows the family to go to one location rather than traveling to several different clinics for care. The CF team can work with the family and the primary care physician to meet the needs of the patient and family.

Respiratory Relief. Most new approaches in treatment are focused on the lung. The targeted outcomes are improved airway clearance, thinning of secretions, treatment of infections, and reduction of inflammation. **Antibiotics** may be given as a preventive measure against respiratory infection; however, this treatment is subject to controversy. Full dosages of antibiotics are given in an acute infection. The physician determines the particular antibiotic to be used on the basis of the results of throat and sputum cultures. The route may be oral or intravenous. Intravenous medication may be given via **heparin lock** or, in some cases, a **Broviac catheter** or **implanted port.** This can be used successfully in both inpatient and outpatient settings. The child's respiratory status can be monitored through the pulmonary function test, which indicates the lung's capacity.

Intermittent aerosol therapy is administered to provide medication and water to the lower respiratory tract and to promote evacuation of secretions. DNase, an enzyme, has been approved for use with CF. It is administered by inhalation and results in decreasing the viscosity of the sputum. A new inhaled antibiotic, TOBI, has been marketed as a maintenance prophylactic to be used with CF. Bronchodilators are used to increase the width of the bronchi, allowing free passage of air into the lungs.

Postural drainage, chest clapping, and breathing exercises are also important. These are performed by the respiratory therapist during hospitalization. When postural drainage and chest clapping are done properly, the secretions in the chest are moved up and out. During latent periods or in mild cases, the patient may not raise sputum. This should be explained to the parents so that they do not discontinue this valuable procedure when the child goes home. Instructions may need to be repeated frequently to encourage full cooperation of the parents and child. These procedures should be done after nebulization and at least 1 hour after eating. General exercise is good for the patient because it stimulates coughing. Somersaults, headstands, and wheelbarrow play within the child's endurance are therapeutic.

Preventing respiratory tract infections is important. The child should be isolated from patients and per-sonnel who may harbor infections. The period of hospitalization is kept brief, if possible, to avoid cross infection. The patient must be given the necessary immunizations against childhood diseases. Appropriate boosters should be given so that the immunity obtained is kept up to date.

Diet. Adequate nutrition is essential. The diet should be high in calories, as much as 50% more than normal. There should be increased protein and moderate amounts of fat in conjunction with pancreatic extracts. Simple sugars are easy to digest, and banana products are particularly good. Fruits, cottage cheese, vegetables, and lean meats, which are high in protein and low in fat and starches, are recommended. Restrictions on ice cream, peanut butter, butter, french fries, and mayonnaise are advised. Extra salt may be provided with pretzels and salted bread sticks and crackers. Discrepancies in the diet may be allowed by the physician to keep meals from becoming drab and to provide a more normal atmosphere. At such times, the child is allowed to eat what is desired and is given extra digestive enzymes. Some institutions have a **gastrostomy button** placed so that the child can receive addition nutritional supplements at night.

Supplements of vitamins A, D, and E in a water-miscible base are given each day in double the recommended dose. Vitamin K may also be given when indicated. Salt tablets may be given to the older child during hot weather. Forcing fluids may be ordered because larger amounts of fluid are lost in the stools. The nurse may be asked to weigh the child daily.

The nurse feeding the infant with CF must be calm and unhurried. The baby may cough, have difficulty breathing, and vomit. Careful burping is necessary to avoid abdominal distention. In general, the appetite is good. Older children need small amounts of food served attractively and frequently. Food piled high on a child's tray is discouraging. The child may have eaten a perfectly good meal for the size, but the nurse who carries the remainder of the tray to the kitchen charts "poor appetite." The nurse records the fluid intake at the end of the meal. The child's reaction to new foods and any variations in stools resulting from the food are noted. The food refused and the type, character, and amount of vomiting, if any, are also noted.

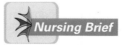

Nursing Brief

Because mealtime is a social time, the nurse should remain with the child if the parents are not present. Try to make the meal more satisfying by giving good companionship mixed with a little encouragement.

General Hygiene. The nurse must pay special attention to the skin of the child with CF. The diaper area should be cleansed after each bowel movement. An ointment to protect the skin is advisable because the character of the stool subjects the diaper area to irritation. The buttocks are exposed to air when a rash occurs. Careful attention to bony areas is necessary to prevent decubitus ulcers. Because the patient has little fat and muscle, it is important that the position be changed frequently, especially if the child is weak and cannot get out of bed. This also prevents pneumonia. The patient wears light clothing to avoid becoming overheated; it should be loose to allow freedom of movement. Good oral hygiene is necessary because the teeth may be in poor condition from dietary deficiencies. Mouth care is given after postural drainage because foul mucus may be raised, leaving an unpleasant taste in the patient's mouth.

Long-Term Care. Today the child with a lengthy illness spends most of the time at home and is hospitalized mainly for diagnosis, relapses, and complications. This burden, which the family willingly assumes, is extremely taxing financially, physically, and emotionally. Somehow the mother must distribute her time and energy within the family yet give careful attention to her sick child or, in the case of CF, sometimes children. How does she keep from spoiling the child? Does she limit the normal activities of the remaining children to spare her sick one? What about birthday parties, camping, Cub Scouts, pets, epidemics at school? What does a trip to the shore or mountains entail? When do the husband and wife find time for themselves? These seemingly overwhelming problems are being faced daily by many people in every community. Parent groups are helpful in promoting exchange of ideas and in providing support. The National Cystic Fibrosis Research Foundation disseminates useful information. The nurse should become familiar with the local chapter to guide parents to reliable sources of information.

Communication Alert

Parents of patients with CF need encouragement and reassurance. When you meet them in the clinic or hospital, be kind and attentive. If a child looks obviously well cared for, mention this to the parents. If you are asked direct questions about the illness you might say, "Dr. Parker is a fine pediatrician. What did he tell you about Bobby's illness?" This encourages the parents to express themselves and gives you an idea of what the patient and parents have been told.

Parents need explicit instructions regarding diet, medication, postural drainage, prevention of infection, rest, and continued medical supervision. Plan teaching periods and provide printed materials for reinforcement so that parents are not overwhelmed. Many families require the assistance of a social worker to secure funds for equipment and drugs. Parents should be told that help is available as the need arises.

The mother, who is usually more directly involved, may benefit from these added hints:

- She needs rest herself; the family must take over some of the responsibilities of the household. Relatives may care for the child periodically so that she can "get away from it all." Respite care is another alternative; it is helpful if she can develop at least one outside interest of her own.
- An alarm clock set for medication time reminds her of this task.
- A downstairs bedroom for the child is preferable.
- Extra spoons and a pitcher of water on the bedside stand save steps.

Emotional Support. The child who is chronically ill finds it hard to accept restricted activity. The amount and kinds of diversion required vary in CF because the disease affects children of all ages, with variations in severity.

It is believed that children benefit from simple straightforward answers about the illness. An uncomplicated diagram might be helpful. Children who understand why they are being restricted from certain activities are more cooperative. They should know why they must take medications with each meal, use the nebulizer, undergo postural drainage, and so on. They should see and handle the unfamiliar equipment necessary for their care.

The young child finds it difficult to be separated from the parents during hospitalization. Even when the prognosis is grave, a child's courage is sustained if the parents are there. Parents are encouraged to stay with the child when possible. Close contact by mail with school, church, and clubs is important for school-age children. It is helpful for patients to develop an activity at which they are good, such as piano or art. This increases their feeling of worth and provides outlets for emotions. Consideration must be given to ways of fostering love, acceptance, trust, fair play, security, freedom of choice, creativity, and self-identity.

Nurses should learn the patient's likes, dislikes, fears, and interests. They should observe them with their families and note the types of relationships that exist. They then can form their own impressions about the patients and are not misled by labels given them by those with less understanding. Patients have to be allowed to communicate in a manner that is meaningful to them. Sometimes children are able to express feelings; sometimes they are not. Drawing with children may stimulate conversation. It is important that nurses be aware of children's facial expressions, posture, eyes, and how they play. What are they saying to their toys, their playmates? Nurses' observations of children's behavior should be incorporated into nursing care plans.

Nurses and parents must not show undue concern for a patient's illness. Overindulging children has a tendency to make them demanding. Patients may then exaggerate small problems. The children's impressions of themselves and their illness are determined a good deal by how they feel physically, how the family feels about their condition, and how others behave toward them.

Development of new approaches in treatment has changed the outlook for CF families. Advancements in airway clearance techniques, new medications, gene therapy, and lung transplantation have encouraged optimism toward improvement of lifestyle for the patient with CF. The nurse should assist in keeping families informed of new, available therapies (Nursing Care Plan 8-2).

GASTROINTESTINAL SYSTEM

INGUINAL HERNIA
Description

An inguinal hernia is a protrusion of part of the abdominal contents through the inguinal canal in the groin. The condition is more common in boys than in girls. It is also seen frequently in premature infants. Hernias may be present at birth (congenital) or may be acquired and can vary in size. A hernia is termed **reducible** if the abdominal contents can be put back in place with gentle pressure; if this cannot be done, it is called an **irreducible** or an **incarcerated** (constricted) **hernia.**

Signs and Symptoms

The infant with a hernia may be relatively free of symptoms. Irritability, fretfulness, and constipation are sometimes evident. The diagnosis is made when physical examination shows a mass in the inguinal area that reappears from time to time, particularly when the child cries or strains (Figure 8-11). A **strangulated hernia** occurs when the intestine becomes caught in the passage and the blood supply is diminished. This happens more frequently during the first 6 months of life. Vomiting and severe abdominal pain are present. Emergency surgery is necessary if strangulation occurs, and in some cases a bowel resection is performed.

Treatment and Nursing Care

Inguinal hernias are repaired successfully with the surgical operation called a **herniorrhaphy.** This is a relatively simple procedure that is tolerated well by the child. Most patients are scheduled for same-day surgery units. The benefits of this method are both economical and psychological. Parents remain with the child during the entire time except for the actual procedure. They are encouraged to assist in routine postoperative care if they choose. Often no dressing is applied to the wound. Sometimes a waterproof collodion dressing may be used. Postoperative care is directed toward keeping the wound clean. Diapers are left open for this purpose. Wet diapers are changed frequently. The child is discharged in about 2 to 3 hours, when fluids are tolerated. Activity is not limited.

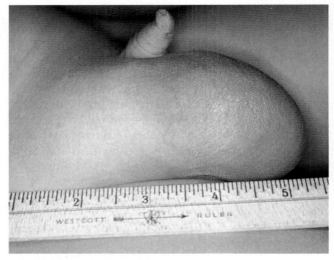

FIGURE **8-11** Inguinal hernia in a male may occur with crying and straining.

Parents are provided with written instructions about home management. Follow-up telephone calls may be made by nursing personnel, and return appointments are scheduled.

Patients with incarcerated hernias are hospitalized. After surgery, vital signs are carefully monitored. Nasogastric (NG) suctioning and intravenous fluids are maintained until bowel function returns. The nurse measures and records the patient's intake and output. The child is turned frequently to avoid respiratory complications. The nurse observes the child carefully for signs of peritonitis or bowel obstruction.

UMBILICAL HERNIA
Description

An umbilical hernia is a protrusion of a portion of intestine through the umbilical ring (an opening in the muscular area of the abdomen where the umbilical vessels passed through; Figure 8-12). This type of hernia appears as a soft swelling, covered by skin that protrudes when the infant cries or strains. Most of the small umbilical hernias disappear spontaneously during the first year of life. This type of hernia is not known to become strangulated or to cause other complications.

Treatment

Generally, surgery is not advised unless the hernia causes symptoms, becomes enlarged, or persists until the child is 3 to 5 years of age. The use of tape or coins in an attempt to reduce the hernia is ineffective.

PYLORIC STENOSIS
Description

Pyloric stenosis (narrowing of the pylorus) is a disorder of the digestive tract. The pylorus, the lower end of the stomach, becomes partially blocked so that food does not empty properly into the duodenum

NURSING CARE PLAN 8-2

The Child with Cystic Fibrosis

NURSING DIAGNOSIS *Ineffective airway clearance related to accumulation of mucus*

Goals/Outcome Criteria	Nursing Interventions	Rationales
The child has improved aeration, as evidenced by: • Absence of dyspnea and tachypnea • Ability to expectorate mucus • Respiratory rate appropriate for age • Heart rate appropriate for age (O_2 saturation = 93% on room air)	Assess lung sounds: rate and depth.	Provides information on how the patient is doing.
	Assess O_2 saturation. Assess heart rate.	As oxygen is needed, the heart speeds up to help the body compensate.
	Provide adequate hydration.	Fluids are needed by the body to help thin secretions.
	Assist patient with aerosol therapy.	Bronchodilators and an increase in the inspired humidity aid the functioning of the respiratory system and aid in expectorating mucus.
	Assist with chest physiotherapy and postural drainage.	Aids in expectorating mucus by dislodging mucous plugs and, with the addition of gravity, aids in removal of mucus from the body.
	Administer medications and explain their use.	Important for the family to know the effects of the medication and the side effects. Aids in compliance.
	Teach patient the importance of breathing exercises.	Breathing exercises increase the body's ability to compensate. The muscles needed to compensate are strengthened.
	Monitor the effectiveness of medication and respiratory treatments.	As the child grows and as the body's needs change, adjustments are needed in the course of treatment. It is also important for the family to know how to monitor the effectiveness of the treatment.

NURSING DIAGNOSIS *Imbalanced nutrition: less than body requirements related to malabsorption from absence of pancreatic enzymes*

Goals/Outcome Criteria	Nursing Interventions	Rationales
The child has adequate nutrition, as evidenced by: • Ability to eat $1\frac{1}{2}$ to 2 times the recommended dietary allowance for age • Weight gain or lack of weight loss • Increase in muscle mass • Maturation in growth and development	Assess baseline nutrition.	Indicates what information is needed for the patient and the family.
	Administer pancreatic replacement enzymes.	The body lacks the ability to excrete the pancreatic enzymes needed to digest fats and proteins.
	Administer water-miscible, fat-soluble vitamins.	Fat-soluble vitamins are given in a water-soluble form to aid in the absorption of these vitamins.
	Monitor serum electrolytes.	Electrolytes, particularly sodium, are lost in large amounts during periods of heavy perspiration (fever, hot weather, exercise).
	Provide a diet high in calories and proteins and normal in fat.	Because of the body's inability to absorb nutrients, it is necessary for there to be an abundance. Extra energy is also used by the respiratory system.
	Provide between-meal treats.	Adds additional calories and nutrients.
	Monitor caloric count.	A calorie count is needed to ensure that the child is getting the needed calories and nutrients.
	Teach child and caregiver the importance of daily evaluation of diet.	Allows the family to function in an independent manner; adjustments can be made more easily.
	Weigh daily and record while in the hospital.	Diet and activity can be adjusted according to needs.
	Monitor and record characteristics of stool.	Because it is difficult for the body to digest fats, the stool record aids in identifying needed adjustments to the diet and medication regimen.

Continued

NURSING CARE PLAN 8-2—cont'd

The Child with Cystic Fibrosis—cont'd

NURSING DIAGNOSIS *Imbalanced nutrition: less than body requirements related to malabsorption from absence of pancreatic enzymes—cont'd*

Goals/Outcome Criteria	Nursing Interventions	Rationales
	Consult with the dietitian.	A dietitian is an integral part of the team in the treatment and management of the patient. A dietitian can provide information for the patient and the family and aid them in their selections.

NURSING DIAGNOSIS *Deficient knowledge related to the diagnosis and condition of the child*

Goals/Outcome Criteria	Nursing Interventions	Rationales
The parents have an understanding of what is occurring, as evidenced by • Repeating information correctly that has been given to them • Asking questions • Describing the home care regimen • Discussing the need for medical follow-up • Ability to express fears • Accepting referrals for outside assistance	Assess parents' understanding of the disease process and its future outcome.	Allows the nurse to know where to begin.
	Provide emotional support for the parents and the child.	The parents may find it difficult to deal with all that is going on. Make sure both the parents' and the child's needs are met.
	Allow the parents to ask questions.	Parents may feel overwhelmed by the situation. Make sure they feel comfortable asking questions. If they are not asking questions, use open-ended statements with them.
	Answer questions or provide the parents with resources to answer their questions.	The nurse may not have all the answers to the questions asked, but it is important that resources be used. Find out for the parent or direct the parent where to go (e.g., "That is a good question. Let's write it down so you can ask your doctor when he comes in.").
	Help parents understand and support the child through various activities.	If parents can support the child in the hospital, they are more likely to be successful in a home setting.
	Encourage parents' participation in the care of the child.	Parents who participate in care can show their concern for the child and feel they are team players in the management of the child.
	Assess the home environment for long-term care.	Allows for home-care plans to be made.
	Initiate referral to aid the parents.	Often, parents need extra resources to meet the needs of this child.
	Teach parents and child the signs and symptoms of respiratory distress.	If these are known, the family can make changes to correct further deterioration. Also, knowing what to do is helpful and aids in their independence.
	Consultation or referral with social service.	The family may need additional services, such as financial advice and equipment, and need the aid of a social worker.

NURSING DIAGNOSIS *Risk for infection related to invasion of respiratory system by bacterial organisms*

Goals/Outcome Criteria	Nursing Interventions	Rationales
The child is free of infection, as evidenced by: • Remaining afebrile • Respiratory rate appropriate for age • Clearing of mucus after regular and routine respiratory treatments • Following proper procedure when doing treatments	Assess vital signs.	Early recognition of changing vital signs alerts nurse to the possibility of an infection.
	Use and know the importance of handwashing. Teach parents, child, and visitors proper technique.	Done properly, handwashing can decrease the spread of organisms.
	Encourage proper pulmonary hygiene.	By getting rid of mucus and secretions, there is less opportunity for harmful organisms to multiply and spread.
	Teach proper handling and disposal of secretions and sputum.	Helps decrease the possibility of reinfecting the body.

Goals/Outcome Criteria	Nursing Interventions	Rationales
	Teach or review with the child and parents why the pulmonary system is at risk for infection.	Information helps the child and family understand the need to be careful and follow recommendations; aids with compliance in treatment.
	Give reassurance and praise when procedures are done correctly by the child or parents.	Shows that nurse recognizes the child or family has learned and gives them more motivation to learn. The more motivated the child and family are to learn, the more compliant they are in following procedures.
	Provide guidance related to being independent.	Independence increases self-esteem. As learning increases, the child is able to be more independent and self-esteem is greater.

CRITICAL THINKING QUESTION

- A newly diagnosed 5-year-old with CF refuses to take pancreatic enzymes with meals. The mother is frustrated and is threatening the child. What interventions could the nurse use in attempting to obtain compliance with this child? How can the nurse help the mother become more effective in dealing with the situation?

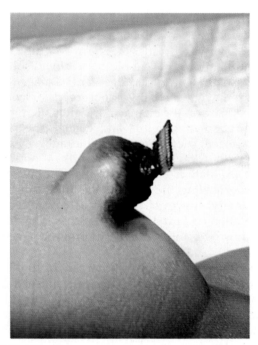

FIGURE 8-12 Umbilical hernia. The predominant umbilical hernia was noted at birth.

(Figure 8-13). Pyloric stenosis is caused by an overgrowth of the circular muscles of the pylorus. The stomach muscles above the obstructed area also enlarge in their attempt to force material through the narrowed passage. An abnormal increase in the size of an organ or part, such as this, is called **hypertrophy.** This condition is commonly classified as a congenital anomaly; however, its symptoms do not appear until the baby is 2 or 3 weeks old. Pyloric stenosis is the most common surgical condition of the digestive tract in infancy. Its incidence is higher in boys than in girls, with a tendency for it to be inherited.

Signs and Symptoms

Vomiting is the outstanding symptom of this disorder. The force progresses until most of the food is ejected a considerable distance from the mouth. This is termed **projectile** vomiting and occurs before and after feedings. The nonbilious vomitus contains mucus and may be blood streaked. The baby is constantly hungry and eats again immediately after vomiting has occurred. Dehydration—as evidenced by a sunken fontanel, poor turgor, and decreased urination—may occur. An olive-shaped mass may be felt in the right upper quadrant of the abdomen. Ultrasonography is commonly used today for diagnostic purposes because it is noninvasive and accurate. In severe cases, the outline of the distended stomach and peristaltic waves are visible during feedings (Figure 8-14). The urine and blood are alkaline because the fluid being lost from the body is mostly hydrochloric acid from the stomach juices. Bowel movements gradually diminish because little or no food passes into the intestine.

Treatment

The surgery performed for pyloric stenosis is called **pyloromyotomy** (*pyloro,* gatekeeper; *myo,* muscle; *tomy,* incision of). This procedure can either be laparoscopic or open. The surgeon incises the pyloric muscle in such a way that the opening is enlarged and food may again pass easily through it.

Nursing Care

If the infant is not dehydrated, surgery is usually performed as soon as possible. The dehydrated infant is

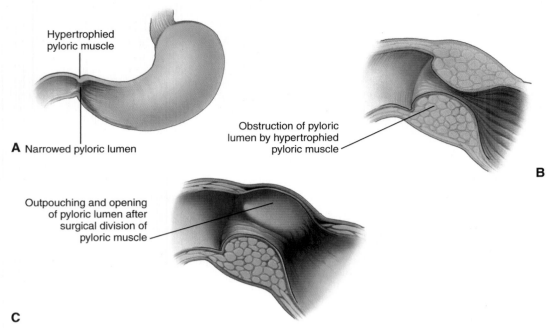

A Narrowed pyloric lumen

Hypertrophied pyloric muscle

Obstruction of pyloric lumen by hypertrophied pyloric muscle

B

Outpouching and opening of pyloric lumen after surgical division of pyloric muscle

C

FIGURE **8-13** In pyloric stenosis, the pyloric muscle hypertrophies and obstructs the passage of stomach contents into the intestines. Surgically splitting the muscle relieves the obstruction.

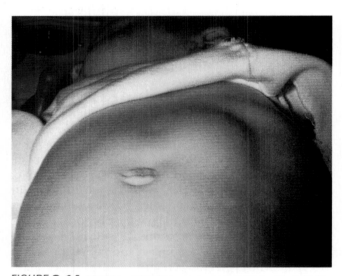

FIGURE **8-14** Visible peristaltic waves associated with pyloric stenosis.

given intravenous fluids before surgery to restore fluid and electrolyte balance. If this is not done, shock may be an issue. The infant may be NPO to prevent further losses from vomiting. Monitoring of intravenous fluids intake, accurate urine output, and emesis should be important nursing actions. Comforting the infant and supporting and alleviating the parental anxiety are also important actions.

The postoperative care of the patient includes such procedures as careful observation of vital signs and intravenous administration of fluids. The wound site is inspected frequently for bleeding. Signs of shock are an increase in the pulse rate and respiration rate;

pale cool skin; and restlessness. An NG tube may or may not be in place; it should be removed soon after surgery so that oral feedings can begin. After the tube is removed, the baby is observed for vomiting. Place the baby on the stomach or right side to prevent the aspiration of vomitus and change the position gently. Current views are that the infant may resume full-strength formula or breast milk 4 hours after surgery (Miniati & Albanese, 2004). The nurse must avoid overfeeding the patient. Vomiting can be seen after surgery; however, it is not as severe as before the operation and gradually diminishes. The diaper is placed low over the abdomen to prevent infection of the wound.

The infant is generally discharged 24 to 48 hours after surgery. Normal feedings are reestablished. Parental instructions should include feeding schedule and wound care. Parents should have instructions regarding symptoms of complications such as wound infection, recurrent vomiting, and dehydration. Follow-up care is stressed.

INTUSSUSCEPTION
Description

Intussusception (*intus*, within; *suscipere*, to receive) is a slipping of one part of the intestine into another part just below it (Figure 8-15). The condition is frequently seen at the ileocecal valve, where the small intestine opens into the ascending colon. The **mesentery,** a double fan-shaped fold of peritoneum that covers most of the intestine and is filled with blood vessels and nerves, is also pulled along. Edema occurs. At first this telescoping of the bowel causes intestinal

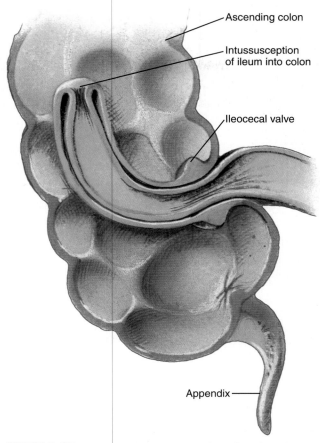

FIGURE **8-15** In intussusception, a portion of the bowel telescopes into itself, causing signs and symptoms of intestinal obstruction.

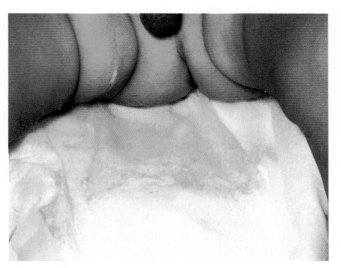

FIGURE **8-16** "Currant jelly" stools are a classic sign of intussusception.

obstruction, but as peristalsis forces the structures tighter, strangulation takes place. This portion may burst, causing peritonitis.

Intussusception generally occurs in male infants who are otherwise healthy. It can occur at any age but typically affects children under the age of 2, with the highest incidence rate between 4 and 9 months. The exact cause is still in question. Occasionally, the condition corrects itself without treatment. This is termed a **spontaneous reduction.** However, because the patient's life is in danger, the physician does not wait for spontaneous reduction. The prognosis is good when the condition is treated within 24 hours.

Signs and Symptoms

In typical cases the onset is sudden. The infant feels severe pain in the abdomen, evidenced by loud cries, straining efforts, and the kicking and drawing of the legs toward the abdomen. At first the child is comfortable between pains, but the intervals shorten and the condition becomes worse. The child vomits. The stomach contents are green or greenish yellow in color because of bile stain, and the contents are described as **bilious.** If the condition is left untreated, fecal vomiting ensues. Bowel movements diminish,

and little flatus is passed. Stools of blood and mucus that contain no feces are common about 12 hours after the onset of the obstruction; these are termed **currant jelly stools** (Figure 8-16). The child's fever may run as high as 106° F (41.1° C), and signs of shock such as sweating, weak pulse, and shallow grunting respirations appear. The abdomen is rigid.

Treatment

Intussusception is an emergency situation, and because of the severity of the symptoms, most parents contact a physician promptly. The diagnosis is determined from the history and physical findings. The physician may feel a sausage-shaped mass in the right upper portion of the abdomen during bimanual rectal and abdominal palpation. Abdominal films may also indicate the mass. Hydrostatic reduction materials such as barium, air, oxygen, saline, and aqueous contrast materials have proven successful to reduce the intussusception (Keating, 2006). Intussusception may recur after the reduction. For this reason, the child is kept for observation after any of these procedures. Surgery may be the only corrective measure.

During the operation a small incision is made into the abdomen, and the wayward intestine is "milked" back into position. The intestine is inspected for gangrene, and if all is well, the abdomen is sutured. Barring complications, recovery is straightforward. If the intestine cannot be reduced or if gangrene has set in, a resection is done and the affected bowel is removed. The cut end of the ileum is joined to the cut end of the colon; this is called an **anastomosis.**

Nursing Care

Preoperative. The patient is admitted to the hospital for procedures to prepare for surgery and to prevent postoperative complications. Treatment is aimed at combating shock and restoring blood, fluids, and electrolytes. The physician or charge nurse obtains written consent for surgery from the parents or guardians of the child. It is wise for the admitting nurse to confirm this by checking the appropriate sheet in the patient's chart. This procedure takes on even greater importance in emergency situations.

Gastric suction is necessary to prevent stomach distention. This may be continued for some time after surgery, particularly if a resection is done. The nurse applies elbow restraints to the patient to prevent dislodgment of the nasal tube, if this has not already been done for intravenous therapy. The child's identification band is checked to see that it is secure, and voiding before surgery is recorded. Preoperative medication is given to relax the patient and to prevent the aspiration of secretions. Once the child has been medicated, the surrounding activity should be kept to a minimum. The medical record accompanies the child. Proper safety precautions are taken during transit.

More than likely, this is the first surgery the child has undergone. The parents need to be supported, and explanations concerning the procedures and care of the child are important to them. Make sure the parents' needs are also addressed. If at all possible, let them accompany the child to the surgical area. Make sure they know where the family can stay during the surgical procedure. Information provided in a timely manner is consoling and respectful to the family.

Postoperative. After surgery, care is mainly symptomatic. Vital signs are checked frequently, the child's position is changed often, and careful attention is given to the skin. Mouth care is essential because the patient receives little or nothing by mouth for a while. The nostrils need cleaning and lubricating because the nasal tube can be irritating. If a urinary catheter has been inserted in the operating room, it is observed for kinks that could hamper the flow of urine. The drainage from the catheter is measured and described in the nurse's notes. The operative site is kept clean and dry. Promptly report any odor from the incision. Be on the alert for abdominal distention. Clear fluids are given when bowel sounds are heard. The passage of gas, liquids, or solids through the rectum is of particular significance because it indicates peristalsis.

Gastric suction keeps the stomach and upper intestine empty. The gastric tube is attached to suction and is run on low to avoid damage to the lining of the stomach. Small saline irrigations are usually ordered to prevent clogging of the tube. The amount used is recorded on the patient's fluid balance sheet. Drainage in the bottle is measured and recorded every 8 hours or more frequently if necessary. Accurate recording of fluid drainage is essential because this type of drainage removes salts and hydrochloric acid from the stomach, which must be replaced by intravenous fluids.

The patient and the family are given supportive help throughout this ordeal. A pacifier may soothe the young child who is deprived of feeding by mouth.

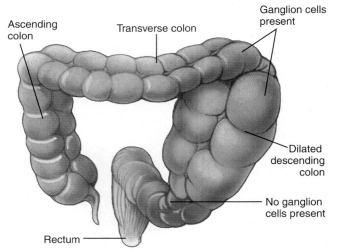

FIGURE 8-17 In Hirschsprung's disease, dilation of the colon occurs proximal to the aganglionic section.

Some of these patients are at an age when fear of strangers is prevalent; thus their need for the security of parents is paramount. Parents need assurance that their child is in good hands and that their presence is not a hindrance to the hospital staff.

HIRSCHSPRUNG'S DISEASE
Description
Hirschsprung's disease, or **aganglionic megacolon,** is characterized by the absence of ganglion nerve cells in the colon (Figure 8-17). This causes abnormal peristalsis and resulting chronic constipation. The affected segment of the colon is in constant contraction and obstructs the flow of stool. The portion of the colon proximal to the affected colon becomes distended (megacolon). The results can be decreased blood flow, ischemia, and breakdown of the intestinal walls. Inflammation (enterocolitis) and infection can result in a life-threatening situation. It is a rarely seen disorder.

Signs and Symptoms
Newborn infants may not pass meconium within 48 hours of birth. Abdominal distention with ribbon-like stools and vomiting can be present. Older children have a history of chronic constipation with foul-smelling, pellet-like stools, ribbon-like stools, or liquid stools. They have abdominal distention and may have failure to thrive. Parents may have tried a variety of methods to treat the constipation. Diagnosis is made with a barium enema and rectal mucosa biopsy. Rectal manometry can be used to measure the strength of the internal rectal sphincter.

Treatment and Nursing Care
Nursing interventions include parent education and support during the testing procedures. The disease requires the surgical removal of the affected portion of the colon and anastomosis of the normal bowel to

the rectum. Past treatment by surgical correction of the affected colon included a stepped approach with a colostomy in the first few weeks followed by corrective surgery in 3 to 6 months. Currently, the approach is to perform a complete repair without a colostomy on the infant in the first few weeks of life (Halter et al., 2004).

Before surgery, the child is NPO and undergoes gastric decompression. Fluids and electrolytes are administered and monitored. Abdominal distention should be monitored with repeated measurements. Antibiotics may be administered if enterocolitis is suspected. Depending on the age of the child, both child and parents need support and education regarding ostomy care if necessary.

Postoperative care is similar to that of any abdominal surgery. The child is NPO and often has an NG tube to suction. All fluid output is measured and documented. A Foley catheter may be in place to prevent contamination to the wound site. Assessment of bowel function is monitored and indicates the readiness for oral feedings. If a colostomy was performed, the nurse follows routine ostomy care. Parents should be encouraged to participate in the care of the child in preparing for home discharge. Additional supervision and education of the family may be met with involvement of a home health care agency.

VOMITING
Description
Vomiting, a common symptom during infancy and childhood, is the result of sudden contractions of the diaphragm and the muscles of the stomach. It must be evaluated in relation to the child's total health status. Occasional vomiting is to be expected. Persistent vomiting requires investigation because it results in dehydration and electrolyte imbalance. The continuous loss of hydrochloric acid and sodium chloride from the stomach can cause alkalosis. In this condition, the acid-base balance of the body becomes disturbed because of a loss of chlorides and potassium. This can result in death if left untreated.

The well child vomits from various causes. Some of them stem from improper feeding techniques. The nurse should ask the following questions when an infant vomits: Was the baby fed too fast? Too much? Was the infant burped frequently and properly positioned after the feeding? Has there been a recent formula increase or change? Were any previous feedings vomited? Sometimes the difficulty lies with the formula. If the fat content is too high, it can slow down the emptying process of the stomach. The introduction of foods of a different consistency may also precipitate this symptom. Infants sometimes instigate vomiting by gagging themselves with fingers or objects of play.

Other factors that cause vomiting are ear, nose, and throat infections. Vomiting is seen in the primary stages of many communicable diseases. Specific disorders, such as Reye's syndrome, peptic ulcer disease,

increased intracranial pressure, strangulated hernia, and various bowel obstructions, are also responsible. In these conditions, the vomiting is not necessarily associated with feedings. When the cause of the illness is discovered and properly treated, the symptom disappears. Aspiration and aspiration pneumonia are serious complications of vomiting. Vomitus becomes drawn into the air passages on inspiration and causes immediate death in extreme cases.

Treatment and Nursing Care
To prevent vomiting, the nurse must carefully feed and burp the baby, especially an ill child. Treatments are avoided immediately after feedings. The baby should be handled as little as possible at this time. To prevent aspiration of vomitus, the nurse places the infant on the right side after feedings. When an older child begins to vomit, the head is turned to one side and an emesis basin and tissues are provided. The infant's hands and face are bathed with warm water. Particular attention is given to the creases of the neck and behind the ears. To change position, the nurse turns the patient slowly and gently because motion tends to increase nausea. A clean gown is applied, and the bed linen is changed if necessary.

The nurse may estimate the amount of material vomited by filling a similar basin with water to about the same level as the vomitus and measuring the water. Factors to be charted include time, amount, color (bloody, bile-stained), consistency, force, frequency, and whether or not vomiting was preceded by nausea or feedings. The diet after vomiting is prescribed by the physician. In the hospital, intravenous fluids may be given (see Parenteral Fluids, Chapter 17). Oral fluids are withheld for a short time to allow the stomach to rest. Gradually, sips of water are given according to the infant's tolerance and condition. The patient's intake and output are carefully recorded so that the physician is able to compare the urine output with the total fluid intake.

When vomiting is persistent, drugs such as trimethobenzamide (Tigan) or promethazine (Phenergan) may be prescribed. They are available in rectal suppository form. The nurse lubricates the suppository and inserts it well into the rectum, where it dissolves. Slight pressure is exerted over the anus for a short time to ensure that the suppository is not expelled. Charting includes the time, name of suppository, and whether or not relief from vomiting was obtained.

FLUID IMBALANCE
Dehydration
When a person is in good health, fluid intake and output balance and homeostasis (a uniform state) exist. This is accomplished by appropriate shifts of fluids and electrolytes across cellular membranes and by elimination of those products of metabolism that

Table 8-3	*Signs of Isotonic, Hypertonic, and Hypotonic Dehydration*		
	SIGNS OF DEHYDRATION		
BODY RESPONSES	**ISOTONIC**	**HYPOTONIC**	**HYPERTONIC**
Level of consciousness	Irritable to lethargic	Lethargic to coma	Lethargic, hyperirritable with stimulation
Skin turgor	Diminished turgor, feels dry	Diminished to absent turgor, "tenting"	Fair turgor, feels thickened, "doughy"
Skin temperature	Cold	Cold	Cold to hot
Eyeballs	Sunken	Sunken	Sunken
Tearing and salivation	Absent or decreased	Absent or decreased	Absent or decreased
Mucous membranes	Dry	Dry to slightly moist	Parched
Fontanel	Sunken	Sunken	Sunken
Body temperature	Afebrile to febrile	Afebrile to febrile	Afebrile to febrile
Respiration and pulse	Rapid	Rapid	Rapid
Blood pressure	Normal to low	Normal to low	Very low

are no longer needed or that are in excess. The volume of blood plasma and interstitial and intracellular fluid (ICF) remains relatively constant. Dehydration occurs whenever fluid output exceeds fluid intake, regardless of the cause.

Disorders of fluids and electrolytes (sodium [Na], potassium [K], calcium [Ca], and magnesium [Mg]) are more complex in children who are growing. A newborn infant's total weight is approximately 77% water, compared with 60% in adults. This varies with the amount of fat. Also, the daily turnover of water in an infant is equal to almost 24% of total body water, compared with about 6% in adults. An infant's body surface in comparison with weight is three times that of the older child; therefore the infant is subject to greater evaporation of water from the skin. The younger the patient, the higher the metabolic rate and the more unstable the heat-regulating mechanisms. (Elevations in temperature are also higher, increasing the rate of water loss.) Rapid respirations speed up this process, and when diarrhea is present, additional fluid is lost in the stools. Immaturity of the kidneys impairs the infant's ability to conserve water. Preterm and newborn infants are also more susceptible to dehydration from variations in room temperature and humidity. Cessation of intake alone can result in significant depletion. When this is coupled with higher fluid losses, life-threatening deficits can occur in a few hours.

Problems of fluid and electrolyte disturbance require evaluation of the type and severity of dehydration, clinical observation of the patient, and chemical analysis of the blood. Types of dehydration are classified according to the amount of **serum sodium,** which depends on the relative losses of water and electrolytes. These types (Table 8-3) are usually termed **isotonic** (the child has lost equal amounts of fluids and electrolytes), hypotonic (the child has lost more electrolytes than fluids), and hypertonic (the child has lost more fluids than electrolytes).

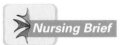
Nursing Brief

Mild dehydration = 3% to 5% loss of body weight
Moderate dehydration = 6% to 9% loss of body weight
Severe dehydration = 10% or more loss of body weight

These classifications are important because each form of dehydration is associated with different relative losses from intracellular fluid (ICF) and extracellular fluid (ECF) compartments, and each requires certain modifications in treatment. **Maintenance therapy** replaces normal water and electrolyte losses, and **deficit therapy** restores preexisting body fluid and electrolyte deficiencies. The replacement of a deficit may take several days, and the deficit continues unless adequate maintenance therapy is also provided. The physician calculates the volume of fluids to be administered through the use of various formulas on the basis of caloric expenditures because daily physiological water losses are directly proportional to caloric expenditure. The patient's temperature and activity (coma, restlessness) must also be considered. **Basal calories** are determined by the weight of the child. Volume is calculated on a 24-hour basis. Isotonic dehydration is the most common form in children.

Adjustments in fluid therapy are made constantly, according to the condition of the patient. The higher daily exchange of water that occurs in infants leaves less volume reserve with dehydration. Shock (hypovolemia) is the greatest threat to life in isotonic dehydration. The electrolyte content of oral fluids is particularly significant in the care of infants and small children with disorders of fluid balance and those receiving infusions. Commercially prepared electrolyte solutions are available by bottle; however, the nurse should ascertain whether they are to be given freely or by physician's order only. Patients with hypotonic dehydration—that is, excess water with sodium electrolyte depletion—are at risk for water intoxication. This can also occur if tap water enemas are given to small children. Loss of potassium occurs in almost all states of dehydration. Replacement potassium is administered only after normal urinary excretion is established.

Overhydration

Overhydration results when the body receives more fluid than it can excrete. This can occur in patients with normal kidneys who receive intravenous fluids too rapidly. It can also occur in a patient receiving acceptable rates of fluid, especially when the patient's illness is related to disorders of fluid mechanism. These disorders include kidney disease, burns, cardiovascular disease, protein deficiencies, and certain allergies. Hormonal therapy also may disrupt fluid mechanisms.

Edema is the presence of excess fluid in the interstitial spaces. Trauma to or infections of the head can cause cerebral edema, which can be life-threatening. A constrictive dressing may obstruct venous return, causing swelling, particularly in dependent areas. Early detection and management of edema are essential. Taking accurate daily weights is indispensable, as is close attention to body weight changes. Vital signs, physical appearance, and changes in urine character or output are noted. Edema in infants may first be seen about the eyes and in the presacral, occipital, or genital areas. In **pitting edema,** after exerting gentle pressure with the finger, the nurse should notice an impression in the skin that lasts for several seconds.

NERVOUS SYSTEM

BACTERIAL MENINGITIS

Meningitis is an inflammation of the **meninges,** the membranes covering the brain and spinal cord. Different organisms cause bacterial meningitis in different age groups (Table 8-4). Organisms may invade the meninges indirectly by way of the bloodstream from such centers of infection as the teeth, sinuses, tonsils, and lungs or directly through the ear (otitis media), from neurological procedures, or from a fracture of the skull. Bacterial meningitis is often referred to as **purulent** (pus-forming) because a thick exudate surrounds the meninges and adjacent structures. This can lead to certain sequelae such as subdural effusion and, less frequently, hydrocephalus. The peak incidence for bacterial meningitis is between 6 and 12 months of age. It is less frequently seen in children older than 4 years. The nursing care for all types is similar.

Signs and Symptoms

The symptoms of purulent meningitis result mainly from intracranial irritation. The onset of the illness generally follows two courses. Most often the disease is preceded by an upper respiratory infection or gastrointestinal problem. Nonspecific symptoms such as

Table 8-4 *Organisms That Cause Bacterial Meningitis in Various Age Groups*

AGE	ORGANISM
Birth to 2 mo	Enteric bacilli
	Group B streptococci
2 mo to 12 yr	*H. influenzae* b
	S. pneumoniae
	Neisseria meningitidis (meningococci)
Over 12 yr	*N. meningitidis*
	S. pneumoniae

irritability and lethargy may follow. The other course is sudden rapid onset with shock, **purpura,** changes in level of consciousness, and disseminated intravascular coagulation (DIC). Other nonspecific reactions include headache, drowsiness, delirium, irritability, restlessness, fever, vomiting, and stiffness of the neck and spine (Figure 8-18). The infant may have a characteristic high-pitched cry and a bulging tense fontanel. Convulsions are common. Coma may occur fairly early in the older child. In severe cases, involuntary arching of the back from muscle contractions is seen. This condition is called **opisthotonos** (*opistho,* backward; *tonos,* tension). The presence of **petechiae,** small hemorrhages beneath the skin, is suggestive of meningococcal infection.

Treatment

At the first indication of meningitis, the physician performs a spinal tap for laboratory analysis (see Assisting with a Lumbar Puncture, Chapter 17). In the early stages of the illness, the fluid may be clear, but it rapidly becomes full of pus. The pressure is increased, and further laboratory analysis indicates many white cells, sometimes too numerous to count. There is an increase in protein and a decrease in glucose.

Isolation is used until the patient has received at least 24 hours of antibiotic therapy. An intravenous line is established. The fluid serves as a vehicle for the administration of antibiotics, which need to be quickly assimilated, and also aids in the restoration of fluids and electrolytes. Antibiotics are given in combination and are adjusted on the basis of culture and sensitivity reporting. The initial choice is dictated by the cerebrospinal fluid gram-stained smear and the patient's age. Antibiotics are given according to the patient's progress but are always administered for a minimum of 10 days. With increasing antibiotic-resistant bacteria, medical management has changed to use of third-generation cephalosporins (cefotaxime or ceftriaxone) in combination with vancomycin. Neonates may be treated with ampicillin, gentamicin, and third-generation cephalosporins. An anticonvulsant such as Dilantin may also be necessary if the child is having seizures.

Most children with bacterial meningitis have the **syndrome of inappropriate antidiuretic hormone (SIADH)** develop. To determine the presence of SIADH, body weight, serum electrolytes, and serum

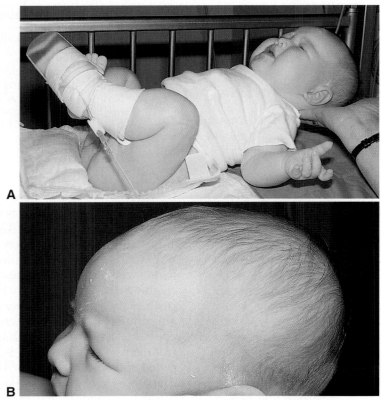

FIGURE **8-18** **A,** An infant shows nuchal rigidity with meningitis. Attempts to flex the neck result in the infant grimacing with pain, neck stiffness, and flexed knees and hips. **B,** A quiet infant shows a bulging fontanel that indicates increased intracranial pressure.

and urine osmolarities should be measured at the time of hospital admission. If detected, the syndrome is best treated with fluid restriction.

Initially, the patient is given nothing by mouth. An accurate record is kept of fluid intake and output, and vital signs and pupils are checked hourly. Strict isolation is maintained for 24 hours after the start of medications. (It is uncommon for others in the family to contract the disease, but the physician orders preventive medicines if necessary.) New or persistent fever requires reevaluation. Computed tomographic (CT) scan may be helpful in pinpointing secondary sites of infection.

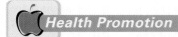
Health Promotion

Decreasing Risks for Meningitis

- The number of cases of meningitis related to *H. influenzae*, *Neisseria meningitidis*, and *Streptococcus pneumoniae* have been decreased with the use of the Hib, pneumococcal, and meningococcal vaccines.
- Immunization should be encouraged for all children.

Nursing Care

The nursing care of the child with meningitis is extensive. The isolation room is prepared in accordance with hospital procedure. Disposable equipment is used whenever possible. The room is kept cool and as clean and orderly as time permits.

Because the patient is overly sensitive to stimuli, indirect lighting should be used. Shades are drawn on a bright day. The nurse carefully raises and lowers the crib sides to avoid jarring the bed. Padded side rails ensure that the patient is not injured in the event of a convulsion. The nurse avoids startling the patient by using a gentle touch when waking the child and by speaking in a low voice. This need is also explained to the parents.

The patient is placed on the side to avoid aspiration of vomitus. Because handling must be kept to a minimum during the acute stage, it is important that the nurse organize care so that the patient is disturbed as little as possible yet still receives the treatment necessary for survival and recovery. Frequent changes of position are necessary to prevent pneumonia and to avoid breakdown of the skin. However, careful planning and consolidation of nursing procedures can minimize activity about the patient. As the child's condition improves, nursing care should include range-of-motion exercises (easily done during bath time) to prevent the development of painful contractures. In patients with long-term conditions, splinting of the extremities may also be necessary to avoid this complication.

Frequent monitoring of the patient's vital signs is necessary. Fever may be controlled with antipyretics, sponge baths, and the use of a hypothermia blanket. The nurse observes the child for signs of increased intracranial pressure, especially a change in alertness, or muscle twitching. The joints are also observed for swelling, pain, and immobility. Oxygen is given as needed.

The patient's intake and output are carefully observed and recorded. **Careful attention is given to maintaining the intravenous line.** If SIADH occurs, there may be fluid restriction. Good oral hygiene is essential during this stage when the patient is receiving nothing by mouth. As the patient's condition improves, the diet progresses from clear fluids to regular diet. A special formula may be given when NG feedings are necessary. The nurse promptly reports a decrease in output of urine, which could signal **urinary retention.** Bowel movements are recorded each day to detect constipation and avoid fecal impaction (an accumulation of feces in the rectum). Watch for signs of residual effects from the disease, such as weakness of limbs, speech difficulties, mental confusion, behavior problems, and hearing problems.

The diagnosis of meningitis is frightening to parents, as is the prospect of the child undergoing a spinal tap. Early recognition, appropriate antibiotic therapy, and supportive care have decreased the mortality of the illness. There is also concern for the health of other members of the family. The nurse should direct attention to the parents. Parents should be encouraged to stay.

GENITOURINARY SYSTEM

HYDROCELE

A hydrocele (*hydro*, water; *cele*, tumor), an excessive amount of fluid in the sac that surrounds the testicle, causes the scrotum to swell. Its appearance in the neonate is not uncommon, and in many cases, the condition corrects itself as the baby grows.

If a chronic hydrocele persists in the older child, it is corrected with surgery. Routine postoperative nursing care is given. Same-day or outpatient surgery may be arranged.

UNDESCENDED TESTES (CRYPTORCHIDISM)
Description

The **testes** are the male sex glands. These two oval bodies begin their development in the abdominal cavity below the kidneys of the embryo. Their function is to produce spermatozoa (male sex cells) and male hormones, particularly testosterone. Toward the end of the fetal period, they begin to descend along a pathway into the scrotum. If, for reasons that are still unclear, this descent does not take place normally, the testes may remain in the abdomen or inguinal canal. This condition is common in about 30% of low–birth

weight infants. When one or both testes fail to descend into the scrotum, the condition is termed **cryptorchidism** (*kryptos*, hidden; *orchi*, testis). The unilateral form is seen more frequently. Because the testes are warmer in the abdomen than in the scrotum, the sperm cells begin to deteriorate. If both testes are affected, sterility can result. Other complications include increased exposure to injury, an increase in tumor formation, and emotional problems, particularly in the school-age boy, who may be ridiculed by his peers. An **inguinal hernia** often accompanies this condition. Secondary sex characteristics such as voice change, growth of facial hair, and so on are not affected because the testes continue to secrete hormones directly into the bloodstream.

Treatment and Nursing Care

Occasionally, spontaneous descent of the testis or testes occurs during the first 6 months of life. If this does not happen, treatment is recommended at 9 to 15 months. The testes can be brought down to the scrotum with a surgical intervention called **orchiopexy** (*orchio*, testicle; *pexy*, fixation). Although orchiopexy improves the condition, the fertility rate among these patients, even when only one testis is undescended, may be reduced. For boys with congenital absence of a testis, a testicular prosthetic may be psychologically important. In addition, although testicular tumors are rare, their incidence is increased in these patients during adulthood. Parents are told to teach the growing child the importance of self-examination of the testes.

The psychological approach of the nurse to the patient and his family is of importance because of the embarrassment involved in cases of this nature. People may ask the child why he is having surgery when there is no visible evidence of trauma. This problem is frequently compounded by the fact that the older child has been told not to discuss his condition. In addition, his understanding of his problem and just what is going to happen in surgery really may be vague. Therefore it is important that the nurse caring for the child knows just what he has been told and how he feels about his operation to give emotional support during his care. Terminology needs to be clarified. The nurse assures the child that his penis will not be involved in the surgery.

The parents too may have anxieties that they cannot verbalize. It is difficult for many of them to communicate with their child in matters such as these. They may also fear that the child will become homosexual or less virile. A thoughtful, sensitive nurse who tries to anticipate these and other related feelings and fears is a definite asset to the patient's adjustment.

HYPOSPADIAS AND EPISPADIAS
Description

Hypospadias is the most common congenital anomaly of the penis. The opening of the urinary meatus appears on the ventral or underside of

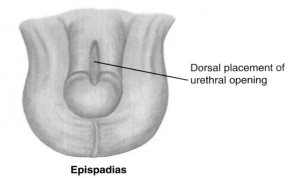

Epispadias

Dorsal placement of urethral opening

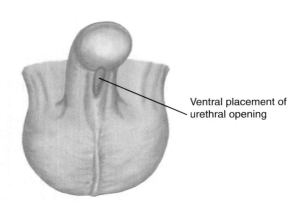

Hypospadias

Ventral placement of urethral opening

FIGURE **8-19** Possible locations of the urethral meatus in the child with hypospadias and epispadias.

the shaft of the penis. Epispadias has the urethral opening on the dorsal or upper surface of the shaft (Figure 8-19). **Chordee,** a downward curvature of the penis, is the result of a tight fibrous band and may be seen with hypospadias. The displacement of the urinary meatus opening should not interfere with continence.

Treatment and Nursing Care

The nurse may discover the defect while the infant is in the nursery. Treatment is determined by the location of the defect. The ultimate goals are for the child to be able to void standing up, to prevent any possible psychological problems, and to avoid potential difficulties with sexual function. Surgical repair is usually performed between 6 and 12 months of age. New microsurgery techniques may allow for an earlier repair. Repair may be done in stages. Circumcision is avoided because the foreskin may be needed in reconstruction. After surgery, a urinary catheter or **urethral stent** may be placed to allow for healing of the meatus. A pressure dressing may be on the penis and is removed by the physician. Parents need instruction for home care of such devices.

Fluid intake is important, and increased amounts are necessary to decrease the risk for infection. Antibiotics and

medications for bladder spasms may be administered. Before discharge, parents should be instructed to observe for signs of urinary infections such as cloudy urine or foul smell. The child's temperature should be monitored.

Surgical correction may occur at a developmental stage that involves fear of separation and anxiety of mutilation. These concerns should be included in providing care for the child. Parents should be instructed to the possible fears that the child may experience.

SPECIAL TOPICS

SUDDEN INFANT DEATH SYNDROME

Sudden infant death syndrome (SIDS) is defined clinically as the sudden, unexpected death of an apparently healthy infant less than 1 year of age for which a routine autopsy fails to identify the cause. It is also referred to as **crib death** or **cot death.** Although precise data are not available, it is estimated that in the United States, SIDS kills about 3000 infants per year. In industrialized countries, SIDS is one of the leading causes of death in early infancy; the peak incidence is between 2 and 4 months of age. It is more common in low–birth weight babies, in boys, in families with crowded living conditions, and during the winter months. Autopsy may reveal slight respiratory infection or otitis media, petechiae over the pleura, and pulmonary edema. Two clinical features of the disease remain constant: (1) death occurs during sleep, and (2) the infant does not cry or make other sounds of distress. In some cases, the baby is found in one corner of the crib with blood-tinged froth coming from the nose.

Theories concerning the cause of SIDS are numerous. Although there appears to be an increased incidence among siblings, no genetic pattern has been determined. The risk for SIDS is increased in twins.

Many theories concerning cause, such as suffocation, aspiration allergy, and hormone deficiency, have been disproved. The exact cause is not known. Some researchers propose that crib death results from an interruption of some basic function in the central or autonomic nervous system that causes apnea. Carotid bodies located in the neck and involved in the control of breathing have been found to be abnormal in victims of SIDS. Current opinion holds that SIDS has more than one cause.

The death rate has continued to decrease, and the focus is on decreasing risk factors that contribute to SIDS. The "Back-to-Sleep" program has produced positive results. Co-sleeping has been identified as an increased risk of SIDS even if mothers did not smoke or if they breast-feed. Health care providers should encourage a separate crib or bassinet for sleeping (Hunt, 2006).

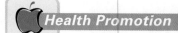

Health Promotion

Guidelines for Prevention of SIDS

- Always place infant on his or her back to sleep and do **NOT** use side-lying position.
- Use firm sleep surfaces with safety-approved crib mattress.
- Keep soft objects and loose bedding out of infant's sleep area.
- Avoid overheating, keeping head uncovered.
- Do not smoke during pregnancy or near babies.
- Avoid co-sleeping but keep infant's sleep area close. Keep infant's bedroom door open.
- Avoid respiratory or cardiac monitors to reduce SIDS risk.
- Avoid devices that claim to maintain sleep position to reduce SIDS.
- Consider offering clean, dry pacifier (controversial).
- Provide tummy time during awake periods.
- Stress that all care providers for infant follow the guidelines (AAP, 2005).

Community Cue

African-American infants are twice as likely to be put to sleep on their stomachs, and parents may need more instruction (Pollack & Frohna, 2002).

Babies with **infantile apnea** (also called near-miss infants) and subsequent siblings of babies with SIDS are often monitored at home until they are past the age of danger. Monitors can be leased. Parents are provided with ongoing education and support during this period. Parents are taught cardiopulmonary resuscitation before having their child monitored.

In dealing with grieving parents after the death of their infant, the nurse must convey some important facts: that the baby died of a disease entity called *SIDS*, that this disease currently cannot be predicted or prevented, and that they are **not** responsible for the child's death. Grieving parents need time to say good-bye to their child. They should be encouraged to hold and rock their infant, shed tears, and assist in burial preparations. This process, not common in the past, is conducive to the resolution of grief (see also Chapter 18). One mother who was denied this experience stated that *5 years later*, while visiting a florist's shop, she noticed a heart-shaped wreath intended for an infant. She unexpectedly burst into tears and wept.

Parents of a child who dies of SIDS experience a great deal of guilt and are catapulted into a totally unexpected bereavement, requiring numerous explanations to relatives and friends. Often needless blame has been placed on one parent by the other or by relatives. The family babysitter and physician may also be targets of attack. Emergency department personnel need to be especially sensitive and supportive during this crisis. There have been occurrences of SIDS for which parents have been charged with child abuse and have even been jailed because of lack of public knowledge about the disease.

Sudden infant death syndrome can occur in the hospital, and many nurses and physicians have personal experience of the suffering that losing a child to SIDS can cause. Group therapy with other parents of SIDS victims is recommended. Two nationally supported organizations are the Compassionate Friends, Inc, and the National Sudden Infant Death Syndrome Foundation. These groups have local chapters in most states.

FAILURE TO THRIVE
Description

Failure to thrive is now used to describe infants and children who, without superficially evident cause, fail to gain, and often lose, weight **(nonorganic).** Although this condition can be caused by organic abnormalities as well, this discussion is limited to environmental causes. Infants who fail to thrive are frequently admitted to the hospital for evaluation with presenting symptoms of weight loss or failure to gain, irritability, and disturbances of food intake such as anorexia, pica, or abnormal consumption of food. Vomiting, diarrhea, and general neuromuscular spasticity sometimes accompany the condition. Patients fall below the 5th percentile in growth (Figure 8-20). Their development as ascertained by the Denver Developmental Screening Test and other means is delayed. These children seem apathetic, some have a rag doll limpness about them (hypotonia), and they often appear wary of their caretakers. Others appear stiff and unresponsive to cuddling. The personality of the baby may be one that does not foster maternal attachment.

Although causality is sometimes obscured, there appears to be a disturbance in the mother-child or caretaker-child relationship. The situation is complex and is often associated with marital discord, economic pressures, parental immaturity and low stress tolerance, and single parenthood. Alcohol and drug abuse are often present. Many mothers feel deprived and unloved and have conflicting needs. The infant suffers from the inability to establish a sense of trust in caretakers. Coping abilities are affected by a lack of nurturing. Outward neglect and physical abuse are not uncommon.

Treatment and Nursing Care

Prevention of environmental failure to thrive consists chiefly of instituting social measures such as parenting classes, family planning, and early recognition and support of families at risk. Treatment involves a multidisciplinary approach in accordance with the circumstances; physician, nurse, social worker, family agency, and counselor may all participate. If no progress can be made, temporary or permanent placement of the child or children in a foster home may be necessary.

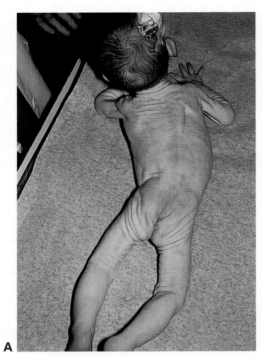
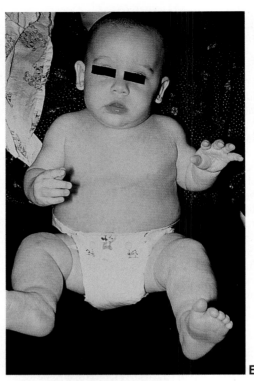

FIGURE **8-20** **A,** A 4½-month-old who is well below her birth weight and shows severe developmental delay. Note the loss of subcutaneous tissue manifested by wrinkled skin on the buttocks, shoulder, and upper arms. **B,** Same infant after 3½ months in foster care. Note that the infant is well nourished and is caught up developmentally.

Treatment of the child who fails to thrive requires maturity on the part of the nurse. It is vital to support rather than reject the mother. Maternal attachment can be facilitated by listening to her and helping her get in touch with her feelings and frustrations and explore her choices. Encourage her to assist with the daily care of her child. Stress the baby's uniqueness and responses to the mother. Point out developmental patterns and provide anticipatory guidance in this area. Avoid lecturing. Try to understand her situation and needs. Take the initiative. Frequently, the mother's "lack of interest during visiting hours" stems from her own insecurities and feelings of rejection by hospital staff that seem critical to her. Provide parents with a 24-hour telephone number and encourage them to use it when stress mounts. Parents Anonymous and parent aides are other resources.

A consistent caregiver should be provided so that the child develops trust in the individual. The caregiver should model appropriate parenting behaviors. The parent should be praised for positive parenting.

Interaction between the parent and child should be observed and documented. Nurses must be diligent about charting only objective observations. Behaviors observed and statements made by the parents meet these criteria. Nurses cannot chart their feelings or instincts about the parent-child relationship.

When the child is hospitalized, nursing measures are similar to those cited for child abuse and neglect (discussed subsequently). Hospitalization often leads to dramatic improvement in weight gain and improved social response. The nurse should feel free to discuss ambivalent feelings toward the parents during staff conferences. Feeling angry is natural. However, expressing anger to parents is damaging and limits their cooperation. If a nurse is having particular difficulties, reassignment should be considered because body language could be detrimental to the parents' progress.

The prognosis of this condition is uncertain. Emotional abuse, particularly in the early years, can be psychologically traumatic. Inadequacies in intelligence, language, and social behavior have been documented in children who fail to thrive.

CHILD ABUSE AND NEGLECT
Description

Because of the scope of the problem, no one definition seems entirely satisfactory, but efforts are being made to reduce ambiguity. The term *battered child syndrome* was coined by C. Kempe in his landmark paper published in 1962 in the *Journal of the American Medical Association*. The term refers to "a clinical condition in young children who have received serious physical abuse, generally from a parent or foster parent." The impact of Kempe's research was considerable and focused the attention of physicians on unexplained fractures and signs of physical abuse (Figure 8-21). Today most authorities consider this definition rather

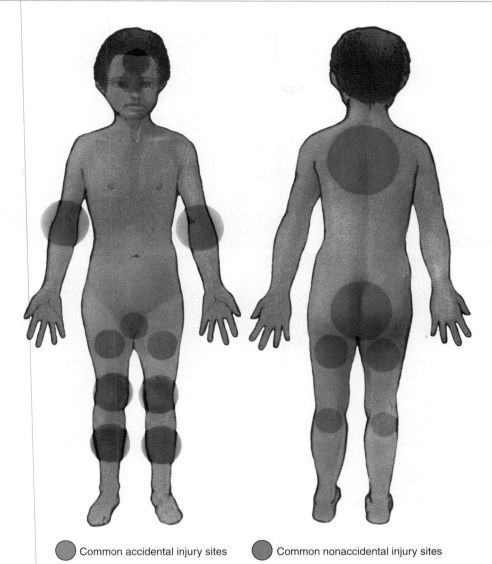

⬤ Common accidental injury sites   ⬤ Common nonaccidental injury sites

FIGURE **8-21** Accidents typically cause injuries in specific sites *(purple areas).* The nurse should suspect physical abuse in children with injuries in nonaccidental sites *(red areas).*

narrow and have broadened it to include neglect and maltreatment. Differences of opinion about what constitutes child abuse exist from state to state and in the criteria of various agencies concerned with this problem. Nurses must become aware of the mandates of the states and institutions in which they practice.

Statistics show that 11.9 of every 1000 children are victims of abuse or neglect (U.S. Department of Health and Human Services, 2003). The exact number is unknown because many cases go unreported. Three children die each day as a result of abuse or neglect and one half of all deaths are in children under 1 year of age (Box 8-2).

Federal Laws and Agencies

By 1963, the Children's Bureau had drafted a model mandatory state reporting law that has been adopted in some form in all 50 states. This law aids in establishing statistics and is based on the need to provide therapeutic

---

Box 8-2 *Risk Factors for Child Abuse and Neglect*

PARENTAL/CARETAKER RISK FACTORS
- Victim of abuse/neglect as a child
- Social isolation
- Low self-esteem, poor impulse control, antisocial behavior
- Inaccurate knowledge about child development/unrealistic expectations
- Young parent
- Mental illness/depression/anxiety
- Substance abuse
- Domestic violence/marital conflict/single parent
- Poverty/unemployment
- Stress
- Harsh discipline

CHILD RISK FACTORS
- Infants and young children
- Adolescence (for sexual abuse)
- Physical, cognitive, and emotional disabilities
- Behavior problems, attention deficit

Data from Office on Child Abuse and Neglect (2003).
Goldman J, Salus MK, Wolcott D, Kennedy KY, Office on Abuse and Neglect: *A Coordinated Response to Child Abuse and Neglect: The Foundation for Practice.* User Manual Series. Washington, DC, Child Welfare Information Gateway, 2003.

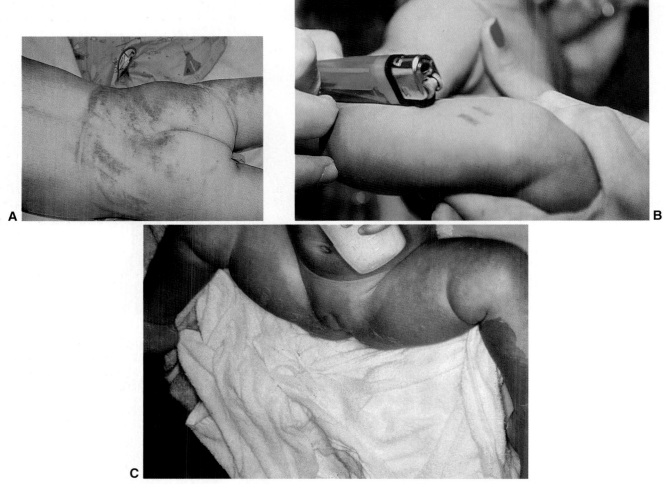

FIGURE **8-22** **A,** Lesions caused by hand, hairbrush, and a belt. **B,** Lesions caused by heated cigarette lighter wheels. **C,** Child was dipped in scalding water as a lesson for a toileting accident.

help to both the child and the family. Immunity from liability is provided for persons reporting suspected cases. Most states have penalties for failure to report child abuse. Originally, only physicians were held responsible for reporting suspected cases; however, many states now include all professionals who are in contact with children, such as nurses, social workers, teachers, and clergy. Other laws state specifically that anyone may report an offense. Referrals usually go to Child Protective Services, where a caseworker is assigned to the case.

Identification and Types

The types of child abuse and means of identification are listed in the Health Promotion box. In the past, much of the treatment of child abuse was provided after the fact. Current literature stresses the need for prevention and early intervention.

Child abuse can be physical, sexual, or emotional (Figure 8-22). It may entail neglect. It is often difficult to determine whether an injury or situation reflects abuse. Jurgrau (1990) suggests that injuries can happen

by accident—but rarely more than once. The nurse should be suspicious if there is a severe injury without evidence of a traumatic event, if there is a pattern of "accidents," or if an injury does not match the history given.

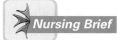

A citizen can report suspected child abuse or neglect by contacting the Child Protective Services in the Yellow Pages of the telephone directory under Social Service Organizations. This can be done with or without the use of the caller's name. After obtaining the facts, the agency informs the parents that a report is being filed and checks the condition of the child. A visit must be initiated within 72 hours. In most cases, this is accomplished within 48 hours or earlier if the situation is life threatening. All persons who report suspected abuse or neglect are given immunity from criminal prosecution and civil liability if the report is made in good faith. Many professionals, such as physicians, nurses, social workers, and so on, are mandatory reporters of child abuse.

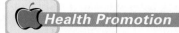

How to Recognize Child Abuse and Neglect

TYPE	CHILD'S APPEARANCE	CHILD'S BEHAVIOR	PARENT'S OR CARETAKER'S BEHAVIOR
Physical abuse (injury inflicted by caretaker for any reason)	Bruises, welts, burns, bite marks, intraabdominal injuries, or fracture Injury history does not explain or fit the injury History of suspicious injuries	Displays negative behavior as viewed by caretaker May have history of prolonged neonatal hospitalization Developmentally delayed Displays a "trigger" behavior such as crying, incontinence	May have been abused as a child May use harsh discipline May misuse alcohol or other drugs Poorly prepared for child rearing Unrealistic expectation of child Low self-esteem; lacks resources
Shaken baby syndrome	Irritable, vomiting, bulging fontanel, seizures, retinal hemorrhages	Lethargic; eating poorly	Same as physical abuse
Neglect (physical, emotional)	Failure to thrive; developmentally delayed Physically dirty; tired, and lethargic Comes to school without breakfast; often does not have lunch or lunch money Lacking in essential necessities Often left alone for extended periods of time Lacking medical attention	Is frequently absent from school Displays negative or unacceptable behavior May use alcohol or drugs Engages in vandalism or sexual misconduct	Misuses alcohol or other drugs May have disorganized, upset home life Noncompliant with medical treatments Fails to seek medical care May have a history of neglect as a child Isolated with few resources
Emotional abuse (often verbal)	Signs less obvious than in other forms of mistreatment	Passive and withdrawn to aggressive and acting out	Fails to provide child verbal and behavioral expressions of love and affection Determined to destroy child; poor parental self-image Unable to tolerate parental stresses
Sexual abuse	Pain or itching in the genital area Painful urination; bruising Venereal disease Pregnancy	May display regressive behavior or overly adult behavior Depends on age of child Overly mature or regressive behavior Sleeping or eating disorders Poor school performance Runs away from home	Perpetrator may have been molested as child Usually known by child May use drugs and alcohol May threaten child if child reveals
Munchausen syndrome by proxy	History of unexplained illnesses, near-death experiences	Nondocumented symptoms only seen by caretaker	Usually caused by mother Even-tempered person with some medical education Gives false information regarding child's illness

Child abuse is not limited to abuse by parents, but parents account for 80% of the offenders. Abuse can be inflicted by babysitters, boyfriends, relatives, or casual acquaintances. Drug or alcohol abuse increases the risk for child abuse. Abuse occurs at every socioeconomic level and is often precipitated by a stressful situation within the family (unemployment, marital problems, chronic illness, poverty).

Sexual abuse is a topic that is not easy to discuss; however, it is estimated that 10% to 25% of girls and 8% to 10% of boys have been sexually abused (Kellogg, 2005). Family members and adolescent acquaintances are the most common offenders. Rarely are strangers the offenders, yet many parents focus on "bad strangers" and "good and bad touch," which can leave many children unprotected (Nelms, 2003).

Nursing Care

Prevention of child abuse is of utmost importance. One approach currently taken is identification of high-risk infants and parents during the prenatal and perinatal periods. Predictive questionnaires are used as screening tools in some clinics. Many hospitals also provide closer follow-up of mothers and neonates. The process of **maternal-infant bonding** and its significance to later parent-child relationships have recently been explored.

Nurses in obstetrical clinics have the opportunity to casually observe parents and their abilities to cope. The history of the patient, the desirability of the pregnancy, the number of children already in the family, the financial and personal stability of the family, the types of support systems they have, and other factors may have a bearing on how the parents accept the new offspring. Pertinent observations include a description of parent-newborn infant interaction. Both verbal and nonverbal communications are important, as is the amount of body and eye contact. Lack of interest, indifference, or negative comments about the gender, looks, or temperament of the baby could be significant.

In other areas, a cooperative team approach is necessary. This includes providing a wide range of services such as family planning, protective services, daycare centers, homemakers, education for parenthood classes, hotlines, self-help groups, family counseling, emergency shelters for children, child advocates, and a massive effort to reduce the incidence of preterm birth. Other related areas include financial assistance, employment services, transportation, emotional support and encouragement, and long-term follow-up. More research and data services are required, as are evaluation and reduction of violent behaviors that are prevalent in our society.

Individual nurses can help detect child abuse by maintaining a high level of suspicion in their work settings. Record keeping should be factual and objective. Pediatric nurses should make a point of reviewing old records on their patients, which may reveal repeated hospitalizations, radiographs of multiple fractures, persistent feeding problems, history of failure to thrive, and chronic absenteeism from school. Delay or neglect in seeking medical attention for a child or failure to obtain immunization and well-child care is sometimes significant. Children who seem overly upset about being discharged need to be brought to the attention of the physician.

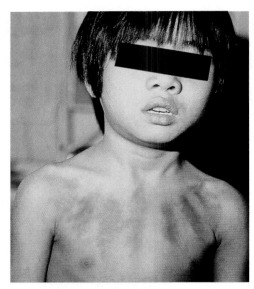

FIGURE **8-23** Oil is applied using vigorous stroking of the skin of a child with a fever. This produces a bruising pattern called coining and may be incorrectly interpreted as abuse.

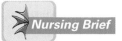
Community Cue

Although it is important to detect potential injuries, it is also important to avoid reporting innocent families. Health care providers should be aware of cultural healing practices. For example, Southwest Asians practice coin rubbing as a means of treating fevers (Figure 8-23).

Nursing Brief

Bruises heal in various stages according to color (0 to 2 days, swollen, tender; 0 to 5 days, red; 5 to 7 days, green; 7 to 10 days, yellow; 10 to 14 days, brown; 14 to 28 days, clear). Does this bruise match the caretaker's explanation of what happened?

The abused child should be approached quietly, and preparation for treatments should be carefully explained in advance. The number of caretakers should be kept to a minimum. The child may be able to express some hostility and fear through play. It is not unusual for these patients to be either unresponsive or openly hostile or to show affection indiscriminately. Keep direct questioning to a minimum. Use praise when appropriate. Encourage activities that promote physical and sensory development. Avoid speaking to the child about the parents in a negative manner. Consult with other professionals about setting limits for poor behavior.

The nurse must acknowledge that in cases of child abuse there are always two victims: the child **and** the abuser. Because of personal problems, the abuser often leads an isolated life. Some were themselves battered or neglected children. Many have unrealistic expectations regarding the child's intelligence and capabilities. There may be a role reversal, in which the child becomes the comforter. Although removing the child from the home is one answer, many authorities believe that this can be more detrimental in the long run. Being open to parents in this type of crisis is difficult but essential if the nurse wishes to be part of the solution rather than part of the problem. When placement in a foster home is necessary, parents experience feelings of grief, loss, and remorse. The child also mourns the loss of the family even if there has been abuse. The nurse should be aware of the child's needs and facilitate expression of feelings of loss. The nurse who recognizes the potential for violence that lies in all persons is better able to deal with this complex problem.

In dealing with sexual abuse, parents should understand that a good parent-child relationship that fosters open communication is essential. Parents should learn good listening skill and be willing to spend time listening to their child. Parents should discuss with their child the idea of keeping secrets and that no one should have the child keep a secret from their parent. Parents should be aware of all individuals who spend time with their child. Many offenders are either related or a close acquaintance. The child should know that he or she can tell the parent and that the parent will protect him or her and stop the abuse.

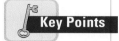

Key Points

- Nursing care of a child with atopic dermatitis includes frequent moisturizing of the skin.
- Cow's milk consumption should be decreased with iron-deficiency anemia; solid and iron-enriched foods should be encouraged.
- Parental knowledge of precipitating factors that can cause a sickle cell crisis (infection, dehydration, stress, or exposure to cold) is necessary in home care management.
- Anatomical differences in the respiratory system predispose infants and children to respiratory distress.
- Respiratory distress should be identified early to prevent respiratory failure.
- Children infected with RSV should be placed in contact isolation.
- Bronchopulmonary dysplasia occurs primarily in premature and low–birth weight infants who have needed mechanical ventilation for a prolonged period of time.
- Aggressive pulmonary therapy, including antibiotics and intermittent aerosol therapy, has increased the life expectancy of children with CF.
- Infants and children are at greater risk for dehydration than are adults.
- Monitoring of hydration status includes intake and output, vital signs, and level of consciousness.

- Educating families regarding preventive measures for bacterial meningitis should include Hib.
- When interviewing parents of an infant who died of suspected SIDS, avoid implications of guilt.
- Incompatibility between the history and the injury is probably the most important indicator for suspected child abuse.
- Mandatory reporting of suspected child abuse is required for all professionals involved with children.
- Good parent-child relationships that include open communication and parental vigilance with all individuals who interact with their child are necessary to reduce the risk for sexual abuse.

 Go to your Companion CD-ROM for an Audio Glossary, video clips, and more.

evolve   Be sure to visit the companion Evolve site at http://evolve.elsevier.com/Price/pediatric/for WebLinks and additional online resources.

ONLINE RESOURCES

American SIDS Institute: http://www.sids.org

Child Abuse Prevention Network: http://child-abuse.com

Child Welfare Information Gateway http://www.childwelfare.gov

Directory of Health, Medicine, and Human Life Sciences: http://www.medlina.com

Eczema: http://www.vh.org

National SIDS Resource Center: http://www.sidscenter.org

SIDS Alliance: http://www.sidsalliance.org

SIDS Network: http://sids-network.org

Objectives

Upon completion of this chapter, the student will be able to:

1. Define the vocabulary terms listed
2. Describe the physical and psychosocial development of children from 1 to 3 years of age, listing age-specific events and guidance when appropriate
3. Discuss how adults can help small children combat their fears
4. Identify five strategies that aid in meeting a toddler's nutritional needs
5. Identify the principles of toilet training (bowel and bladder) that assist in guiding parents' efforts to provide toilet independence
6. Discuss questions to use in evaluation of daycare centers
7. Discuss the use of car seats with toddlers
8. Identify four potential safety hazards specific to the toddler and anticipatory guidance for caretakers in preventing such accidents

Key Terms

Be sure to check out the bonus material on the Companion CD-ROM, including selected audio pronunciations.

autonomy (ăw-TAWN-ŏ-mē; p. 178)
baby bottle tooth decay (p. 181)
cariogenic (KĀR-ē-ō-JĔN-ĭk; p. 181)
defecation (děf-ĭ-KĀ-shĭn; p. 178)
Denver II (p. 180)
egocentric (Ē-gō-SĔN-trĭk; p. 176)
epidemiological framework (ĔP-ĭ-DĒ-mē-ŏ-lŏj-ĭ-kăl; p. 193)
fluorosis (FLOO-ō-RŌ-sĭs; p. 182)
negativism (NĔG-ă-tĭv-ĭsm; p. 176)
parallel play (p. 187)
phagocytosis (făg-ō-sī-TŌ-sĭs; p. 178)
physiological anorexia (fĭz-ē-ō-LŎJ-ĭ-kăl ăn-ŏ-R ĔK-sē-ă; p. 183)
ritualism (p. 176)
temper tantrum (p. 176)

GENERAL CHARACTERISTICS AND DEVELOPMENT

Children between the ages of 1 and 3 years are referred to as toddlers. They are able to move about on their own and are no longer completely dependent persons. By 1 year of age, they have generally tripled their birth weights and gained control of head, hands, and feet.

The remarkably rapid growth and development that occurred during infancy begins to slow. The toddler period presents different challenges for parents and children. This chapter discusses what toddlers are like as people and some of the obstacles they face (Table 9-1).

Toddlers are curious explorers who get into everything. As each month passes, they gain more control of their bodies. Soon they are walking, running, jumping, and climbing (Figure 9-1). They enjoy repeating these new skills, and with practice, they become less clumsy and awkward. Their desire to touch, taste, smell, and smear lead them into trouble. They quickly discover that much of their conduct alarms their parents. Unlike when they were infants, toddlers find that their parents no longer accept their actions willingly and without question. Toddlers cannot understand the need for restrictions, and as a result, they revolt. Temper tantrums are common, and behavior is not consistent. Negativism is reflected in unreasonable behavior and by saying "no" frequently. Ritualism is characteristic of toddlers. By making simple tasks into rituals, they increase their sense of security and self-mastery. Dawdling serves essentially the same purpose, and egocentric thinking predominates.

DEVELOPMENTAL TASKS

The developmental tasks seen during this period are based on a continuum of trust established during infancy. Physicians and nurse practitioners can readily focus on age-related tasks at the toddler's well-visit. Toddlers are now ready to give up total dependence. They become autonomous and seek independence (see Erikson, Table 2-2). They begin to differentiate themselves from others, particularly from their mother. They learn to delay gratification and to incorporate rudiments of socially acceptable behavior as determined by the limits of their family's culture. Important self-regulatory functions include toilet independence, eating, sleeping, and perfection of new-found physical skills.

Separation continues to be a major issue with this age group. Toddlers are beginning to separate somewhat from their parents but can tolerate only brief periods of independence and still remain very

| Table 9-1 | **Summary of Toddler Growth and Development** | | | | |

AGE	PHYSICAL	GROSS MOTOR	FINE MOTOR	VOCALIZATION	SOCIALIZATION
15 mo	Steady growth in height and weight Head circumference, 48 cm (19 in) Weight, 11 kg (24 lb) Height, 78.7 cm (31 in)	Walks without help Cannot throw a ball without falling	Builds tower of two cubes Releases a pellet into a narrow-necked bottle Uses cup well	Says four to six words, including names Understands simple commands Uses "no" while agreeing to request	Less likely to fear strangers Begins to imitate parents, such as cleaning house Has temper tantrums Kisses and hugs parents
18 mo	Physiological anorexia from decreased growth needs Anterior fontanel closed Physiologically able to control sphincters	Runs clumsily, falls often Walks up stairs with one hand held Throws ball overhand without falling Pulls and pushes toys	Builds tower of three to four cubes Turns pages of a book two or three at a time	Says 10 or more words Points to a common object, including two to three body parts	Takes off shoes and socks; unzips Beginning awareness of "my" toy, etc. May develop dependency on transitional object such as blanket
24 mo	Head circumference, 49.5 to 50 cm (19 to 20 in) Chest circumference exceeds head circumference Usual weight gain, 1.8 to 2.7 kg (4 to 6 lb) Usual gain in height, 10 to 12.5 cm (4.5 to 5 in) Adult height, approximately double height at 2 yr May have achieved readiness for beginning control of bowel and bladder Primary dentition of 16 teeth	Goes up and down stairs alone with two feet on each step Runs fairly well, with wide stance Picks up object without falling Kicks ball forward without overbalancing	Builds tower of six to seven cubes Aligns two or more cubes like a train Turns pages of book one at a time In drawing, imitates vertical and circular strokes Turns doorknob, unscrews lid	Has vocabulary of approximately 300 words Uses two-word and three-word phrases Says "I," "me," "you" Understands directional commands Gives first name; refers to self by name Verbalizes need for toileting, food, or drink Talks incessantly	Stage of parallel play Has sustained attention span Temper tantrums decreasing Pulls people to show them something Increased independence from mother Dresses self in simple clothing
30 mo	Birth weight quadrupled Primary dentition (20 teeth) completed May have daytime bowel and bladder control	Jumps with both feet Jumps from chair or step Stands on one foot momentarily Takes a few steps on tiptoe	Builds tower of eight cubes Good hand-finger coordination Draws cross	Gives first and last name Refers to self by appropriate pronoun Uses plurals Names one color	Separates more easily from mother Helps put things away Begins to notice gender differences; knows own gender May attend to toilet needs without help except for wiping

Modified from Hockenberry, M., & Winkelstein, M. (2007). *Wong's nursing care of infants and children* (8th ed.). St. Louis: Mosby.

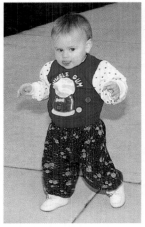
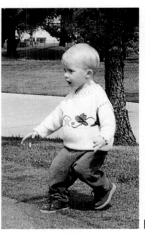

FIGURE **9-1** **A,** At 13 months, the child walks and toddles quickly. When moving fast, the child brings the arms to the upper chest area to maintain stability. **B,** By 15 months, the child can run with arms extended outward.

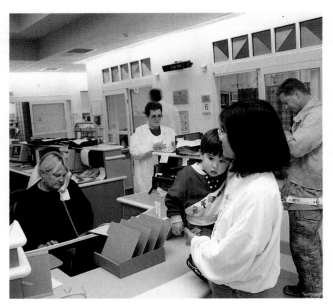

FIGURE **9-2** The hospital can be frightening to a toddler. A parent's presence is often reassuring.

interested in knowing where their parents are (Figure 9-2). Their greatest fear is separation from their parents. They need to be reassured that when their parents leave, they will return. The younger toddler might exhibit night waking as a response to fear of separation. This same child might use a transitional object (blanket, toy) for consolation when separated from the parent. By 2 years of age, the child still gets upset when separated from the parents, although not as much as before. The nurse should be reminded that separation fears are increased when a child is under stress. So the hospitalized child needs to be supported if the parents are unable to stay. Parents should never "sneak out" on a child. Mastering separation is a normal developmental process. The gradual control of these activities provides toddlers with a sense of mastery and contributes to their positive self-concept.

Erik Erikson (psychosocial development) defines the developmental task of the toddler age as learning autonomy versus shame or doubt. Toddlers need to be encouraged to become independent, and the caregiver should not do everything for them. The toddler who is happy and is allowed gradually increasing independence also develops a sense of security.

Lawrence Kohlberg (moral development) believes the toddler begins to formulate a sense of right and wrong but obeys only because the parent tells the toddler to. Moral development continues throughout childhood.

Sigmund Freud (personality development) described the toddler as being in the "anal phase" because elimination has taken on a new meaning. The child learns in this phase to control urination and defecation.

PHYSICAL GROWTH

Certain physical changes foster the growth process. Weight gain slows to about 4 to 6 pounds (1.81 to

2.72 kg) per year, and height increases about 5 inches (12 cm) a year during the toddler period. Toddlers' bodies change proportions. Legs and arms lengthen from ossification and growth in the epiphyseal areas of the long bones. The trunk and head grow more slowly. The growth of the brain decelerates. The increase in head circumference during infancy is 4 inches (10 cm). During the second year, the increase is only 1 inch (2.5 cm). Chest circumference continues to increase. Head circumference equals chest circumference at 6 months to 1 year. The size and strength of muscle fibers increase. Myelination of the spinal cord is practically complete by 2 years, allowing for control of anal and urethral sphincters. Respirations are still mainly abdominal but shift to thoracic as the child approaches school age. The stomach capacity increases to the point where the child can eat three meals a day. Appetite decreases, but it remains important that the toddler get adequate intake of all nutrients. (Nutrition is discussed subsequently in this chapter.)

The toddler is more capable of maintaining a stable body temperature than is the infant. The shivering process in which the capillaries constrict or dilate in response to body temperature has matured. The skin becomes tough as the epidermis and dermis bond more tightly, protecting the child from fluid loss, infection, and irritation. The defense mechanisms of the skin and blood, particularly phagocytosis, are working more effectively than during infancy. The lymphatic tissues of the adenoids and tonsils enlarge during this period. Eruption of deciduous teeth continues. By age 3 years, all 20 deciduous teeth are generally present (see Chapter 7).

The senses of toddlers do not function independently of one another or of their motor abilities. Two-

Table 9-2 *Behavior Problems of Toddlers*

BEHAVIOR	CAUSES	PARENTING TIPS FOR CORRECTING BEHAVIOR
Biting	Teeth are established. Child wants attention. Child is angry.	Establish "no biting" rule. Firmly tell child "no" while looking straight in the eye. Suggest alternative safe behavior. Put child in time out.
Bedtime resistance or refusal	Child does not want to go to bed. Child awakens several times at night. Child has already established history of being allowed to sleep with parent.	Describe the new rule of sleeping in own bed. Establish a pleasant bedtime routine. Escort child back to bed.
Hitting and spitting	Children fight when angry or they become jealous. They see this behavior in playmates or on television.	Establish "no hitting" rule because it hurts people. Teach children "Spitting doesn't look nice." Tell child to handle with words; ignore bullies. Use time out. Never hit your child for hitting someone else. Praise friendly behavior.
Nightmares	Relate to developmental challenges (toddlers fear separation from parents).	Reassure and cuddle child. Talk about the dream during the day. Avoid frightening movies or television programs (applies more to older children).
Temper tantrums	Child is angry (may be precipitated by wanting something but not getting it).	Ignore child but monitor safety. Take child to his or her room for 2 to 5 min. Avoid spanking (conveys you are out of control).
Sibling quarrels	Occurs because of nature of being siblings. Quarrel over possessions, etc. Want to gain parents' attention.	Encourage them to settle their own arguments; if children come to you, keep an open mind when resolving and avoid getting in the middle. Intervene if argument gets too loud. Do not permit hitting. Avoid showing favoritism. Praise cooperative behavior.

Modified from Schmitt, B. (2005). Patient Education Handouts. McKesson Corporation.

year-old toddlers reach, grasp, inspect, smell, taste, and study objects with their eyes. Their attention becomes centered on those characteristics of their surroundings that capture their interest. They can correlate sight with sound, as in the ringing of a bell. Binocular vision is well-established by the age of 15 months. By 2 years, visual acuity is about 20/40. Memory strengthens; toddlers can compare present events with stored knowledge. They assimilate information through trial and error plus repetition. They try alternative methods of accomplishing a goal. Thought processes advance, preparing the way for more complex mental operations. Language development parallels cognitive growth. The increase in the level of comprehension is particularly striking and exceeds their verbalization. (Language development is further discussed subsequently in this chapter.)

GUIDANCE AND DISCIPLINE

Toddlers' emotions fluctuate greatly. They show ambivalence. They love one minute and hate the next. They cry, kick, and slap when they decide to play outdoors longer than the parent wants and then turn around and kiss that same parent for giving them a drink of water. It may be difficult for parents to understand these mood swings. Toddlers are usually trying to assert their independence. It may be best to ignore this behavior as long as children are not hurting themselves or someone else. After the tantrum, parents should divert toddlers to some pleasant activity. Table 9-2 summarizes behavior problems that may occur during early childhood, causes

of those problems, and parenting tips for correcting the problems.

One of the objectives in the management of toddlers is to help them establish limits for themselves and find socially acceptable outlets for their behavior. Parents who direct all their child's activities cannot expect the toddler to develop self-confidence or autonomy.

Rituals play an important part in toddlers' ability to achieve independence. They provide them with known routines and people and places to come back to for support and security. Children's rituals (as at bedtime) should be incorporated into the hospital routine.

 Communication Alert

Whenever possible, children should be given choices: "Would you like to take your medicine from a medicine cup or from the syringe?" or "Would you like Mommy to put the medicine in your mouth?" Never say, "Do you want to take your medicine?" If the child replies "no," the nurse has created a communication block.

Toddlers need a certain amount of discipline. They get into many situations that are "over their head." When adults make a firm decision for them, the problem is at least for the time being resolved. Children feel secure because parents have helped them escape from their own primitive natures. There is controversy concerning spanking children. A time-out period is effective (Figure 9-3). The general rule is 1 minute per year of the child's age, up to 5 minutes. Time out can

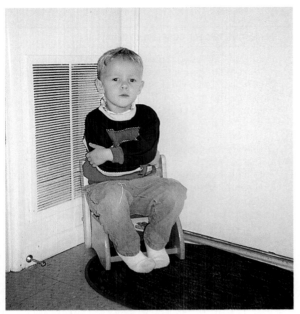

FIGURE **9-3** Time outs are a disciplinary measure used to remove the child from an activity and allow him or her to calm down and consider what was wrong in his or her actions.

change almost any disruptive childhood behavior and is most effective if the child is over 2 years of age.

Children, like adults, seek approval. Providing this approval is effective and helps increase their self-confidence. Take the positive approach as much as you can. Assume that the toddler is going to be good rather than bad. For instance, "Thank you, Johnny, for giving me the matches," will make the matches arrive in your hand more quickly than saying in a threatening tone, "Give me those matches right now."

Positive parenting steps also include spending time alone with the toddler, praising the toddler for good behavior ("You were such a good boy to help put your toys away"), and making the child feel safe and secure through discipline and love.

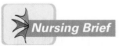

Caregivers need to provide safe areas for the toddler to explore. They need to watch carefully before saying no.

COMMUNICATION

LANGUAGE DEVELOPMENT

At about the end of the first year, the baby begins to make noises that sound like "bye-bye," "ma-ma," and "da-da." When toddlers see a happy response to these sounds, they repeat them. This is true throughout the toddler period. For small children to want to learn to talk, they must have an appreciative audience. At first, children refer to animals by the sounds the animals

make. For example, before saying "dog," toddlers repeat "bow-wow." Soon they can say short phrases, such as "daddy gone car." The 2-year-old can speak in simple two-word noun-verb sentences. Three-year-olds generally speak in three-word sentences and so on. Toddlers respond also to tone of voice and facial expression. If an adult sounds threatening, toddlers may answer "no" and then "no" again in a louder voice. Toddlers also use "no" to express their developing autonomy. It is good to remember that toddlers who talk remarkably well and understand more than they say still cannot comprehend much of adult conversation. Sometimes when adults forget this, they scold the child merely for being too young to understand what is requested of them. Imagine yourself being punished in a foreign country because you are unable to speak or understand the language well enough to defend yourself. Adults who show empathy to small children can help minimize their frustrations. A guideline for vocalization appears in Table 9-1.

Toddlers who have just learned to walk may practically give up repeating words because they are so overjoyed at being able to get about independently. As soon as their initial fascination becomes less pronounced, they take up speech again. Delayed speech does not necessarily indicate that a child is mentally slow. The temperament and personality of the child and the family play an important role. No two toddlers have the same vocabulary at the same age; however, generalities are found in language development. If a parent is concerned about a child's delayed speech, it can be discussed with the pediatrician during one of the child's routine physical examinations. This allows the concern to be evaluated in light of the child's total physical growth and development. Late talkers may be perfectly normal children who prefer listening to active participation.

Developmental norms in the use of language have been established. One widely used tool is the Denver II (Appendix G), a revision of the Denver Developmental Screening Test (DDST). This test is used to assess the developmental status of children during their first 6 years. It evaluates according to four categories: personal-social, fine motor-adaptive, language, and gross motor. It is neither an intelligence test nor a neurological test. A low score merely indicates a need for further evaluation. The test is designed for both professionals and paraprofessionals to use, and because it is a standardized test, proper administration and interpretation are crucial. Specific instructions for administering the test, scoring of the results, and a further description of the test are included in a manual that may be purchased from the publisher.

COMMUNICATING WITH TODDLERS

Adults must keep their everyday conversation with small children simple. Offering them too many choices confuses them. When talking to a toddler, adults should position themselves so that they are at eye level with the child. In this way, adults seem less overwhelming. This is of particular importance when the child is in a fear-provoking environment such as the hospital.

Adults should also use the "I message" when communicating with a child. Saying "I feel angry when you hit your sister" does not blame or criticize in the way that "You are a bad boy to hit your sister" does. "Bad" also demoralizes the child and makes him or her feel guilty. This can leave a lasting impression.

HEALTH PROMOTION AND MAINTENANCE

DAILY CARE

Toddlers need proper nutrition, plenty of fresh air and exercise, and sufficient rest. They also need structure and routine. By the time a child is a toddler, the mother has usually found it easier to give the bath in the evening rather than in midmorning. A flexible schedule organized around the needs of the entire household is best. This routine, however, can vary during the summer months because outdoor water play may make a tub bath optional. Parents may need to be reminded to never leave a toddler alone in the bathtub because at this age drowning and burns from hot water are still a concern.

The clothing of toddlers should be simple and easy for them to put on and take off. Pants with elastic waists are convenient for them to pull down when they go to the toilet. All clothing must be fairly loose to provide freedom of movement for jumping and other strenuous activities. Children should wear shoes with flexible soles. Tennis shoes are good choices once children are walking well. Shoes should fit the shape of the foot and be one-half inch longer than the big toe. The heels must fit securely. Children should wear their usual shoes at their periodic checkups because these show how the shoes have been worn, which indicates to the doctor how the children are using their bodies. Parents need to check the fit every few months because shoe size changes frequently as toddlers grow. Whenever possible, toddlers may go barefoot because this strengthens the foot muscles (Schmitt, 2005a).

In the summer months, children may sunburn quickly and should be protected by clothing/sunscreen so as to prevent future skin damage. Sunscreen should be applied at least 30 minutes before going outside. Sunscreen should be used even on cloudy days. According to the American Academy of Pediatrics, the SPF (sun protection factor) should be at least 15.

Sleep needs gradually decrease as children grow older. For example, they may enter toddlerhood sleeping 12 hours a night with two daytime naps. By the time they reach the preschool years, this amount may decrease to 8 hours of sleep at night and one nap. Establishing a routine for bedtime and naptime is also helpful advice.

Parents may need advice on how to get the child out of the crib and into a regular bed. During the adjustment period, be sure there is a railing or chair placed next to the bed at night. The toddler's mattress should be firm.

Adapt the toddler's environment accordingly. The chair and play table should be adjusted to their size (Figure 9-4). In some cases, this can be easily accomplished by placing a few magazines in the seat of the chair. A sturdy, small stool placed in the bathroom allows a toddler to stand at the proper height for brushing the teeth. These simple actions help to promote independence.

DENTAL HEALTH

By the time they are 30 months, most toddlers have a complete set of 20 deciduous teeth. An easy way to remember how many teeth young children should have is the age of the toddler in months minus 6. This approximation is a helpful rule to teach parents. Care of the toddler's teeth begins in infancy when teeth begin to erupt. Parents need to realize that access to a bottle of milk or juice exposes tiny teeth to hours of sugary acids that can cause severe damage (baby bottle tooth decay). The Health Promotion box lists important reminders for dental health.

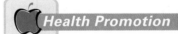

Health Promotion

Care of the Teeth

- Encourage fruits, protein foods, and calcium-rich foods
- Promote low-cariogenic snack foods
- Avoid sucking on lollipops and chewing sugary gum
- Examine labels for sugar content (cereals, etc).
- Avoid using the bottle as a daytime or nighttime pacifier
- Encourage toddlers to drink from a cup instead of a bottle

Good dental health is essential to the growing child. Attractive, healthy teeth promote self-esteem and contribute to physical well-being. Today techniques are available to prevent dental problems in most children. Unfortunately, many poor children seldom visit the dentist's office. More children today are uninsured for health services than in earlier years. When parents have limited income, they fall behind in dental health practice. These factors have an impact on preventive and acute health care. Nurses must realize that although most middle-class children see their dentist regularly, tooth decay is still rampant among the poor. Nurses can play an important role in decay detection, nutrition education, and teaching oral hygiene. They also can direct parents to dental clinics (and dental schools) serving low-income clientele.

Prevention of dental problems consists of good nutrition (a diet high in calcium, phosphorus, and appropriate vitamins), proper brushing and flossing of the teeth, and regular dental care. It is also important

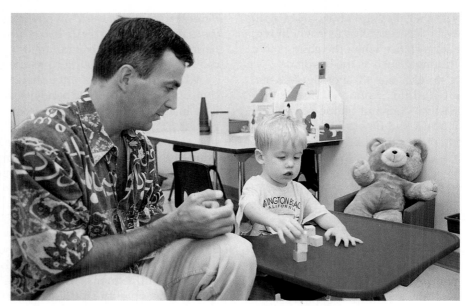

FIGURE **9-4**   A child's play area should have furniture adapted to his or her size.

after 6 months of age to administer fluoride by mouth. City water typically contains fluoride. The recommended level according to the American Dental Association is 0.7 to 1.2 parts fluoride per million parts water. Local testing can determine whether the content is adequate. Fluoride supplements can be given if water levels are not sufficient. Supplements should be given until about age 12 years, when the last permanent tooth erupts.

The 2-year-old enjoys putting toothpaste on a brush. However, the use of too much toothpaste must be avoided; only a small amount (pea-sized) is necessary. Children can ingest fluoride from toothpaste, leading to a total fluoride intake higher than recommended. Too much fluoride can cause fluorosis, or mottling of the teeth. In addition, during brushing, allow the toddler to experience and handle frustration. Technique improves with practice. To ensure effectiveness, parents need to assist the child until at least the end of toddlerhood. Teeth should be brushed at least twice daily.

The American Academy of Pediatrics Dentistry and the American Dental Association recommend children should see a dentist within 6 months of the eruption of the first primary tooth and no later than 12 months of age. When the child visits the dentist, the visit includes an examination of teeth, gum tissue, and bone structure. It also includes educating parents about proper nutrition, feeding patterns, tooth-cleaning procedures, and fluoride treatments.

NUTRITION COUNSELING

A toddler's need for food is not as great as that of an infant. This is because, despite an increased activity level, a toddler's growth is not as rapid. Often the growth patterns for toddlers are described as step-like

because of periodic growth spurts. Children need an adequate protein intake to meet maintenance needs and to provide for optimal growth. Toddlers need a total of about 13 grams of protein per day because muscle and other body tissues are growing rapidly (Food and Nutrition Board, Institute of Medicine, 2002). The protein is provided mainly by milk, other dairy products, meat, and eggs. Milk should be limited to 2 to 3 cups per day (16-24 ounces). Whole milk is recommended until age 2 years because the fat content of regular milk is needed for brain growth. After age 2 years, children can be given low-fat or skim milk. Too few solid foods can lead to dietary deficiencies of iron. Children between the ages of 1 and 3 years are high-risk candidates for anemia. Drinking too much milk satiates their appetite and decreases their intake of solid foods that are rich in iron.

Fruit juice should not be introduced into the diet before 6 months of age and should be limited to 4 to 6 ounces per day for children 1 to 6 years old. High intake of juice can contribute to diarrhea, overnutrition or undernutrition, and the development of dental caries (American Academy of Pediatrics, Policy Statement, 2001, 2006).

Vitamins and minerals are necessary for normal growth and development. Insufficient intake can result in impaired growth and deficiency diseases. Calcium is needed for adequate mineralization and maintenance of growing bone; vitamin D is needed for calcium absorption and for deposition of calcium in the bones and teeth (Behrman et al., 2004.) The child who is healthy does not need vitamin supplementation; a balanced diet consisting of a variety of foods is more likely than a vitamin preparation to supply all the necessary nutrients for growth. Vitamin and mineral supplements can help infants and toddlers with special nutrient needs or marginal intake achieve adequate balance, but care is needed to avoid excessive intake (Briefel et al., 2004). A well-nourished toddler shows steady proportional gains on height and weight charts and has good bone and tooth development.

The toddler is noted for having a fluctuating appetite and strong food preferences. **Physiological anorexia** is a phenomenon of toddlerhood that occurs because of decreased appetite and decreased nutritional need. These children have appetite fluctuations and may show a preference for one particular food for a period of time. Remind parents that any nutritious food can be eaten at any meal: for example, soup for breakfast, eggs for supper. Serving size is important. Servings that are too large are discouraged because they can overwhelm the child and lead to later overeating problems. Generally, a toddler will eat one fourth to one third of an adult portion. A quiet time before meals provides an opportunity for the child to wind down. Toddlers may refuse to eat because they are fatigued or because they are not particularly hungry. They may eat one food with vigor one week and refuse it completely the next. A flexible schedule designed to meet the needs of the toddler and those of the rest of the family must be worked out by the individual family. Forcing toddlers to eat only creates further difficulties. They are quick to sense parental frustration and may then use mealtime as a tool to obtain attention by behaving poorly and refusing to eat. Discipline and arguments during mealtime only upset everyone's digestion. Two or three healthy snacks during the day help to ensure a balanced diet.

Toddlers are fond of ritual. This is frequently seen at mealtime. They may want a particular dish, glass, and bib. It is best to go along with these wishes, as long as they do not become too pronounced. These rituals give them a sense of security and, in the long run, saves time and energy for the adult.

Toddlers have a brief attention span. They may be able to sit still for only about 15 minutes. They may try to stand in the highchair or wander away from the table. If they have eaten a fair amount of the meal, excuse them; otherwise, distraction of some type is necessary. Some restaurants that cater to families provide crayons and a special place mat to keep the small child occupied until adults finish their dinners. In the hospital, the toddler who is fed in a highchair needs to have the safety straps and tray secured. The nurse also needs to remain with the patient while he or she is in the chair.

Toddlers are at risk for choking on foods such as grapes, frankfurters, and raw vegetables. Injury prevention can be achieved by simply cutting foods into small pieces or thin strips and cooking raw vegetables until slightly soft. All food portions should be small and separated. Foods should be served at moderate temperatures. Candy, cake, and soda between meals are to be avoided. Offer a variety of foods and try to plan contrast in colors and textures. Finger foods such as crackers or cereal can be introduced at 8 to 10 months of age. Toddlers will continue to eat finger foods and can begin using a spoon at 12 months. By 15 months, many are feeding themselves.

MyPyramid (Figure 9-5) was introduced by the U.S. Department of Agriculture in 2005 to encourage people to make healthy food choices and to be active every day. Healthy food choices include emphasis on fruits, vegetables, whole grains, and fat-free or low-fat milk and milk products. Lean meat, poultry, fish, beans, eggs, and nuts are also promoted. The diet should be low in saturated fats, trans fats, cholesterol, salt, and added sugars. Parents should follow the guidelines of the pyramid by placing greater emphasis on the grains, fruits/vegetables, and milk products—the food groups that have wider color stripes. The wider base of the stripe stands for foods with little or no solid fats or added sugars. The narrower top area represents foods containing more added sugars or solid fats. The more active someone is, the more of these foods can fit into their diet. According to the guidelines, 2- and 3-year-olds require from 1000 to 1400 calories, depending on whether their lifestyle is sedentary or active. The guidelines then discuss how many servings of each group are required to meet the calorie level. For example, a child requiring 1000 calories per day would need 1 cup each of fruits and vegetables, 3 ounces of grains, 2 ounces of meat/beans, 2 cups of milk, 3 tsp of oil, and a discretionary calorie allowance of 165 calories.

Children like colorful dishes, which must be made of an unbreakable substance. Washable plastic bibs and placemats are convenient. Protect the floor around the highchair with newspapers. Silverware should be small enough so that it can be handled easily. Adjust seating equipment so that the child is comfortable and maintains good posture. Allow children to eat outdoors if weather permits. A picnic is enjoyable at any age (Figure 9-6).

TOILET INDEPENDENCE

There are many approaches to toilet training. Much depends on the temperament of the individual child and the person guiding him or her. Readiness is important. Voluntary control of anal and urethral sphincters occurs at about 18 to 24 months. If the child wakes up dry in the morning or after a nap, this is an indication of maturity. Children must also be able to communicate in some fashion that they are wet or need to urinate or defecate. They must be willing to sit on the potty for at least 5 to 10 minutes. The parent can place the child on the potty chair or toilet at regular intervals, such as when the child wakes up in the morning, after naps, before meals, and at bedtime. Toddlers seek approval and like to imitate the actions of their parents. They wander into the bathroom and are curious about what

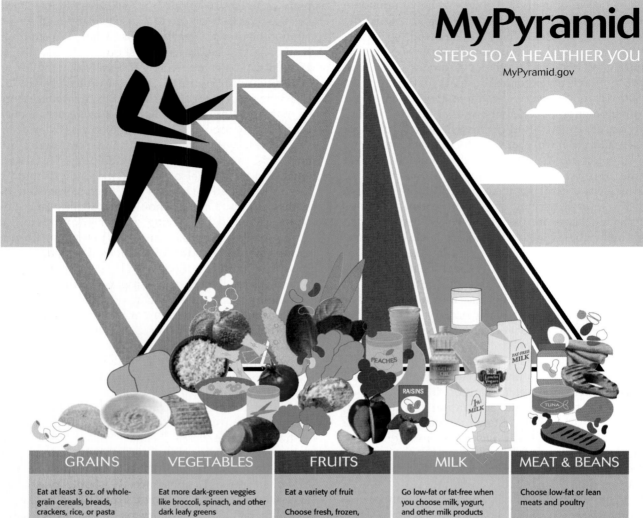

MyPyramid
STEPS TO A HEALTHIER YOU
MyPyramid.gov

GRAINS	VEGETABLES	FRUITS	MILK	MEAT & BEANS
Eat at least 3 oz. of whole-grain cereals, breads, crackers, rice, or pasta every day 1 oz. is about 1 slice of bread, about 1 cup of breakfast cereal, or ½ cup of cooked rice, cereal, or pasta	Eat more dark-green veggies like broccoli, spinach, and other dark leafy greens Eat more orange vegetables like carrots and sweet potatoes Eat more dry beans and peas like pinto beans, kidney beans, and lentils	Eat a variety of fruit Choose fresh, frozen, canned, or dried fruit Go easy on fruit juices	Go low-fat or fat-free when you choose milk, yogurt, and other milk products If you don't or can't consume milk, choose lactose-free products or other calcium sources such as fortified foods and beverages	Choose low-fat or lean meats and poultry Bake it, broil it, or grill it Vary your protein routine — choose more fish, beans, peas, nuts, and seeds

For a 2,000-calorie diet, you need the amounts below from each food group. To find the amounts that are right for you, go to MyPyramid.gov.

Eat 6 oz. every day	Eat 2½ cups every day	Eat 2 cups every day	Get 3 cups every day; for kids aged 2 to 8, it's 2	Eat 5½ oz. every day

Find your balance between food and physical activity
- Be sure to stay within your daily calorie needs.
- Be physically active for at least 30 minutes most days of the week.
- About 60 minutes a day of physical activity may be needed to prevent weight gain.
- For sustaining weight loss, at least 60 to 90 minutes a day of physical activity may be required.
- Children and teenagers should be physically active for 60 minutes every day, or most days.

Know the limits on fats, sugars, and salt (sodium)
- Make most of your fat sources from fish, nuts, and vegetable oils.
- Limit solid fats like butter, stick margarine, shortening, and lard, as well as foods that contain these.
- Check the Nutrition Facts label to keep saturated fats, *trans* fats, and sodium low.
- Choose food and beverages low in added sugars. Added sugars contribute calories with few, if any, nutrients.

MyPyramid.gov
STEPS TO A HEALTHIER YOU

U.S. Department of Agriculture
Center for Nutrition Policy and Promotion
April 2005
CNPP-15

FIGURE **9-5** The U.S. Department of Agriculture's new MyPyramid *(www.MyPyramid.gov)* symbolizes a personalized approach to healthy eating and physical activity. Children as young as 2 years of age can follow the MyPyramid guidelines. MyPyramid for kids is adapted for 6- to 11-year-olds *(www.usda.gov/cnpp/KidsPyra/index.htm)*. The toll-free telephone line is 800-687-2258.

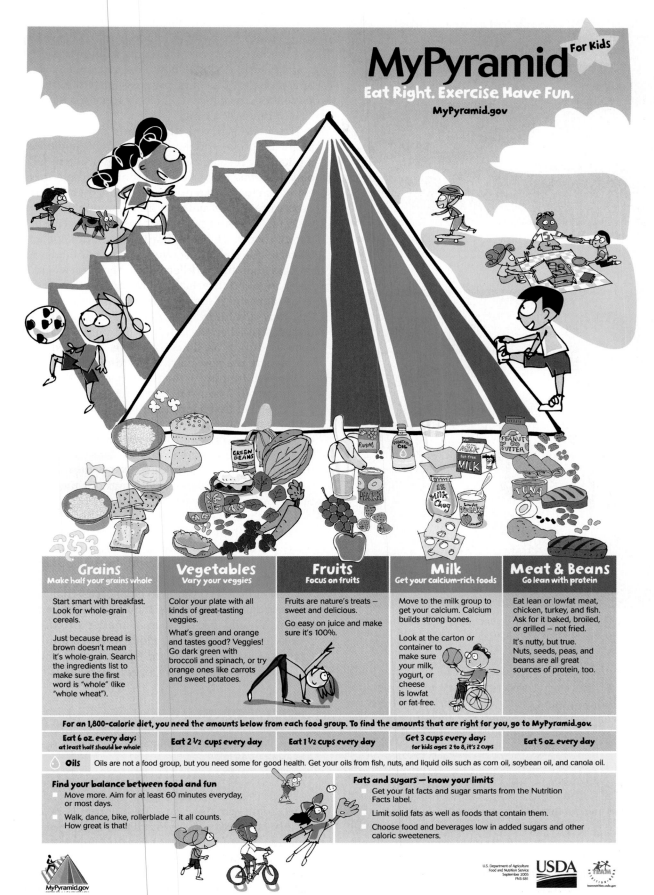

FIGURE 9-5 cont'd. For legend see opposite page.

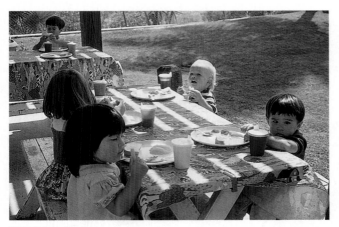

FIGURE **9-6** Children enjoy picnics. Keep servings small and nutritious.

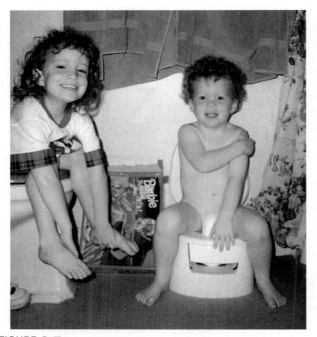

FIGURE **9-7** The toddler may be encouraged to use the toilet by watching and following the lead of an older sibling.

is taking place there. If parents feel that their child will respond to training at this time, they might first put the toddler in training pants (e.g., Pull-Ups). These can be removed quickly and easily, and the child becomes more aware of being wet. The use of a child's potty chair or a device that attaches to an adult seat is a matter of personal preference. A potty chair may make a toddler feel more secure because it is smaller-sized (Figure 9-7). The child's feet should touch the floor. The child needs time to become accustomed to this new piece of equipment. Toddlers may want to climb in and out of it and drag it about before they actually try to use it. If a potty seat is not available, a child can sit on a regular toilet facing the toilet tank back. This sitting in reverse gives the child a greater feeling of security.

Bowel training is generally attempted first; however, some toddlers become bladder-trained during the day because they enjoy listening to the "tinkle" in the potty. If toddlers have bowel movements at the same time each day, they may progress fairly rapidly. Do not leave them on the potty chair or toilet for more than 5 to 10 minutes at a time.

If a child's bowel movements are not regular, it might be good to delay training for a while because the toddler resents being constantly interrupted from play and taken to the bathroom. Toddlers generally enjoy having a parent remain with them during the procedure. Most parents find some phase of toilet training discouraging. Perhaps it is because some parents work at it too hard. They think of it as an obstacle that they must overcome rather than a normal process that the toddler easily masters when ready. Spankings and threats do more damage than good. Life is less stressful if the parent remains patient and keeps this new adventure pleasant. Training should not be undertaken when the family or the child is under stress, such as during an illness, a move to a new home, or when there is a new baby in the family.

Bladder training is begun when the toddler stays dry for about 2 hours at a time. One morning a mother may discover that her toddler has gone the entire night without wetting. At this point, it is logical to put the child on the potty chair and praise his or her success. Bladder training varies widely, particularly during the night. Restricting fluids before bedtime may help. Getting the child up half asleep and putting him or her on the potty chair accomplishes little.

If the child does not seem to catch on after a couple of weeks, parents need to accept that the child is not ready yet and they should not make the child feel bad. It is perfectly acceptable to continue to use diapers and then to try again after a month or so.

Most children continue to have occasional accidents until the age of 4 or 5 years. If the toddler has a mishap, parents should accept it as a matter of course and merely change the child's clothes. When adults show continuous affection toward their children and accept the bad and the good days, everyone benefits.

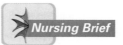

Nursing Brief

Nurses can help parents identify readiness for toilet independence.

The word that toddlers use to signal their need to defecate or urinate should be one that is recognized by others besides the immediate family. Sometimes, a parent may forget to inform the babysitter or the nursery school teacher of the word that the child uses. This causes children unnecessary frustration because no one can understand what they are trying to say.

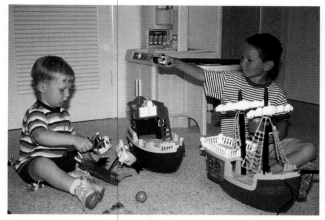

FIGURE **9-8** During parallel play, children may play side by side but do not influence each other's play activities.

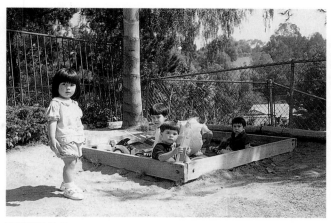

FIGURE **9-9** Cooperative play begins as toddlers approach the preschool years. Socialization is becoming important.

Toddlers who are toilet-trained at home should continue to use the potty in the hospital setting. They may be embarrassed if they have "accidents."Nurses regularly consult parents about their child's habits so as to make young patients feel more at home. Attentive nurses quickly respond to a toddler's pleas and consider whether or not the patient needs to urinate. Although regression in bowel and bladder control is common during hospitalization, personnel often contribute to this regression by not taking the time to investigate children's needs.

PLAY

Toddlers spend much of the day playing. In this way they develop coordination, which contributes to physical well-being. Play also contributes to mental health by bringing relief from emotional tension. At first, toddlers enjoy **parallel play**, playing near other children but not with them (Figure 9-8). This is the beginning of socialization. Gradually, as they learn to communicate more easily and become more skilled in handling toys, cooperative play takes place (Figure 9-9). They learn to give and take and begin to sense moral values of right and wrong. Play also has educational value. Toddlers learn continuously as they explore, and they delight in having many new play experiences.

It takes time for small children to learn to share. They clutch their toys, shouting "Mine!" Once in a while, they voluntarily offer a toy to a playmate. Parents should not force toddlers to share their possessions. This comes at a later stage of development. If they are constantly corrected for hoarding, they may eventually give up their toys when they are supervised but then seldom share when left to their own devices.

Toddlers need adult supervision during play, especially when other children are involved. The oldest in the group must be distracted from pushing,

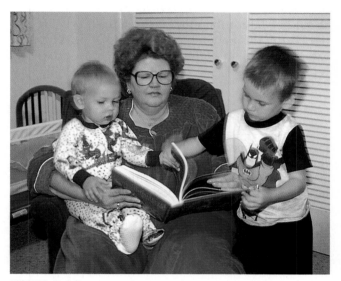

FIGURE **9-10** The toddler enjoys examining pictures in books and listening as stories are read.

hugging, and directing the play of others. The youngest child needs protection from being bullied. Toddlers feel secure when they know they will be rescued from alarming experiences. It is unfair to expect them to rise to situations beyond their capabilities.

The type of toy the toddler selects for play depends on age. The young toddler is content with pots and pans from the mother's kitchen and enjoys repeating acts such as removing clothespins from a bucket and replacing them. The toddler likes certain books and looks at the same pictures over and over again (Figure 9-10). Some children become attached to a certain stuffed toy or blanket. Two-year-olds like to unlace their shoes and remove them frequently. They are fond of water play and may resent being removed from the tub. They enjoy playing in a sandbox, scribbling with a crayon, and prancing to rhythmic music. It is not long until toddlers discover the stairs. Most small children start up them on all fours. As children become more accomplished in walking upright, they shift to the method of placing one foot on the stairs and drawing the other foot up to it, supporting themselves with the handrail. Eventually they can climb the stairs by using their feet alternately, as in walking.

Toddlers like puppets, puzzles, stuffed animals, and clay or Play-Doh. They enjoy imitative toys (lawn mowers, carpenter kits, housekeeping toys)—anything that looks like what their parents use. In addition, toys do not need to be expensive. Toddlers need to use their imaginations when they play.

Toys that can be pedaled, such as a tricycle, should be adapted to the size of the child. Wind-up toys, as a rule, cannot be fully enjoyed by toddlers because they cannot manipulate them by themselves. Objects that can be pushed or pulled delight the small child. Toys with small, removable parts are dangerous because of the risk for aspiration. As a rule, toys should be larger than the size of a toddler's fist. See the Health Promotion box "Choosing Toys" on p. 232 for additional guidelines on toys appropriate for toddler play.

DAYCARE

Daycare has become a way of life for many children under the age of 6 years. For school-age children, it also provides before-school and after-school care. More mothers are not only working, but also returning to work sooner after their children are born. Today most mothers of childbearing age work at least part time outside the home. It is clear that alternative methods of child care are necessary. These arrangements must meet families' personal preferences, cultural perspectives, and financial and special needs. Parents must take an active role in ensuring high-quality care. Nurses need to serve as resource persons and family advocates because finding adequate daycare can be stressful.

There are basically two types of child care: home-based and center-based. In home-based care, caregivers either give care in their own homes or come to the home of the child. These caregivers may be relatives, neighbors, friends, or those who have advertised their services. There is little research available on these types of private arrangements and few standards of quality control. With registered family homes, there are minimum standards published at the state and national levels.

Community Cue

The Maternal and Child Health Bureau has established the National Resource Center for Health and Safety in Child Care and Early Education *(http://nrc.uchsc.edu)*. The link "State Licensing and Regulation Information" lists child care licensure regulations.

Center-based care providers care for several children at once. These centers are usually private businesses run for profit. They too are subject to state regulations regarding physical makeup, number of children per caretaker, education of personnel, and so on. Child care centers run by businesses for their employees are becoming common. Sick-child care centers are also available in some areas for children who have minor illnesses that would prevent them from attending conventional types of daycare. Often these centers are located in hospitals that provide pediatric services. Parents need to determine their child's needs when choosing daycare. The philosophy of the center and the attitudes of the caregivers need to be evaluated. Parents should also consider the precautions taken by the daycare center to prevent disease transmission. The fewer the number of children to be cared for, the lower the incidence of infectious disease. Inspection and monitoring of child care facilities in terms of health (physical and mental) and safety standards are paramount. Parents should inquire whether the center is licensed and what the staff members' qualifications are. Additional criteria for evaluating a daycare center are similar to those discussed for preschools or nursery schools (see Chapter 11).

Ideally, all future daycare programs might include comprehensive health services and health education programs. Health care resources would be readily available to children, and the concept would tremendously increase the access of small children to health care.

INJURY PREVENTION

Accidents kill and cripple more children than any human disease and are the leading cause of childhood deaths. Although we do not have a preventive weapon, we do have a defensive one. This is knowledge. If parents understand their child's activities at certain ages, they can take the necessary precautions and prevent many serious injuries. For example, when statistics indicate that poisonings or burns are particularly prevalent at a specific age, parents can take measures to guard against them.

Most accidents occur in or near the home (Figure 9-11). Toddlers are especially vulnerable because they have a natural curiosity for investigating their environment. Parents must allow them some natural experiences, which teach them to look out for their own safety. They should also strive to teach toddlers what is and what is not safe. Toddlers are at the highest risk for accidents involving motor vehicles, drowning, and burns. Many of these accidents are preventable; parents and caregivers need to become aware of these dangers, which are directly related to toddlers' ability to be mobile, their need for independence, their lack of knowledge of danger, and their curiosity.

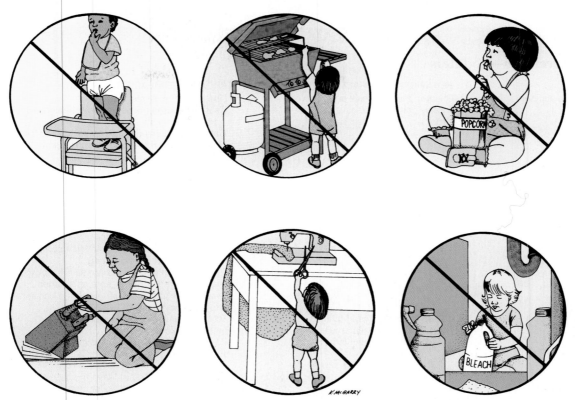

FIGURE **9-11** Safety measures should be taken to protect toddlers from these household hazards.

Nurses can demonstrate safety measures to patients and their families. This is most effectively done by good example. Measures pertinent to the pediatric unit are discussed in Chapter 3. Nurses in the community often can contribute indirectly to the welfare of others by the example they set and by being aware of emergency medical facilities available in the community.

 Community Cue

Nurses in clinics and schools need to promote safety through anticipatory guidance.

The federal government and concerned private agencies have attempted to regulate some of the variables surrounding certain accidents. A few examples are the use of nonflammable material for children's sleepwear, childproof caps on medicine bottles and certain household products, and the establishment of maximum temperatures for home hot water heaters. The U.S. Consumer Product Safety Commission has established regulations for crib slats, locks and latches, and mattress size and thickness. Safety warnings on the crib's carton advise buyers to use a snug mattress only.

Motor vehicle accidents are the number one cause of childhood death from injury after age 1 year. Laws have been passed in all states requiring infants and small children to be restrained while riding in automobiles

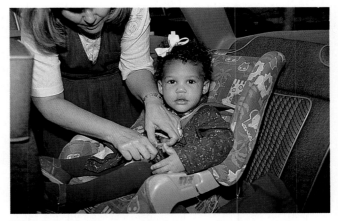

FIGURE **9-12** When an older infant reaches 1 year and 20 pounds, the car safety seat can be adjusted to a forward-facing, upright position. The safety straps should fit snugly. The seat should be placed in the back seat, ideally in the middle.

(Figure 9-12). Children under 1 year of age and less than 20 pounds are to be in rear-facing car seats, placed in the middle of the back seat of the automobile. These seats should be reclined at a 45-degree angle to receive full protective benefit. Children over 1 year and at least 20 pounds (up to 40 pounds) are able to sit forward in a convertible safety seat. Children weighing between 40 and 80 pounds should be restrained by a belt-positioning booster seat. Children age 12 years and under should *never* ride where there is an airbag. All child seat restraints must follow standards

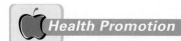

Injury Prevention—Toddlers

HAZARD	BEHAVIORAL CHARACTERISTIC	PREVENTIVE MEASURE
Motor vehicle accidents	Children are impulsive and unable to delay gratification, have increased mobility, and are egocentric.	Use car safety seats. Caution children not to run from behind parked cars or snow banks. Hold toddler's hand when crossing the street. Never allow to ride on/never carry on tractor or riding mower. Supervise tricycle riding; allow toddler to ride as a passenger on adult bike *only* with special seat and helmet. Do not allow children to play in a car or leave them alone in it. Do not allow children to ride in the back of open trucks. Drivers must look carefully in front of and behind vehicles before accelerating. Teach children what areas are safe for playing. Watch children under 3 years at all times. Teach never to run into street after a ball and never to ride toys in street.
Burns	Children are fascinated by fire. The toddler can reach articles inaccessible to the infant.	Teach the child the meaning of "hot." Install smoke detectors. Put matches and cigarettes out of reach and sight. Turn handles of cooking utensils toward the back of the stove. Avoid scaldings; do not leave the bathroom when hot water is being drawn or after the tub is filled. Treat burns with cold water; call doctor or emergency number. Teach child to turn on "cold" first. Avoid tablecloths that overhang. Keep appliances such as coffee pots, electric frying pans, and food processors out of reach. Test food and fluids heated in microwave ovens to ensure that portions are evenly warmed and not too hot. Keep hot foods and liquids out of reach; never carry such items around a child. Beware of hot barbecue grills. Never smoke near a child. Use snug fireplace screens. Teach child to stop, drop, and roll until fire is extinguished. Devise a fire escape plan and practice what to do in case of a fire in your home. Mark children's rooms to alert firemen in an emergency.
Falls	Toddlers like to explore different parts of the house. They can open doors and lean out open windows. Their depth perception is immature. Their capabilities change quickly. Although they may seem quite grown up at times, they still require constant supervision at home and on the playground.	Never underestimate climbing ability. Never leave alone on changing table, etc. Use safety straps. Teach children how to go up and come down stairs when they show a readiness for this task. Fasten crib sides securely and leave them up when child is in the crib. Lock basement doors, use safety knobs, or use gates at top and bottom of stairs. Mop spilled water from floor immediately. Do not wax floors heavily. Avoid use of baby walkers. Keep scissors and other pointed objects away from the toddler's reach. Use window screens or guards that cannot be pushed out. Fill in under playground equipment with sand or other soft material.

HAZARD	BEHAVIORAL CHARACTERISTIC	PREVENTIVE MEASURE
Suffocation and choking	Explores with senses, likes to bite on and taste things. Eats on the run.	Do not allow small children to play with deflated balloons because they can be sucked into windpipes. Keep powders out of reach; do not use when changing child's diaper. Inspect toys for loose parts. Remove small objects, such as coins, buttons, and pins, from children's reach. Store toys in a toy box without a dropping lid. Avoid popcorn, nuts, small hard candies, chewing gum, hard vegetables. Cut food into small pieces. Debone fish, chicken. Learn Heimlich maneuver. Inspect width of crib slats (should be no more than 2⅜ inches apart). Keep plastic bags away from small children; do not use as mattress cover. Use snug-fitting, firm mattress; do not allow young children to sleep on water beds. Do not lift child from crib if vomiting; turn on his or her side. Avoid nightclothes and play clothes with drawstring necks; allow no cords near crib. Discard old refrigerators (have door removed). Be sure playpens have sturdy sides.
Poisoning	Ingenuity increases, can open most containers. Increased mobility gives child access to cupboards, medicine cabinets, bedside stands, interior of closets. Looks at and touches everything. Learns by trial and error.	Store household detergents and cleaning supplies out of reach; install safety latches. Lock cabinet if toddler is particularly fascinated by items. Do not put chemicals or other potentially harmful substances into food or beverage containers; store in separate cabinets. Keep medicines in a locked cabinet; put them away immediately after using them. Use child-resistant caps and packaging. Dispose of old medicine. Follow physician's directions when administering medication. Do not allow one child to give another medicine. Do not refer to pills as "candy." Keep mouthwash away from small children to avoid potential alcohol poisoning. Keep telephone number of poison control center available. Explain poison symbols to child (Mr. Yuk stickers) and to parents not fluent in English. When painting, use paint marked "for indoor use" or one that conforms to standards for use on surfaces that may be chewed by children. Wash fruits and vegetables before eating. Obtain name of any new plant purchased and record. Alert family of location of poisonous plants on or around property.
Injuries from firearms		Unload and lock away all firearms separate from the ammunition.
Cuts		Pad sharp corners of furniture (and fireplaces). Use safety latches on drawers. Never allow children to play near running lawnmowers or power tools.
Drowning	Lacks depth perception. Does not realize danger. Loves water play.	Watch child continuously while at beach or near a pool or pond (including frozen ponds or lakes in winter). Empty wading pools when child has finished playing. Cover wells securely. Never allow to swim unsupervised. Wear recommended life jackets in boats. Begin teaching water safety early. Lock fences surrounding swimming pools. Supervise hot tubs; be aware that a young child can drown in an inch or two of water.

Continued

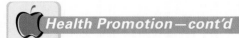

Health Promotion—cont'd

Injury Prevention—Toddlers

HAZARD	BEHAVIORAL CHARACTERISTIC	PREVENTIVE MEASURE
Electrical shock	Pokes and probes with fingers.	Cover electrical outlets. Cap unused sockets with safety plugs. Water conducts electricity; teach child who is wet not to touch electrical appliances; keep appliances out of reach.
Animal bites	Immature judgment.	Teach child to avoid stray animals. Do not allow toddler to abuse household pets. Supervise closely; do not allow child to play near pet that is eating or has a bone.
General		Keep first aid chart and emergency numbers handy. Know location and how to access local emergency care system. Become trained in child CPR.

established by the Federal Motor Vehicle Safety Department. Installment guidelines come with the automobile and the car seat. Many hospitals also have car seat installation checks that are free to the public. This service should be recommended for parents with young children, especially for first-time parents. Unfortunately, many parents still do not understand the importance of safety seats and neglect to use them. This is an essential area of patient teaching and begins with the first ride home from the hospital. Most hospitals have a car seat loan program and mandate the use of car seats for any young child leaving the hospital.

Community Cue

SafetyBeltSafe U.S.A. *(www.carseat.org)* is a national child safety seat resource that offers a help line, materials, training, recall lists, and answers to questions. The phone number is 800-745-SAFE or 800-747-SANO (Spanish language).

Legislation mandating car seats has reduced the risk for injury while toddlers are in cars. However, toddlers remain at risk for being hit by a car while playing in their own driveways. Before drivers start the car, they must be aware of any nearby children and pay attention to the children's locations.

New homes are required to have smoke detectors. Consumers who live in older homes and apartment complexes are also encouraged to install them. Various other safety codes are mandatory for public buildings, with additional measures required for buildings that are specifically for the disabled. The problems of surveillance and upkeep are, nevertheless, considerable. Many children live in substandard housing with little supervision. The education of parents is of monumental importance in decreasing death and disability.

Anyone who cares for children should be aware of the danger posed by any standing body of water. This includes bathtubs, toilets, swimming pools, hot tubs, and even small containers holding water. Parents should be instructed *never* to turn their back on a child, whether in a tub or standing near a body of water. Turning their back could result in tragedy. All parents should be trained in CPR.

Scald burns are the most common type of burn injury in children. Toddlers can pull liquids down on themselves by tugging at tablecloths, cords, and handles. Parents need to watch for toddlers underfoot, especially when working in the kitchen. Knobs, handles, and cords should be placed out of the child's reach. The temperature of the water coming from the hot water faucet should be monitored. Hot water heaters should be set no higher than 120° F to prevent scald burns. Small children can turn on the hot water while playing in the bathtub or while playing with the knobs. Always teach toddlers to turn on the cold water first.

Matches and lighters can cause devastating accidents. They should be stored out of reach of children. Parents should teach children the dangers of playing with them. Electrical outlets should have safety guards so as to prevent harm.

With their natural curiosity and new-found mobility, toddlers can find and swallow plant leaves, cleaning materials, medication, and anything else that catches their attention. All potentially dangerous substances should be placed out of the child's reach. A lock should be attached. Although most medications now have a safety cap, many children have been able to remove these caps. Parents should have the nearest poison control center number readily available. Specific treatment and care of the poisoning victim are covered in Chapter 10.

Choking is a concern with the young child. They do not understand that they should not put small items in their mouths. Coins, pins, removable toy parts, deflated balloons, and hard foods are common causes of choking. Nuts, popcorn, and hard candy should

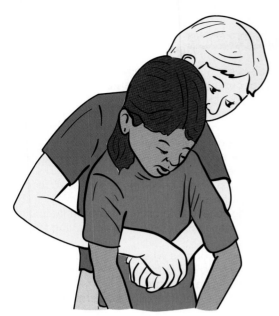

FIGURE **9-13** Abdominal thrusts (the Heimlich maneuver) are used for choking victims over 1 year of age.

never be given to young children. Abdominal thrusts (Heimlich maneuver) are the treatment of choice for the conscious choking person older than 1 year of age (Figure 9-13). In conscious infants younger than 1 year of age, back slaps and chest thrusts are used to dislodge the object (Figure 9-14). Specific instructions on how to relieve a foreign body airway obstruction are taught in a CPR class.

Playground injuries are another cause for concern. The toddler loves to run and climb and often disregards the danger associated with these activities. Children should be taught how to safely play when on playground equipment or riding toys.

For prevention of falls, doors, windows, and gates should be kept closed or guarded with a screen. When the child begins to climb out of the crib, parents should consider moving the child to a bed.

EPIDEMIOLOGICAL FRAMEWORK

An epidemiological framework for accident prevention is a means of providing a systemic method of evaluation. It consists of three parts: the characteristics of the host (the child), the agent (the direct cause: for example, poisonous plants), and the environment.

Host and Agent

The individual characteristics of the child must be assessed by the nurse. Particular attention is paid to the parents' description of the child. Some children are much more active, independent, and inquisitive than others. Evaluate carefully children who are aggressive and stubborn and show low frustration tolerance. Children who appear accident-prone may be calling attention to themselves in an attempt to reconcile parents (parents usually communicate when an accident happens to a child) and for many other reasons. Children are less receptive to parental advice when they are tired and hungry. The child's age and developmental stage influence the types of accidents that occur. Providing anticipatory guidance is important. Nurses must closely assess children with special needs in terms of safety considerations. Parents who have children with handicaps, such as visual, motor, or intellectual impairments, convulsive disorders, or diabetes, require extended instruction according to the child's particular needs. Immobile children need to be protected from sunburn and inclement weather. Adults also must guard

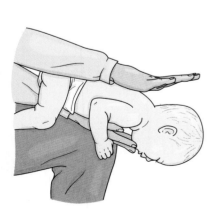

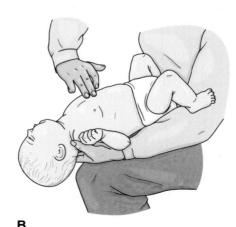

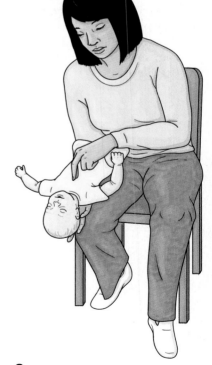

A   **B**   **C**

FIGURE **9-14** Infants up to 1 year of age who are choking are positioned with the head lower than the trunk. Back slaps are initiated **(A)**, followed by chest thrusts **(B)**. Both may be perfomed while seated; chest thrusts are shown here **(C)**.

these children from mosquitoes and other vectors. Control of the agent refers to some of the methods mentioned in the section on parent education. These include childproof caps on medication containers, regulations concerning children's furniture, and so on.

Environment

The physical, economic, and social environments of the child are also important in accident prevention. Families may be poor, overcrowded, fatigued, and dysfunctional. Children reared in households burdened by significant stress appear to be more at risk for accidents. A new parent (or babysitter) may underestimate the developmental capabilities of the child. The reverse may occur when a new baby arrives and an older child is given tasks beyond her or his abilities. Some suggest that the time of day has a bearing on accidents; morning rush hour, after-school hours (particularly for latchkey children), and evening have been cited. Family nationality and lifestyle also are considerations.

Vacations and relocations, which place small children in strange environments, are also potentially dangerous. The nurse is often the person in close contact with families and can be helpful in determining specific environmental hazards. Discussing potential hazards in the home and reviewing the locations of those hazards can be helpful for the parents. Emphasize that the kitchen and bathroom are the two most dangerous rooms in the house as far as accidents are concerned. A discussion of the neighborhood environment, such as playgrounds, schoolyard, and street lighting, may also be relevant. Because children absorb parental attitudes and behaviors, explain the need for proper "modeling" of safety precautions. Use community resources such as the library, fire department, and police. Give priority to problem solving, repeat the information, and evaluate its effectiveness.

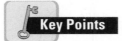

Key Points

- Toddlers are developmentally ready to give up total dependence and seek autonomy and independence.
- Weight gain slows as body proportions change.
- Thought processes and language development become more advanced.
- Daily care becomes easier as toddlers become more independent.
- Good dental health becomes essential; routine dental care is established.
- Physiological anorexia occurs; appetite fluctuations are best managed by providing nourishing foods and snacks.
- Toilet training occurs when the child becomes physically able, can communicate the need, and has patience to sit on the potty.
- Play is the work of the child; toddlers enjoy parallel play.
- Daycare is a part of many toddlers' lives; parents need to visit daycare facilities and evaluate the philosophy of the center and the attitudes of the caregivers.
- Accidents are the leading cause of death in childhood; safety precautions must be upheld at all times by all toddler caregivers.

 Go to your Companion CD-ROM for an Audio Glossary, video clips, and more.

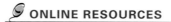 Be sure to visit the Companion Evolve site at http://evolve.elsevier.com/Price/ for WebLinks and additional online resources.

ONLINE RESOURCES

American Academy of Pediatrics: http://www.aap.org

National Safe Kids Campaign: http://www.safekids.org

U.S. Department of Agriculture: http://www.usda.gov/cnpp

evolve http://evolve.elsevier.com/Price/pediatric/

Objectives

Upon completion of this chapter, the student will be able to:

1. Define the vocabulary terms listed
2. List and define the more common disorders of the toddler period
3. Differentiate two types of hearing loss
4. Outline the nursing observation and care necessary for a 2-year-old child with croup
5. Identify two ways in which the bones of the toddler differ from those of the adult
6. List various types of pediatric fractures
7. Discuss care of the child in traction
8. Describe the signs of increased intracranial pressure in a child with a head injury, including nursing observations necessary to establish a baseline of information
9. Discuss preoperative and postoperative care of the child with Wilms' tumor
10. Discuss care of the autistic child
11. Describe treatment for acetaminophen poisoning in children
12. List screening measures to prevent lead poisoning

Key Terms

Be sure to check out the bonus material on the Companion CD-ROM, including selected audio pronunciations.

ataxia (ă-TĂK-sē-ă; p. 209)
audiometry (ăw-dē-ŎM-ě-trē; p. 196)
compartment syndrome (p. 202)
corrosive (p. 216)
dysarthria (dĭs-ĂR-thrē-ă; p. 209)
hydrocarbon (p. 199)
intention tremor (p. 209)
laryngotracheobronchitis (lă-RĬNG-gō-TRĀ-kē-ō brŏn-KĬ-tĭs; p. 197)
nephroblastoma (NĚF-rō-blăs-TŌ-mă; p. 214)
ototoxic (ō-tō-TŎK-sĭk; p. 195)
pica (PĪ-kă; p. 218)
tripod position (p. 199)
tympanography (TĬM-păh-nŏ-gră-fē; p. 196)

The toddler's world is one that expands from the intimacy of the family. Toddlers' motor skills are improving, which puts them at high risk for fractures, head injuries, and ingestions. This age group may have more exposures to respiratory diseases. With the improvement in motor function, neurological deficits may be recognized. Although the diseases and problems discussed in this chapter may occur frequently during the toddler period, they are not limited to this age group.

EARS

DEAFNESS
Description

Deaf children present special challenges to the nursing team. They may be hospitalized for direct evaluation and treatment of hearing loss, or they may have other medical or surgical problems that are—or are not—related to the deafness. The nurse should have a basic knowledge of the problems that confront deaf children to give them comprehensive nursing care.

The inner ear is fully formed during the first months of prenatal life. If an expectant mother contracts German measles (rubella) or takes medications such as the antibiotic streptomycin, the child may be born with a hearing loss, which is termed **congenital deafness.** Deafness can also be **acquired.** Infectious diseases such as measles, mumps, chickenpox, or meningitis can result in various degrees of hearing loss. Ototoxic (injurious to the ear) medications or ear infections may also be responsible. Deafness can also be temporary, as a result of wax accumulation that blocks the ear canal.

Hearing loss falls into two major categories. **Sensorineural** hearing loss results from damage to the structures of the inner ear or auditory nerve. This can result from congenital defects of the inner ear or from the effects of certain conditions such as kernicterus (Chapter 5) or infection. Complications can also arise from ototoxic drugs such as streptomycin, kanamycin, neomycin, and others. In addition, sensorineural hearing loss can be caused by noise pollution, such as loud rock music or target shooting. Symptoms include buzzing in the ears and muffled dull sounds immediately after exposure. Most people with sensorineural deafness benefit to some degree from hearing aids. With an interruption in the transmission of sound waves (from structural problems) from the external or middle ear, **conductive** hearing loss occurs. Common causes of conduction deafness are otitis media (ear infections), injury, foreign bodies, and wax build-up. Many children with this type of deafness can be helped with treatment for infection, surgery, or other measures to remove a blockage. Some children have **mixed** hearing loss, which is a combination of conductive and sensorineural causes.

Signs and Symptoms

It is important that parents know whether their child has hearing problems, especially when the child is young. Early intervention becomes critical for successful childhood development. Parents need to be alert for signs of hearing loss and notify their doctor if their baby:

- Does not startle with sudden loud sounds.
- Does not turn his or her head toward a sound by 3 or 4 months.
- Does not begin babbling by 6 months of age.
- Does not respond by interacting to music around 8 months of age.
- Does not attempt to speak syllables such as "da" by around age 1 year.

The various degrees of deafness range from complete hearing loss bilaterally to a loss so mild that the problem is never discovered. **Bilateral** deafness affects both ears. If this is complete, the child misses all the pleasures that sound brings to life and has difficulty communicating because children learn to talk by imitating what they hear. Behavior problems arise because the children do not understand directions. They may become aggressive with other children in their attempts to communicate. If children are ridiculed by playmates, their personality development is affected. Without help, these children become socially isolated and unable to attend school.

Partial bilateral deafness may be responsible for behavior problems and poor progress in school. This may be caused by chronic infections such as otitis media or by blockage of the eustachian tube. It may be a warning signal of more serious defects in later life. Children who are deaf in one ear are less disabled if the hearing in the other ear is normal.

Treatment and Nursing Care

The nurse must stress the importance of proper immunization during childhood to prevent many of the communicable diseases that contribute to acquired deafness. Vaccines against measles (rubeola), mumps, and German measles (rubella) are available, as is the vaccine against *Haemophilus influenzae* type b (a cause of meningitis in childhood). The child should be taken to the doctor for periodic health examinations. Early diagnosis and early intervention are important in the treatment of the deaf child to prevent adverse physical and mental complications.

Complete bilateral deafness is usually discovered during infancy. As discussed in Chapter 4, the Joint Committee on Infant Hearing (JCIH) recommends universal screening of hearing loss in newborns before hospital discharge. Two measures, the auditory brainstem response (ABR) and the otoacoustic emissions (OAE), provide identification of infants with hearing losses. These noninvasive, computerized tests can be performed in a short period of time. Early detection of hearing loss results in a child being able to develop speech and language skills along with peers.

Partial deafness may be unrecognized until the child begins school. Many hearing problems are detected then with standard hearing tests. A machine called an **audiometer** is used. The measurement of hearing as with an audiometer is called audiometry. The child puts on an earphone that is connected to the audiometer. When the audiometer is turned on, it makes various noises and pitches of sound. The child raises a hand on hearing the tones. The results of these tests are interpreted by specialists in this field. A child should be screened two times before a referral is made to avoid unnecessary referrals. Another test used to assess hearing problems in children is tympanography. The tympanogram measures the movement of the eardrum in response to sound waves. Decreased movement of the eardrum causes temporary hearing loss. This happens primarily when children have fluid in the middle ear as a result of an ear infection. Children who fail hearing tests should be referred to an otolaryngologist (specialist in ear, nose, and throat [ENT]) or audiologist for further testing.

Community Cue

The American Speech-Language-Hearing Association (ASHA) can refer parents to an audiologist in their area via their Consumer Helpline (800-638-8255).

Members of the health team concerned with the child who is hard of hearing include the physician, otolaryngologist, audiologist, speech therapist, specially trained teacher, social worker, psychologist, nurse, and the child's family. Children with a severe loss of hearing may need more extensive help from personnel at special hearing and speech centers. Whether the child should be placed in special classes in a regular school or should attend a school for the deaf is decided on an individual basis. Some children who spend a few years in a school for the deaf can be transferred to a regular school. These children need to begin their education early to help them catch up on what they have missed since infancy.

The deaf child in the hospital needs the same opportunities to develop a healthy personality as the child with normal hearing. The nurse who uses a relaxed manner with the patient creates an atmosphere that others will follow. Remember the following points when communicating with a deaf child:

- Smile when approaching a deaf child.
- Face the child when you speak.
- Position yourself so that you are at eye level with the child.
- Use short sentences rather than separate words.
- Speak clearly in a natural tone.
- Use appropriate gestures to accompany your speech.
- Try to talk to the child in an area that is free of background noise (television, radio, loud conversation).

The older child who is able to write can use this as a means of communication. Have the patient read aloud what has been written. In this way you become better accustomed to the child's speech. Regression in speech patterns may occur during hospitalization. Do not assume that because a child is not talking a great deal he or she does not understand what is being said. Repeat or reword certain statements as you would with any child.

Various methods are used to bring the child into the world of sound. Lip reading, sign language, writing, closed captioning (on television), computers, visual aids, music, and amplified sound are but a few examples.

Safety needs have to be addressed also. Flashing lights can be attached to a telephone or doorbell to indicate its ringing. Hearing ear dogs can also be of great assistance for older children and adults. Telecommunications devices for the deaf (TDD or TDY) also help older children and adults. Through these special teletypewriters, deaf persons can communicate with each other over the telephone.

Babies (usually over 3 months of age) can be successfully fit with hearing aids. Through education, the parent knows that the hearing aid is working correctly. If a hearing aid is indicated in an older child, the child and parent are taught how to use it. A hearing aid is expensive and invaluable to the patient. It should be kept in a safe place when it is not in use. Be sure the parent safeguards the hearing aid if their child ever has surgery. Regular checkups ensure that the device is working properly. A malfunctioning hearing aid may cause a child to lose interest in its use. Surgical procedures with cochlear implants are also used. These devices have met with success in profoundly deaf children with sensorineural hearing loss. Amplification technology is critical so that sound can get to the child's developing brain as soon as possible. This enables children to develop at or nearly at a normal rate, enabling them to keep up with peers as much as possible.

Because preventing deafness is so important, the nurse should take advantage of opportunities to demonstrate and teach proper hygiene of the ears to the child and family. No objects should be inserted into the ear canal when cleaning. If a foreign object gets into the ear, the child should be seen by a doctor.

Do *not* try to remove any object from the ear yourself. If assisting with an ear examination, have the parent hold the young child in his or her lap with the head pressed against the parent's chest. The parent can hold one hand on the child's forehead and the other securely around the body. The child can also lie on his or her side on the examination table. The parent or nurse may assist in holding the child still. The head is held still so that the delicate ear canal is not injured by the **otoscope.** The doctor may need cotton swabs or other instruments to remove excess secretions from the external ear. The ear **speculum** (a funnel-shaped device that is attached to the otoscope and comes in direct contact with the ear) must be disinfected after each use.

RESPIRATORY SYSTEM

CROUP
Description

Respiratory infections are common in pediatric patients, especially in children less than 5 years of age. Children have smaller air passages than adults and experience more narrowing with inflammation. Acute infections of the larynx are common in the toddler. Involvement of other parts of the respiratory tract is frequent. A wide variety of organisms cause croup, but most often the infectious agent is a virus. The patient's history is valuable in the diagnosis because there appears to be a familial tendency. Although this respiratory infection can occur at any age, it is most common in children between the ages of 6 months and 3 years.

Croup (**laryngotracheobronchitis**) is the most common infection of the middle respiratory tract. The cause is generally viral. The chief symptom is a brassy (croupy) "barking" cough and varying degrees of inspiratory **stridor.** When the larynx is involved, the picture becomes more serious because of possible alterations in respiratory status (such as airway obstruction, acute respiratory failure, or hypoxia). Bacterial tracheitis is usually caused by *S. aureus* and involves high fever with cough and stridor. These children are usually intubated and receive antibiotic therapy. Figure 10-1 illustrates the pathophysiology of croup.

Signs and Symptoms

Croup usually begins with an upper respiratory infection with or without fever. The child begins to develop hoarseness and a harsh, barking, "croupy" cough. As the subglottic area becomes obstructed by edema and exudate, the child develops **stridor,** a harsh, high-pitched sound when breathing. Cough and stridor are usually worse at night. Although croup is alarming to the child and parents because the child is distressed, most cases are mild, and it is not communicable. Signs of pallor, increased respiratory

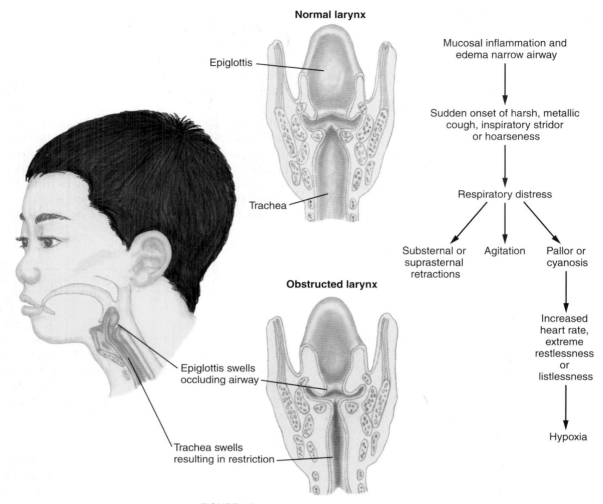

FIGURE 10-1 Pathophysiology of croup.

effort, and restlessness indicate that the child should be seen by a physician because respiratory distress is increasing.

Treatment and Nursing Care

Most children can be managed at home. Use of steam from a shower or hot bath in a closed bathroom can often stop the acute respiratory distress and laryngeal spasm. Parents should be instructed to use a cool mist humidifier in the child's room. The machine must be disinfected regularly. Steam vaporizers are usually avoided because of the danger of scalding. Exposure to cold air also relieves stridor. Many a parent has carried a child out into the cold night on the way to the emergency room only to have the child appear quite comfortable on arrival at the hospital. This may be caused by the colder atmospheric air cooling the upper airway mucosa and decreasing local edema (Behrman et al., 2004). Clear fluid intake should also be increased.

Children with croup should be hospitalized if there is progressive stridor, respiratory distress, or suspected epiglottitis (Behrman et al., 2004).

The toddler admitted to the hospital with respiratory distress is anxious and fatigued. A calm, reassuring approach by the nurse can relieve the child's and family's anxiety. As the parents become more relaxed, the child also becomes less apprehensive.

A mist tent with low-dose oxygen might be used if the child is hypoxic. Having someone remain with the child while he or she is in the tent is desirable to prevent distress if the child is frightened. Be sure to allow the child to have a familiar toy or transitional object in the tent.

Medications used in the treatment of croup include corticosteroids and inhaled racemic epinephrine. Corticosteroids have proved helpful in avoiding intubation in seriously ill children by decreasing subglottic edema. Racemic epinephrine is inhaled via a face mask. It decreases edema by vasoconstriction and provides immediate relief, although this may be temporary. Racemic epinephrine may be repeated in several hours if necessary. A single inhaled dose peaks in 10 to 30 minutes, with an overall duration of 2 hours. **Close observation is necessary because some patients may have a relapse, with return of symptoms when the**

medication effect has worn off. For this reason, many children who have received racemic epinephrine are admitted to the hospital for observation.

The nurse observes and records temperature, pulse, respirations, and blood pressure, if ordered. Particular attention is given to the type and rate of respirations. The child's color and degree of restlessness and anxiety are also observed. An increase in respiratory distress is reported immediately because complications may arise that necessitate endotracheal intubation or tracheostomy (see Data Cues). Specific nursing care is indicated in such cases (see Chapter 17 for tracheostomy care).

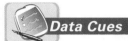

Data Cues

For the Child with Increasing Respiratory Distress

- Increased respiratory rate
- Increased pulse
- Pallor
- Restlessness
- Nasal flaring
- Retractions, or pulling of the skin under or above the sternum or between the ribs

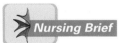

Nursing Brief

Spasmodic croup is similar to acute laryngotracheobronchitis, except that the history of illness may be absent. This child (primarily toddlers) awakens at night with the characteristic barking cough and may appear anxious. The child is usually afebrile, and the symptoms diminish during the daytime. The attacks may continue for another night or two. Allergies may play a role in spasmodic croup. Treatment and nursing care are managed as indicated previously.

Administer the child's favorite clear, cool, oral fluids if the child does not have severe respiratory distress. Intravenous (IV) fluids may be started to provide intake and conserve energy. Care should be planned to allow time for uninterrupted rest.

EPIGLOTTITIS
Description

Epiglottitis is a swelling of the tissues **above** the vocal cords—that is, **supraglottic** (Figure 10-2). This results in narrowing of the airway inlet with the possibility of total airway obstruction. It is most frequently caused by *H. influenzae* type b infection and occurs most often in children from 2 to 6 years of age. It can occur in any season. Unlike croup, which progresses over a period of days, the course is rapid and progressive (airway obstruction can occur in a period of hours). Epiglottitis is a life-threatening medical emergency.

Signs and Symptoms

The child with epiglottitis appears acutely ill with a sudden sore throat, high fever, drooling, muffled voice, and rapid respirations with difficulty breathing. Stridor is a late, *ominous* sign with epiglottitis. Nearly complete airway obstruction is most likely occurring if stridor is heard. The child with epiglottitis prefers to sit upright, leaning forward with the chin up and mouth open while leaning on the arms (**tripod position**). Blood gases fluctuate, and there is leukocytosis. Bacteremia is often present.

Treatment and Nursing Care

If epiglottitis is suspected, do not examine the pharynx (back of the throat) because laryngospasm may occur, followed by respiratory arrest. It is important for the nurse to display a calm, soothing, and reassuring attitude toward the child while being alert for respiratory complications. Endotracheal intubation equipment must be readily available. Epiglottitis requires endotracheal intubation to maintain the airway. Occasionally, a tracheostomy may be necessary. Children who have been intubated are cared for in an intensive care unit. The child generally receives oxygen, IV therapy, and antibiotics. The incidence of epiglottitis has decreased since *H. influenzae* type b vaccine has been administered routinely beginning at age 2 months.

BRONCHITIS

Bronchitis refers to *bronchial* inflammation. The bronchi are the two lower divisions of the trachea that branch off to the lungs. This condition is usually preceded by a viral upper respiratory tract infection. It is more common in the winter.

The child may initially have a cold followed by a cough that may or may not be productive. Low-grade fever may be present. Crackles and wheezing may be detected on auscultation. As with all respiratory disorders, fluids are important. Bronchitis is generally self-limiting and resolves in 2 to 3 weeks. Antibiotics, cough suppressants, antihistamines, and expectorants are not indicated (Behrman et al., 2004).

PNEUMONIA
Description

Pneumonia is an infection of the lower respiratory tract in which the *alveoli* (air sacs) become filled with exudate. As the infection progresses, the exudate becomes solidified (consolidation). The affected portion of the lung does not receive enough air. Breathing is shallow. As a result, the bloodstream is denied sufficient oxygen. *Pneumonitis* is a general term for lung inflammation and may or may not be associated with consolidation.

About 80% of pneumonia is caused by viruses, and 20% by bacteria. Aspiration of foreign substances such as talcum powder, peanuts, or popcorn may result in pneumonia. Aspirated **hydrocarbons** (kerosene, furniture polish, paint thinner) damage the lung cells

Clinical manifestations

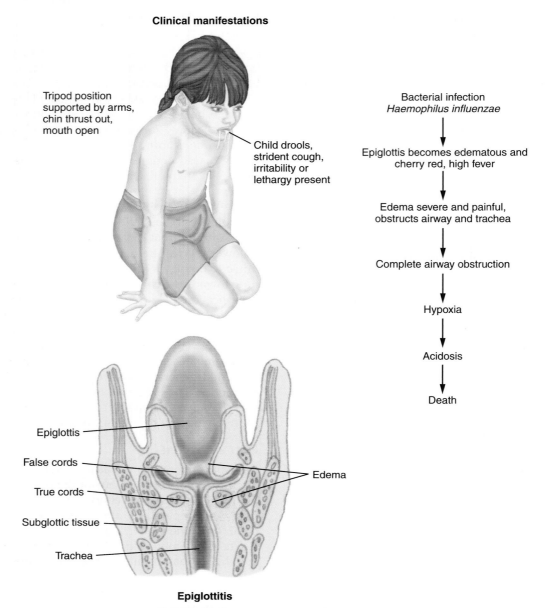

Tripod position supported by arms, chin thrust out, mouth open

Child drools, strident cough, irritability or lethargy present

Bacterial infection
Haemophilus influenzae

↓

Epiglottis becomes edematous and cherry red, high fever

↓

Edema severe and painful, obstructs airway and trachea

↓

Complete airway obstruction

↓

Hypoxia

↓

Acidosis

↓

Death

Epiglottis
False cords
True cords
Subglottic tissue
Trachea

Edema

Epiglottitis

FIGURE **10-2** Pathophysiology of epiglottitis.

by impairing the surface tension. Gastroesophageal reflux may result in the aspiration of gastric contents, resulting in pneumonia.

Viral pneumonia can be caused by respiratory syncytial virus (RSV), influenza, and adenovirus. This occurs more frequently during the winter months. Bacterial pneumonia generally causes a more severe infection. The common bacterial organisms are *S. pneumoniae*, group A streptococcal, *Staphylococcus aureus*, and *H. influenzae*. Additional agents may cause pneumonia. Severe acute respiratory syndrome (SARS) spread worldwide in 2003. Avian flu, or bird flu, is a highly contagious disease of poultry and other birds that is caused by influenza A (H5N1). A high mortality rate is associated with bird flu, and there is concern of a worldwide pandemic.

Pneumonia might occur as the initial or **primary** disease, or it can complicate another illness, in which case it is termed **secondary** pneumonia. Secondary pneumonia may accompany various communicable diseases or may follow surgery. It is more serious than primary pneumonia because the child is in a weakened condition.

Signs and Symptoms

The symptoms of pneumonia vary with the age of the child and the causative organism. They may develop suddenly or be preceded by an upper respiratory tract infection. The cough is dry at first but gradually becomes productive. Fever rises as high as 103° F to 104° F (39.5° C to 40° C) and may fluctuate widely over a 24-hour period. The respiration rate may increase to 40 to 80 times per minute in infants, and in older children to 30 to 50 times per minute. Rhonchi and faint crackles may be heard with breath sounds. Respirations are shallow as the patient attempts to reduce the chest pain. Sternal retractions may be seen as the assisting muscles of respiration are brought into use. Flaring of the nostrils may appear. The child's color may vary from pale to cyanotic. The child is listless and has a poor appetite. The patient tends to lie on the affected side.

Treatment and Nursing Care

The child is given a complete physical examination. A tuberculosis skin test is administered if the child is at risk or if the child has not been tested recently. The doctor pays particular attention to the examination of the child's chest. Radiographs confirm the diagnosis and determine whether there are complications. A differential white blood cell count is routinely done. Blood specimens show a marked increase in the number of white blood cells (greater than $20,000/mm^3$). Obtaining blood specimens can be traumatic to the toddler, and crying can increase coughing spells. The nurse or parent should hug and calm the child afterward.

Treatment depends on the severity of the disease and the causative organism. Children who are in severe respiratory distress, dehydrated, vomiting, or are immunocompromised are treated in the hospital. Bacterial pneumonia is treated with antibiotics. Treatment for viral pneumonia is supportive. The nurse checks the vital signs at regular intervals. When a child is flushed with fever, remove heavy clothing and blankets and administer antipyretics. The nurse may be asked to give the child tepid sponge baths to help reduce a high fever (see Chapter 17). Oxygen is administered for dyspnea or cyanosis and needs to be monitored with pulse oximetry (Figure 10-3). Rest and conservation of energy are an important part of the treatment of this disease. The nurse needs to organize work so that the child is not disturbed unnecessarily. An increase in fluid intake is important. Encouraging children to increase oral fluid intake is often a goal. Besides water, offer the child Gatorade, juice, or a Popsicle, depending on preference. IV fluids are administered if the child cannot retain fluids because of vomiting or will not take fluids by mouth. They are also given to replace insensible fluid loss from tachypnea and fever. The appetite of the child improves as the condition does. Most cases of pneumonia in healthy children can be managed outside of the hospital.

Reposition the child frequently. Although this is painful, it is paramount to total recovery. The child probably prefers the affected side (if pneumonia is unilateral) because it splints the chest on that side and therefore decreases the discomfort. Administer prescribed analgesics to increase the patient's comfort. The nurse assists and encourages the patient to walk about the room and in the hallways when such activity is prescribed. Small children can exercise their lungs

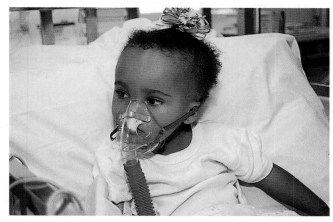

FIGURE **10-3** Child receiving oxygen via a face mask.

by blowing bubbles through a straw. The respiratory therapist may provide chest percussion and postural drainage exercise.

Although recovery from uncomplicated pneumonia is dramatic today, recuperation takes time. When the child is discharged from the hospital, parents should receive written instructions concerning diet, activity, medication, return appointments, and so on. It is helpful if the parents repeat these instructions to the nurse to determine whether they have interpreted them correctly.

GASTROINTESTINAL SYSTEM

PINWORMS
Description

Of the several varieties of worms that affect humans, the most common is the pinworm *Enterobius vermicularis* (*enteron*, intestine; *bios*, life; *vermis*, wormlike). Pinworms can affect individuals of all ages but are more common in young children. Crowded living conditions, institutions (schools and daycare centers), and pinworm infestation in the family are factors of high risk. The child infects himself or herself by handling contaminated toys or soiled linen. The route of entry is the mouth. The pinworm looks like a white thread about a third of an inch long. It lives in the lower intestine but comes out of the anus to lay its eggs, generally during the night. Hand-to-mouth activity contributes to reinfection.

Signs and Symptoms

Signs and symptoms include the child scratching the bottom, complaining of itchiness, and becoming irritable and restless. Weight loss, poor appetite, and fretfulness during the night may develop. The rectal area may become irritated from scratching. Worms may be seen on the surface of stools or around the anus. A special pinworm diagnostic tape or paddle or a tongue blade covered with cellophane tape, sticky side out, may be placed against the anal region in an attempt to obtain pinworm eggs. This is done early in the morning or after a period of inactivity. The tape is then put on a glass slide. The physician's office examines this with a microscope.

Treatment and Nursing Care

Several effective **anthelmintics** are available. Vermox (mebendazole) is a single-dose chewable tablet, appropriate for children older than 2 years of age. It is generally the drug of choice because it is safe and effective and has few side effects. Antiminth (pyrantel pamoate) is also a taken as a single dose. It is also not recommended for children less than 2 years of age. The medication is repeated 2 weeks later.

If it is determined that a hospitalized child has pinworms, linen and stool precautions are taken. The child must be taught to wash the hands well after bowel movements. The child's fingernails are kept short. A soothing ointment is applied to the rectal area. The patient wears clean underwear that fits snugly and is changed daily.

All other members of the family are treated for this condition to prevent reinfection. In the home, the toilet seat is scrubbed daily. Underwear and bed linens are washed in hot water. Bed linens are handled carefully to avoid spreading the infection. The parents are taught the danger of anthelmintic overdosage.

MUSCULOSKELETAL SYSTEM

FRACTURES
Description

A **fracture** is a break in a bone and is caused mainly by accidents. With children, falls are responsible for a large number of fractures. A fracture is characterized by pain, tenderness on movement, and swelling. Discoloration, limited movement, and numbness may also occur. In a **simple fracture,** the bone is broken but the skin over the area is not. In a **compound fracture,** a wound in the skin leads to the broken bone and there is the added danger of infection. Figure 10-4 depicts the various types of pediatric fractures.

Fractures heal faster in children than in adults. The child's periosteum is stronger and thicker, and there is less stiffness on mobilization. Injury to the cartilaginous **epiphyseal plate,** found at the ends of long bones, is serious if it happens during childhood because it may interfere with longitudinal growth.

Treatment and Nursing Care

Common fracture sites in children include the ulna, tibia, femur, and clavicle. (Femur fractures are discussed separately in the next section.) Children typically have pain, and swelling may be obvious with a fracture. If a fracture is suspected, do not allow the child to use the limb or part and do not move it yourself. If the child is in a safe place, do not move the child. Keep the child warm and prepare for transport via emergency medical services (EMS) to the hospital. An ice pack, covered with a cloth to prevent skin burns and applied to the fracture, may minimize swelling. If the fracture is compound, cover the injury lightly with a sterile dressing.

If it is necessary to move the child, apply a splint. The joints above and below the break are immobilized with a rolled newspaper or bath towels and tied beyond the injury. Commercially made splints are available; for example, a padded board that is bandaged to the extremity or air splints that can be inflated. If the arm is injured, keep it elevated with a sling to reduce swelling and hemorrhage. If a back or neck injury is evident, do not move the child unless the injury is life threatening. Activate the EMS in the area.

Radiography is the most effective method of determining the type of fracture that has occurred. Fractures are treated with closed or open reduction. Closed reduction involves manually aligning the break followed by immobilization. Figure 10-5 shows a child in a long arm cast. Cast care is discussed in Chapter 6. Open reduction involves surgical insertion of fixation devices, such as pins, to maintain alignment while healing occurs. The child is hospitalized and monitored for possible complications, including infection, neurovascular complications, and fat embolism. Any change in general condition or any signs or symptoms of infection, including elevated temperature, pin-site redness, drainage, or odor, need to be reported. Signs of neurovascular compromise also need to be reported. The nurse checks the child's affected extremity frequently to see that toes or fingers are warm and that their color is good. Cyanosis, numbness or irritation from attachments, tight bandages, severe pain, or absence of pulse in the extremities must be reported immediately to the nurse in charge. Refer to Data Cues for specifics on lower extremity neurovascular checks.

Compartment syndrome can occur as a result of pressure on tissues resulting from edema or swelling. Circulation is compromised. Paralysis and necrosis can occur. Neurovascular checks alert the nurse to possible compartment syndrome.

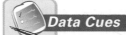 **Data Cues**

Signs Suggesting Lower Extremity Neurovascular Impairment

Circulation: Decreased pedal pulse, pallor, toes feel cool to the touch, slowed capillary refill (pink color slow to return after toe is pressed and released)

Sensation: Child complains of numbness or "pins and needles" sensation, pain

Motion: Toes swollen, not moving well

Pediatric fractures are seldom complete breaks. Rather, children's bones tend to bend or buckle because of increased flexibility. This flexibility is due to a thicker periosteum and increased amounts of immature bone.

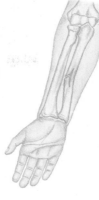

Greenstick

Break occurs through the periosteum on one side of the bone while only bowing or buckling on the other side. Seen most frequently in forearm.

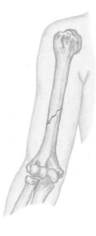

Spiral

Twisted or circular break that affects the length rather than the width. Seen frequently in child abuse.

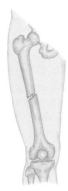

Oblique

Diagonal or slanting break that occurs between the horizontal and perpendicular planes of the bone.

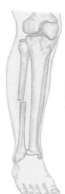

Transverse

Break or fracture line occurs at right angles to the long axis of the bone.

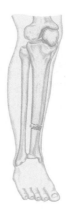

Comminuted

Bone is splintered into pieces. This is a rare occurrence in children.

FIGURE **10-4** Pediatric fractures.

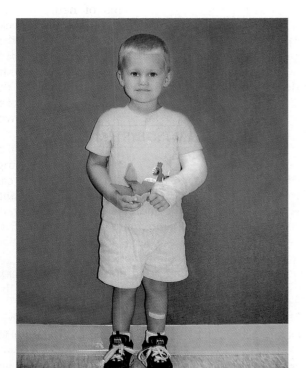

FIGURE **10-5** Most children adapt well to their casts, although they may fear the removal.

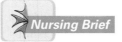

Nursing Brief

Remember the 5 Ps when performing neurovascular checks: pain, pallor, pulselessness, paresthesia, and paralysis.

Fat embolism can occur as a result of orthopedic trauma. Particles of fat escape from the fracture sites and are carried through the circulatory system; they can lodge in the lung capillaries, causing respiratory distress. The child exhibits signs of altered respiratory status and possible altered level of consciousness (LOC). Such condition changes must be reported immediately.

Femur Fractures. The femur (thighbone) is the largest and strongest bone of the body. Fracture of the femur is one of the most common serious breaks that occur during early childhood. Femur fractures usually result from a severe fall or automobile accident. Child abuse may be suspected if spiral fracture has occurred. Skin or skeletal traction is used to reduce the fracture, to keep the bones in proper place, and to immobilize the leg. The type of traction depends on the age of the child and extent of the injury. **Bryant** traction is no longer recommended. This skin traction positioned the child's legs at a 90-degree angle to the body. This type of traction could cause circulatory problems that resulted from constant elevation of the legs (Hockenberry & Wilson, 2007). For children over 6 years, 90-90 skeletal traction with a boot cast on the lower leg and a skeletal Steinmann pin or Kirschner wire through the distal femur is commonly used. Other types of traction that are frequently used in children with lower extremity fractures are split Russell traction and balanced suspension traction with a Thomas ring and Pearson attachment. Various types of traction are shown in Tables 10-1 and 10-2.

Care of the Child in Traction. The nurse observes the traction ropes to be sure that they are intact and in the wheel grooves of the pulleys and that the child's body is in good position. Elastic bandages stabilizing skin traction should be neither too loose nor too tight. The child is to avoid turning from side to side. Do not remove the weights once they have been applied. Continuous traction is necessary. The weights must hang free, and the pull of the weights must not be obstructed by bedroom furnishings such as a chair. The weights are **not** supported when the bed is moved.

Initially, the child might have pain, both from the fracture itself and from the muscle spasms associated with the traction. The pain is spasmodic and can be severe. Pain assessment with age-appropriate pain scales and treatment are essential. Pain assessment and management are discussed in Chapter 3.

The child is bathed daily, and the back is massaged frequently to prevent ulceration. The nurse reaches under the patient's body to rub the back and buttocks. The sheets are pulled taut and kept free of crumbs. Two nurses should be available when the elastic wraps of skin traction are changed, one to hold the adhesive traction tapes in place and one to rewrap the bandages.

The nurse provides pin care to the child in skeletal traction. The purpose of pin care is to keep crusting around the pins to a minimum, to minimize unnecessary pulling of the skin at the pin sites, and to prevent infection. *Osteomyelitis* is the most serious complication associated with skeletal traction. This bone infection manifests itself with localized pain, warmth, swelling, tenderness, or unusual odor. Antibiotics are prescribed if this complication occurs.

The child is encouraged to drink lots of fluids and to eat foods that are high in roughage content to prevent constipation caused by lack of exercise. Stool softeners may be necessary. A fracture pan is used for bowel movements, and a careful record is kept of eliminations. Deep breathing is encouraged through the use of breathing exercises, blowing bubbles, moving a windmill toy, and so on. Diversional therapy is important because hospitalization lasts for a month or longer. Range of motion (ROM) to unaffected extremities is important.

Try to encourage ROM by making it a game whenever possible. Toys may be suspended over the child's head within reach. The older child can use an overhead trapeze to assist with movement in the bed. Videos, computer games, stories, and other forms of entertainment are essential to the total nursing care plan. Parents are encouraged to stay with the child when possible. The prognosis for patients with this condition is good with proper treatment. Children's bones heal faster than those of adults. The care of a child in traction is illustrated in Nursing Care Plan 10-1.

DISLOCATIONS

Dislocations of the elbow (often referred to as "nursemaid's elbow") are seen in young children who have tried to twist their hand out of a parent's hand. The pulling and twisting motion most often dislocates the radial head. Symptoms of a dislocated elbow are immediate and marked. The child splints the affected arm with the unaffected hand and refuses to move it. Often the child cries and appears anxious or in pain. Even when distracted with a toy, the child does not move the affected arm. Treatment of a dislocated elbow is simple and provides immediate relief in most cases. The physician turns the hand and forearm in an upward direction while placing pressure at the elbow until a click is heard or felt. The child is able to move the arm shortly after treatment. Because repeated incidents of elbow dislocation are common, the nurse should advise the parent to avoid placing any pulling motion on the child's arm.

Elbow dislocations may occur in older children as the result of a fall on a hyperextended elbow. There may also be an associated elbow fracture. Reduction is performed under conscious sedation. If stable, it is then immobilized until range of motion exercises are ordered (Burg et al., 2006).

NERVOUS SYSTEM

CEREBRAL PALSY
Description

Cerebral palsy (CP) refers to a group of nonprogressive disorders that affect the motor centers of the brain, causing problems with movement and coordination. Often children with CP have associated language, perceptual, and intellectual deficits. It is one of the most common disabling conditions seen in children, occurring in approximately 1.2 to 2.5 per 1000 live births (Burg et al., 2006).

This condition can be caused by one or more of several factors, which most frequently include the following:

- Congenital problems involving the central nervous system (e.g., hydrocephalus, hemorrhage)
- Conditions of pregnancy or labor that interfere with oxygen reaching the fetal brain (e.g., pre-

Table 10-1 | *Types of Skin Traction*

TYPES	ILLUSTRATION	USES	NURSING CONSIDERATIONS
Cervical		Neck sprains or strains Torticollis Cervical nerve trauma Nerve root compression	Limit of weights of 5 to 7 pounds. Avoid compressing the throat or ears with the chin strap. Elevating the head of the bed 20-30 degrees helps maintain alignment.
Side-arm 90-90		Fractures and dislocations of the upper arm or shoulder	Hand may feel cool because of its elevation. Hand can be covered with sock or mitten if desired.
Dunlop		Supracondylar elbow fracture of the humerus	Avoid pressure over bony prominences or nerves.
Buck extension traction		Hip and knee contracture Legg-Calvé-Perthes disease	Remove boot every 8 hours and assess skin. Leg may be slightly abducted.
Russell traction		Supracondylar femur fracture Stabilize fractured femur until callus forms	Sling may need to be repositioned often; mark leg to ensure proper placement.
Split Russell		Femur fracture Legg-Calvé-Perthes disease	Avoid pressure over bony prominences or nerves. Weights are not added or removed without a physician's order.

Modified from Bowden, V., Dickey, S., & Greenberg, C. (1998). *Children and their families: The continuum of care.* Philadelphia: Saunders; and McKinney, E., James, S., Murray, S., & Ashwill, J. (2005). *Maternal-child nursing* (2nd ed.). Philadelphia: Saunders.

Table 10-2 | *Types of Skeletal Traction*

TYPES	ILLUSTRATION	USES	NURSING CONSIDERATIONS
Cervical (Crutchfield) skeletal tongs		Preoperative spine distraction Fractures or dislocations of cervical or high thoracic vertebrae	A special bed may be used to assist with turning patient. Logroll patient while maintaining straight body alignment.
Halo cast or vest		Postoperative immobilization after cervical fusion Fracture or dislocation of cervical or high thoracic vertebrae	Balance is altered with a halo cast; patients ambulating need close supervision. Cast may need to be sawed in case of emergency; front panel of brace may need to be removed in case of emergency.
Dunlop (side-arm 90-90)		Fracture of upper arm	Turn patient toward the affected side only. Hand may feel cool despite intact neurovascular status; cover hand with mitten or sock if desired.
90-90 femoral traction		Femur fractures	Encourage child to dorsiflex foot often to prevent foot drop or lower leg may be casted. Ensure weights do not catch on bottom of the bed.
Thomas ring with Pearson attachment (balanced suspension)		Femur fracture Hip fracture Tibial fracture	Avoid pressure to the area behind the knee, which could cause popliteal nerve injury. If the system is truly balanced, the splint can be placed at any height and will remain there.

Modified from Bowden, V., Dickey, S., & Greenberg, C. (1998). *Children and their families: The continuum of care.* Philadelphia: Saunders; and McKinney, E., James, S., Murray, S., & Ashwill, J. (2005). *Maternal-child nursing* (2nd ed.). Philadelphia: Saunders.

mature separation of the placenta, prolonged labor)
- Exposure during pregnancy to infections (e.g., German measles or rubella, cytomegalovirus, toxoplasmosis) or toxins

The incidence rate of CP is high in infants weighing less than 2500 g at birth and in multiple births. Untreated high levels of bilirubin from jaundice and Rh incompatibility have also been associated with CP. Head injuries, meningitis, and encephalitis can cause CP in the older child. In some cases, no single cause can be found.

Signs and Symptoms

The symptoms of CP vary with each child and may range from mild to severe (see Data Cues). About two thirds of children who have CP are intellectually impaired (National Institute of Neurological Disorders and Stroke, Cerebral Palsy Information Page, 2006). CP is suspected during infancy when developmental milestones are not met. Diagnostic tests include electroencephalography, computed tomography (CT), and screening for metabolic disorders. Brain tumors must also be ruled out. Early recognition is important so that early intervention can begin.

NURSING CARE PLAN 10-1

The Child in Leg Traction

NURSING DIAGNOSIS *Impaired physical mobility related to restrictions of the traction apparatus and the child's injury*

Goals/Outcome Criteria	Nursing Interventions	Rationales
Child is free of hazards related to immobility, as evidenced by: • Intact skin • Normal elimination patterns for age • Normal respiratory function • Maintenance of muscle tone	Place child on sheepskin or pressure-equalizing mattress.	Equalizing pressure on back reduces pressure areas and skin breakdown.
	Change child's position in bed every 2 hr. Observe for and gently massage reddened areas.	Promotes circulation to the area and prevents skin breakdown.
	Keep crumbs and small toys off the sheets.	Can get underneath the child and cause skin irritation.
	Keep back clean and dry. Use flat fracture bedpan.	Perspiration can cause skin irritation.
	Encourage increased fluids and high-fiber foods. Use stool softeners if ordered.	Promotes adequate elimination.
	Encourage deep breathing and muscle movement through play: singing, blowing bubbles or a pinwheel, bean bag toss, Nerf basketball, simple games.	Deep breathing inflates the lungs, decreasing respiratory compromise.
	Allow child to use overhead trapeze if appropriate and encourage frequent changes of position.	Muscle movement enhances muscle tone in unaffected extremities. Improves tone of upper extremities; keeps child in alignment.
	Encourage child to feed, bathe, and dress within traction limitations; provide foods high in calcium.	Enhances self-care and muscle movement; calcium promotes adequate bone healing.

NURSING DIAGNOSIS *Acute pain related to tissue injury and muscle spasm*

Goals/Outcome Criteria	Interventions	Rationales
Child exhibits relief from pain, as evidenced by the following: • Minimal to no pain on the pain rating scale • Sleeping comfortably • Able to play with others • No crying or expressions of pain	Provide pharmacological pain relief as ordered around the clock for the first 24 to 48 hr.	Giving medication around the clock provides more effective pain control than waiting until the child has pain.
	Monitor the effects of the medication. Note and report any adverse effects.	Proper effectiveness of pain relief depends on achieving the maximum possible relief with the minimum amount of sedation.
	Use age-appropriate rating scale to monitor pain levels.	Rating scales are the most effective way to monitor pain in children.
	Use nonpharmacological methods of pain relief, such as distraction, storytelling, music, play, gentle touch.	Effective use of nonpharmacological methods decreases the number of pharmacological agents necessary.
	Encourage relaxation and deep breathing during muscle spasms.	Conscious muscle relaxation decreases muscle spasms.

Continued

NURSING CARE PLAN 10-1—cont'd

The Child in Leg Traction—cont'd

NURSING DIAGNOSIS *Fear related to injury, traction apparatus, hospitalization*

Goals/Outcome Criteria	Nursing Interventions	Rationales
Child adjusts to being in traction, as evidenced by: • Cooperating with plan of care • Sleeping well, no nightmares • Playing appropriately with others • Exhibiting behavior consistent with usual temperament	Use imaginary play frequently in care. Bring the child to the playroom if hospital policy permits; wheel the whole bed in. Continue regular routine. Review with parents and child the purpose of the traction, keeping alignment, and what they can do to help.	Helps the toddler deal with fear and loss of control. Seeing other children decreases fears. Following routines and rituals helps adjustment. Knowledge increases cooperation with care.

NURSING DIAGNOSIS *Risk for infection related to skin irritation at pin sites*

Goals/Outcome Criteria	Nursing Interventions	Rationales
Child remains free of infection, as evidenced by: • Intact skin • No redness, tenting, swelling, or purulent drainage at site	Monitor pin sites at least once a shift; document condition of skin around pin entry sites. Monitor vital signs. Provide pin care according to hospital protocol.	Frequent monitoring allows for more rapid recognition of infection. Elevated temperature can signify infection; elevated pulse and respiration can indicate subtle pain. Keeping the site clean can prevent infection.

NURSING DIAGNOSIS *Risk for peripheral neurovascular dysfunction related to edema and traction apparatus*

Goals/Outcome Criteria	Nursing Interventions	Rationales
Child maintains adequate peripheral perfusion, as evidenced by: • Strong pedal pulse • Good movement of toes • No numbness or tingling • Toes warm, pink, good capillary refill	Monitor peripheral circulation, sensation, and motion every 4 hr when stable. Note edema of toes or feet. Encourage child to move the toes of the affected foot frequently. Remove and reapply elastic bandages of skin traction as ordered (use another person to stabilize traction adhesive tapes).	Frequent monitoring detects problems for early intervention. Edema contributes to decreased peripheral circulation. Movement increases circulation locally. Periodic removal of tight bandages promotes circulation to the extremity.

NURSING DIAGNOSIS *Risk for injury related to traction apparatus and confinement to bed*

Goals/Outcome Criteria	Nursing Interventions	Rationales
Child remains free from injury: • Remains quietly in bed • Cooperates with plan of care	Check traction apparatus frequently: • Weights swing freely • Ropes on pulleys • Child in straight alignment • Affected leg supported properly in sling, if used. Cover sharp pin sites with foam or tape. Keep side rails up. Keep snacks, toys, and TV or call buttons within child's reach.	Frequent monitoring of traction apparatus and alignment ensures appropriate traction on the affected extremity. Sharp pin edges can lacerate the unaffected extremity. Prevents falls. Reduces the chance that the child will lean too far and fall.

⁇CRITICAL THINKING QUESTION

■ How would the nurse design a routine for the toddler or young child in traction to avoid boredom, overcome fear, and maintain mobility of nonimpaired extremities? Consider pain control, risk for injury, and prevention of complications.

NURSING CARE PLAN 10-1—cont'd

The Child in Leg Traction—cont'd

CRITICAL THINKING
SNAPSHOT

In evaluating this child in traction, what would be documented regarding the traction set-up? What precautions need to be taken for the child in traction? What would the nurse evaluate and document regarding the child? What are the signs and symptoms if this child has complications from infection? What information would be reported to the physician?

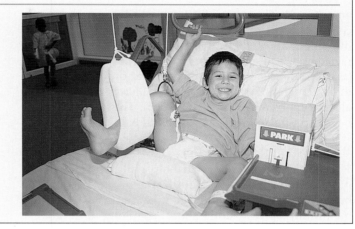

Data Cues

For the Child with CP

- Apgar score of less than 5
- Seizures, usually within 48 hours of birth
- Delay in reaching developmental milestones: sitting, crawling, creeping, standing, reaching for objects
- Difficulty with fine motor skills such as holding feeding utensils, writing, using scissors
- Feeding difficulties: poor sucking and swallowing, drooling, persistent tongue thrust
- Involuntary movements such as uncontrolled writhing motions of the hands
- Increased muscle tone: infant may be rigid when pulled to a sitting position, infant reflexes do not disappear at the normal time

Children may have symptoms of more than one type of CP. **Spastic** CP affects between 70% and 80% of patients. It is characterized by tension in certain muscle groups. The stretch reflex is present in the involved muscles. When the child tries to move the voluntary muscles, jerky motions result, and eating, walking, and other coordinated movements are difficult to accomplish. The lower extremities are usually involved. The legs cross and the toes point inward **(scissoring).** Toe walking can occur from muscle tightness (Figure 10-6). Upper extremities, or upper and lower extremities on only one side of the body, can be affected. With **athetoid or dyskinetic** CP, the child has uncontrolled, slow, writhing movements that can increase during periods of emotional stress and disappear during sleep. About 10% to 20% of patients are affected. These abnormal movements usually affect the hands, feet, arms, or legs and, in some cases, the muscles of

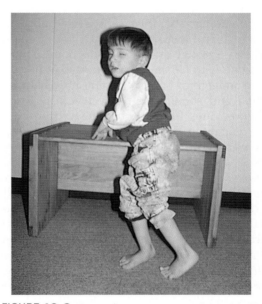

FIGURE **10-6** Toe walking in a young child with CP.

the face and tongue, causing grimacing or drooling. Problems can also occur with the coordination of muscle movements needed for speech (dysarthria). Ataxia, or lack of muscle coordination, can be shown by disturbances of balance and depth perception. A wide-based gait accompanied by unsteadiness is generally present. Intention tremor may also be present. When beginning a voluntary movement, such as reaching for a book, there is a resultant trembling that affects the body part being used and worsens as the individual gets nearer to the desired object. Emotional problems sometimes present more difficulties than the physical disability. This disorder affects 5% to 10% of the patients. **Mixed** CP is usually a combination of spastic and athetoid movements; however, other combinations of symptoms are possible.

According to the National Institute of Neurological Disorders and Stroke, "Doctors will often describe the type of cerebral palsy a child has based on which limbs are affected. The names of the most common forms of cerebral palsy use Latin terms to describe the location or number of affected limbs, combined with the words for weakened (*paresis)* or paralyzed (*plegia).* For example, *hemiparesis (hemi* = half) indicates that only one side of the body is weakened. *Quadriplegia (quad* = four) means all four limbs are paralyzed" (2006). Thus a child may have "spastic quadriplegia" cerebral palsy.

Treatment and Nursing Care

The goal of treatment is to help children make the most of their assets and guide them into becoming happy, well-adjusted adults who perform at their maximum ability. Both short and long-term goals must be realistic and attainable. Parents work with a multidisciplinary team including a physician, such as a pediatrician, an orthopedist, a physical therapist, an occupational therapist; a speech and language pathologist; and a social worker. A psychologist may become a necessary referral at some point as well.

Children with CP are usually treated at home unless they are undergoing surgery. Parents need help to accept the child and should not be deceived into expecting miraculous cures from the treatment. The sooner the child is diagnosed, the fewer the physical and emotional problems. Parents need to be informed of community resources available to them. The family's religious affiliation should not be overlooked in this respect because it can become a source of support and help during times of stress. The long course of this disability is a financial burden, and contact with social service agencies can assist in this regard. Caretakers need respite care from time to time so that they can refresh their outlook on life. It is not uncommon for the parents of children with CP to become the experts in caring for their child, and therefore it behooves nursing personnel to listen to and incorporate parents' suggestions when developing nursing care plans.

The specific treatment is highly individualistic, depending on the severity of the disease. Treatment often includes physical and occupational therapy to assist with activities of daily living, special education and communication devices, and recreational activities designed for the child's developmental level and adapted to functional limitations. Sometimes surgery is necessary to correct deformities, improve function, or reduce spasticity. The speech therapist helps with communication. Many children with cerebral palsy cannot produce intelligent speech.

Medications may improve overall function in children with CP. Dantrolene reduces calcium release, thereby decreasing excitation-contraction in skeletal muscle.

Skeletal muscle relaxants such as baclofen may decrease spasticity. Intrathecal baclofen delivered via a pump reservoir can help with spastic quadriparesis. Botulinum toxin type A (Botox) has also been successfully used to reduce spasticity (Burg et al., 2006). Antianxiety agents may relieve excessive motion and tension, especially in the athetoid child. Anticonvulsants are prescribed for children with seizures.

Many of these children wear braces and splints, and assessing the skin is essential. The nurse should observe for areas of redness or pallor. The child might find it helpful to wear a light shirt under a body brace. The bedclothes must be kept clean, dry, and free of wrinkles.

All precautions are taken to prevent the formation of **contractures** (degeneration or shortening of the muscles because of lack of use). The damage may be permanent, resulting in loss of function of the part involved, such as a leg, arm, or finger. A common expression in relation to this is, "What you don't use, you lose." Knowing this, the nurse represses a natural desire to help patients and encourages them to do as much as they can for themselves. When patients take their own baths in the morning, they put muscles and joints through their normal ROM. When nurses give the bath, they put *their* muscles through the necessary movements, not the patient's. Of course, nurses must use their judgment in assessing each patient's capabilities.

Other measures necessary to prevent deformities include frequent changes of position, the use of splints, and the carrying out of passive range-of-motion and stretching exercises. The nurse must also ensure that the patient maintains good posture while in bed. This is done through the proper positioning of pillows and other comfort devices. The principles involved in preventing contractures can be applied to the nursing care of all long-term patients. The physical therapist spends many hours with the patient. His or her instructions must be carried out by unit personnel to ensure continuity of care.

Feeding problems may occur because of swallowing and sucking difficulties. During infancy, the child should be fed slowly to prevent aspiration. The child may need jaw support to facilitate chewing and swallowing. As children grow older, they should be fitted with a chair with good foot support. The child should be taught as soon as possible to manage special feeding equipment. High-caloric diets are necessary to replace calories used by the constant muscle tension.

The disabled child needs opportunities to play alone and with other children. Games suited to abilities, such as finger painting, are fun and allow freedom of expression. Activities that require the use of fine muscular movements of the hand cause frustration in the child whose arms and hands are affected by the disease. The nurse can learn a great deal from the parents in regard to types of play enjoyed by the child.

Children with CP tire easily but find it difficult to relax. They are under a constant strain to accomplish the simplest of tasks. The nurse must see that they take frequent naps in a quiet room. They should not become overexcited before bedtime.

When possible, the child should attend regular school. Children with CP may need speech and physical therapy, and this can often be provided within the school setting. Communication devices, such as communication boards or computers with voice synthesizers, help the child who has difficulty speaking or writing. Mental ability is difficult to evaluate because the type of brain injury associated with CP interferes with both verbal and motor expression. The family should be referred to the United Cerebral Palsy Association.

Community Cue

The United Cerebral Palsy Association (http://www.ucp. org) can be reached at 1600 L. Street, NW, Suite 700, Washington, DC 20036. The telephone number is 800-USA-5UCP (800-872-5827).

Mental Health Needs of the Disabled Child. The requirements for good mental health in disabled children do not differ greatly from those for all persons. They need to have their basic human drives satisfied, and they need people who are genuinely interested in them. As children grow, they need social experience with both genders to help them adjust to adolescence. The disabled child needs to participate to the fullest extent in family, school, and community activities. Friendships with other disabled and nondisabled peers are encouraged. Extended family and the community may be important resources or sources of stress. Frequently families are isolated or stigmatized because of fear and lack of knowledge on the part of the public. Educational programs are attempting to integrate disabled individuals more fully into the community. Barrier-free buildings and modifications that improve accessibility contribute positively to these efforts.

Attitudes of the Nurse. Inexperienced nurses may find that they are not immediately attracted to children who are disabled. Nurses may feel inadequate and may not know how to approach or assist these children. Fear of the unknown is natural. The nurse's first problem may be to think of what to say to the child. The best advice is the easiest: be natural and treat the child as you would any child of that developmental level. Watch the parent interact with the child. Let the child do as much independently as possible. Be there to assist if necessary but do not wait on the child hand and foot. The child is happier without pity. Limit setting is essential and provides security. Even patients with the most serious defects can grow up to be happy and self-reliant if they are accepted for who they are and encouraged to perform the tasks they are capable of doing. Disabled children want to be treated like other children of their age and to be loved and accepted as individuals.

HEAD INJURIES

Children suffer from head injuries that may occasionally result in brain damage. Falls, motor vehicle injuries, and bicycle injuries account for a large number of these statistics. Toddlers especially are famous for the number of blows received to the head. Fortunately, most of these injuries are not serious, but they are alarming to parents. The skulls of infants and young toddlers are more pliable and absorb much of the impact to the head. By 2 years of age, both fontanels have completely closed, and the cranium no longer has the same pliability in response to force.

Description

Types of head injuries are discussed in Table 10-3.

Complications

The major complications of head injury are hemorrhage, infections, cerebral edema (swelling of the brain), and compression of the brainstem. The brain and its interrelated compartments are tightly confined by the skull, more so after closure of the fontanels. Enlargement of any intracranial component (brain or subarachnoid, venous, or arterial space) can produce **increased intracranial pressure (ICP),** which can lead to permanent brain damage or death.

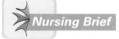
Nursing Brief

Shaken baby syndrome can result in increased ICP. The shearing force that results from brain movement as the baby is vigorously shaken may tear small arteries and cause cerebral edema. Always be alert for signs of ICP in children with the possibility of this diagnosis.

Treatment and Nursing Care

Frequently a child who has had a blow to the head is brought to the hospital for observation to rule out or confirm the diagnosis. Initial care of the child with a head injury includes assessment of the ABCs (airway, breathing, circulation), assessment for spinal cord injury, and documentation of baseline vital signs. The patient may have all or some of the following symptoms: headache (manifested by fussiness in the toddler), drowsiness, blurred vision, vomiting, and dyspnea (see Data Cues). In severe cases, the patient may be completely unconscious or having seizures. **Decerebrate** (indicating injury to the midbrain) or **decorticate** (indicating injury to the cerebral cortex) **posturing** may be evident (Figure 10-7). A careful history is obtained to determine any preexisting conditions and to ascertain the exact circumstances of the accident. Of particular importance is the patient's state of consciousness immediately after the occurrence. Radiography, CT, and magnetic resonance imaging (MRI) can be used to diagnose the specific head injury.

Table 10-3 | *Types of Head Injuries*

	SKULL AND SCALP INJURIES	FRACTURES	CONCUSSION	CONTUSION	HEMATOMA
Etiology	Falls, blunt trauma, penetrating	Falls, blunt trauma	Blunt trauma	Blunt trauma	Falls, motor vehicle accidents
Manifestations	Lacerations, bleeding, hematoma	Linear: thin, clear line usually with no symptoms; suspect child abuse Depressed: indentation of skull; may have fragments in brain tissue Basilar: fracture at base of skull; symptoms include hemorrhage of nose, nasal pharynx, middle ear, over mastoid bone (Battle's sign), and around eyes (raccoon eyes)	Alterations in mental status, with or without loss of consciousness, headache, nausea, vomiting, dizziness, irritability, seizures, retrograde amnesia (of events up to and including the injury)	Bruising or tearing of the brain, usually temporal or frontal sites; focal symptoms depending on area of injury; altered LOC, from confusion and disorientation to obtunded; focal seizures	Lacerations of arteries or veins in the brain; momentary unconsciousness Epidural: usually arterial, may be fatal; sleepiness, headache, bulging fontanel, paresthesias, papilledema, fixed pupils, increased ICP Subdural: usually venous; change in LOC
Treatment	Usually observation at home	Observation, supportive, or surgical intervention	Observation, supportive, and usually at home unless unconscious for more than 5 min or if there is amnesia of event	Observation and supportive	Observation or surgical intervention with evacuation of hematoma

ICP, Intracranial pressure; *LOC,* level of consciousness.

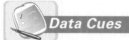

Data Cues

For the Child with Increasing ICP

- Behavior changes; disorientation with an older child
- Restlessness, fussiness; older child may have headache
- Dizziness, ataxia
- Increasing systolic blood pressure; widening pulse pressure
- Changes in respiratory pattern, decreasing pulse
- Several episodes of vomiting
- Pallor
- Listlessness, followed by increasing difficulty in arousing
- Changes in pupil size and reactions to light
- Seizures

Should the child be alert, without significant symptoms, and the parents reliable, the child can be sent home with instructions for observation.

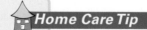

Home Care Tip

Guidelines for a Child with a Minor Head Injury

Monitor the child and alert the physician if the child exhibits any of the following:

- Severe headache or vomiting
- Blurred or double vision
- Unequal pupils
- Slurred speech
- Watery fluid from nose or ears
- Gait problems or unusual weakness in extremities
- Any seizure activity
- Will not awaken from sleep
- Becomes confused or is acting unusual
- Any other symptoms that are worrisome

Decorticate Posturing

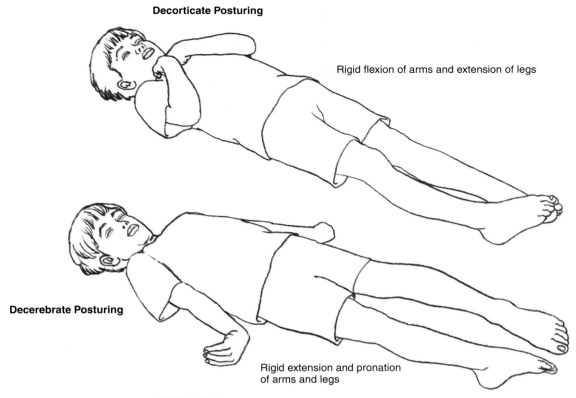

Rigid flexion of arms and extension of legs

Decerebrate Posturing

Rigid extension and pronation
of arms and legs

FIGURE **10-7** Decorticate and decerebrate posturing.

Further assessment includes the level of consciousness (LOC); changes are particularly meaningful and require immediate medical attention. Changes in behavior can be an *early* sign of increasing ICP. Response should be correlated with the developmental age of the patient. Parents can be helpful in providing information about the child's usual capabilities. In general, patients should be oriented to person, time, and place (may not be accessible in the toddler). Ask "What is your name?" and "Where are you?" Older children may know the day of the week. The patient should recognize the parents. Point to the mother and ask "Who is this?" When the patient does not respond to verbal stimuli, pinch the upper arm gently and observe the response. Note the presence or absence of crying or speech. It is not unusual for the child to fall asleep, but he or she should be easily aroused. Record changes in sleeping pattern, posture, movements of extremities, and any signs of tremors or restlessness.

The Child Coma Scale (Table 10-4), based on the adult Glasgow Coma Scale, is valuable in determining various LOCs. It consists of three parts: eye opening, motor response, and verbal response. A numerical value is assigned to each part. The lower the score, the deeper the coma.

Evaluation of pupil and eye movement requires documentation of size, shape, and equality of pupils and their reaction to light and extraocular movements. (Have the patient follow your finger from side to side and up and down to detect movement.) Strabismus, nystagmus, "sunset" eyes (eyes deviated downward), and inability to move eyes in all four quadrants indicate abnormality. If ICP is increasing, pupils become sluggish to light stimulus, dilated, and eventually fixed; this is an indication of a medical emergency.

Advanced ICP causes an increase in systolic blood pressure with a widening **pulse pressure** (the diastolic blood pressure usually decreases), a decrease in pulse, and altered respiratory pattern. This is referred to as the **Cushing triad.** Temperature is routinely monitored. Never take oral temperatures in children prone to seizures. Elevations may result from inflammation, systemic infection, or damage to the hypothalamus, which regulates body temperature. Body temperature may be reduced by administering antipyretics or by using a hypothermia blanket. Mild elevations in temperature are not uncommon in the first 2 days after trauma. Any seizure activity is treated with anticonvulsants.

The quality and strength of muscle tone should be observed in all four extremities. The patient should be able to squeeze the nurse's hands. The grip should be equal in both hands. The patient should be able to move the legs and push against the examiner's hands with both feet. The face should be symmetrical, and the patient should be able to smile and frown. Drooping of the eyes, ptosis, inability to close the eyes tightly, and drooping of the corner of the mouth are considered adverse signs. The child should be able to raise the

Table 10-4 *Glasgow Coma Scale Modified for Children*

SCORE*	CHILD	INFANT
EYES		
4	Opens eyes spontaneously	Opens eyes spontaneously
3	Opens eyes to speech	Opens eyes to speech
2	Opens eyes to pain	Opens eyes to pain
1	No response	No response
	——— = Score (Eyes)	
MOTOR		
6	Obeys commands	Spontaneous movements
5	Localizes (pain)	Withdraws to touch
4	Withdraws	Withdraws to pain
3	Flexion	Flexion (decorticate)
2	Extension	Extension (decerebrate)
1	No response	No response
	——— = Score (Motor)	
VERBAL		
5	Oriented	Coos and babbles
4	Confused	Irritable cry
3	Inappropriate words	Cries to pain
2	Incomprehensible sounds	Moans to pain
1	No response	No response
	——— = Score (Verbal)	
	——— = Total Score (Eyes, Motor, Verbal)	

*Reprinted from James, H.E., Anas, N.G., & Perkin, R.M. (1985). *Brain insults in infants and children*. Orlando, FL: Grune & Stratton. Scores range from 3 to 15.

arms and turn the palms up and down. Abnormal posturing should be described and recorded.

Record the type and amount of any drainage from the ears and nose. Leakage of cerebrospinal fluid from a fractured skull is seen as clear drainage from the ears or nose. Head circumference (FOC) should be monitored in infants, as should tension of the fontanels and the presence of a high-pitched cry.

Fluids are carefully monitored to control cerebral edema. Overhydration increases the amount of cerebral fluid. Feeding difficulties should be noted as the child's diet is increased. Patients should be observed for signs of shock, which can also occur.

Children whose conditions have remained stable are discharged. Parents are instructed about any additional observations and follow-up care.

It is important to teach parents about preventing head injury. Encourage parents of infants *never* to leave the child unattended on a changing table or bed.

Childproofing the home with stairway gates decreases falls. Teaching the toddler and preschooler not to run out in the street is an important safety measure. As the child becomes older and more active, a helmet should be worn during activities that provide risk, such as biking, rollerblading, and contact sports.

GENITOURINARY SYSTEM

WILMS TUMOR
Description
Wilms tumor, or **nephroblastoma**, is one of the most common malignant diseases of early life. It is a renal tumor arising from embryonic tissue. Nephroblastoma is now known to be associated with certain congenital anomalies, particularly of the genitourinary tract. The fact that it commonly occurs in siblings and twins indicates a genetic component.

Signs and Symptoms
During the early stages of growth, as with some other malignant diseases, there are few or no symptoms. It usually occurs in children between 2 and 5 years of age. A mass in the abdomen is discovered, generally by the mother or by the physician during a routine checkup. CT scan can confirm the origin and extent of the tumor and whether the other kidney is affected. Chest radiographs to identify possible metastases (the lungs are the most common site of metastasis in this disease), ultrasonography, bone surveys, liver scan, and urinalysis may be indicated. Wilms tumor seldom affects both kidneys.

Treatment and Nursing Care
The cornerstone treatment consists of surgery, unless there is involvement in both kidneys, the patient only has one kidney, or resection is not possible. Chemotherapy and radiation therapy postsurgery are based on the extent of the tumor and the histologic appearance of the tumor (Burg et al., 2006). The kidney and tumor are removed as soon as possible after the diagnosis has been confirmed. It is important to prepare the parents and the child for the extent of the incision, which is considerable. The National Wilms Tumor Study lists several categories of effective treatment. Five stages of tumor activity are cited, and appropriate refinements in chemotherapy and radiation are suggested. Children with stages I to III (tumor is confined to kidney or abdomen) have a cure rate varying from 88% to 98% (Behrman et al., 2004). The prognosis also depends on the histological character of the tumor and evidence of recurrence.

Nursing care is supportive before surgery. When the diagnosis of Wilms tumor has been made or is suspected, the *abdomen should not be palpated* because trauma to the mass could release cancer cells into the system. This is explained to the parents, and a sign is placed on the crib or child: "Do not palpate abdomen." The nurse must consider this extremely important.

In addition to preoperative teaching, the nurse teaches the parent and child about side effects from the chemotherapy and irradiation. Drugs and irradiation may cause reactions such as nausea, vomiting, anorexia, and general malaise. Ulceration of the mouth, hair loss, and peeling of the skin may also be seen. The nurse should anticipate such problems and should immediately report their appearance to the team leader or the nurse in charge of the unit.

The postoperative care of the child includes routine postoperative observations and specific monitoring for signs of intestinal obstruction from chemotherapy. These signs include vomiting, decreased or absent bowel sounds, and abdominal distention. Chemotherapy depresses the immune system, so the nurse must closely monitor the child for signs of infection. Bloody urine and elevated blood pressure are other symptoms that should be reported immediately.

The nurse needs to provide the family with information about protecting the remaining kidney as the child grows. Avoiding activities that risk kidney trauma is essential. Otherwise, the child should participate in activities normal for age and developmental level. Depending on the prognosis, helping the family and patient face the possibility of a fatal illness is an important nursing function (see Chapter 18).

SPECIAL TOPICS

AUTISM

Autism is described as a complex developmental disorder of the brain, most likely caused by abnormalities in brain structure or function. It is now viewed as a *spectrum disorder* and affects social interaction, language, and communication, as well as behavior (Burg et al., 2006). It is estimated that about 2 to 4 per 1000 children have autism. Autism typically appears in the first 3 years of life. The exact cause is unknown, although many theories abound. One theory is that the measles-mumps-rubella (MMR) vaccine has led to autism in some children. As discussed in Chapter 7, sufficient proof does not exist to support this theory. The Centers for Disease Control and Prevention have also done research in this area and current evidence does not show a link between the two. Other theories include genetic involvement, environmental factors, pregnancy complications, and possible related medical conditions.

Parents suspect something is wrong with their child but they do not know what it is. Autistic children may exhibit bizarre characteristics. They like things to stay the same; disruption of order in their world can upset them. They may have temper tantrums. Autistic children do not interact well with others; they prefer to be alone. These children often do not maintain eye contact with another person. They may play with toys in an unusual manner and live in their "own little world." Children with autism often exhibit a delay in or lack of language development. They may use repetitive language and exhibit repetitive motor movements such as rocking. Often there is some degree of mental retardation. On the other hand, autistic children, have been known to be particularly talented in certain areas such as music, memory, or mathematics.

The prognosis is not promising. Some children can acquire language skills. Many require lifelong care. Providing a structured routine is one of the best things parents can do for autistic children. These children need positive reinforcement. They also need to learn a social awareness of others and communication skills. Autistic children can and do show affection in the right environment. Research has also promoted programs for parents that enable them to work with children on improving communication.

This condition may be difficult for the family to accept. Parents may feel guilty and that they are to blame for the disorder. The family is in need of counseling once the diagnosis is determined. The Autism Society of America (ASA) can provide information about education, treatment programs, and resources for parents.

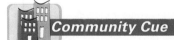 **Community Cue**

The Autism Society of America (http://www.autism-society.org) can be reached at 800-3AUTISM or 301-657-0881.

POISONINGS

Because toddlers are naturally curious and particularly mobile, they are prone to accessing places and items that are dangerous. Poisoning incidents are a particular risk for children at this developmental level (Figure 10-8).

Prevention

Nurses play a major role in the prevention of poisoning in children. As nurses use their knowledge of growth and development in teaching anticipatory guidance, they must focus the attention of the parent on the dangers of each age. Children are naturally curious, and as they become mobile, they can climb and reach any hiding place and open almost any bottle. The use of safety caps has been effective in reducing the number of ingestions. Parents are encouraged to have the local poison control center telephone number posted in a prominent place and are advised to call this number *first* before treating the child. The use of syrup of ipecac has become controversial. From the Brazilian plant *caephalis ipecacuanha*, this over-the-counter medicine has been kept in the medicine cabinets of families for years. Its purpose was to induce vomiting after a poisoning, when recommended by the Poison Control Center.

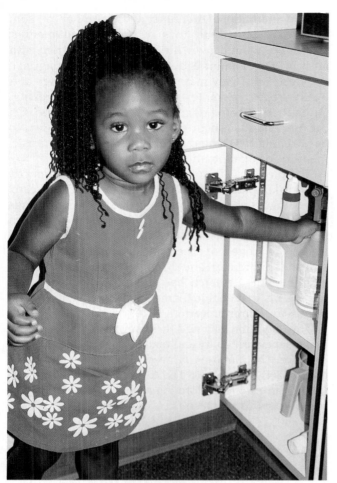

FIGURE **10-8** Children can easily discover poisons that are not in childproof cabinets.

Recently, concern about misuse of syrup of ipecac by those with bulimia has arisen. There is also controversy over exactly how effective this medicine really is. The American Academy of Pediatrics currently recommends "syrup of ipecac should not be used routinely as a poison treatment intervention in the home" (2004).

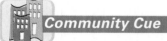

Community Cue

Teach parents that the American Association of Poison Control Centers' nationwide poison control hot line is 800-222-1222.

Emergency Care

Most poisonings can be managed in the home with the advice of the poison control center. If a child is not breathing after ingesting a poison, EMS (911) should be called. When a poisoned child is brought to the emergency department, certain steps should be taken. The nurse initially assesses the child for any signs of either impending or current respiratory or cardiac distress (ABCs). Cardiorespiratory support is initiated if needed.

Removal of toxins has historically been done with the use of emesis with syrup of ipecac, gastric lavage, and activated charcoal. Gastric lavage is currently still used for toxic substances that must be removed from the stomach. However, it has little, if any, benefit when performed beyond 30 minutes after ingestion. Activated charcoal use has increased since its effectiveness has been proven. It binds with most poisonous compounds; exceptions are metals, ethanol, caustics, and many hydrocarbons (Burg et al., 2006).

Depending on the poison, the nurse can anticipate the need for follow-up tests or treatments (such as electrolyte studies, IVs, temperature control measures, cardiac monitoring, respiratory treatments, and dialysis). When the child has ingested a corrosive substance such as toilet cleaner or bleach, tissue injury can interfere with breathing or swallowing. Corrosives are to be diluted with water or milk; vomiting is never to be induced. Vomiting redamages the mucosa. Some children need a tracheostomy to maintain an airway. Children with esophageal strictures may need a permanent gastrostomy. Hydrocarbons such as gasoline or paint thinner cause gagging, choking, coughing, and vomiting. The immediate danger is aspiration, and respiratory symptoms such as tachypnea and cyanosis are to be observed for. Changes in sensorium can also occur. Inducing emesis is also contraindicated with hydrocarbon ingestion. Gastric lavage is generally not performed because of the aspiration risk. Chemical pneumonia is treated with high humidity, oxygen, hydration, and antibiotics for secondary infection (Hockenberry & Wilson, 2007).

The Family

The nurse should give special attention to the family. The parents may feel guilty and blame themselves for the child's condition. The nurse must not reinforce this belief through either verbal or nonverbal communication. The parents should be kept informed about their child's condition, allowed to be with the child if at all possible, and given a chance to vent their feelings. The nurse should listen and support them through this difficult period. Preventive teaching should not be done until the acute stage has passed.

Acetaminophen Poisoning

Description. Acetaminophen (Tylenol) has become the most common drug poisoning in children because aspirin is used to treat children less frequently. Because acetaminophen has replaced aspirin in the medicine cabinet, children are accidentally ingesting this medication. Acetaminophen poisoning occurs from acute ingestion, not long-term overdose as may be seen in aspirin toxicity. Acetaminophen is metabolized in the liver. Therefore hepatic damage is the major concern. Children under 6 years of age are much less likely to have significant toxic effects from acetaminophen

Table 10-5	*Stages in the Clinical Source of Acetaminophen Toxicity*	
STAGE	**TIME AFTER INGESTION**	**CHARACTERISTICS**
I	0.5-24 hr	Anorexia, nausea, vomiting, malaise, pallor, diaphoresis
II	24-48 hr	Resolution of above; upper quadrant abdominal pain and tenderness; elevated bilirubin, prothrombin time, hepatic enzymes; oliguria
III	72-96 hr	Peak liver function abnormalities; anorexia, nausea, vomiting, malaise may reappear
IV	4 days to 2 wk	Resolution of hepatic dysfunction or complete liver failure

From Behrman, R., Kliegman, R., & Jenson, H. (2004). *Nelson's textbook of pediatrics* (17th ed.). Philadelphia: Saunders.

ingestion than are older children and adults (Behrman et al., 2004).

Signs and Symptoms. Four stages occur in the clinical course of acetaminophen poisoning (Table 10-5). Signs and symptoms may be vague, and the diagnosis may be delayed. Most children recover if treated promptly and correctly. Death may result if treatment is delayed in severe overdosage.

Treatment and Nursing Care. The stomach is emptied by lavage. *N*-acetylcysteine (Mucomyst) is the antidote and is given as soon as possible after ingestion but may be started 24 to 36 hours after the ingestion in severe cases. It is administered according to the serum acetaminophen level. Active charcoal absorbs acetaminophen and should be given within 1 to 2 hours of the ingestion (Behrman et al., 2004).

If the antidote is given, the nurse assists and supports the child in taking the offensive-smelling Mucomyst (smells like rotten eggs). It may be given with nasogastric tube or mixed with a carbonated drink. *N*-acetylcysteine may also be given IV; however, there is a higher incidence of anaphylaxis. Vital signs are monitored, intake and output are observed and recorded, and laboratory results (particularly liver functions) are monitored and reported if abnormal.

Salicylate Poisoning

Description. Because of the risk of Reye's syndrome (Chapter 14), aspirin should not be given to children unless recommended by a physician. Although salicylate poisoning has decreased since childhood fever has been treated more often with acetaminophen, it is still a problem. Aspirin is used by adults in most homes and often is stored carelessly on bedside stands or in mother's purse. This drug acts rapidly but is excreted slowly. Aspirin toxicity can occur from a single toxic-level ingestion or from repeated small therapeutic doses. Salicylates are also an ingredient in some over-the-counter antihistamines and decongestants. Pepto-Bismol (*bismuth subsalicylate*) even contains salicylate. Parents should be taught to read the labels and to use caution when giving these drugs.

Signs and Symptoms. The symptoms of salicylate poisoning vary depending on whether the toxicity is from an acute or chronic ingestion. The peak action occurs about 1 to 2 hours after a single toxic dose. Poisoning may manifest with ringing in the ears, dizziness, anorexia, sweating, nausea, vomiting, and diarrhea. **Hyperpnea,** faster and deeper respirations, is an early symptom of more serious trouble. This is because the respiratory center is stimulated by the drug. When carbon dioxide is eliminated, respiratory alkalosis quickly follows. Dehydration, metabolic acidosis, high fever, convulsions, and coma may follow. Bleeding is sometimes seen because excessive levels of aspirin inhibit the formation of prothrombin, which is necessary for normal blood clotting. Hypokalemia often accompanies this condition because salicylates directly affect the renal tubular mechanism.

Treatment and Nursing Care. There is no specific antidote for salicylate poisoning; therefore treatment is aimed at gastric emptying, preventing further absorption, and relieving the patient's symptoms. Activated charcoal is important in the treatment. A blood sample is taken to detect the level of salicylate poisoning and to determine electrolyte and blood gas status. Urine pH and output are monitored frequently. The doctor may request that the child be admitted to the hospital for observation. A sponge bath may be given to reduce fever. The patient's vital signs are closely observed and recorded. When IV fluids are necessary to correct electrolyte imbalance and rid the body of toxins, the child's intake and output of fluid are charted hourly.

Vitamin K may be administered to correct bleeding tendencies. IV infusions of fluids with sodium bicarbonate and potassium help correct imbalances. With severe intoxication, dialysis may be necessary.

As with acetaminophen poisoning, the psychological needs of the family are a top priority.

Ibuprofen Poisoning

Ibuprofen (Motrin, Advil) is commonly used as an analgesic and antipyretic. Seizures and coma can occur with toxic levels. Nausea, vomiting, epigastric pain, drowsiness, lethargy, and ataxia (unsteady gait) are common effects of overdosage. Renal function studies and acid-base balance need to be monitored with ingestion of large doses. There is no antidotal therapy; however, activated charcoal can be administered (Behrman et al., 2004).

Lead Poisoning (Plumbism)

Description. Lead poisoning results when a child repeatedly ingests or absorbs substances containing lead. Because of public awareness and health concerns, lead content from gasoline, paints and ceramic products, caulking, and pipe solder has been dramatically reduced in recent years. Children may, however, be exposed to lead through the use of health care products or folk remedies that contain lead (azarcon and greta), which are use for upset stomach; and paylooah, which is used for rash on fever.

Another major source of lead in the environment is soil contaminated with lead (usually paint from a deteriorating house), ingestion of paint chips, or inhalation of paint dust from lead-painted surfaces. In addition, lead solder was used in house plumbing in some sections of the country until 1978. The lead leached into the drinking water in these homes. The highest prevalence of lead poisoning is among inner-city, underprivileged children who live in deteriorating pre-1970s housing containing lead-paint surfaces.

Lead poisoning is more common in the summer months. Children chew on windowsills and stair rails. They ingest flakes of paint, putty, or crumbled plaster. They play outside in soil contaminated with lead. Food, particularly fruit juices consumed from improperly glazed earthenware, is another source.

Community Cue

Lead poisoning among Mexican Americans may be caused by azarcon, a bright orange powder containing approximately 93.5% lead. This folk remedy is given for diarrhea. Another folk remedy containing lead used for diarrhea among Mexican Americans is Greta, a yellow-orange powder.

Signs and Symptoms. Lead exposure can affect unborn children. Harmful effects include premature births, smaller babies, decreased mental ability and learning difficulties in children, and reduced growth in young children. Children may also develop anemia, stomach aches, and muscle weakness. Radiographs of the long bones may show deposits of lead.

The patient's history might reveal pica. This is a condition in which a child has a perverted appetite, eating a variety of things that most persons consider unpalatable, such as sand, grass, wool, glass, plaster, coal, animal droppings, and paint from furniture. This tendency is sometimes seen in neurotic children and is common in the mentally retarded. An underlying nutritional disturbance and family dysfunction may also account for it.

Treatment and Nursing Care. Preventing lead poisoning is foremost. Lead paint should not be used on children's toys or furniture. Instead use paint that is marked for indoor use. Close observation of children in this age group also acts as a deterrent. The nurse and the parents should provide safe objects such as a teething ring or washcloth for the toddler to suck and chew on

during the oral stage of development; this meets the normal sucking and chewing needs.

The Centers for Disease Control and Prevention (CDC) recommends that children who may be exposed to lead have their blood tested. The CDC considers children to have an elevated level of lead if the amount of lead in the blood is at least 10 mcg/dL. Medical evaluation and environmental investigation and remediation should be done for all children with blood lead levels equal or greater than 20 mcg/dL. Medical treatment may be necessary in children if the lead concentration in blood is higher than 45 mcg/dL.

The treatment approach selected for the child and parent depends on the result of the blood lead test. In addition to more frequent screening, educational materials that describe how lead exposure can be decreased in the home and environment may be the only intervention necessary. In some cases, a professional environmental assessment is warranted. The child should not remain in any home where renovations involving lead paint are taking place.

Treatment is generally initiated in the child with moderate-to-severe lead poisoning (blood lead level greater than 45 mcg/dl. Reducing the concentration of lead in the tissues and blood becomes important when levels get this high. First, the child is removed from the source of lead and is closely supervised. Family members should also be tested. Chelating agents that render the lead nontoxic and allow it to be excreted in the urine are given. All chelating agents can have potentially serious side effects. Calcium disodium edetate (CaEDTA) and British antilewisite (BAL) are the two most commonly used drugs. CaEDTA may be given either with deep intramuscular injection or with IV drip. BAL is given with deep intramuscular injection. Succimer, an oral chelating agent, can be used for children with blood lead levels of 45 to 69 mcg/dL. The child may need repeated courses of chelating therapy before normal lead levels return.

The prognosis depends on the degree and duration of the lead ingestion. Some children do not have any residual effects; others may have severe encephalopathy.

The nurse should stress the importance of continued treatment to prevent the recurrence of lead poisoning symptoms. Infectious disease in these youngsters must be treated promptly to avoid reactivation of the process. Parents are taught to be suspicious of changes in the disposition of their child. Siblings and playmates should also be screened. All residents should be removed from homes being de-leaded to avoid exposure. Parents living in apartments owned by uncooperative landlords may need assistance in relating to the housing authority. Appropriate literature and explanations are provided at the "therapeutic moment" and thereafter.

Nursing care is symptomatic. Unnecessary handling of the patient is avoided to prevent stimulating the central nervous system. Injection sites are rotated, and the skin is evaluated for thickness of fibrous lumps. Therapeutic syringe play is advised. Observation and charting of convulsions are discussed in Chapter 12. Indications of respiratory distress are reported immediately. The services of the public health nurse are valuable in investigating the physical and emotional environment of the child and in continuing the education of the parents.

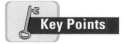

Key Points

- Children with hearing impairments need special preparation and orientation to the health care setting.
- Infants and children under the age of 3 years are at increased risk for respiratory infections because of their immature immune system and narrow airways.
- Symptoms of drooling, high fever, muffled voice, and rapid respirations require immediate medical attention.
- The typical hand-to-mouth behavior of young children makes them prone to pinworm infestation.
- Neurovascular assessments should be performed on children in casts and in traction.
- Children in skeletal traction require diversional therapy and physical outlets for their lack of physical activity.
- Children with CP should be involved in stimulation programs that assist them in achieving their highest level of functioning.
- Level of consciousness assessment is the most important evaluation of neurological status in children.

- Palpation of a Wilms tumor can lead to trauma of the tumor, resulting in the release of cancer cells; therefore children with Wilms tumor should not have their abdomen palpated.
- Families of children with autism need education and support.
- Nursing intervention for the ingestion of poison should begin with the ABCs.
- Injury prevention is an important role of the pediatric nurse. Using anticipatory guidance and injury prevention information, nurses can assist caretakers in identifying potential risks. Motor vehicle injuries, head injuries, poison ingestions, and falls can largely be prevented.

 Go to your Companion CD-ROM for an Audio Glossary, video clips, and more.

evolve Be sure to visit the companion Evolve site at http://evolve.elsevier.com/Price/pediatric for WebLinks and additional online resources.

ONLINE RESOURCES

Alexander Graham Bell Association for the Deaf and Hard of Hearing: http://www.agbell.org/information/brochures_faq.cfm

Cerebral palsy website: http://www.ninds.nih.gov/health_and_medical/disorders/cerebral_palsy.htm

Head injury website (Virtual Children's Hospital): http://www.vh.org/pediatric/patient/pediatrics/cqqa/headinjuries.html

Poison prevention website: http://www.aapcc.org

The Preschool Child

Objectives

Upon completion of this chapter, the student will be able to:

1. Define the vocabulary terms listed
2. Describe the physical and psychosocial development of children from 3 to 5 years of age, listing age-specific events and guidance when appropriate
3. Describe the characteristics of a good preschool facility
4. Discuss the value of play in the life of a child
5. Designate two toys suitable for the preschool child and provide the rationale for each choice
6. Identify the developmental characteristics that predispose the preschool child to certain accidents and suggest methods of prevention for each type of accident

Key Terms

Be sure to check out the bonus material on the Companion CD-ROM, including selected audio pronunciations.

animism (ĂN-ĭ-mĭsm; p. 220)
artificialism (ĂR-tĭ-FĬSH-ăl-ĭsm; p. 222)
centering (p. 222)
domestic mimicry (MĬM-ĭk-RĒ; p. 222)
egocentrism (Ē-gō-SĔN-trĭsm; p. 220)
enuresis (ĕn-ū-RĒ-sĭs; p. 228)
identification (p. 223)
modeling (p. 226)
play therapy (p. 233)

GENERAL CHARACTERISTICS AND DEVELOPMENT

The child from ages 3 to 5 years is often referred to as the preschool child. This period is marked by a slowing down in the child's growth. By 1 year, infants have tripled their birth weight, whereas by the age of 6 years, these same children have only doubled their 1-year weight. For instance, the boy who weighs 20 pounds on his first birthday will probably weigh about 40 pounds on his fifth. Weight gain during the preschool years is about 5 pounds per year. The child between 3 and 5 years of age grows taller and loses the chubbiness that is seen during the toddler period. Height increases approximately 2.5 to 3 inches per year. Appetite fluctuates widely. The normal pulse rate is 90 to 110. The rate of respirations during relaxation is about 20 per minute. The systolic blood pressure is about 92 to 95 mm Hg; the diastolic is about 56 mm Hg.

By the preschool years, at least 90% of brain growth is achieved and handedness begins to become apparent. A summary of preschool growth and development is presented in Table 11-1.

Preschool children have good control of their muscles and participate in vigorous play activities. As each year passes, they become more adept at using old skills. They can swing and jump higher. Their gait resembles that of an adult. They are quicker, and compared with toddlers, they have more confidence in themselves. Although preschool children may seem more or less quiet and steady with respect to physical development, certain difficulties do arise from an increase in independence, social participation, interaction, and cognitive ability.

THEORIES OF DEVELOPMENT

The thinking of the preschool child is unique. Piaget called this period the preoperational phase. This phase comprises the ages of 2 to 7 years and is divided into two stages: the preconceptual stage, from 2 to 4 years; and the intuitive thought stage, from 4 to 7 years. The increasing development of language and symbolic functioning is important in the preconceptual stage. Symbolic functioning can be seen when children play and pretend that an empty box is a fort; this creates a mental image, which stands for something that is not there.

Preoperational thinking also implies that children cannot think in terms of operations, or the ability to logically manipulate objects in relation to each other. They base their reasoning on what they see and hear. They also believe they have magical powers that can cause events to occur. For example, a child might wish that someone or something would die. If the death does occur, the child feels at fault because of the "bad" thought that made it happen.

Another characteristic of this period is egocentrism, a type of thinking in which children have difficulty seeing any point of view other than their own. Children's knowledge and understanding are restricted to their own limited experiences, and as a result, misconceptions arise. One of these misconceptions is animism. This is a tendency to attribute life to inanimate objects. Another

| Table 11-1 | *Summary of Preschooler Growth and Development* |

AGE	PHYSICAL	GROSS MOTOR	FINE MOTOR	VOCALIZATION	SOCIALIZATION
3 yr	Usual weight gain of 1.8 to 2.7 kg (4 to 6 pounds) Average weight of 14.6 kg (32 pounds) Usual gain in height of 7.5 cm (3 inches) Average height of 95 cm (37.25 inches) May have achieved night-time control of bowel and bladder	Rides tricycle Jumps off bottom step Stands on one foot for a few seconds Goes up stairs using alternate feet; may come down using both feet on step Broad jumps May try to dance; balance may not be adequate	Builds tower of 9 to 10 cubes Adeptly places small pellets in narrow-necked bottle Copies a circle, imitates a cross, names what has been drawn; cannot draw a stick figure but may make circle with facial features	Has vocabulary of approximately 900 words Uses complete sentences of 3 to 4 words Repeats sentence of 6 syllables Asks many questions Begins to sing songs	Dresses self almost completely Has increased attention span Feeds self completely; can prepare simple meals, such as cold cereal and milk Can help to set table May have fears (of dark or going to bed) Knows own gender and gender of others Play is parallel and associative; begins to learn simple games but often follows own rules; begins to share
4 yr	Growth rate is similar to that of previous year Average weight of 16.7 kg (36.75 pounds) Average height of 103 cm (40.5 inches) Length at birth is doubled Maximum potential for development of amblyopia	Skips and hops on one foot Catches ball; throws ball overhand Walks down stairs using alternate footing	Uses scissors successfully Can lace shoes Copies a square, traces a cross and diamond, adds 3 parts to stick figure	Has vocabulary of 1500 words or more Uses sentences of 4 to 5 words Questioning is at peak Tells exaggerated stories Knows simple songs May be mildly profane if associates with older children Names one or more colors	Very independent Tends to be selfish and impatient Aggressive physically and verbally Takes pride in accomplishments Has mood swings Shows off dramatically, enjoys entertaining others Still has many fears Play is associative; imaginary playmates are common Sexual exploration and curiosity shown through play, such as being "doctor" or "nurse"
5 yr	Average weight of 18.7 kg (41.25 pounds) Average height of 110 cm (43.25 inches) Eruption of permanent dentition may begin Handedness is established (approximately 90% are right-handed)	Skips and hops on alternate feet Throws and catches ball well Jumps rope Skates with good balance Walks backward with heel to toe Jumps from height of 12 inches Balances on alternate feet with eyes closed	Ties shoelaces Uses scissors, simple tools, and pencil well Copies a diamond and triangle; adds 7 to 9 parts to stick figure; prints a few letters, numbers, or words, such as first name	Has vocabulary of approximately 2100 words Uses sentences of 6 to 8 words Names coins Names 4 or more colors Knows names of days of week, months, and other time-associated words	Less rebellious and quarrelsome More settled and eager to get down to business Independent but trustworthy; not foolhardy; more responsible Has fewer fears; relies on outer authority to control world Eager to do things right and to please; tries to "live by the rules"; has better manners Cares for self with only occasional assistance Play is associative; tries to follow rules but may cheat to avoid losing

Modified from Hockenberry, M., & Wilson, D. (2007). *Wong's nursing care of infants and children* (8th ed.). St. Louis: Mosby.

is artificialism, the idea that the world and everything in it is created by human beings (Table 11-2).

Evolving from preconceptual thinking to intuitive thinking involves a shift from egocentric thought to a social awareness and ability to consider another's point of view. This is considered to be closely associated with superego or conscience development.

Another distinctive characteristic of intuitive thinking is centering, the tendency to concentrate on a single outstanding characteristic of an object while excluding its other features. With time and experience, more mature conceptual awareness is established. The process is highly complex, and the implications for practical application are numerous. In addition, through intuitive thinking, play becomes more socialized and words are used to express ideas and thoughts.

According to Erik Erikson's theories, preschoolers acquire a sense of initiative. They believe learning is fun and try new activities and experiences. Conflict arises when initiative is criticized or punished; then they develop a sense of guilt. This guilt can carry over later in life and affect their ability to make decisions or solve problems.

It is important to provide preschoolers exposure to a wide variety of experiences and play materials to enhance their learning. They need to be allowed to play with finger paints, build sand castles, play with clay, and engage in activities that enhance their imaginations.

Preschoolers enjoy dressing up and pretending to be real and make-believe characters (Figure 11-1). They love to imitate people around them and often mimic what they see their parents doing. Playing "store" or "office" or doing household chores such as "lawn-mowing" or "doing the dishes" are activities that preschoolers enjoy. Toy companies manufacture many toys that encourage the preschooler to engage in this domestic mimicry.

Lawrence Kohlberg emphasized moral development and moral judgment. Preschoolers are at a preconceptual stage of moral development. Young children learn whether an action is good or bad depending on whether the action is rewarded or punished. Preschool children progress to a stage where they can carry out actions to satisfy their own needs but not society's in general. They do something for another if that person does something for them.

Table 11-2   *The Nature of Early Childhood Thought*

SAMPLE QUESTION	TYPICAL ANSWER
ECOCENTRISM	
Why does the sun shine?	To keep me warm.
Why is there snow?	For me to play in.
Why is grass green?	Because that is my favorite color.
What are television sets for?	To watch my favorite shows and cartoons.
ANIMISM	
Why do trees have leaves?	To keep them warm.
Why do stars twinkle?	Because they are happy and cheerful.
Why does the sun move in the sky?	To follow children and hear what they say.
Where do boats go at night?	They sleep like we do.
ARTIFICIALISM	
What causes rain?	Someone emptying a watering can.
Why is the sky blue?	It has been painted.
What is the wind?	A man blowing.
What causes thunder?	A man grumbling.

From Helms, D., & Turner, J. (1978). *Exploring child behavior: Basic principles* (p. 447). Philadelphia: Saunders, with permission.

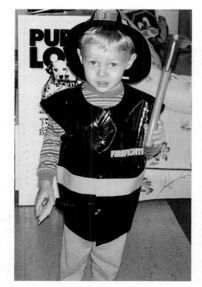
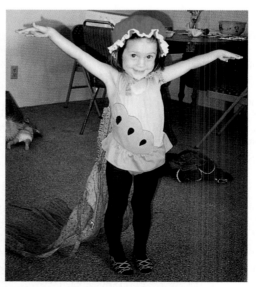

FIGURE **11-1** Preschoolers have vivid imaginations and enjoy playing "dress-up."

Children at this age are just beginning to learn right from wrong. Spiritual development is strongly linked to development of the conscience (Hockenberry & Wilson, 2007). The preschooler is just beginning to understand spiritual matters. Rudimentary knowledge is provided by parents or significant others. Their concrete thinking allows them to perceive God as an imaginary friend. Children this age enjoy hearing Bible stories and reciting simple prayers. If hospitalized, saying prayers as part of their routine can actually help with the stressors of hospitalization.

Sigmund Freud emphasized that early childhood is critical in the socialization of the individual. Freud believed that during the preschool years, the child focuses on the genital area. He referred to this as the phallic phase. According to Freud's theory, the child fantasizes about satisfying phallic desires by identification with the parent of the opposite gender and thus conflict results with the parent of the same gender. This is known as the Oedipal complex (boys) and the Electra complex (girls). Freud also stated that once the conflict is resolved, the child identifies with the same-gender parent.

PHYSICAL, PSYCHOSOCIAL, AND COGNITIVE DEVELOPMENT

THE 3-YEAR-OLD CHILD

Most 3-year-olds are a delight to their parents. They are helpful and can participate in simple household chores. They obtain articles on request and return them to the proper place. Three-year-olds come very close to the ideal picture that parents have in mind of their child. They are living proof that their parents' guidance during the "terrible twos" has been rewarded. Temper tantrums are less frequent, and in general, the 3-year-old is a pretty good youngster. Of course, they are still their individual selves, but they seem to be able to direct and control their primitive instincts better than before. They can help dress and undress themselves, use the toilet, and wash their hands. They eat independently, and their table manners have improved.

The 3-year-old talks in longer sentences and can express thoughts such as "What are you doing?" or "Where is Daddy?" They also provide more company to their parents because they can verbally share their experiences with them. They are imaginative, talk to their toys, and imitate what they see about them. Soon they begin to make friends outside the immediate family. Because they can now converse with playmates, they find satisfaction in joining their activities. Three-year-olds do not play cooperatively for long periods of time, but at least it's a start. Through associative play, they begin to share with other children; playing with other children their own age teaches them socialization skills. Much of their play still consists of watching others, but now if they

have the need, they can offer verbal advice. They can ask others to "come out and play." If 3-year-olds are placed in a strange situation with children they do not know, they commonly revert to parallel play because it is more comfortable.

At this time, there is a change in the relationship between the child and the family. Preschoolers begin to find enjoyment away from Mom and Dad. However, they want them to be right there when needed. They begin to lose some of their interest in their mother, who up to this time has been more or less their total world. Their father's prestige begins to increase. Romantic attachment to the parent of the opposite gender is seen during this period. Johnny wants to "marry Mommy" when he grows up. They also begin to identify themselves with the parent of the same gender. This behavior reflects Freud's beliefs. It is important for parents to remember to help the child fully develop his or her potential.

Preschool children have more fears than the infant or the older child. Some of the many causes of this are increased intelligence, which enables them to recognize potential dangers; the development of memory; and graded independence, which brings them into contact with many new situations. Toddlers are not afraid of walking in the street because they do not know any better. Preschool children realize that trucks can injure them, and therefore they worry about crossing the street. This type of fear is well founded, but many others are not. The fear of bodily harm is particularly peculiar to this stage. The little boy who discovers that his baby sister is made differently worries that perhaps she has been injured. He wonders if this will happen to him. Masturbation is common during this stage as children attempt to reassure themselves that they are all right. Other common fears include fear of animals, fear of the dark, and fear of strangers. A little night wandering is typical for this age group.

Preschool children become angry when others attempt to take their possessions. They grab, slap, and hang on to them for dear life. They become very distraught if toys do not work the way they should. They resent being disturbed from play. They are sensitive, and their feelings are easily hurt. It is good to bear in mind that much of the disturbing social behavior seen during this time is normal and necessary to the children's total pattern of development.

 Communication Alert

Preschool children sometimes believe that they are being punished for something they thought or did. Thus when a painful procedure is performed on the child, the nurse might say, "I am sorry that it hurt when I put the needle in your arm. I did that so we can give you medicine to make you feel better, not to hurt or punish you."

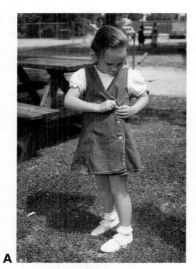

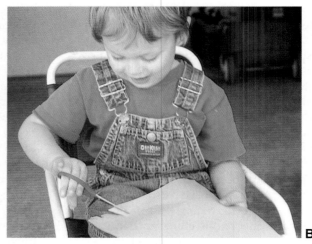

FIGURE **11-2** The child progressively achieves mastery of fine motor skills and cognitive abilities, such as **(A)** buttoning clothes and **(B)** using scissors.

THE 4-YEAR-OLD CHILD

Four is a stormy age. Children are not as eager or willing as they were at 3 years. They also are more aggressive and like to show off. They are eager to let others know that they are superior and are prone to pick on their playmates. They often take sides and make life difficult for any child who does not measure up to their standards. Four-year-olds are boisterous, tattle on others, and may begin to swear if they are around children or adults who use profanity. Personal family activities are repeated with an amazing sense of recall, but they still forget where they left their bicycle. At this age, children become interested in how old they are and want to know the exact age of each playmate. It bolsters their ego to know that they are older than someone else in the group. Their ego is also bolstered by being a "big brother" or "big sister" to a younger sibling. They are able to help care for and protect them. The relationship of one person to another interests them as well. For example, Timmy is not only a brother but also is Daddy's son.

Four-year-olds can use scissors successfully. They can lace their shoes and do simple buttons (Figure 11-2). Vocabulary has increased to about 1500 words. They run simple errands and can play with others for longer periods of time. Many feats are done for a purpose. For instance, they no longer run just for the sake of running. Instead, they run to get someplace or to see something. They are imaginative and like to pretend they are firefighters or cowboys. Much of their play time is spent pretending. They may even have an imaginary friend. The friend may "exist" until the child starts school. They also begin to prefer playing with friends of the same gender rather than with those of the opposite gender.

The preschool child enjoys simple toys. They love to color pictures and have mastered the use of large

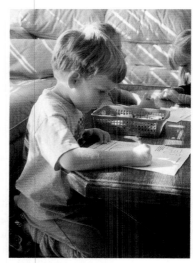

FIGURE **11-3** The preschooler enjoys coloring. Preschoolers often play *cooperatively*.

crayons (Figure 11-3). Raw materials are more appealing than toys that are ready-made. An old cardboard box that can be moved about and climbed into is more fun than a dollhouse with tiny furniture. A box of sand or colored pebbles can be made into roads and mountains. A small mirror becomes a lake. "Dress up" becomes more dramatic, especially with the 4-year-old. Parents should avoid showering their children with ready-made toys. Instead they can select materials that are absorbing and that stimulate the child's imagination.

Stories that interest young children depict their daily experiences. If the story has a simple plot, it must be related to what they understand to hold their interest. They also enjoy music; they like songs that they can march around to and simple instruments that they can shake or bang. Make up a song about their daily life and watch their reaction.

Children's curiosity concerning sex continues to heighten. If the parents have answered questions simply, they should not be alarmed to find their children checking up on them. It is common for children of this age to take down their pants in front of friends of the opposite gender. They discuss their differences with their friends. It is important that parents provide simple explanations when sexual questions are asked. Older children who are more sensitive about their bodies should be told that this is a natural curiosity among small children. This may help to get rid of any guilty feelings that they might have, particularly if they also participated in similar activities during the preschool period. Children are as matter-of-fact about these investigations as they would be about any other learning experience and are easily distracted to more socially acceptable forms of behavior.

Between ages 3 and 4 years, children begin to wonder about death and dying. They may be the hero who shoots the intruder dead or they may witness a situation in which an animal is killed. Their questions are very direct: "What is dead? Will I die?" There are no set answers to these inquiries. Preschoolers may see death as a kind of sleep. They may not believe the dead person no longer breathes or eats. They cannot understand the true concept of death. The religion of the family plays an important role regarding the interpretations of this complex phenomenon.

Perhaps children can become acquainted with death through objects that are not of particular significance to them. For instance, the flower dies at the end of the summer. It does not bloom any more. It no longer needs sunshine or water because it is not alive. Usually young children realize that others die but do not relate this to themselves. If they continue to pursue the question of whether or not they will die, parents should be casual and reassure them that people do not generally die until they have lived a long and happy life. Of course, as they grow older, they will discover that sometimes children do die. The underlying idea, nevertheless, is to encourage questions as they appear and gradually help them accept the truth without undue fear. Chapter 18 discusses additional end-of-life issues.

THE 5-YEAR-OLD CHILD

Five is a comfortable age. Children are more responsible, enjoy doing what is expected of them, have more patience, and like to finish what they start. Five-year-olds are serious about what they can and cannot do. They talk constantly and are inquisitive about the environment. They have a vocabulary of about 2100 words. They want to do things right. They also seek answers to their questions and go to those who they think are knowledgeable. Five-year-olds can begin to play games governed by rules. They are less fearful

because they feel that their environment is controlled by authorities. The worries they do have are not as profound as they were at an earlier age. They may play with and talk to a best friend.

The physical growth of 5-year-olds is not particularly outstanding. Their height may increase 2 to 3 inches, and they may gain 3 to 6 pounds. The variations in height and weight of a group of 5-year-olds are remarkable. They may begin to lose their deciduous teeth at this time. They can simultaneously run and play games, jump three or four steps at once, and tell a penny from a nickel or a dime. They like games with numbers or letters. They can name the days of the week and can understand what is a weeklong vacation. They usually can print their first name.

Five-year-olds can ride a tricycle around the playground with speed and dexterity. With training wheels, they also can begin riding two-wheelers as well. They can use a hammer to pound nails. Adults should encourage them to develop motor skills. Adults should not continually remind them to "be careful" because this practice enables children to compete with others during the school-age period and increases confidence in their own abilities. As with any age level, children should not be scorned for failure or for not measuring up to adult standards. Overdirection by solicitous adults is damaging. Children must learn to do tasks themselves for the experience to be satisfying.

The amount and type of television programs that parents allow preschool children to watch is a topic of current discussion. Although children enjoy television at 3 or 4 years of age, it is usually for short periods of time. They cannot understand much of what is happening. Five-year-olds have better comprehension and may spend a great deal of time watching television. The plan of management differs for each family. Whatever is decided needs to be discussed with the children. Television should not be allowed to interfere with good health habits, such as regular sleep, meals, and physical activity. Most parents find that children do not insist on watching television if there is something better to do.

GUIDING THE PRESCHOOL CHILD

DISCIPLINE, SETTING LIMITS

Much has been written on the subject of discipline, which over time has changed considerably. Today authorities place a great deal of importance on the development of a continuous, warm relationship between the child and the parents. This, they believe, helps prevent many problems. The following is a brief discussion that may help the nurse to guide parents.

Discipline and punishment are not one and the same: "Discipline includes all methods that are used to change behavior. Punishment is a very specific procedure that is used to decrease behavior that will be described under basic principles" (Larsen & Tentis, 2003). Children need to have limits set on their behavior. Setting limits makes them feel secure, protects them from danger, and relieves them from making decisions that they may be too young to understand. Expectations, however, must be appropriate to the age and understanding of the child. Parents need to encourage children to make acceptable choices. Children who are taught acceptable behavior have more friends and feel better about themselves. They live more enjoyably within the neighborhood and society. The manner in which discipline or limit setting is carried out varies from culture to culture. It also varies among different socioeconomic groups. Individual differences occur among families, between parents, and according to the characteristics of each child. The purpose of discipline is to teach and to gradually shift control from parents to the child, that is, to promote self-discipline. The Health Promotion box lists discipline techniques.

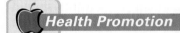

Health Promotion

Discipline for Young Children

- Establish rules for safety by 8 months of age
- Explain rules clearly and concretely ("Don't push your brother")
- State acceptable behavior ("Walk, don't run")
- Do not constantly criticize
- Use rules that are fair and attainable for the child's age
- Apply rules consistently
- Remember that yelling teaches the child to yell back
- Logical consequences occur as a result of misbehavior (removal of possession or privilege)

Schmitt, B. (2006). Discipline basics. Pediatric Advisor. McKesson Corporation. Retrieved from www.med.umich.edu/1libr/pa/pa_bdisbasc_hhg.htm.

Timing, Time Out

Most researchers agree that to be effective, discipline must be given at the time the incident occurs. It should also be adapted to the seriousness of the infraction. The child's self-worth must always be considered. Warning the preschool child who appears to be getting into trouble may be helpful. Too many warnings without follow-up, however, lead to ineffectiveness. Spankings, for the most part, are not productive. The child associates the fury of the parents with the pain rather than the wrong deed because anger is the predominant factor in the situation. In addition, the parent serves as a role model for aggression. Whether a parent is affectionate, warm, or cold (uncaring) also plays a role in the effectiveness of child rearing. Time-out periods (discussed in Chapter 9), such as sitting for 5 minutes in a chair or corner, are one alternative to inappropriate behavior. Parents need to be taught to resist using power and authority for its own sake. As the child understands more, privileges can be withheld. The reasons for such actions should be carefully explained.

Rewarding Positive Behavior

Rewarding the child for good behavior is a positive and effective method of discipline. This can be done by the use of hugs, smiles, tone of voice, and praise. Praise can always be tied to the act: "Thank you, Sara, for picking up your toys." The encouragement of positive behavior eliminates many of the undesirable effects of punishment.

Consistency and Modeling

Consistency is difficult for parents. However, they should try to be consistent as much as possible. Consistency must exist between parents and within each parent. It is suggested that parents establish a general style in terms of what, when, how, and to what degree punishment is appropriate to misconduct. Parents who are lax or erratic in their discipline and alternate such procedures with punishment have children who experience increased behavioral difficulties. The influence of *modeling,* or good example, has been widely explored. Such studies show that adult models significantly influence the education of children. Children identify and imitate adult behavior, both verbal and nonverbal. Parents who are aggressive and repeatedly lose control demonstrate the power of action over words. Those who communicate, show respect and encouragement, and use appropriate limit-setting serve as more positive role models. Finally, parents need assistance in reviewing their own childhood in regard to parental discipline to recognize destructive patterns that they may be exhibiting.

Spanking

The American Academy of Pediatrics has made the following statement regarding spanking: "Because of the negative consequences of spanking and because it has been demonstrated to be no more effective than other approaches for managing undesired behavior in children, the American Academy of Pediatrics recommends that parents be encouraged and assisted in developing methods other than spanking in response to undesired behavior" (AAP Policy Statement, 2004). The role of the nurse is to encourage parents to use other forms of discipline with their children. By explaining the use of timing, time out, consistency, modeling, etc., parents become empowered and can make positive choices when raising their children.

BAD LANGUAGE

Parents express astonishment at the words that flow from the mouths of their sweet little children during the preschool period. Bad language is inevitable. Caretakers should suppress their desire to emphatically shout their disapproval. The small child delights in attention, and it does not matter, unfortunately, whether this attention is good or bad. Swearing at this age is not particularly meaningful because children are merely imitating what they hear and it does not have any real significance to them. They use swearing as a way of identifying themselves with the older children in the neighborhood and to shock adults. One mother dealt with this problem by saying, "Johnny, Mommy does not mind if you hear or know what that word means, but we do not use it in our home any more than you would think of going outdoors without your clothes on." Johnny felt free to discuss what he heard with his mother and shortly thereafter his interest was taken up by other subjects.

JEALOUSY AND SIBLING RIVALRY

Jealousy is a normal response to actual, supposed, or threatened loss of affection. Children or adults may feel insecure in their relationship with the person they love. The closer children are to their mothers, the greater their fear of losing mother. Young children may envy a new baby. They love the sibling but at the same time resent its presence. They cannot understand the turmoil that is taking place within themselves. Jealousy of a new baby is strongest in children less than 5 years of age and is shown in various ways. Children may be aggressive and may bite or pinch. They may be rather discreet and hug and kiss the baby with a determined look on their faces. Another common situation occurs when children attempt to identify with the baby. They may revert to something they outgrew such as thumb sucking or wetting the bed. Some 4-year-olds even try the bottle, but it is usually a big disappointment to them.

Preschool children may be jealous of the attention that their mother gives their father. They may also envy the children they play with if those children have bigger and better toys than they do. School-age children more often are jealous of those who are more athletic or popular. There is less jealousy in only children because they are the center of attention and have only a minimum of rivals. Children of varied ages in one family are apt to feel that the younger ones are "pets" or that the older ones have more special privileges. These feelings of sibling rivalry present new challenges for the parents.

Parents can help reduce jealousy with the early management of individual occurrences. Preparing young children for the arrival of the new baby lessens the blow. They should not be made to think that they are being crowded. If the new baby is going to occupy their crib, it is best to get older children happily settled in a large bed before the baby is born. Children should feel that they are helping with the care of the infant. Parents can inflate their ego from time to time by reminding them of the many activities they can do that the new baby cannot. Parents also need to attend to the older child's needs first if both children have needs at the same time (Anderson, 2006). If it is convenient, the new baby is given a bath or feeding while the older child is asleep. In this way the older sibling avoids one of the occasions on which the mother shows the newborn infant affection for a relatively long period of time. Special time should also be spent with the older child while the new baby is asleep. Some people believe that giving the child a pet to care for at this time helps. Many hospitals offer sibling courses that assist parents in helping the child to overcome jealousy.

If the child indicates an intention to hit the baby or another child, the children must be separated. It is important to remember that the one who has caused or is about to cause the injury needs as much, if not more, attention than the victim. Aggressiveness similar to this is seen when the child is made to share toys. It is even more difficult to learn to share the mother, so the child must be given time to adjust to the new situation. Children should be assured that they are loved but should also be told that they are not allowed to injure others. Use of the "I message" is helpful when correcting this type of behavior: "I feel angry that you hit your brother (or sister), and hitting is not allowed because it can hurt people."

THUMB SUCKING

From 1914 to 1921, the U.S. Children's Bureau pamphlet entitled *Infant Care* cautioned mothers that thumb sucking would deform the mouth and cause drooling. Today we recognize that thumb sucking is an instinctual behavioral pattern that can be considered normal. It is often used as a comforting measure and does not necessarily mean the child is insecure. Finger sucking or thumb sucking does not have a detrimental effect on the teeth as long as the habit is discontinued before the second teeth have erupted. Most children give up the habit by the time they reach school age, although they may regress during periods of stress or fatigue. Management includes education and support of the parents so as to relieve their anxiety and to help prevent secondary emotional problems in their children. The child who is trying to stop thumb sucking is given praise and encouragement.

MASTURBATION

Masturbation is common in both genders during the preschool years. The child experiences pleasurable sensations, which lead to repetition of the behavior. It is beneficial to rule out other causes of this activity, such as rashes or penile or vaginal irritation. Masturbation is also exhibited in the child who feels emotionally isolated or anxious. A variety of interpretations of masturbation have been postulated; however, it appears that there are still many questions left unanswered regarding the significance of this behavior for the child. One common anxiety in boys that should be explored is fear of castration. Masturbation at this age is considered harmless if the child is outgoing, sociable, and not preoccupied with the activity. However, if masturbation is "compulsive" or "interferes with the child's normal activities" or involves "acting out of sexual intercourse in doll play or with other children," the possibility of sexual abuse must be explored (Behrman et al., 2004).

Education of the parents consists of assuring them that this behavior is normal and not harmful to the child, who is merely curious about sexuality. The cultural and moral background of the family must be considered when assessing the degree of discomfort in relation to this experience. A history of the time and place of masturbation and the parental response is helpful. Punitive reactions are discouraged because these can be potentially harmful to the child. Parents are advised to try to ignore the behavior and to distract the child with some other activity. If the parent calls unnecessary attention to this behavior, the child's anxiety level and masturbation activity may increase. The child needs to know that masturbation is not acceptable in public; however, this must be accomplished in a nonthreatening manner. Children who masturbate excessively and who have experienced a great deal of disruption in their lives benefit from ongoing counseling.

ENURESIS
Description

The term enuresis is derived from the Greek word *enourein*, to void urine. There are two types: primary and secondary. **Primary enuresis** refers to bedwetting in the child who has never been dry. **Secondary enuresis** refers to a recurrence of bedwetting in a child who has been dry for a period of 1 year or more. Diurnal, or daytime, wetting is less common than nocturnal episodes. It is more common in boys than in girls, and there appears to be a genetic influence. In many children, a specific cause is never determined. Most children who wet the bed overcome the problem between 6 and 10 years of age. Some organic causes of nocturnal enuresis are urinary tract infections, diabetes mellitus, diabetes insipidus, seizure disorders, obstructive uropathy (uncommon cause), abnormalities of the urinary tract, and sleep disorders. Sudden onset may be the result of psychological stress, such as a death in the family or divorce. Reduced antidiuretic hormone production at night and genetic factors are also likely causes of nocturnal enuresis. Other causes include small bladder, inability to delay voiding, not awakening to the sensation of a full bladder, and maturational delay of the nervous system.

Treatment and Nursing Care

A detailed history is obtained. Such factors as the pattern of wetting, number of times per night or week, number of daytime voidings, type of stream, dysuria, amount of fluid taken between dinner and bedtime, family history, stress, and the reactions of the parents and child are documented. It is also important to determine any medications that the child may be taking and the extent to which social life is inhibited by the problem, such as a child's inability to spend the night away from home. Developmental landmarks, including toilet training, are reviewed. If there appears to be an organic cause,

appropriate blood and urine studies are undertaken. In most cases, physical findings are negative.

Education of the family is extremely crucial to prevent secondary emotional problems. It is important to reassure parents that many children experience enuresis and that it is self-limited in nature. Power struggles, shame, and guilt are fruitless and destructive. Reassurance and support from the nurse greatly help.

Therapies for bedwetting are subject to controversy. Some methods include counseling, hypnosis, behavior modification, and pharmacotherapy. Imipramine (Tofranil) has been found to decrease enuresis in controlled studies. It is administered before bedtime and is used only on a short-term basis. Imipramine has a variety of side effects, including mood and sleep disturbances and gastrointestinal upsets. Overdose can lead to cardiac arrhythmias, which may be life-threatening. Therefore dosage and administration should be closely supervised. Imipramine should not be given to children under 6 years of age. Desmopressin acetate (DDAVP) also has been used with some success. It is an antidiuretic hormone that inhibits urine production. These drugs may be especially beneficial when short-term control is desired such as for slumber parties, camping trips, or vacations.

See the Health Promotion box for bedwetting tips. A spontaneous cure may occur with little or no intervention or after other types of treatment have failed. The nurse prepares the parents for relapses, which are common.

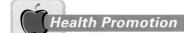

Health Promotion

Tips for Bedwetters

- Use moisture-activated conditioning devices (with alarm when the child wets).
- Encourage bladder training exercises (strengthen bladder muscle).
- Try to have bedroom close to the bathroom (bathroom should have a nightlight).
- Have the child help in clean up if the bed is wet.
- Promote more fluids during the daytime hours.
- Never punish a child for bedwetting.

LANGUAGE AND SPEECH IMPAIRMENT

The child communicates through speech and language skills. Speech is defined as the utterance of vocal sounds conveying ideas; language is a defined set of characters that, when used alone or in combinations, form a meaningful set of words and symbols that are used for communication.

Parents need to be aware of delays in language development as the child matures. Most children say 10 words by 18 months, 50 words and two-word phrases by 24 months, and so on. Language delay is often a symptom of a larger developmental disorder. Possible

Table 11-3 | *Warning Signs of Speech or Language Disorders*

AGE RANGE	SIGNS
First 12 mo	Does not smile at familiar faces or voices by 2 mo
	Does not try to imitate any sounds by 4 mo
	Does not babble by 8 mo
	Uses no single words by 12 mo
	Does not use gestures such as waving "bye-bye" or point to pictures/objects by 12 mo
12 to 24 mo	Does not use at least 15 words by 18 mo
	Does not use two-word utterances by 2 yr
	Does not imitate words or actions by 2 yr
	Does not follow simple instructions by 2 yr
24 to 36 mo	Does not combine words into short phrases/sentences by 3 yr
	Frequent expression of frustration in communicative situations
	Does not interact or play with others
	Unable to understand and answer simple questions
4 yr	Unable to be understood by people outside of family
	Cannot retell simple stories or recall recent events clearly
	Sentences seem unorganized, with a lot of errors

Modified from Kelly, D., & Janine, S. In Levine, M., Carey, W., Crocker, A. (1999). *Developmental-behavioral pediatrics* (3rd ed.). Philadelphia: Saunders.

causes include hearing loss, mental retardation, learning disabilities, severe emotional disturbances, and certain genetic or organic problems. It is important to recognize milestone achievements. Any signs of problems in language or speech development need to be evaluated (Table 11-3).

Speech impairment can include articulation problems (distorting consonants or omitting consonants), voice disorders (deviations in pitch, loudness, or quality), and rhythm disorders (stuttering and stammering). Stuttering is the involuntary repetition of words or speech sounds, whereas stammering includes an involuntary pause in the formation of words. Speech therapy may be necessary for each of these problems. Remember to provide support to families as well.

HEALTH PROMOTION AND MAINTENANCE

DAILY CARE

Preschoolers are able to provide self-care almost totally, especially as they reach 5 years of age. They like to do things for themselves. Simple clothes make it easy for them to dress. A hook on the door within easy reach is helpful. They should dress and undress themselves as much as they can. A simple hairstyle is easily managed by the preschooler. Mother or father can assist with daily care but should not take over. Preschoolers may still need supervision with hygiene and may need to be reminded to use the toilet from time to time. Some 3-year-olds may still need assistance to get up onto the seat. A stool kept next to the bathroom sink enables them to wash their hands. They need to be reminded to do this after use of the toilet.

Brushing teeth still needs supervision. Children must be reminded to brush their teeth regularly. Parents still need to check that all tooth surfaces are cleaned and they should floss the child's teeth. The child needs to visit a dentist regularly, at least every 6 months. Children generally have all 20 of their deciduous teeth by 3 years of age. The first dental visit should have occurred by the first birthday. The deciduous teeth are important for the proper formation of the permanent teeth and should not be neglected. The child's diet should continue to emphasize milk, vegetables, and fruits. Excess sweets, which contribute to dental decay, are restricted. The child should still drink fluoridated water or receive a prescribed oral fluoride supplement.

Preschool children need simple, nourishing meals, prepared with foods according to the basic food groups (see MyPyramid, Figure 9-5). Like toddlers, preschoolers do not like foods mixed together. They also have varying interest in food, and their appetites go up and down. Preschoolers require about 1600 kcal/day (U.S. Department of Agriculture, 2006). It is also important to provide protein, calcium, iron, and plenty of vitamins A and C. Continue to limit juice intake to 4 to 6 ounces per day. Too much juice can provide excess kilocalories or limit milk intake. Their appetites fluctuate, and they should not be bribed, scolded, or coaxed. Encourage children to try different foods as they get older. If they did not like it in the past, they may like it now. Focus positively instead of negatively. Mealtimes should be happy. Parents who use good table manners set an example. The milk glass must be unbreakable and not filled completely. A waterproof tablecloth is useful. Children are included in the conversations but should not be not allowed to take over. A nourishing dessert such as a custard pudding eases apprehension about what has been left on the child's plate.

Preschool children need periods of active play both indoors and outdoors. Parents who see that their children are having a particularly good time should ask themselves whether it is necessary to interrupt them right at that moment. When children have verbal arguments, parents should avoid rushing in to defend their child. Growth can be painful, but children need to do it at their own rate.

Sleep habits at this time vary. Toward the end of this stage, children may balk at taking a nap. Instead of insisting that they sleep, parents should see that they engage in something interesting but restful, such as reading a story together or playing with a simple puzzle. They need an opportunity to relax. Bedtime rituals are still important, and children may use these to put off going to bed. In addition, preschool children may wake up frightened during the night. Everyday items in the bedroom become frightening at night because of the child's imagination. Parents should attend to their needs and reassure them that they are safe and that the parents are close by. A night light may be helpful. If the children continue waking up and are usually frightened, parents should talk to the doctor during one of the checkups. Children of this age should have a complete physical examination each year. Booster injections of various immunizations are given when required.

Community Cue

Bright Futures (http://www.brightfutures.org) is a national health promotion initiative that provides an array of publications to health care clinicians. One such publication is an activity book (also available in Spanish) that teaches young children about health and safety. Children can color, draw, fill in the blanks, tell stories, and talk about staying healthy and being safe. They learn about nutrition, fitness, self-expression, safety, and oral health.

PRESCHOOL

The change from home to preschool or nursery school is a big step toward independence. At this age, the child is adjusting to the outside world and to the family group. Some children have the complicating factor of a new baby in the house. The child also finds at this time that parents are beginning to expect more in regard to neatness and cooperative play with others. This transition period is troublesome. A good preschool provides the child with opportunities to get rid of some pent-up emotions. There is plenty of room to run and shout. The toys are sturdy, and children can manipulate them because they are their own size. Because they are not their own, they find it easier to share toys. Children are not as emotionally involved with the teacher as they are with their parents. They are more willing to express their negative and positive feelings because the teacher is able to be more objective. The teacher expects the child to decide what materials to play with and with whom to play. Children take responsibility for their own belongings.

Children are accepted into preschools between the ages of 2 and 5 years. Most sessions last about 3 hours.

This may be a child's first exposure to different cultures. A good nursery school should challenge the child's imagination and creativity (Figure 11-4). It should also attempt to acquaint children with the new social world in such a way that it adds to their security and increases independence. Parents can help with the transition to daycare or preschool attendance by having the child take a family picture, favorite toy, or stuffed animal for comfort. Always discuss the experience at the end of the day and ask the teacher for feedback as well. The Health Promotion box examines guidelines for daycare or preschool.

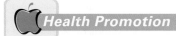
Health Promotion

Child Care Guidelines

Parents who are considering preschool for their child should evaluate the following factors:
- Are the teachers trained in CPR?
- How many children are there per teacher?
- Are the teachers prepared in early childhood education?
- Are the physical facilities adequate?
- What is the cost? Is the child ready for preschool?
- Parents should also visit the school and talk with the person in charge before the child starts the program. They may also wish to talk with parents whose children are attending the program. Parents should feel free to drop in to a daycare or preschool *at any time* unannounced.

The student nurse may have the opportunity to visit a preschool during studies of the well child. This can be a rewarding experience if nurses use their powers of observation. When observing an individual child, nurses should compare him or her with others in the age group and not merely with one other child. The types of behavior to be observed are outlined in Box 11-1.

PLAY IN HEALTH AND ILLNESS

VALUE OF PLAY

It has often been said that play is the work of children. Investigations stress the importance of play to both the well and the sick child's physical, mental, emotional, and social development. Children climbing on a jungle gym develop coordination of muscles and exercise all parts of the body. They use up energy and develop feelings of self-confidence. Their imaginations may take them to a jungle where they are swinging from limb to limb. They mentally face fears and solve problems that would be much more trying, if not impossible, in reality. They communicate with the other children and take a further step in the development of moral values, such as learning to take one's turn and learning consideration for others. Other types of play help them learn colors, shapes, sizes, and textures and teach them to be creative.

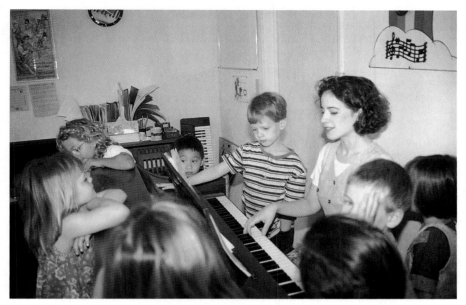

FIGURE **11-4** In the preschool setting, children are exposed to a variety of activities to enhance development of multiple intelligences.

Box 11-1   *Observing the Preschool Child*

Objective: To observe the behavioral characteristics of the preschool child
Watch for and evaluate the following in terms of a child's security and independence:

PHYSICAL DEVELOPMENT
Ability to walk, run, jump, use play equipment
General health: easily fatigued, etc.

EMOTIONAL DEVELOPMENT
Easily excited
Whines, cries frequently
Evidence of temper tantrums
Persistence in a task
Aggressive
Shy
Reaction to failure

SOCIAL DEVELOPMENT
Talkative
Quiet
Plays with others
Plays near others
Special friends
Tends to lead
Tends to follow

Friendly toward other children and adults
Ability to share
Ability to take turns
Behavior when an object or attention of the teacher is desired

DEGREE OF INDEPENDENCE
Removing coat, hat, boots; putting them away
Attending to toilet needs
Getting a drink
Amount of time going from one activity to another
Dependence on adult suggestions and help

RELAXATION
Relaxes during rest periods
Sits and listens to stories
Is restless, in constant motion

SPECIFIC ROUTINES
Music period: Sings, plays games
Snacks: Eats lunch, takes other children's food, wanders about, disturbs others, plays with food
Free play period: Toys preferred, amount of skill using hands, span of interest, evidence of destructive play, plays with others or alone, has imaginary friend

This natural and readily available outlet must be tapped by institutional personnel. Preschool children may be unfamiliar with every facet of the hospital, but they know how to play, and playing is a good way for the nurse to establish rapport with them.

THE NURSE'S ROLE

Some hospitals have well-established Child Life programs supervised by play therapists (see Chapter 3).

Play experience may be included during the nurse's education. It is not necessary to be an expert in manual dexterity, art, or music. To be of assistance, one must be able to understand the needs of the child. Play is not just the responsibility of those who are assigned to it, nor is it confined to certain times or shifts.

Many factors are involved in providing suitable play for children of various ages in the hospital. The patient's state of health has to be considered. This

Health Promotion

Choosing Toys

AGE	TOYS	GENERAL CONSIDERATIONS
Infant	Soft stuffed animals and dolls Cradle gym Soft balls Bath toys Rattles Pots and pans	Baby likes to pat and hug. Toys should be brightly colored, of different textures, washable. Large enough so that they cannot be aspirated. Smooth edges. Attention span is short. The infant looks at, reaches, grabs, chews.
Toddler	Nest of blocks Push-pull toys Dolls Toy telephone Rocking horse or chair Wooden pegs and hammer Cloth books Pots and pans Ball	May have favorite toy. Enjoys exploring drawers and closets. Likes to place things in containers and dump them out. Parallel play. May injure others.
Preschooler	Crayons Simple puzzles Paints with large brushes Finger paints Dolls Dishes, housekeeping equipment Sandbox, playground equipment Floating boats for water play Trucks Horns, drums, simple musical instruments Books about familiar circumstances CDs; audiocassettes	Shifts from solitary to parallel to beginning cooperative play. Exchanges ideas with others. Active play: climbs, runs, and hammers. Imitative play: firefighter, teacher. Imaginative play: let's pretend. Creative and dramatic play. Toys that do not require fine hand coordination. Games that teach safety in everyday life.
School age	Dolls and doll house Toy housewares Handicrafts Jump rope Skates Construction sets Trains Dress-up materials Table games Books for self-reading Bicycles Puppets Music Videogames/computer games	Attention span increases. Play is more organized, more competitive. Interested in hobbies or collections of things.
The convalescent child	(Many toys previously listed are also applicable) Telephone Easy puzzles Large beads to string Tape player Goldfish bowl Miniature autos, trains, dolls, farm animals Stick'ems, paper dolls Hand puppets Lap blackboard Alphabet boards Cutouts VCR; videos to watch	Play should not require a great expenditure of energy. Offer a wide variety because the child's interest span is decreased. Consider bed limitation. Toys should not require long, continuous focusing of eyes. Consider toys that are a little easier than those liked when well. Pay attention to special interests of individual child.

determines the amount of activity in which the child can participate. The nurse can provide many activities that relieve stress and provide enjoyment for the patient on bed rest. Overstimulation, nevertheless, is hazardous for the severely ill child, such as the child with a heart disorder, because he or she needs to conserve strength. Nurses should always be on guard for signs of fatigue or pain in a patient and should use their judgment accordingly. Basically, toys should be safe, durable, and suited to the child's developmental level. Children love to go to the hospital playroom. If they are unable (isolation, etc.), toys may be brought to their rooms. Proper cleaning is required of any toy used by any child in the hospital before it is returned to the playroom or used by other children.

Toys should not be sharp or have parts that can be easily removed and swallowed. Too many toys at one time confuses the child. Complicated toys are frustrating and disappointing. Well-selected toys, such as balls, blocks, and dolls, are useful throughout the years. Three-year-olds participate in simple games, and four-year-olds have longer attention spans and can participate in group activities. Preschoolers of all ages enjoy coloring and "reading" books. Each child needs sufficient time to complete the activity. In general, quiet play should precede meals and bedtime for both the well and the sick child. Investigations have shown that the toys that are enjoyed by both boys and girls are more similar than dissimilar.

The nurse can entertain the child during routine procedures with nursery rhymes, stories, nonsense games, songs, or finger play. Simple crafts are fun. Collections of scrap material containing bright ribbons, bits of string, tongue depressors, paper bags, newspapers, or bits of cotton can be kept on the unit. Scrapbooks are also entertaining. The child may even want to make a storybook or keep a diary (older children) about the hospital experience. To encourage ambulation, a scavenger hunt on the nursing unit can be made into a fun activity. With the fairly high turnover of patients, many projects can simply be repeated with different children.

Music is provided by the radio, tape, or CD player. Older children enjoy sending electronic messages to friends. Most hospitals have VCRs available as well, and many pediatric units keep a supply of children's videos. Video and computer games are also often available. Drawing materials, finger paints, and modeling clay foster expression and creativity. They require merely a flat surface such as the over-bed table and the particular medium. The bedridden child can participate in messy projects, too. The bed linens can be protected with plastic or extra linens. Children in cribs need adequate back support for such projects. This is done by elevating the mattress or using pillows.

Nurses can encourage children to play together in the hospital if their condition warrants. Children need playmates to promote social development. Children who are ambulatory can visit other children in the playroom. The 1-year-old plays near other children. The 2-year-old grabs, pushes, and cannot share but in an individual way acknowledges other children. The older preschool child shows a beginning readiness for cooperative play. The ability to play with others increases during the school years and in late elementary years; girls prefer to play with girls, and boys prefer to play with boys. This preference changes during adolescence. It is important for children of all ages to socialize as much as possible with other children while in the hospital.

OTHER ASPECTS OF PLAY
Therapeutic Play

Play and toys can be of therapeutic value in the retraining of muscles, in the improvement of hand-eye coordination, and in helping children crawl and walk (push-pull toys). A musical instrument such as the clarinet promotes flexion and extension of the fingers. Blowing is an excellent prerequisite for speech therapy. Therapists supervise such activities. They should leave specific instructions if they wish their work reinforced on the unit.

The nurse can ask the child to draw a picture or make up a story; this allows the nurse to assess fears the child may be experiencing. What children *say* about what they draw can also be important in understanding a child's concerns and is an important communication technique (Driessnack, 2006).

Play Therapy

The nurse may also hear the term **play therapy** used. This technique is used for the child under stress. A well-equipped playroom is provided. The child is free to play with whatever articles he or she chooses. A counselor may be in the room observing and talking with the child, or the child may be observed through a one-way glass window. With this method and other methods, the therapist obtains a better understanding of the patient's struggles, fears, resentments, and feelings toward self and others. When the child acts out feelings through "dramatic play," those feelings are externalized and provide a relief from tension. Child behavior is complex and requires a great deal of time, study, and sensitivity before it can be fully understood.

Art Therapy

Art has been defined by Elinor Ulman as "the meeting ground of the world inside and the world outside." Art therapy is a process that is useful in communicating with children and adults. It is becoming more widely used. The art therapist is specially trained to assist children to express their feelings through drawings, clay, and other media. Some hospitals with inpatient mental health units have art therapy departments.

Role of the Nurse

The nurse who is with a child daily can describe his or her behavior. This is helpful if the child has emotional or social problems. It is important to describe good and poor behavior, conversations that you may feel are pertinent, and the relationships with other children in the hospital. What is the approach to play? Do they join in freely or linger outside the group? Do they prefer active or quiet activities? Do they seem to be able to tolerate frustrations? Can they talk with their playmates and communicate their ideas? What kind of attention span do they have? This type of charting is meaningful and should be used to describe the activities of pediatric patients so that they may be better understood.

INJURY PREVENTION

Accidents are still a major threat during the years from 3 to 5. Preschoolers need to follow the same injury prevention guidelines as toddlers (see the Health Promotion box titled Injury Prevention—Toddlers in Chapter 9). At this age, children may also suffer injuries from a bad fall. Preschool children hurtle up and down stairs. They climb trees and stand up on swings. They play hard with their toys, particularly those they can mount. Stairways must be kept free from clutter. When buying toys, parents must be sure the toys are sturdy and can take a beating. Preschool children should *never* be asked to do anything that is potentially dangerous, such as carry a glass container or sharp knife to the kitchen sink.

Automobiles continue to be a threat. The use of car seats or booster seats needs to be enforced (depending on age and weight; see Chapter 9). Children should be taught where they can safely ride their tricycles. Once they begin to ride a two-wheeler, they need to wear a helmet every time they use the bike. This prevents brain injury and even death. They also need to be taught where they can safely play. For example, they should not be allowed to use a sled on streets that are not blocked off for this purpose. They must not play in or around the car. Whether they are asleep or awake, children this age must *never* be left alone in the car. In an attempt to "drive like Mommy," they can quickly set a car into motion. Accidents also have been caused by children left in cars who find matches or play with the cigarette lighter. When crossing a street or when in a parking lot, they need to hold hands with a grownup. They should not operate an electronic garage door.

The potential for drowning is a danger. Do not leave children alone in a bathtub, swimming pool, or near any body of water. They can begin to learn to swim with supervision (Figure 11-5).

Burns that occur at this age are frequently caused by children's experimentation with matches. Children are also intrigued by cigarette lighters. These items are common hazards for this age group; they should be kept well out of reach, and their dangers should be explained.

Poisoning is still a danger. Children try to imitate adults and are apt to sample pills, especially if they smell good or look like candy. Their increased freedom brings them into contact with many interesting containers in the garage or basement. Poisons should *never* be put into used milk cartons or other household containers that would confuse children. Containers should be marked in such a way that the child knows it is a poison.

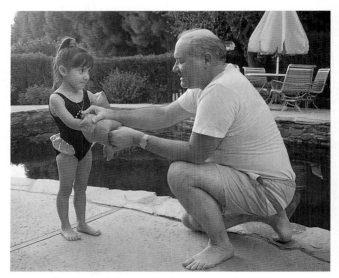

FIGURE **11-5** The preschooler should wear safety equipment while swimming and be accompanied by an adult.

Trampoline injuries have been on the rise. The American Academy of Pediatrics does not advocate the use of home trampolines and further states that trampolines should not be regarded as play equipment. Trampolines have no place in outdoor playgrounds or in schools for routine physical education (AAP Policy Statement, 1999, 2006).

Preschool children should also be taught the dangers of talking to or accepting rides from strangers. They need to know that a stranger is someone they do not know, not just someone who is odd-looking. If they are stopped by a driver, they should run to a house where they know the people. Parents should make it clear to children in preschool that they will *never* send a stranger to see them or to pick them up. Children must know the dangers of playing in lonely places and of accepting gifts from strangers. Children should always know where to go if their mother or father cannot be found.

Preschool children still require a good deal of supervision to protect them from dangers that arise from their immature judgment or social environment.

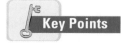

Key Points

- The preschool period is marked by a slowing of the growth process and more well-developed muscle control.
- Preoperational thinking predominates, and preschoolers base their reasoning on what they see and hear. They also believe they have "magical" powers and can only understand their own viewpoint.
- Preschoolers' sense of initiative empowers them to try new activities and experiences. They still need to be supervised to prevent injury.

- Encouraging positive behavior helps eliminate the undesirable effects of punishment. When necessary, time out is an effective method of discipline.
- Common problems of preschoolers (bad language, jealousy, thumb sucking, masturbation, and enuresis) can be easily dealt with through gentle explanation or correction of behavior and reassurance.
- The attainment of milestones for speech and language needs to be evaluated with the preschooler.
- The older preschooler becomes almost completely independent in dealing with daily care.
- Preschools should be evaluated through parental visits and the evaluation of the facility.
- Play of preschoolers often involves the beginning of cooperative play and imaginative and imitative play.

 Go to your Companion CD-ROM for an Audio Glossary, video clips, and more.

 Be sure to visit the Companion Evolve site at http://evolve.elsevier.com/Price/pediatric/ for WebLinks and additional resources.

ONLINE RESOURCES

Bright Futures: http://www.brightfutures.org

Objectives

Upon completion of this chapter, the student will be able to:

1. Define the vocabulary terms listed
2. List and describe the causes, symptoms, and treatment of disorders most frequently seen in the preschool child
3. Identify two methods of evaluating burn injury
4. Differentiate amblyopia and strabismus
5. Demonstrate comfort measures for a child undergoing chemotherapy
6. Describe the nursing care for preschool children undergoing surgery for removal of tonsils and adenoids
7. Discuss the nursing care of a child with celiac disease
8. Describe nursing care for a child with Duchenne muscular dystrophy
9. Differentiate the types of generalized and partial seizures and describe the nursing measures necessary for a child during and after a tonic-clonic seizure
10. Discuss the nursing care of the child with a urinary tract infection
11. Compare and contrast acute glomerulonephritis and nephrotic syndrome
12. Discuss common communicable diseases in children
13. Describe two diseases associated with bioterrorism
14. Demonstrate a positive attitude when caring for developmentally disabled children and their families

Key Terms

Be sure to check out the bonus material on the Companion CD-ROM, including selected audio pronunciations.

anuria (ăn-ŪR-ē-ă; p. 258)
aura (AW-ră; p. 253)
blasts (p. 241)
cover test (p. 241)
eschar (ES-kăr; p. 239)
glomerulus (glō-MĔR-ū-lŭs; p. 258)
gluten (GLŪ-těn; p. 249)
hemarthrosis (hē-măr-THRŌ-sĭs; p. 244)
idiopathic (I-dē-ō-P AH- ik; p. 252)
ketogenic diet (KĒ-tō-JĔN-ĭk; p. 255)
neutropenic (NŪ-trō-PĒ-nĭk; p. 244)
occlusion (ō-KLŪ-zhun; p. 241)
oliguria (Ō-lig-Ū-rē-ă; p. 258)
postictal (pōst-ĬK-tăl; p. 253)
prodromal symptoms (prō-DRŌ-măl; p. 260)
transfusion (p. 242)
uncover test (p. 241)

The preschooler shows initiative and independence. Many children of this age are in daycare, which predisposes them to communicable diseases. Because they are becoming more worldly, they begin to experience a higher incidence of accidents. Many of their health issues deal with their new ability to explore their environment.

SKIN

BURNS
Description

Burns are a leading cause of accidental death in children. Most burns are minor and can be treated on an outpatient basis. However, some burns are quite severe and require hospitalization either locally or at a burn center. Toddlers may pull hot liquids down on themselves. Older children sometimes misuse matches and flammable materials. One common preventable burn is caused by a curling iron. Burns are categorized as thermal, radiation, electrical, or chemical. Severe burns cause fluid and electrolyte imbalances and can affect every body system. Infection, scarring, and functional disabilities are major complications of severe burns.

Signs and Symptoms

The burn wound is classified according to percentage of body surface involved, depth, location of the injury, and association with other injuries. The age of the child and the presence of respiratory involvement are also important factors.

A method for determining the percentage of skin surface area in children at various ages is presented in Figure 12-1. The "rule of nines," which is used with the older adolescent and the adult, is not applicable in the infant and small child because of the difference in body proportions.

Depth of burn injury is described in Table 12-1. Burns are described as superficial, partial-thickness (superficial and deep), and full-thickness. Some references differentiate full-thickness and deep full-thickness; deep full-thickness would include fascia and muscle with potential for bone and tendon damage. Superficial burns heal in 3 to 7 days, whereas partial-thickness burns can take weeks to months, provided there is no infection. This is

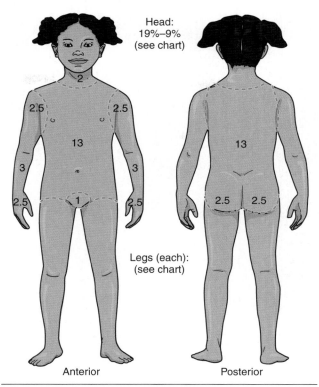

Head:
19%–9%
(see chart)

Legs (each):
(see chart)

Anterior   Posterior

Child Burn Size Estimation Table
(percent total body surface area)

Age in Years

	<1 yr	1	5	10	15	Adult
Head	19	17	13	11	9	7
Neck	2	2	2	2	2	2
Ant Trunk	13	13	13	13	13	13
Post Trunk	13	13	13	13	13	13
Buttock	2.5	2.5	2.5	2.5	2.5	2.5
Genitalia	1	1	1	1	1	1
Upper arm	2.5	2.5	2.5	2.5	2.5	2.5
Lower arm	3	3	3	3	3	3
Hand	2.5	2.5	2.5	2.5	2.5	2.5
Thigh	5.5	6.5	8	8.5	9	9.5
Leg	5	5	5.5	6	6.5	7
Foot	3.5	3.5	3.5	3.5	3.5	3.5

FIGURE **12-1** Calculating total body surface area (TBSA) burned in children. The standard "rule of nines" and standard body surface charts must be adapted because of the difference in body proportions between adults and children. (From Deitch, E. & Rutan, R. [2001]. *The challenges of children: The first 48 hours.* Chicago: American Burn Association.)

because partial-thickness burns involve the epidermis and the dermis. Full-thickness burns generally do not heal without skin grafting. Scarring is present in deep partial-thickness and full-thickness burns. Full-thickness burns (Figure 12-2) involve total destruction of the epidermis and dermis and underlying tissues. The wound is leathery, tan, dark red or brown, and not as painful as the partial thickness burn. Although the patient may not have pain at the actual wound site, there is pain along the edges of the wound where nerve endings are intact. Unless they are very small, full-thickness burns require debridement, topical antimicrobials, and grafting; they are managed at a burn

center. The child with a burn covering more than 10% of total body surface area, inhalation burns, chemical burns with serious threat of functional or cosmetic impairment, or electrical burns should be treated in a specialized setting. Box 12-1 describes the American Burn Association's burn unit referral criteria.

Treatment and Nursing Care

ABCs. The primary goal in the initial treatment of major burns is the maintenance of an airway and the prevention of shock *(airway, breathing, circulation).* Airway obstruction should be suspected if the child has inhaled smoke or the burn involves the face.

Table 12-1 *Depth of Burn Injury*

| NORMAL SKIN | SUPERFICIAL (FIRST-DEGREE) | PARTIAL-THICKNESS (SECOND-DEGREE) | | FULL-THICKNESS (THIRD-DEGREE) |
		SUPERFICIAL	DEEP	
Normal skin				
Morphology	Destruction of epidermis; physiology functions remain intact	Destruction of epidermis and some dermis	Destruction of epidermis and dermis	Destruction of epidermis, dermis, underlying tissue; may include fascia, muscle, tendon, bone
Blister formation	After 24 hr (e.g., from sunburn)	Within minutes; thin-walled, fluid-filled	May or may not appear as fluid-filled blisters; often they are flat, dehydrated, and like tissue paper; body fluids lost through burn tissue must be replaced	Rare; may appear as a tissue paper-like layer that is flat and dehydrated
Appearance	Peels after 24-48 hr	Red to pale ivory, moist surface	Mottled, waxy white, dry surface	White, cherry red, or black
Healing time	3-7 days	7-21 days if no infection develops	30 days to several months if no infection; if infected, this type of burn may convert to full-thickness	Will not heal; skin grafting required; very small areas may heal from edges after a period of weeks
Patient reaction	Moderate discomfort, pain; chills; nausea; vomiting	May cause considerable pain	Severe pain on exposure to air or water because nerve endings are intact	No pain in area of full-thickness burn because nerve endings are destroyed; surrounding areas of lesser depth are painful
Scarring	None	Minimal; influences by genetic predisposition	Greatest because the slow healing of these burns increases scar tissue; scar formation influenced by genetic predisposition	Autograft scarring is minimizes by early excision and grafting; scar formation influenced by genetic predisposition

Modified from McKinney E et al. (2005). *Maternal child nursing* (2nd ed.). Philadelphia: Saunders.

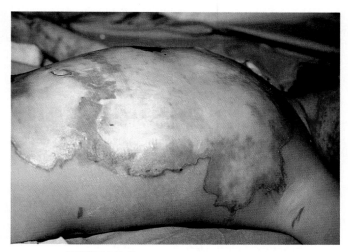

FIGURE **12-2** Full-thickness thermal injury.

Oxygen is administered, and oxygenation is monitored closely. An endotracheal tube is inserted if the child is in respiratory distress. After assessment of the airway and respiratory status, fluid resuscitation is the next priority. *Burn shock* occurs with major burns as a result of massive capillary leakage of circulating fluid into the surrounding tissues. The fluid loss resulting from major burns must be replaced to prevent shock. An intravenous (IV) infusion is started, and fluid volume restoration is initiated. Ringer's lactate solution is often used for initial resuscitation. The Parkland formula recommends 4 mL/kg per percentage of TBSA burned. The total calculated is administered over the first 24 hours; half is given within the first 8 hours from the time of the injury, and the remaining half is given over the next 16 hours. Blood pressure, capillary refill, heart rate, and urine output must be monitored. A Foley catheter is placed; 1 to 2 mL/kg/hr of urine output serves as the guideline for ensuring successful fluid volume restoration (Duffy et al., 2006). After initial stabilization, the child with a major burn is transferred to a burn treatment facility.

Wound Management. A superficial burn does not require topical antimicrobial medication. Cool compresses and soothing lotions may be used for superficial burns. An antimicrobial agent such as bacitracin is best used for a superficial partial-thickness burn that is expected to heal within 2 to 3 weeks. Bacitracin may also be used on the face. Silvadene is an antimicrobial cream that has bactericidal activity and is commonly used on partial- and full-thickness burns to prevent wound sepsis. It should not be used on children with known sulfa sensitivity. Sulfamylon is similar, yet effective against *Pseudomonas aeruginosa*; it is used as a topical antimicrobial for a partial- or full-thickness burn (Duffy et al., 2006). Burn wounds may be treated as open (wound uncovered) or covered with a range of thin gauze to bulky gauze. Dressings are changed one to three times daily. Hydrotherapy can be used to remove old dressing and clean the wound and the

child. Range-of-motion exercises can be done during this time. Hydrotherapy can be done in a tub or shower. Debridement is done to remove dead tissue. Burned tissue called **eschar** must be removed to prevent infection. Breaking blisters is controversial. Pain management during dressing change is essential. The goal of care is to prevent infection in the wound. Tetanus prophylaxis should be given if the child is not current in this immunization.

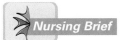
Nursing Brief

New silver-based antimicrobial sheets may be applied to burn wounds and left in place for several days, following initial debridement. These pads deliver medication and also absorb exudate from the wound. They may be left in place a few days, reducing the need for frequent dressing changes. These products are currently being evaluated at burn centers.

In full-thickness burns where re-epithelialization does not take place, grafting (skin transplant) is necessary. Temporary grafts, such as biological or synthetic skin coverings, may be needed until permanent grafting can take place. Permanent grafts are obtained from an undamaged area of the patient's body (autografts).

Wound care is extremely painful and causes emotional consequences in children if the pain is not addressed. Adequate use of pharmacological and non-pharmacological pain relief approaches is essential. Maintenance of strict sterile technique reduces the chance of infection.

Scarring can be minimized through application of continuous pressure to the scar during the rehabilitative phase. If scarring is extensive, especially around joints, joint limitation and contractures can result. Physical therapy and surgery to release contractures may be necessary.

Pain Control. Morphine sulfate is the drug of choice for severely burned patients. It should be given intravenously. Special attention should be given to respiratory rates when morphine is given. Acetaminophen with codeine may be given for less severe pain.

Nutritional Management. The child may be on nothing by mouth (NPO) restriction for the first 24 to 48 hours if the burn is severe and bowel sounds are absent. A nasogastric tube may be inserted.

Metabolism increases and severe protein and fat wasting occurs in response to severe burns. The child requires a high-protein, high-calorie diet. Oral feedings are preferred, although it may be necessary to supplement with nasogastric feedings. Many of these children have poor appetites, and facilitating adequate intake is a challenge. Small, frequent feedings of favorite foods should be provided. Supplements may be added to foods to meet the high protein and calorie needs. Parents may be able to bring favorite foods from home. Daily weights and intake and output are recorded.

Social and Emotional Issues. The nurse must always be aware of the psychological needs of the family and the child at this time. Families may be dealing with guilt, anger, grief, denial, and fear. Body image concerns become paramount for the older child as recovery progresses. Encourage parents to spend as much time as possible with the child. Because this may be a long-term admission, they may not be able to be with the child at all times. Activities appropriate for the child's age and condition should be provided. Schooling needs should be met when the child is of school age. Encourage the child to help with bath, dressing change, feeding, and other self-care activities. Provide opportunities for family and child to talk about feelings and changes in body appearance. Provide for visits by siblings and friends. Accept negative behaviors expressed by the child. Assist in ventilating negative feelings through play therapy and the use of a play therapist, social worker, or psychologist.

EYES

Preventing and detecting early vision problems in infants and children can improve long-term visual health. Adequate vision is necessary for normal growth and development. Taking a careful history during every well-infant examination with observations on visual tracking and recognition of parent faces is important. Children should have a thorough ophthalmic examination by the age of 3 to 4 years. These are crucial years for detecting and treating eye problems that may possibly lead to permanent vision loss.

The nurse should stress the importance of continued proper care of the eyes. Young children who are beginning to read need books with large type and letters spaced far apart. The lighting provided must be adequate and without glare. Chairs and desks must be of proper height.

Symptoms that may indicate eye strain include inflammation, aching or smarting of the eyes, squinting, a short attention span, frequent headaches, difficulties with schoolwork, or inability to see the blackboard. They may occur suddenly. The child between 6 and 10 years of age often becomes nearsighted and has to hold books close to the eyes to read. If this occurs, an eye examination and, in some cases, a complete physical examination are indicated.

Determining visual acuity for children under the age of 3 years can only be done indirectly. By 3 years, most children can cooperate to obtain a full assessment. The standard Snellen E test is modified and available for nonreaders. A kindergarten eye chart with familiar shapes is also available. Directions for testing are standardized and must be carefully adhered to for proper results.

AMBLYOPIA

Description

Amblyopia is a decrease in or loss of vision, usually in one eye. The vision loss is not caused by structural eye damage but results from the brain "turning off" confusing visual images. This condition occurs when the visual image does not fall on the retina. The prognosis depends on how long the eye has been affected and the age of the child when treatment is begun. Because critical visual development occurs from birth until age 6 years, treatment should begin as early as possible to prevent permanent vision loss.

Signs and Symptoms

The condition is not usually noticed until the child's first vision screening at approximately 3 to 4 years old. An observant parent might notice that the child sits closer to the television or appears to have difficulty seeing. Conditions such as congenital cataract or strabismus can alert the ophthalmologist to the possibility of amblyopia.

Treatment and Nursing Care

The goal of treatment is to obtain normal and equal vision in each eye. Treatment consists of glasses for significant refractive errors (hyperopia, myopia) and

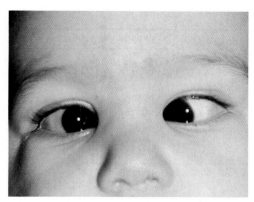

FIGURE **12-3** Infantile esotropia with asymmetrical corneal light reflexes.

occlusion of the unaffected eye. Patching the unaffected eye forces the affected eye to function better. In most cases an adhesive patch covers the eye throughout the waking hours. Some older children respond better to an opaque contact lens on the unaffected eye (Behrman et al., 2004).

Occlusion therapy may be difficult to maintain. Many families tolerate it well, however. The nurse can help by explaining the importance of the procedure and offering support. The child may be subject to ridicule by peers. Listening to children express their feelings is important in promoting healthy self-esteem.

STRABISMUS
Description
Strabismus ("cross-eye") refers to ocular misalignment and is a condition in which the child is not able to direct both eyes toward the same object. If the malalignment is not corrected, the weak eye becomes "lazy" and the brain eventually suppresses the image produced by that eye. Amblyopia can result. There are several kinds of strabismus. Most children with strabismus have **esotropia,** or an inward deviation of one or both eyes (Figure 12-3). Some children have **exotropia,** which is outward turning. Strabismus may be present at birth or may be acquired after a disease.

Signs and Symptoms
Simple tests can be done to detect strabismus. With the **corneal light reflex,** the examiner shines a light into the child's eyes. With the child looking directly into the light, the reflection should be at the same point in each pupil. In the uncover test, the eyes are observed for compensatory or adjustment movements. The eye is covered and the child looks at a light source; when it is quickly uncovered, the eye should not move. This indicates alignment. If the eye has to shift to focus on the light, malalignment is present. In the cover test, one eye is covered and the movement of the uncovered eye is observed while the child looks at a distant object (preferably 6 m or 20 ft). If the uncovered eye does not move, it is aligned. **Epicanthal folds,** the

vertical folds of skin on either side of the nose that are frequently seen in children of Asian descent, can give a false impression of strabismus. Transient strabismus is normal in very young infants (less than 4 months). If present after 4 months, infants should be referred to an ophthalmologist.

Treatment and Nursing Care
Depending on the type of strabismus, eye exercises and glasses may be effective ways of treating the condition medically. Occlusion therapy is used for strabismic amblyopia treatment. Surgery is reserved for patients in whom nonsurgical methods are likely to be unsuccessful (Ticho, 2003).

The child undergoing surgery for strabismus is hospitalized for only a brief period. Some doctors prefer not to have the child restrained after surgery because it is frightening and the child's struggles may increase. The surgery involves structures outside the eyeball; therefore the child is allowed to be up and about after surgery. Eye dressings are kept at a minimum, and elbow restraints may be all that are needed to keep the child from touching the dressings.

If the doctor believes that it is necessary to cover the eyes and restrain the patient's movements after surgery, the patient is told this before surgery and is assured that the bandages and restraints will be removed as soon as possible. Because this is frightening for young children, it is best that the parents remain with them. Because they cannot move or see, diversions such as stories are necessary.

HEMATOLOGIC SYSTEM

LEUKEMIA
Description
Leukemia (*leuko,* white; *emia,* blood) is a malignant disease of the blood-forming organs of the body that results in an uncontrolled growth of immature white blood cells (WBCs). It is the most common type of cancer in children. There are several types of WBCs. Many are produced in the bone marrow; others are produced in the spleen and lymph nodes. The immature cells are called blasts (*blastos,* germ or formative cell). About 80% of childhood cases are **acute lymphoblastic leukemia (ALL),** 15% to 20% are **acute myeloid leukemia (AML);** remaining types are rare. The survival rate of ALL is around 85%.

The initial WBC count may range from 5000 to as high as 100,000 cells/mm^3. In some cases, the overall WBC count is normal but the differential count may show a predominance of blast cells. The pathology of the disease comes from its ability to infiltrate and compete for metabolic elements. The reticuloendothelial system (liver, spleen, lymph glands) is most severely affected.

Generally speaking, the child's prognosis is most clearly related to age at diagnosis and initial WBC count.

Table 12-2 | *Some Prognostic Features of ALL in Children*

PROGNOSTIC FACTOR	POSITIVE PROGNOSIS	LESS POSITIVE PROGNOSIS
Age at diagnosis	1-10 yr	<2 or >10 yr
Initial WBC count	<100,000/mm^3	>100,000/mm^3
Morphology	L$_1$	L$_2$ or L$_3$
Immunological surface markers	Pre–B-cell with CALLA	T-cell or B-cell
Cytogenetics	>50 chromosomes per cell	Presence of chromosome translocations
Other	Absent mediastinal mass or CNS involvement at diagnosis	Presence of mediastinal mass or CNS involvement at diagnosis

ALL, Acute lymphoblastic leukemia; *CALLA,* common acute lymphocytic leukemia antigen; *CNS,* central nervous system; *WBC,* white blood count.

Other important factors include the structure of the leukemic cells **(morphology)**, their reaction to different chemical agents **(cytochemistry)**, their genetic makeup **(cytogenetics)**, and the type of cell-surface antigens they exhibit **(immunological markers)**. A classification system that identifies three major subtypes of ALL on the basis of morphology and cytochemistry (L$_1$ to L$_3$) is called the French-American-British (FAB) system. The classification of childhood leukemia has aided in the identification of prognostic factors and methods of treatment (Table 12-2).

The incidence rate of leukemia is highest in children between 3 and 4 years of age, and the disease is more common in boys than in girls. The cause of the disease is unknown. Research on the relationship of viruses to leukemia is under way. There also seems to be a genetic correlation because the incidence rate of leukemia is higher in children with Down syndrome and in twins. Investigators have associated leukemia with disorders of the immune mechanism of the body.

All tissues of the body are affected, either by direct infiltration of cancer cells or by the change in the blood that is carried to them. Because leukemia affects the bone marrow, there is also a reduction in the number of red blood cells (RBCs), which produce anemia. In addition, the platelet count is reduced, and because platelets are essential for the clotting of blood, hemorrhage occurs. Intracranial bleeding, if it occurs, can cause immediate death. Hemorrhage from other vital organs may occur. Bone and joint pain are experienced because of increased pressure within the bone marrow as blast cells continue to reproduce. Physiological fractures may occur.

Leukemia that occurs outside the bone marrow is referred to as **extramedullary**. The most common sites for this are the central nervous system (CNS) and the testicles. More cases of extramedullary leukemia are being seen because children with this disorder are surviving longer.

Signs and Symptoms

The most common symptoms during the initial phase of the illness are low-grade fever, pallor, a tendency to bruise, leg and joint pain, listlessness, and enlargement of the lymph nodes. Abdominal pain, often attributed to other illnesses or even constipation, is a common symptom of leukemia. These symptoms may develop gradually or may be sudden in onset. As the disease progresses, the liver and spleen become enlarged. **Petechiae** (pinpoint hemorrhagic spots beneath the skin) and **purpura** (hemorrhage into the skin) may be early objective symptoms. Anorexia, vomiting, weight loss, and dyspnea are also common. The kidneys and testicles may become enlarged, and hematuria may develop.

Because the WBCs are not functioning normally, bacteria easily invade the body. Strict attention must be paid to infection control. Anemia becomes severe despite transfusions. The child may die as a direct result of the disease or of secondary infection. The symptoms are the same regardless of the type of WBC affected, yet they vary widely with each patient, depending on the parts of the body involved.

The diagnosis of leukemia is made on the basis of the history and symptoms of the patient and the results of extensive blood tests that show the presence of leukemic blast cells in the blood, bone marrow, or other tissues. Because the bone marrow is where many WBCs and RBCs are formed, bone marrow aspiration is performed. Bone marrow is removed from the sternum or iliac crest with a special needle and is studied in the laboratory. Chest radiographs show a mediastinal mass. After the diagnosis has been confirmed, a spinal tap determines any CNS involvement. Kidney and liver function studies are also performed because normal function of these organs is absolutely necessary for chemotherapy to be used in treating the disease.

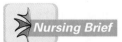 **Nursing Brief**

Repeated blood tests, especially in infants and small children with anemia, can deplete blood volume, which can lead to hypoxia and shock unless the withdrawn blood is replaced.

Treatment and Nursing Care

The development of specific chemotherapeutic agents for treatment of ALL has changed the survival time significantly. In most cases of ALL, it is now possible to induce remissions (no evidence of leukemic cells), which are sustained for prolonged periods even after therapy is discontinued. Other varieties of leukemia show a less predictable response to therapy. Untreated leukemia results in death from infection or hemorrhage in about 6 months. Treatment of ALL consists of three phases: (1) induction, (2) consolidation, (3) and maintenance, which serves to maintain the remission phase. Therapy directed at the central nervous system is a part of each treatment plan (Burg et al., 2006).

The goal of induction therapy is to induce remission and restore normal hematopoiesis. This phase usually lasts 28 days. Chemotherapy drugs include glucocorticoids, vincristine, and L-asparaginase. Consolidation is a period of intensified therapy that uses drugs based on protocol. Methotrexate is frequently used. Maintenance is less intensive chemotherapy and includes methotrexate and 6-mercaptopurine (Burg et al., 2006).

Chemotherapy. Glucocorticoids such as prednisone have the side effects of masking the symptoms of infection, increasing fluid retention, inducing personality changes, and causing the child's face to appear moon-shaped. Methotrexate is useful in maintaining remission because it acts against chemicals vital to the life of the WBC. These powerful medications produce side effects of varying degrees, such as nausea, diarrhea, rash, hair loss (alopecia), fever, anuria, anemia, and bone marrow depression. Peripheral neuropathy may be signaled by severe constipation resulting from decreased nerve supply to the bowel. Footdrop and difficulty with coordination may be seen. These complications are reversed once the offending drug is discontinued. The nurse should consult a pharmacology text for information on the particular drugs used for the patient to anticipate potential problems.

Intrathecal chemotherapy is given for CNS prophylaxis. All children with leukemia are at risk for invasion of the CNS by the leukemic cells. Because medications cannot cross the blood-brain barrier to affect the CNS, chemotherapeutic agents must be injected directly into the spinal fluid through a lumbar puncture.

The various drugs used in treating leukemia may be given in cycles. Antibiotics are administered to prevent or control infection, and transfusions of whole blood or packed cells are given to correct anemia. Sedatives necessary for the patient's comfort are also administered. A pain reliever such as acetaminophen, codeine, or morphine may be ordered if the disease worsens. Medications should be administered before the pain becomes too severe. Pain control is discussed in Chapter 3.

Bone Marrow Transplants and Immunotherapy. Bone marrow transplantation is not recommended for children with ALL during the first remission because of the excellent prognosis with chemotherapy. However, it is a consideration for children with AML during their first remission and for children with ALL who have had a relapse and are in their second remission.

Improvements in transplantation and supportive care, which involve specialized nursing care, have increased the number of long-term survivors of this procedure.

Immunotherapy, although still in the research stages, is another area of therapeutics. Immunotherapy may be passive or active, specific or nonspecific. The main goals of treatment are to strengthen the immune response of the patient to cancer cells and, it is hoped, to prevent cancer with use of immunization.

The child with acute leukemia has many needs, both physical and psychological. These vary in intensity according to exacerbations and progression of the disease. The diagnosis has such an impact on the patient's family members that they are unable to focus on anything other than the child and the illness. Suppression of their own needs mounts if the disease is prolonged and can lead to illness and marital strain. Support groups, such as those provided by Ronald McDonald House and various hospice programs, aid parents in expressing and examining their concerns and give both the child and the family freedom to hurt but still remain whole.

Children's anxieties often center on their symptoms. They fear that the treatments necessary to correct their problems may be painful, as indeed some of them are (e.g., venipunctures, bone marrow aspirations, and blood transfusions). Bone marrow aspiration is depicted in Figure 12-4. Their trust in others is in precarious balance. It is important that nurses inform preschoolers of what they are about to do and why it is necessary. Child Life employees are excellent at explaining procedures to children and allowing them to "play" through their feelings (see Chapter 3). All explanations should be given in terms the children understand.

Communication Alert

It may be the nurse of whom the child asks the inevitable question, "Am I going to die?" One suggested response is to reply with a question, such as "Why do you think you may be dying?" This may encourage the child to verbalize feelings.

The pediatric nurse who gives a patient permission to discuss concerns finds opportunities to clear up misconceptions and decrease the child's feelings of isolation. The element of hope is conveyed because it is indispensable to continued functioning, although the nature of hope may change from that of being cured to that of additional time to live. Further information on the holistic care of the dying child is discussed later in Chapter 18. The following discussion focuses on the intense physical care necessary for the child with leukemia.

Preventing Infection. On establishment of diagnosis, induction therapy is begun. The goal is to reduce the number of leukemic cells and, preferably, to eradicate

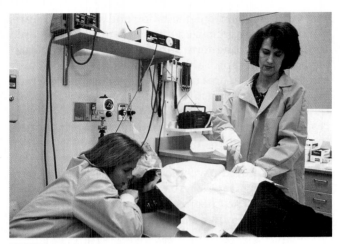

FIGURE **12-4** Child with leukemia undergoing a bone marrow aspiration.

Table 12-3   *Some Infectious Agents Hazardous to the Child with Leukemia*

TYPE	ORGANISM
Bacterial	*Pseudomonas, E. coli, S. aureus, Klebsiella, Proteus*
Viral	Cytomegalovirus, varicella-zoster (chickenpox)
Protozoan	*P. carinii* (prophylactic drugs: Septra, Bactrim)
Fungal	*Candida albicans, Histoplasma*

NOTE: Overwhelming infection can lead to death in children with leukemia. The possibility of infection is high during induction therapy, immediately after radiation therapy, and during maintenance.

them. Careful explanations should be given to the child and family before any procedure is initiated. The disease and many of the necessary medications cause myelosuppression, which depresses the normal function of the bone marrow in addition to destroying cancer cells. The patient becomes anemic, may hemorrhage, and is highly susceptible to infection, even from normally harmless environmental flora. Some of the organisms that may be hazardous to the child with leukemia are listed in Table 12-3. The choice of medication used to combat these infections varies according to the physician's protocol and the causative organism. When fever occurs, broad-spectrum antibiotics are begun until the offending agent is identified. Septra or Bactrim is administered to prevent the development of *Pneumocystis carinii* pneumonia, which is life threatening. WBC transfusions may also be used. Laminar flow patient isolation (LFPI) rooms are available in some centers. These provide a protective environment for the highly susceptible patient.

In most hospitals, patients are placed in a private room for their own protection. The nurse limits visitors and any auxiliary or medical personnel who appear unhealthy. All persons must meticulously adhere to handwashing techniques. Teaching parents concurrently

helps prepare them for home care—that is, protecting the patient from children with communicable diseases, using proper handwashing techniques, and so on. Fresh flowers or plants are not permitted if the child is neutropenic. The nurse explains to the child the purpose for the various procedures used.

Observe the patient frequently for signs of infection. Particular attention should be paid to potentially infected sites, such as the patient's mucous membranes and puncture breaks in the skin from laboratory or therapeutic procedures. Exudates from infection (pus) do not form if WBC counts are low, so it is important to observe frequently for inflammation and fever. Ulcerations develop about the mucous membranes of the mouth and anal region and have a tendency to bleed. Chemotherapy attacks all rapidly growing cells, and the skin and gastrointestinal system are both ordinarily composed of rapidly growing cells. Vital signs are observed for subtle variances because steroid therapy may mask these indicators. Turn the patient often and observe for skin breakdown, particularly in the perianal area. Offer nutritious meals and supplemental feedings high in protein and calories. Teach parents and the child what to look for and to report. Chickenpox and other communicable diseases can be a particular hazard to the immunocompromised child. **Varicella zoster immune globulin (VZIG)** is given within 96 hours of an exposure to chickenpox if the patient has not yet had the disease or the vaccine. Open communication among the school nurse, family, clinic nurse, and physician is paramount.

Managing Bleeding. Thrombocytopenic bleeding is a frequent complication of leukemia. The nurse observes the patient's skin for petechiae and ecchymosis. Nosebleeds are common and are treated with application of cold and pressure.

The mouth is inspected daily for ulcerations and hemorrhage from the gums. Alcohol-based mouthwashes, milk of magnesia, hydrogen peroxide, and lemon glycerin swabs are to be avoided. Administer antifungal drugs as ordered to prevent dissemination in immunosuppressed children. A Water-Pik is helpful in massaging and toughening the gums. A soft sponge toothbrush is helpful. If the platelet count is low, the nurse may also gently clean food particles from the patient's teeth with a piece of gauze wrapped around the finger. Apply lip balm or petroleum jelly to dry, cracked lips.

Hemorrhagic cystitis is not uncommon because some drugs irritate the mucosa of the bladder. The nurse should be alert to symptoms of burning on urination or feelings of pressure, which may indicate infection. Attention is given to providing plenty of fluids and encouraging frequent voidings. The physician is notified of complications immediately so that proper adjustment in medications can be made.

The nurse observes the patient for gastrointestinal bleeding. This is evidenced by **hematemesis** (bloody vomiting) and bloody or tarry stools. Hemarthrosis, or effusion of blood into a joint cavity, may develop. This makes moving about painful; therefore nursing intervention is necessary for the comfort of the patient whether in or out of bed. Scanning the patient's unit for environmental hazards is also of importance. Emergency procedures for control of bleeding are reviewed.

Transfusions. Platelet and packed RBCs may be given to patients with anemia and thrombocytopenia (decrease in platelets in blood). Hemolytic reactions caused by mismatched blood are rare. Nevertheless, the registered nurse should positively identify donor and recipient blood types and groups on labels and the patient's chart with another professional. Blood is administered **slowly.** The patient is observed for signs of transfusion reaction, which include chills, itching, rash, fever, headache, and pain in the back or elsewhere. If such reactions occur, the student nurse clamps off the tubing immediately and reports to the nurse in charge. Save subsequent voiding of urine for hemoglobin determination.

Transfusions with piggyback set-ups are preferred. Blood and normal saline or other suitable IV solutions are connected by a stopcock. When blood must be stopped, tube patency can be maintained by opening the saline line. Necessary emergency medications can thus be administered and the vein preserved for future infusions. Most facilities use an IV pump) to deliver blood products. The line is flushed with normal saline solution before and after the infusion.

Circulatory overload is always a danger with children. Dyspnea, precordial pain, rales, cyanosis, dry cough, and distended neck veins are indicative of this complication. Apprehension can also be a warning signal of air emboli or electrolyte disturbance. The nurse must maintain a high level of alertness for such signs, particularly in children whose conditions warrant repeated transfusions. If a reaction occurs, save the blood bag and tubing and return them to the blood bank. Most transfusion reactions occur within the first 10 minutes of administration; nevertheless, the patient is carefully monitored throughout this treatment.

Establish baseline data (temperature, pulse, respiration, and blood pressure [BP]) before transfusion and monitor for changes. Always follow hospital or institution policy for blood or blood product administration. It is helpful if the parents can remain with the child during this time. Suitable diversions minimize boredom.

Elimination. Constipation is a common side effect of vincristine. Special care to promote normal bowel patterns is essential during the period children receive the drug.

Skin and Hair Care. The skin should be bathed daily and whenever necessary. Observe thoroughly for petechiae and bruising. Careful attention should be given to the rectal mucosa, which is observed for fissures and ulcerations. Cleanse well after each bowel movement. Avoid use of a rectal thermometer. Stool softeners may be necessary for relief of constipation, which frequently accompanies chemotherapy. Sitz baths promote relaxation and may lessen discomfort.

The child's hair is combed daily and whenever necessary. Hair loss (**alopecia**) from drug therapy is not unusual. Psychological preparation of the child and family lessens its impact. Hair returns in 3 to 6 months; meanwhile a wig or hat suitable to the child's preference and age may be worn. Cleaning the scalp prevents cradle cap from forming.

Positioning. Repositioning of the patient is necessary to promote circulation and avoid pressure sores. Bone pain can be acute, and whenever possible, coordinating administration of pain relievers with posture change is helpful. The patient should be handled gently. A bean bag chair, a water bed, or a flotation mattress may be used for comfort. Physical therapy can help prevent footdrop caused by peripheral neuropathy.

Controlling Nausea and Vomiting. One of the more undesirable side effects of chemotherapy in children is vomiting. In addition to monitoring the child for signs of dehydration, the nurse should administer antiemetic medications as ordered during chemotherapy. Non-pharmacological approaches for pain control discussed in Chapter 3 can also be implemented to manage nausea and vomiting. Maintaining IV fluids as prescribed maintains hydration.

Nutrition. The patient should be served well-balanced meals consisting of preferred foods. Because food may not be appealing to children with leukemia, nurses must use their ingenuity to interest them. Mealtimes should be kept pleasant. The companionship of a nurse or attendant is preferable. The nurse should note individual preferences and report them to the dietitian. Food from home may be relished. When the child is too tired or irritable to eat, between-meal feedings are given. When parents understand this, they are less anxious about what the child consumes at a particular meal. Steroid therapy often increases the appetite, which is heartening but temporary. High-calorie commercial foods are tasty and can be used as an adjunct. A low-salt diet may be ordered during chemotherapy cycles that include prednisone to reduce the side effects of the steroid.

Small amounts of fluid are offered frequently. The child who is listless may receive a combination of oral and IV fluids. These children can be expected to have Hickman lines or Mediports for easy access. When parenteral fluids are given, they must be carefully observed (see Chapter 17). A record is kept of all fluid intake and output.

HEMOPHILIA
Description

Hemophilia is one of the oldest hereditary diseases known. It has been called "the disease of kings" because of its occurrence in children of several royal families in Russia and Western Europe. In hemophilia, the blood does not clot normally, and even the slightest injury can cause severe bleeding. The clotting disorder is the result of a deficiency in specific blood clotting factors. A sex-linked genetic pattern causes most cases of hemophilia. Most hemophiliacs are male. Affected males inherit the bleeding disorder from their mothers, who are the carriers. It is possible to determine the level of factor VIII in the blood with a test called the **partial thromboplastin time (PTT).** This aids in the diagnosis and assessment of the child's condition. Women who are carriers and affected fetuses can be identified. Hemophilia can also occur with no family history of the disease, resulting instead from a spontaneous mutation (Wells, 2003). The cause of the mutation is not known, although exposure to excess radiation may be one possibility. Prenatal diagnosis can be made with chorionic villi testing or with amniocentesis.

Two types of hemophilia constitute the highest incidence of the disorder. Factor VIII deficiency, or hemophilia A, is approximately four times more common than factor IX deficiency, hemophilia B. For our purposes, this discussion is limited to classic hemophilia, or hemophilia A, which accounts for about 80% of cases.

The severity of hemophilia A depends on the level of factor VIII in the plasma of the patient's blood. Hemophilia is classified as severe, moderate, or mild. In mild hemophilia, bleeding is usually only a problem after surgery or major trauma. The child with moderate hemophilia can expect bleeding episodes after trauma. Children with severe hemophilia may bleed without apparent cause. The degree of severity tends to remain constant within a given family.

Signs and Symptoms

Hemophilia often is not apparent in the newborn infant unless abnormal bleeding occurs at the umbilical cord, at sites of initial injections, or after circumcision. As the child grows older and becomes more subject to injury, the slightest bruise or cut can induce extensive bleeding. Normal blood clots in about 3 to 6 minutes. In a patient with severe hemophilia, the time necessary for clotting may be an hour or more. Anemia, leukocytosis, and a moderate increase in platelets may be seen in the hemorrhaging child, who may show signs of shock. Hematuria is occasionally seen. Parents may notice it takes a long time to stop bleeding from a cut. Death can result from excessive bleeding anywhere in the body but particularly when hemorrhage occurs into the brain or neck.

An injured knee, elbow, or ankle presents particular problems because of hemorrhage into the joint cavity (hemarthrosis). Hemarthrosis is a cardinal sign in children with hemophilia. The earliest joint hemorrhages appear most commonly in the ankle, from instability of this joint as the toddler assumes an upright posture. Many patients with severe hemophilia develop a "target" joint where repetitive bleeding episodes occur (Behrman et al., 2004). The affected joint is stiff, warm, red, and swollen. Joint limitation occurs. Repeated hemorrhages may cause permanent deformities that could disable the child.

Treatment and Nursing Care

The mechanism of blood formation is complex. Defects in the synthesis of protein may lead to deficiencies in any of the factors in blood plasma needed for clotting to occur. The treatment of each type of hemophilia consists of replacing the deficient factor to ensure clotting. The nursing care for all types is similar.

The child's family history is of particular importance in the diagnosis of hemophilia. When hemophilia is present in the family and the patient has had periods of abnormal bleeding from early childhood, the determination is relatively easy. However, in many cases the family history may be vague or unobtainable. In some instances, even careful scrutiny produces no evidence of the disease in the family.

Current treatment of hemophilia is the administration of highly purified or recombinant factor VIII concentrates to treat bleeding episodes or anticipated bleeding episodes (surgery, tooth extraction). These concentrates are in powder form and may be kept at room temperature or in the refrigerator. They are reconstituted with sterile water before IV administration. In the past, the risk for hepatitis and AIDS was high in this population because concentrates were made from a pool of as many as 20,000 blood donors and were not adequately treated to eliminate viruses. Careful checking of blood donors and new techniques to make concentrate have reduced the risk for children newly diagnosed with hemophilia. Treatment ranges from four times a week (preventive regime) to three times a month.

Parents can be taught at home how to administer factor to their child. Home care and management of bleeding episodes have improved the prognosis and quality of life for children with hemophilia by reducing the cost of treatment and decreasing the risk for psychological trauma. Teaching is done by the physician and nurse in a specialty clinic. Instruction includes an exact explanation of the illness, with emphasis on the signs and treatment of hemorrhage. Specific procedures taught include the storage and preparation of replacement factors, venipuncture, transfusion management and possible reactions, and record keeping. Signs of complications are reviewed, and emergency numbers and other protocols are spelled out. One advantage of home treatment is its immediate availability. The earlier hemarthrosis is treated, the less severe the consequences. The goal is for the patient to become independent and for the health care center to be available as a backup when a need arises. Older school-age children are able to learn self-care. Many children learn more about their disease at hemophilia camp.

Desmopressin (DDAVP) has been found to increase factor VIII levels in children with hemophilia. The increase is not enough to manage hemarthrosis or severe bleeding episodes, but it can be used to treat mild hemophilia. It is less expensive and less invasive than administration of factor VIII concentrate.

Preventing bleeding episodes is an important part of comprehensive care. When the patient with hemophilia is an infant, the crib sides require padding and all toys must be checked for sharp edges. Active toddlers and preschoolers need a safe environment and close supervision in which to practice newly learned gross motor skills. The use of protective equipment such as helmet and joint padding is essential for active children. The older child should avoid contact sports and other activities that have a high risk for injury. Swimming is an excellent competitive sport that also helps strengthen muscles and maintain joint mobility. Walking and bicycle riding are also good ways to exercise. An active, regular exercise program is beneficial. Strong muscles support joints and reduce the numbers of bleeds.

The nurse should teach the parent to carefully observe the skin at bath time for bruises or hematomas. The patient's nails should be kept short. Good oral hygiene is essential. Select a toothbrush with soft bristles. The dentist needs to be consulted early in the preschool years to establish a program of preventive therapy.

The patient needs well-balanced meals. Excessive weight gain is to be avoided because it places additional strain on the joints. A regular exercise program strengthens muscles surrounding the joints, thus decreasing the potential for tissue injury. If the child is receiving medication via injection, or if blood work has been ordered, pressure is applied to the site immediately afterward. The site is carefully observed by the parent or nurse to ensure that all is well. The child's stools and urine are observed for blood. Vital signs are taken routinely to detect concealed bleeding. Patients are instructed to wear a Medic-Alert bracelet. All children should receive routine childhood immunizations, including hepatitis B vaccine.

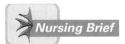
Nursing Brief

Hemophiliacs should receive all injections under the skin (subcutaneously) and not into the muscles. Pressure should be applied for 5 minutes afterward.

An open wound is treated immediately with cold and pressure. When possible, elevate the bleeding area above heart level to decrease blood flow. The child or parents can sometimes sense when a bleed is occurring. Parents should have ice packs available at all times. Nosebleeds can be controlled by tilting the head forward and applying firm pressure to the nose for 15 to 30 minutes. A nasal pack may be necessary.

Mouth bleeding is usually minor, but if it cannot be controlled, an antifibrinolytic agent such as Amicar may be used to promote clot formation.

If hemarthrosis occurs, the deficient factor should be given and the joint immobilized. Hemarthrosis occurs most frequently in the knees, elbows, and ankles. Bleeding is treated with rest, ice, compression, and elevation of the affected part (RICE). Cold packs are applied to decrease the pain, and analgesics such as acetaminophen can be given as ordered. Aspirin and nonsteroidal antiinflammatory drugs (NSAIDs), such as ibuprofen, should be avoided because they have a depressive effect on platelet function. The joint might be placed in a splint for immobilization. Therapy for muscle injuries is essentially the same. When the bleeding has ceased, the child can begin active exercises under the supervision of the physical therapist.

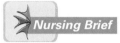
Nursing Brief

Instruct parents of the child with hemophilia to avoid medications that inhibit platelet function, such as aspirin and ibuprofen. Explain the importance of contacting a physician or pharmacist before giving any over-the-counter drugs to the child.

Having a child with hemophilia is a challenge to the family. The family needs to create a positive environment that allows the child to be independent. It is natural for parents to be overprotective. Parents need to understand that they can create a safe environment while still allowing the child to develop his or her full capabilities. The National Hemophilia Foundation (*http://www.hemophilia.org*) is a resource for financial, psychological, and medical support for the family. Research is currently under way to try to find a cure for hemophilia. Gene therapy is one promising area that continues to be explored.

RESPIRATORY SYSTEM

TONSILLITIS AND ADENOIDITIS
Description

The tonsils and adenoids, located in the pharynx, or throat, are made of lymph tissue and act as part of the body's defense mechanism against infection. Group A streptococci are normal flora of the oropharynx and pharynx, and up to 20% of the pediatric population are colonized by this bacteria. However, infectious pathogens such as *Haemophilus influenzae, Staphylococcus aureus, S. pneumoniae, and Moraxella catarrhalis* are also sources of infection. Penicillin is often the drug of choice to treat streptococcal pharyngitis.

The tonsils and adenoids formerly were blamed for causing many assorted illnesses, and for a time it was thought that having them removed was part of growing up. Today, doctors carefully evaluate the need for children to have them removed. A careful physical examination and an evaluation of the patient's history are done to rule out other diseases. Enlargement of the tonsils is not sufficient reason for removal. These structures are normally larger in early childhood than in later years. The current trend is to treat the conditions as separate problems, according to individual criteria. Obstructive sleep apnea syndrome, multiple infections, and peritonsillar abscess are indications for tonsillectomy.

Treatment and Nursing Care

The use of antibiotics during acute infections has reduced the need for surgery. The decision as to whether surgery is necessary is perhaps the single most important factor from a medical standpoint. Ideally, children are beyond toddlerhood when this surgery is performed. They are better able to understand what is happening, and they are more compliant as a result.

Most children are referred to an ear, nose, and throat specialist when contributing conditions become severe. An acute streptococcal infection should be treated prior to surgery. Surgery is usually performed in day surgery units. New surgical tools are being used for tonsillectomy and adenoidectomy. According to Messner (2003), one such instrument is the ultrasonic dissector coagulator, which uses ultrasonic technology to cut and coagulate tissues at lower temperatures than that used with electrocautery. This ultimately minimizes tissue damage (and possibly, postoperative pain).

Preoperative Care. The child is prepared in advance for surgery. Children need to know that the tonsils are two small lumps located far in the back of the mouth. Because they are causing the throat to be sore (or whatever symptoms the child is experiencing) and are not working properly, they need to be taken out. Reassure children that the doctor will not operate on any other part of the body and that it is all right for the tonsils to come out. Children are also informed that they will receive a special medicine that will make them go to sleep and will keep them asleep until the operation is over. Emphasize that after the operation *they will wake up.* After they wake up, they will be sore for several days, but pretty soon they will feel entirely better. Medical personnel and parents must be alert to the young child's fantasies and anxieties and answer questions honestly and at a level suitable to the age of the child.

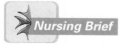
Nursing Brief

In differentiating sleep from death to a young child, the nurse can point out that in sleep the insides of the body slow down, whereas in death they stop completely.

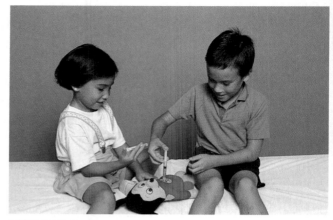
FIGURE **12-5** Playing with syringes provides children with the opportunity to play out fears and concerns.

Many hospitals have special programs to prepare children for surgery. These programs provide videotapes, prehospitalization tours, and opportunities to handle supplies. Familiarization with equipment and the setting reduces fear. Allowing children hands-on play therapy also minimizes fear (Figure 12-5). Children need to know that medical personnel understand their feelings. It is also important that someone they know and trust is close by. Include the child's parents in discussions and encourage them to stay with the child.

A complete physical examination and urinalysis are performed before surgery. Blood work includes hemoglobin, hematocrit, prothrombin time (PT), and PTT. The latter tests are done because bleeding is anticipated. These procedures are usually performed before admission. The child is inspected for loose teeth and signs of upper respiratory tract infection. It is also important to determine any family bleeding tendencies, any history of chronic illness (such as rheumatic fever), elevations in temperature, and recent exposure to communicable diseases.

Instructions are given to the parents regarding the times to stop eating and drinking before surgery. A preoperative checklist is completed. The nurse checks to see that the child's identification band is securely attached to the wrist. The patient should void before going to the operating room. Parents accompany the child to preoperative holding and are encouraged to remain with their child in this area (Figure 12-6).

Many facilities use oral or IV midazolam (Versed) or other preoperative sedation to relax the child before anesthesia induction. Anesthesia induction is usually via inhalation. The child is given a choice what "flavor" is used.

Many hospitals like to have parents in the recovery room to decrease children's anxiety by providing a familiar face and arms to welcome them when they awaken. Review postoperative procedures with the parents, including what to expect when the child

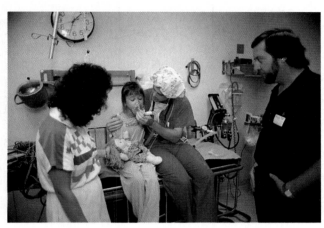

FIGURE **12-6** Parental presence during induction of anesthesia can minimize the child's and parents' anxiety during the preoperative period.

returns to the room (such as color, bleeding, IV fluids, vomiting, and irritability).

Postoperative Care. Nursing care is focused on providing comfort and minimizing potential bleeding. Immediately after surgery, to facilitate drainage, the child is placed partly on the side and partly on the abdomen (prone), with the knee of the uppermost leg flexed to hold the position. The child is watched carefully for evidence of bleeding. Hemorrhage is the most common postoperative complication. The nurse should not assume that because surgery is minor it does not involve certain risks. Because bleeding after this type of surgery is concealed, the nurse must watch carefully for evidence of hemorrhage (see Data Cues). When bleeding is suspected, packing and sometimes ligation are indicated. Lung abscesses and pneumonia are infrequent complications.

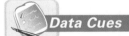

Data Cues

The Child with Possible Posttonsillectomy Bleeding

- Frequent swallowing (a cardinal sign of bleeding)
- Pallor
- Restlessness
- Increased pulse
- Vomiting bright red blood
- Decreasing BP
- Visible blood on careful examination of the throat with a flashlight

An ice collar may be applied for comfort. Some children prefer not to have an ice collar. Most children experience pain and should be medicated. Acetaminophen, with or without codeine, increases comfort and may assist in lessening crying, which can irritate the operative site. Rectal or IV analgesics also may be used.

The child is given fluids intravenously during surgery. It is not uncommon for vomiting to occur. Small amounts of cool, clear liquids are given when the vomiting has ceased. The child usually can tolerate approximately 1 to 2 ounces an hour. Citrus juices, carbonated drinks, and milk products are to be avoided. Avoid extremely hot or cold fluids as they may irritate the throat. A Popsicle may appeal to the child; however, red juices or Popsicles are not to be given because monitoring for bleeding is an important nursing consideration. If clear liquids are well tolerated, progression to a soft diet is begun. The child is kept quiet for the remainder of the day. A small child may nestle on a parent's lap.

Discharge. Written instructions are given to the parents when the child is discharged. The child should be kept quiet for a few days and should receive nourishing fluids and soft foods. After this, children may continue to take a nap or have a rest period so that they have a sufficient convalescent time. Acetaminophen (Tylenol) may be given to reduce discomfort in the throat. The child needs to be protected from exposure to infections. Fresh bleeding, chest pain, or persistent cough should be reported to the physician. Although it occurs rarely, bleeding can occur up to 10 days after surgery from tissue sloughing from the healing process (Hockenberry et al., 2003). The doctor may compare this with a "scab" coming off. Earache may follow a tonsillectomy and/or adenoidectomy, and slight fever (99° F to 100° F, or 37.2° C to 37.8° C) may occur for 2 or 3 days. A follow-up appointment is made because the surgeon will wish to check the operative site after it has healed. The child usually can resume normal activities within 2 weeks.

GASTROINTESTINAL SYSTEM

CELIAC DISEASE
Description

Celiac disease, also known as *celiac sprue* and *gluten-sensitive enteropathy,* is a lifelong, genetic disorder that results in the inability to digest gluten. It is also considered an immune disorder that may be triggered by a virus, major surgery, or extreme stress (Patient Information Collection, 2002). This is a permanent disorder that affects about 1 in 1000 live births in the United States; however, there is a much higher incidence rate in Europe (McKinney et al., 2005).

Signs and Symptoms

Gluten is a protein found in wheat, barley, rye, and oats. Between the ages of 1 and 5, many foods with gluten (pasta, bread, cereals, etc.) are introduced into the child's diet. Gluten breaks down into *gliadin* in the small intestine. In celiac disease, the gliadin cannot be digested and damage to intestinal mucosal cells occurs. Although symptoms may not be noticed initially, malabsorption results and children begin to manifest symptoms that may include failure to thrive, chronic diarrhea, abdominal distention, muscle wasting, anorexia, and irritability. Stools are described as foul-smelling and fatty in appearance because of the malabsorption.

Treatment and Nursing Care

A serum antigliadin antibody (AGA) test may be performed to diagnose celiac disease. The strip AGA test requires only a single drop of blood, so the test can be done quickly and inexpensively. A more definitive test is a small bowel (jejunal) biopsy. Once diagnosed, celiac disease is managed through dietary restrictions. All gluten is to be removed from the diet. Foods containing wheat, barley, rye, and oats should not be eaten. Rice, corn, and soy are safe to eat if no gluten has been added to them. There are many sources of hidden gluten in prepared foods; therefore it is usually necessary to consult a dietitian to design a gluten-free diet. Symptoms may be relieved in as early as 1 week after introducing a gluten-free diet.

This lifelong diet may be difficult to adhere to. It is important to help the child learn the necessary dietary restrictions to avoid later complications. Experimentation with new recipes with suitable ingredients, such as Mexican or Chinese dishes that use corn or rice, helps the family adjust. Vitamin supplements may be necessary. Teenagers may also have difficulty maintaining their diet. Health care professionals and parents play a vital role in teaching children to accept the dietary changes necessary to live a fulfilling life.

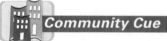
Community Cue

Parents can contact the Celiac Sprue Association/United States of America, Inc, at 877-CSA-4CSA (*http://www. csaceliacs.org*).

MUSCULOSKELETAL SYSTEM

DUCHENNE MUSCULAR DYSTROPHY
Description

The muscular dystrophies are a group of disorders in which progressive muscle degeneration occurs. The childhood form, Duchenne muscular dystrophy (DMD), is the most common type, with an incidence rate of 1:3600 in live-born infant *boys* (Behrman et al., 2004). It is an X-linked recessive trait. Mothers are likely carriers for the disease; however, spontaneous mutations also occur. The gene locus for the disease has been identified, and women at risk may choose to be evaluated and counseled about the carrier state.

Signs and Symptoms

The onset is generally between 2 and 6 years of age; however, a history of delayed motor development during infancy may be evidenced. A waddling gait, slowness in running or climbing, and enlarged rubbery muscles are indicative of this disorder. The calf muscles, in particular, become hypertrophied. Other signs include frequent falling, clumsiness, contractures of the ankles and hips, and the Gower maneuver, a characteristic way of rising from the floor (Figure 12-7).

Laboratory findings show marked increases in blood creatine phosphokinase (CK) levels. An **electromyogram** (**EMG;** a graphic record of muscle contraction as a result of electrical stimulation) shows decreases in amplitude and duration of motor unit potentials. Electrocardiographic (ECG) abnormalities are also common because of progressive cardiomyopathy. A muscle biopsy may be considered. It reveals degeneration of muscle fibers and replacement of these fibers by fat and connective tissue.

The disease becomes progressively worse. With orthopedic bracing, physical therapy, and sometimes surgery, the child may be able to maintain ambulation until the age of 12 years. About a third of boys with DMD have some degree of learning disability, although few are seriously retarded. Death usually results from cardiac failure or respiratory infection.

Treatment and Nursing Care

Treatment at this time is mainly supportive. It consists of passive exercises to prevent joint contractures, bracing, weight control, surgery for joint contractures, and referrals to appropriate social service agencies. Corticosteroid treatment has been explored with these children. The steroids improve muscle strength, but weight gain from steroid use may prove to be more of a problem. Infections are treated with antibiotics. Although cardiac manifestations are usually late events, digoxin and diuretics may be beneficial in the early stages of the disease. Keeping weight down also helps; a low-calorie diet may be encouraged. Psychological considerations have to do with the chronic and progressive nature of the disease and its fatal outcome. Family denial of the diagnosis is common early in the disease, when symptoms are fairly benign.

If the patient is hospitalized for diagnosis, parents and child should be prepared for EMG and possible muscle biopsy. During EMG, small needles are placed in the muscles to record contractions. Muscles examined may ache slightly after the test, but this is temporary. There is no special preparation preceding EMG. Whenever possible, the nurse should plan to remain with the child during the test. During the biopsy, a small piece of muscle is removed for examination. Vital signs and drainage from the incision are monitored after the procedure.

Compared with other children with disabilities, the child with muscular dystrophy may appear passive and withdrawn. Early on, he may become depressed because he is unable to compete with his peers. Social and emotional pressures on the child and his family are great. Financial pressures become magnified as medical and surgical costs escalate. In addition,

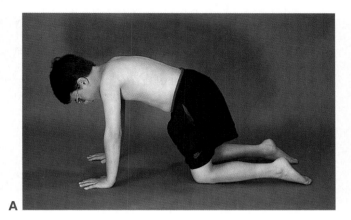
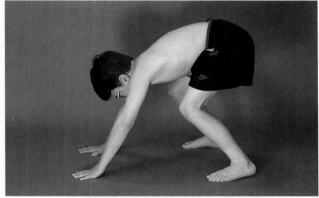
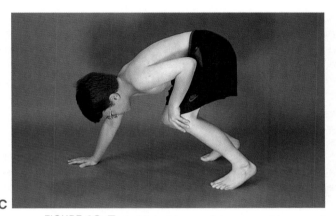
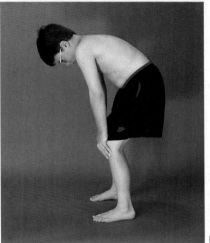

FIGURE **12–7** A child with pseudohypertrophic muscular dystrophy displaying the characteristic Gower sign.

expensive alterations to the family lifestyle, home, and vehicles are sometimes necessary.

Nurses function as team members along with personnel from many other disciplines in the care of the child with muscular dystrophy. They encourage the child to be as active as possible to delay muscle atrophy. Swimming and other activities that promote range of motion and mobility for as long as possible are helpful. Nurses provide support for the many daily issues that occur by placing parents in touch with other parents, camp programs, respite care, the Muscular Dystrophy Association *(http://www.mdausa.org),* public health nurses, home health agencies, family therapists, and eventually hospice care. Although there is no cure at present, different drug therapies, genetic engineering, and stem cell research are beginning to show promise and continue to be investigated.

NERVOUS SYSTEM

ENCEPHALITIS
Description

Encephalitis *(encephalo,* brain; *itis,* inflammation) is an inflammation of the brain parenchyma. It is usually more severe than viral meningitis. This disorder can be caused by arboviruses, enteroviruses (RNA viruses), and herpesvirus types 1 and 2; it can be the aftermath of disorders such as upper respiratory tract infections, German measles, or measles or, rarely, an untoward reaction to vaccinations such as DTP (diphtheria, tetanus, pertussis); or it may result from lead poisoning. Other less common etiological agents are bacteria, spirochetes, and fungi.

This disease also affects horses, and during epidemics, newspapers specify the equine variety if this is the case. If the specific virus is determined, it is given the name of the geographic location in which it is found, such as Eastern (United States), Western (United States), St. Louis, or California. The infection is transmitted to horses and humans by mosquitoes and ticks.

Signs and Symptoms

The symptoms of encephalitis result from the response of the CNS to irritation. In general, the viruses invade the lymphatic system and multiply. The bloodstream becomes affected, and consequently various organs are also involved. Characteristically, the history is that of a headache followed by drowsiness, which may proceed to coma. Because coma is sometimes prolonged, encephalitis is sometimes referred to as "sleeping sickness." Convulsions occur, particularly in infants. Fever, cramps, abdominal pain, vomiting, stiff neck, delirium, muscle twitching, and abnormal eye movements are other manifestations of the disease. The patient's history is of particular significance. Recent illness, injections, travel, and geographic location are recorded.

Treatment and Nursing Care

At this time, no specific treatment with medication is known, with the exception of the use of adenine arabinoside or acyclovir for herpesvirus encephalitis. Parenteral antibiotics are used until a bacterial cause has been ruled out. A brain scan, electroencephalography (EEG), computed tomography (CT), and cerebrospinal fluid analysis may be useful in determining the diagnosis. Intracranial monitoring may also be used.

Treatment is supportive and aimed at providing relief from specific symptoms. Treatment may include sedatives, fluids given intravenously, seizure control, and monitoring for increased intracranial pressure. Catheterization for urinary retention may be necessary. Antipyretics are given as ordered, and seizure precautions are instituted. The nurse provides a quiet dark environment, good oral hygiene, skin care, and frequent change of position. Oxygen is given as needed, and the mouth and nose are kept free of mucus with suctioning. Bowel movements are recorded daily because the patient may be constipated from lack of activity. Preventing this and other secondary effects of immobility is paramount. Physical therapy maintains range of motion. The nurse closely observes the patient for neurological changes.

Fatality rates and residual effects are higher among infants than older children. Speech, mental processes, and motor abilities may be slowed, and permanent brain damage and mental retardation can result. Parents are encouraged to help with the care of the child as soon as the condition is stable. They are instructed in the nursing procedures necessary for home care. In long-term cases, rehabilitation services, the services of the home health care nurse, and related agencies are invaluable.

SEIZURE DISORDERS
Febrile Seizure

Febrile seizures in children occur in association with a fever. They are a common pediatric neurological disorder and are generally transient in nature. Approximately 1 in every 25 children will have at least one febrile seizure, and more than one third of these children will have additional febrile seizures before they outgrow the tendency to have them (National Institute of Neurological Disorders and Stroke, 2006). They usually occur between the ages of 6 months and 5 years and are common in toddlerhood. The cause is uncertain, but research now indicates there may be an association between the fever's causative agent and seizure activity. Viruses, particularly human herpesvirus 6, have been associated with febrile seizures (Warden

et al., 2003). Other theories discuss the height of the temperature (39° C) (102.2° F) as a factor; the seizure generally occurs during the rise rather than after a prolonged elevation (Hockenberry & Wilson, 2007).

Simple febrile seizures are often not present when the child reaches the hospital. Causes other than fever are ruled out. Unless the child has neurological impairments, is younger than 1 year of age, or experiences repetitive or prolonged seizures, epilepsy treatment is not considered. (Epilepsy is discussed in the next section.) Generally, the parents are educated on fever management and seizure precautions, although fever management (such as administering acetaminophen) does not typically reduce the risk for a seizure.

Epilepsy

Description. The term **epilepsy** (chronic recurrent convulsions) comes from the Greek *epilepsia*, which means seizure. It is the name of a very old and misunderstood disease. Epilepsy affects approximately 7 in 1000 people in the general population at any one time and usually begins in childhood (Blume, 2003). Depending on the type of epilepsy, a child may need treatment for only a specified period of time. Others need lifelong treatment.

Epilepsy is characterized by recurrent paroxysmal attacks of unconsciousness or impaired consciousness that may be followed by alternating contraction and relaxation of the muscles or by disturbed feelings or behavior. It is a disorder of the CNS in which the neurons or nerve cells discharge in an abnormal way. These discharges may be focal or diffuse. The site of general discharge can sometimes be ascertained by observing the patient's symptoms during the attack. Types of generalized and partial epileptic seizures are listed in Table 12-4. Treatment is based on accurately diagnosing the type of seizure the child is experiencing. When the cause is unknown, the term idiopathic is used. If a cerebral abnormality is found, the patient may be said to have **organic** or **symptomatic** epilepsy.

Idiopathic epilepsy is the most common cause of recurrent convulsions in children older than 3 years of age. It is possible that some specific genetic defect in cerebral metabolism is responsible in many children. It has been pointed out that EEG abnormalities (cerebral dysrhythmias) are more likely to be found in parents and siblings of affected children than in the population at large.

Organic epilepsy may be caused by a number of conditions or injuries that have impaired the brain. Many genetically determined conditions, such as phenylketonuria (PKU), hydrocephalus, and tuberous sclerosis, are associated with seizures. Convulsions may also occur as a result of brain injury during prenatal, perinatal, or postnatal periods. Acute infections may be responsible for epilepsy in infants and toddlers. There are also contributing conditions that can alter the convulsive threshold. If the patient becomes overtired or overexcited

Table **12-4**   *Generalized and Partial Seizures*

SEIZURE TYPE	CHARACTERISTICS
GENERALIZED SEIZURES	
Generalized tonic-clonic (grand mal)	Sudden loss of consciousness with a cry; fall; rigid muscles followed by muscle jerking; rolling of eyes; pallor or blue skin color associated with slowing or cessation of breathing; possible loss of bowel or bladder control. Seizure lasts a few minutes; then breathing resumes. Child is sleepy and confused and often sleeps 30 min to 2 hr after the seizure. Postictal state may involve vomiting and intense bifrontal headache. Seizure may be preceded by an aura.
Absence (petit mal)	Simple absence seizures are characterized by a sudden cessation of motor activity or speech with a blank facial expression and flickering of the eyelids. Typically last only a few seconds (usually less than 30 sec); are uncommon in children less than 5 yr old; involve possible eyelid and chewing movements during the seizure. Child resumes full activity when seizure ends, although is unaware of what is going on during the seizure. No aura or postictal state. May experience countless seizures daily. Can cause learning difficulties if not recognized.
(Typical) myoclonic	Repetitive seizures consisting of brief muscular contractions with loss of body tone and falling or slumping forward; can cause injuries to face and mouth. Can be associated with generalized tonic-clonic seizures. Onset between 6 mo and 4 yr. May have learning, language, emotional, and behavioral problems; however, more than 50% are seizure-free several years later.
Infantile spasms	Brief symmetric contractions of the neck, trunk, and extremities. Involve sudden *flexion* of the neck, arms, and legs onto the trunk; *extension* of the trunk and extremities; or a combination. Spasms commonly occur while patients are drowsy or immediately on wakening. Onset between 4 and 8 mo. May or may not be associated with underlying neurological disorder or trauma.
Landau-Kleffner syndrome	A rare condition of unknown cause. Mean onset of age is 5½ yr, affecting more boys. Often confused with autism (Chapter 10); loss of language occurs in a previously normal child. Many have an associated seizure disorder. Hearing is normal; behavior problems are common.
PARTIAL SEIZURES	
Simple partial	Motor activity is the most common symptom. Muscle movements involving face, neck, or extremities; can begin in one location and spread to another. Head turning and eye movements are common. Usually lasts 10-20 sec. Child remains aware and may verbalize during the seizure. There is no postictal period. Often preceded by aura ("feeling funny" or "something crawling inside me"). These should not be confused with tics (shoulder shrugging, eye blinking, etc.).
Complex partial	Begins with simple partial seizure with or without an aura; decreased consciousness—child seems dazed; followed by repetitive movements—lip smacking, chewing, swallowing, and excessive salivation; picking and pulling at clothing, rubbing or caressing objects; child may walk or run around randomly and is fearful. Lasts 1 or 2 min. Postictal state with no awareness of the seizure afterward.

Information from Behrman, R., Kliegman, R., & Jenson, H. (2004). *Nelson's textbook of pediatrics* (16th ed.). Philadelphia: Saunders.

or is faced with a stressful situation, a seizure may occur. Bright, flashing lights, or flickering images such as those seen in computer games, can trigger seizures in susceptible people. Alterations in serum and brain concentrations of sodium, potassium, and water resulting from fluid retention can be a precipitating factor. Hormonal changes during puberty, excess fluid intake, and photogenic stimulation have also been suggested as triggers.

Signs and Symptoms. Symptoms vary according to the type of seizure (see Table 12-4). Mixed seizures may also occur in people with epilepsy. Seizures may be convulsive or nonconvulsive. Convulsive seizures usually begin with the **tonic** phase, a phase in which the body stiffens and the patient may lose consciousness and drop to the floor if sitting or standing. The face becomes pale at first and then cyanotic from arrest of respiratory movements. The eyes roll upward or to one side. The child may utter a brief cry as air is forced out of the lungs across tightly closed vocal cords. The head, back, and legs stiffen. Onset is usually abrupt and may be preceded by an **aura**, which is a particular

sensation such as dizziness, visual images, nausea, headache, or an ascending feeling of abdominal discomfort. Children often are unable to describe an aura. The tonic phase lasts about 20 to 40 seconds and is usually followed by the **clonic** phase, which lasts for variable periods. Jerking movements of the trunk and extremities begin. Frothing at the mouth, biting of the tongue, and urinary or fecal incontinence may occur. Muscle contraction and relaxation gradually subside, and the child enters the **postictal** state. The patient appears dazed and confused and generally sleeps for a while. On awakening, patients may have a headache and may perform more or less automatic acts. This is believed to be caused by malfunctioning of the neurons, which may not be fully recovered. The patient has no recollection of the seizure. **Status epilepticus** is a series of convulsions rapidly following one another. The most common cause is abrupt withdrawal of anticonvulsant medication. Families need to be taught to call emergency medical services when this occurs. Status epilepticus is an emergency situation because death can result from respiratory failure and

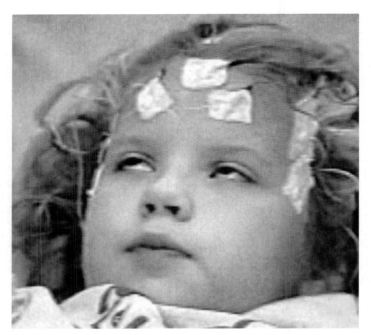

FIGURE **12-8** This absence seizure was recorded during a video electroencephalogram.

exhaustion. Diazepam (Valium) or lorazepam (Ativan) is given IV.

Nonconvulsive seizures take various forms, including lapses in consciousness, loss of muscle tone, distorted sensations, and **automatisms,** or repetitive movements. Most nonconvulsive seizures are not preceded by an aura.

Treatment and Nursing Care. First aid for a child with a convulsive seizure includes protecting the child from harm, loosening clothing around the neck, turning on the side to maintain an airway, and reassuring the child when consciousness returns. Parents need to be taught first aid as well. During a seizure, the nurse observes and records the following: the child's activity immediately before the seizure; body movements; changes in color, respiration, or muscle tone; incontinence; and the parts of the body involved. When possible, the seizure is timed. The child's appearance, behavior, and level of consciousness after the seizure are also documented. Do not place any hard object in the mouth or try to hold the child down during a seizure. Rescue breathing is not necessary unless the child is not breathing when the seizure is finished. Seizure precautions in the hospital setting include padding side rails and having oropharyngeal suction, oxygen, and an oral airway at the bedside. The child's bed should be kept at the lowest position with the rails up at all times.

Initially, treatment of the child with a seizure disorder is aimed at determining the type, site, and cause of the disorder. Diagnostic measures include a complete history and physical and neurological examinations. Skull radiography and CT are used to establish the presence or absence of tumors, skull abnormalities, hematomas, and intracranial calcifications. Magnetic

resonance imaging (MRI) is also used for diagnosis as it is technically superior to CT for this purpose. EEG is also a valuable tool in evaluating seizures. It is especially helpful in differentiating between an absence seizure and a complex partial seizure (Figure 12-8). Video EEG recordings can show more subtle manifestations and provide a permanent record for playback. Prolonged ambulatory EEG monitoring (24 hours) is another advanced technique. Laboratory studies such as a fasting blood sugar, complete blood cell count (CBC), serum calcium, blood urea nitrogen (BUN), and drug screening may detect acute infections, lead poisoning, drug ingestion, or metabolic disorders. A spinal tap may be ordered when encephalitis or meningitis is suspected. If the seizure is related to any such underlying cause, appropriate therapy is begun. Anticonvulsive drug therapy is begun only after all such causes have been excluded.

Some common anticonvulsants and their side effects are listed in Table 12-5. The physician determines the child's medication by the type of seizure and other factors. The goal is to achieve the best control with the minimum dosage and the least number of side effects. Serum anticonvulsant levels should be carefully monitored during initial seizure control stages. Doses are altered accordingly. An important aspect of nursing intervention includes reinforcing the need for drug supervision and compliance. The duration of therapy is individual. Initially the physician prescribes the lowest dose likely to control the seizures. A combination of drugs may be necessary. Drowsiness, a common side effect of many anticonvulsants, can interfere with the child's activities and requires monitoring. Careful recording of seizure activity and adherence

Table 12-5 | *Some Commonly Used Anticonvulsant Drugs*

DRUG	SEIZURE TYPE	SIDE EFFECTS	COMMENTS
Phenobarbital	Generalized tonic-clonic Partial Status epilepticus	Drowsiness, irritability, hyperactivity, behavioral changes	Relatively safe medication; bitter, often combined with other drugs. May cause Stevens-Johnson syndrome. Routine blood tests not indicated.
Primidone (Mysoline)	Generalized tonic-clonic Partial	Aggressive behavior	Similar to phenobarbital; routine blood tests not indicated.
Phenytoin (Dilantin)	Generalized tonic-clonic Partial Status epilepticus	Ataxia, insomnia, motor twitching, gum overgrowth, hirsutism (hairiness), rash, nausea, vitamin D and folic acid deficiencies	Generally effective and safe; regular massaging of gums decreases hyperplasia; is used in combination with phenobarbital or primidone. May be causative agent of Stevens-Johnson syndrome. Many drug interactions.
Valproic acid (Depakene)	Generalized tonic-clonic Absence Myoclonic Partial	Gastrointestinal disturbance, altered bleeding time, liver toxicity	Monitor blood counts; take with food or use enteric-coated preparations; potentiates action of phenobarbital and other drugs.
Clonazepam (Rivotril)	Absence Myoclonic Infantile spasms Partial	Behavior changes, ataxia, anorexia, nystagmus	May increase serum phenytoin concentrations when used together.
Carbamazepine (Tegretol)	Generalized tonic-clonic Partial	Blurred vision, diplopia, drowsiness, vertigo	Anemia, neutropenia, hepatotoxic effects.

Adapted from Behrman, R., Kliegman, R., & Jenson, H. (2004). *Nelson's textbook of pediatrics* (17th ed.). Philadelphia: Saunders.

to the drug regimen are of particular importance in determining a suitable program. Tablet form is preferable to suspensions, which are more expensive and tend to separate if not shaken well. Most small children can ingest the tablet when it is administered in a teaspoon with a small amount of applesauce. Medication is given at the same time each day, generally with meals or at bedtime. Parents need to work with the physician to find the medication that works best for their child. Noncompliance can be a problem because of the side effects (hyperactivity, drowsiness). Parents should be told that children often reach a level where they adjust to the medication and side effects may not be as severe. As with all complicated childhood diseases, using a multidisciplinary approach to treatment generally results in increased compliance and improved outcomes.

If it is necessary for the child to take medication during school hours, the parents sign a consent form so that the school nurse may monitor administration. This provides the child and the nurse opportunities to get acquainted and share their knowledge of the disease. Nurse and teacher response, particularly during and after a seizure, has a significant effect on the attitude of classmates toward the disease.

It is important that medication be reduced gradually under a physician's supervision because abrupt withdrawal of medications is the most common cause of status epilepticus. In the hospital, the nurse consults the physician as to whether anticonvulsants are to be withheld if the patient is to be NPO. As in any long-term drug therapy, periodic blood and urine

tests may be necessary to detect subtle side effects, noncompliance, drug toxicity, and other problems. When children are old enough, they can assume responsibility for their own medications. They should wear a Medic-Alert bracelet. During puberty and adolescence, dosages may have to be adjusted to meet growth needs. Premenstrual fluid retention in girls can sometimes trigger seizures.

The **ketogenic diet** is sometimes prescribed for children who do not respond well to anticonvulsant therapy. It is high in fats and produces ketoacidosis in the body, which appears to have a calming effect. Some children have a reduction in the number of seizures, whereas others may become seizure-free. The diet is difficult to maintain, however, because food has to be carefully measured and controlled and because it is generally unpalatable to children. Research is ongoing with this diet.

Surgery may be considered for some children with intractable seizures that do not respond to medication. Precisely locating the area of seizure activity is critical for a successful outcome. These children need to be monitored carefully after surgery. Other children may be candidates for a vagal nerve stimulator, which is implanted in the chest wall. A reduction of seizure activity with some patients has also been achieved with this device.

Rebellion against medical routine is not uncommon during adolescence. Some states do not allow people with controlled epilepsy to obtain a driver's license, which may be disheartening to the patient. Other states have stipulations about the amount of seizure-free time required before licensing is allowed. In terms of diet, excess intake of fluids, particularly alcoholic beverages, can be a source of contention.

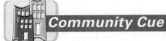

Community Cue

Parents can obtain valuable information and support from the Epilepsy Foundation of America *(http://www. epilepsyfoundation.org)*.

The well-controlled patient can lead a normal life with a few safety restrictions (e.g., using precautions while swimming). Patients can participate in selected athletic and recreational activities. Moderate exercise is encouraged; avoidance of caffeine, alcohol, and trigger factors is recommended. Death or serious injury rarely occurs from a seizure, and a seizure does not cause mental deterioration.

Preventing organic epilepsy includes promoting good prenatal and postnatal care and healthful living for children. Teach parents the importance of providing a safe environment and supervision for small children to prevent injury. Play areas need to be properly supervised, poisonous substances must be stored away from little hands, and proper seat belts should be used in automobiles to prevent head injury. Prevention, early diagnosis, and treatment for such conditions as PKU, meningitis, Reye syndrome, and encephalitis are also crucial in minimizing irreversible brain damage. The abuse of drugs, including alcohol, by teenagers can result in cerebral anoxia and convulsions, and this danger should be stressed in comprehensive health teaching for this age group. It is not possible or desirable to shield children from every stressful situation, but adults can assist growing children by helping them make wise decisions at their level of competency and by being supportive. The response of parents and nurses in stressful situations is also of importance in role modeling. Education of the patient and family is a prime consideration in developing nursing care plans. Children who state that they are subject to seizures indicate that they are aware of their condition, and this encourages others to relate to them in a mature way.

GENITOURINARY SYSTEM

URINARY TRACT INFECTION
Description

Urinary tract infections (UTIs) are caused by bacterial invasion of the upper urinary tract (kidney and ureters) or lower urinary tract (bladder and urethra). Genitourinary anatomy is reviewed in Figure 12-9. They generally occur in children between 2 and 6 years, unless a structural anomaly is the cause. Urinary tract infections are more commonly found in girls because

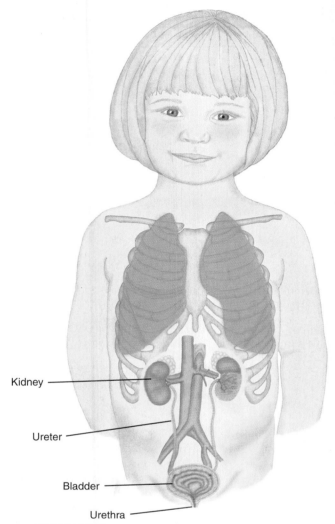

Kidney

Ureter

Bladder

Urethra

FIGURE **12-9** Anatomy of the genitourinary system.

the distance infectious organisms need to travel to enter the bladder is considerably shorter than in boys. Boys have a much longer urethra.

Several factors contribute to the incidence of UTIs in children. These include congenital malformations of the urinary tract and conditions resulting in urinary stasis (ignoring the urge to urinate, neurogenic bladder). In affected infant boys, the incidence is higher in the uncircumcised. Mechanical factors such as tight diapers or underwear, chemical irritation from bubble bath, inflammatory conditions of the external perineal area, and pinworms contribute to UTIs. Although UTI in young girls is not uncommon, repeated UTIs can suggest possible sexual abuse.

Vesicoureteral Reflux. Vesicoureteral reflux (VUR) is a primary contributing factor to upper UTIs. As urine fills the bladder or as the bladder contracts during voiding, the opening to the ureter is normally occluded. With VUR, a malfunctioning valve at the junction of the ureter and bladder allows urine to reflux upward into

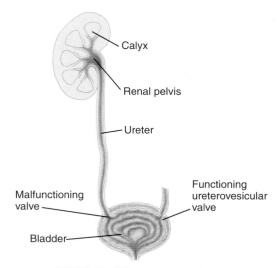

Calyx

Renal pelvis

Ureter

Malfunctioning
valve

Functioning
ureterovesicular
valve

Bladder

FIGURE **12-10** Mechanics of VUR.

the ureters toward the kidney (Figure 12-10). This allows bacteria in the urine to be carried upward, possibly all the way into the kidney. This can cause pyelonephritis and renal damage. In addition, the urine can return to the bladder, creating a residual that becomes a medium for bacterial growth or infection. VUR is graded I to V (1 to 5), with grade V involving a gross dilation of the ureter and pelvis and calyces of the kidney. Diagnosis is generally made after ultrasound and a voiding cystourethrography (VCUG). During a VCUG, contrast medium is injected into the bladder through a urethral catheter; radiographs are taken before, during, and after voiding. This procedure visualizes the bladder outline, urethra, and identifies reflux and other structural complications. All patients (1-10 years) are treated initially with antibiotic prophylaxis. At the end of 1 year, if VUR is not resolved, endoscopy therapy is recommended for children with lower grades of reflux. Open surgery is used if endoscopy is unsuccessful; it may also be used from the outset if children have higher grades of reflux (Greenbaum & Mesrobian, 2006).

Signs and Symptoms

Signs of UTIs in infants and young children are easily missed. The child exhibits poor feeding, fussiness, delayed growth, foul-smelling urine, and incontinence (in a child who has been previously trained). Unexplained fever in infants may be caused by a UTI, and this should be considered when no other source for the fever is found. Many adolescent girls exhibit classic signs of UTI (frequency, urgency, pain on urination, blood in the urine) after the first episode of sexual intercourse. High fever, chills, flank pain, and abdominal pain can indicate kidney infection (pyelonephritis).

Urinary tract infection is diagnosed with urine culture. The specimen is obtained with a clean midstream urine collection in potty-trained children or with cathe-

terization or suprapubic aspiration in infants and untrained children. The culture shows organism growth; usually colony growth exceeding 100,000 of a single organism is diagnostic from a midstream specimen. *Escherichia coli* and other gram-negative organisms are frequently the cause. Antibiotic sensitivities determine the treatment. Blood, protein, and WBC casts might be found in the urine. A complete renal workup to detect urinary tract abnormalities includes ultrasonography, VCUG, and radionuclide cystography, renal nucleotide scans, and CT or MRI.

Treatment and Nursing Care

Treatment of a UTI with older children is a 7 to 14-day course of an appropriate antibiotic, generally sulfamethoxazole/trimethoprim (Bactrim, Septra). Penicillins and cephalosporins may also be ordered. Children who do not improve within 2 days of starting antibiotics for UTI should be re-evaluated with ultrasound and VCUG. Nurses need to teach proper hygiene (no bubble baths or irritating diaper wipes; wiping from front to back).

Explaining procedures using terms with which the child is familiar is important. If a catheterized urine sample is necessary, the nurse needs to reassure the child that the tube does not harm the body but helps find out what is wrong. Practice relaxation breathing exercises with the child before inserting the catheter, and encourage the child to sing or breathe slowly as the tube is being inserted. Sphincter relaxation decreases the amount of discomfort the child might experience.

Other preventive measures include wearing cotton underwear, adequate fluid intake, encouraging children to not put off going to the bathroom when needed, investigating and treating signs of intestinal parasites (pinworms), and avoiding bubble baths. Acidification of the urine with cranberry juice is helpful. Sexually active girls should urinate after sexual intercourse. If urine specimens are obtained at home, teach the parent to bring the specimen immediately to the laboratory. If the parent is unable to get to the laboratory within 30 minutes, the specimen should be refrigerated.

ACUTE (POSTSTREPTOCOCCAL) GLOMERULONEPHRITIS
Description

Acute glomerulonephritis (AGN) occurs as an immune reaction (antigen-antibody) to an infection in the body. The most common of the noninfectious renal diseases in childhood is acute poststreptococcal glomerulonephritis. The infection is generally caused by a Group A betahemolytic streptococci infecting the throat or the skin. It may appear after the patient has had scarlet fever or skin infections (impetigo). The body's immune mechanisms appear to be important in its development. Antibodies produced to fight the invading organisms react against the glomerular tissue. Glomerulonephritis is the most common form of nephritis in children and occurs most frequently in boys between 3 and 7 years of age. It has a seasonal incidence, with peaks in winter and spring. Both kidneys are affected.

The nephron is the working unit of the kidneys. Nephrons number in the millions. Within the bulb of each nephron lies a cluster of capillaries known as the glomerulus. It is these structures that are affected, as the name of the disease implies. They become inflamed and sometimes blocked, permitting RBCs and protein, which are normally retained, to enter the urine. Sodium and fluid are retained, leading to edema and oliguria (decreased urine output). The kidneys become pale and slightly enlarged.

The prognosis is excellent. Patients with mild cases of the disease may recover within 10 to 14 days. Patients with protracted cases may show urinary changes for as long as a year but have complete recovery. Chronic nephritis is seen in a small number of children, with death generally resulting from renal or heart failure. These severe complications, plus hypertensive changes in the blood supply of the brain, necessitate careful observation and care of each patient.

Signs and Symptoms

Symptoms range from mild to severe. From 1 to 2 weeks after a streptococcal infection has occurred in the child, the mother may notice that the urine is smoky brown in color or bloody. This is frightening to the mother and child; medical advice is immediately sought by most parents. **Periorbital edema** (mild swelling about the eyes) may also be present in the morning, and the edema spreads to the abdomen and extremities as the day progresses. The child may have fatigue, headache, abdominal discomfort, and vomiting. After an initial acute phase, the child spontaneously diureses and the symptoms begin to abate. Blood and protein can be found in the urine for several weeks.

Urinary output is decreased. Protein, RBCs, WBCs, and casts may be found on examination. The BUN level can be elevated, as can the serum creatinine and erythrocyte sedimentation rates. The serum complement level is usually reduced. For a definite diagnosis, it may be necessary to have positive confirmation of a streptococcal infection, either with culture or with antibody titer. Mild-to-severe hypertension may be seen. Complications such as renal and cardiac failure and encephalopathy may also occur.

Treatment and Nursing Care

Although the child may feel well, activity should be limited until gross hematuria subsides. The urine should be examined regularly. Every effort is made to prevent the child from becoming overtired, chilled, or exposed to infection. Because renal function is impaired, there is a danger of accumulation of nitrogenous wastes and sodium in the body. A low-sodium diet may be ordered. Parents need to be educated by the dietitian on this diet. Protein restriction is not usually necessary. Fluid restriction may be necessary for some patients. Furosemide (Lasix) may be given if significant edema and fluid overload are present and renal failure is not severe (Hockenberry & Wilson, 2007). Penicillin is given if the streptococcal infection persists, but it usually does not alter the course of the disease. Second attacks of glomerulonephritis are rare.

The nurse should try to make the period of bed rest as pleasant as possible by providing quiet diversions. When the child is allowed up, the nurse observes him or her frequently for signs of fatigue. The child should be protected from contact with persons with infections.

The patient's vital signs are taken regularly, preferably with the same apparatus. A rise in BP is reported immediately. Between readings, the nurse should be alert for symptoms such as headache, drowsiness, vomiting, and blurring of vision. If any of these are noticed, the child is returned to bed and the crib sides or rails are raised. Because convulsions can occur, someone should remain with the child until medication is given. Hypotensive drugs, including short-acting calcium channel blockers such as *nifedipine*, may be ordered by the physician. Parameters for administration are specific. These reduce the BP rapidly, and the cerebral symptoms subside. If cardiac failure is evidenced with an ECG or chest radiograph, sedation, oxygen, and digitalis may be necessary.

The nurse accurately records the patient's daily weight, fluid intake, and urine output. Fluids may be restricted, especially if the urinary output is scant. In this circumstance, the physician orders the oral intake allowed, for example, 650 mL daily. This must be distributed throughout the 24-hour period. Each shift should know the specific amount of fluids the patient is to receive for that shift so that an excess amount is not given. The greater amounts of fluid are allotted to the day and evening shifts, when thirst is more pronounced and when the child is awake. The individual needs of the child should be observed and incorporated into the day's events. Persistent anuria (suppression of urine formation) may necessitate dialysis.

Although glomerulonephritis is generally benign, it can be a source of anguish for parents and child. If the patient is treated at home, the parents must plan activities to keep the child occupied while confined to bed. They must understand the importance of continued medical supervision because follow-up urine and blood tests are necessary to ensure that the disease has been eradicated.

NEPHROTIC SYNDROME (NEPHROSIS)
Description

Nephrotic syndrome refers to a number of different types of kidney conditions that are distinguished by the presence of marked amounts of protein in the urine. Minimal change nephrotic syndrome, idiopathic

Table 12-6 | *Comparison of (Poststreptococcal) Glomerulonephritis and (Minimal Change) Nephrotic Syndrome*

MANIFESTATIONS	APSGN	MINIMAL CHANGE NEPHROTIC SYNDROME
Streptococcal antibody titers	Elevated	Normal
BP	Elevated	Normal or decreased
Edema	Periorbital and peripheral	Generalized, severe
Circulatory congestion	Common	Absent
Proteinuria	Mild to moderate	Massive
Hematuria	Gross to microscopic	Microscopic or none
BUN and serum creatinine	Elevated	Normal
Serum potassium levels	Normal or increased	Normal
Serum protein levels	Minimal reduction	Markedly decreased
Serum lipid levels	Normal	Elevated
Peak age at onset	3-7 yr	2-7 yr
Recurrence	Uncommon	Common

Data modified from Hockenberry, M., Wilson, D., Winkelstein, M., & Kline, N. (2007). *Wong's nursing care of infants and children* (8th ed.). St. Louis: Mosby.

nephrosis, in which the cause is seldom determined, is discussed here because it is the most common type seen in early childhood. Table 12-6 compares poststreptococcal glomerulonephritis and nephrotic syndrome.

The **glomeruli**, the working units of the kidneys that filter the blood, become damaged and allow albumin and other proteins to enter the urine. Proteinuria is massive. There is a fall in the level of protein in the blood, termed **hypoproteinemia**, and a rise in cholesterol content, termed **hyperlipidemia.**

Nephrosis is more frequently seen in boys than in girls and is seen most often in toddlers and preschoolers. The prognosis for children with nephrosis is usually positive. Most children have repeated relapses until the disease resolves itself. Children with types other than minimal change nephrotic syndrome do not have as good a prognosis. They may have renal failure develop and need dialysis or transplantation.

Signs and Symptoms

The characteristic symptom of nephrosis is **edema.** This occurs slowly; the child does not appear to be sick. It is noticed at first about the eyes and ankles but later becomes generalized. The edema shifts with the position of the child during sleep. The child gains weight because of the accumulation of this fluid. The abdomen may become so distended that striae, or stretch marks similar to those that appear on the skin of a pregnant woman, may occur. The child is pale, irritable, and listless and has a poor appetite. The child becomes more susceptible to infection.

The urine appears dark and frothy. Urine output can be decreased. Urine examination reveals albumin. Vomiting and diarrhea may also be present. Renal biopsy may be done.

Treatment and Nursing Care

Control of Edema. Steroid therapy is initiated, and diuresis occurs as the urinary protein excretion diminishes in 7 to 21 days. Prednisone, which comes in liquid form for young children, is the drug of choice.

The drug is continued until the urine is free of protein and remains normal for a prescribed period. The dosage is tapered to discontinuation. Immunosuppressive therapy (e.g., cytoxan, chlorambucil) has shown promise for some steroid-resistant children.

Diuretics are given as ordered to aid in the elimination of excessive fluid. The child is weighed daily to determine changes in the degree of edema. The child is weighed on the same scale each time and at about the same time of day. Abdominal girth (circumference) should also be measured every day.

Albumin may be administered intravenously to help restore normal fluid volume and reduce the amount of edema present. IV furosemide (Lasix) is given following administration of albumin to decrease the chance for fluid volume overload.

Because of the amount of edema in the lower extremities and fluid stasis, cellulitis can occur. Peritonitis can also develop; therefore oral penicillin is frequently given to reduce the risk for such infections.

Diet. A well-balanced diet high in protein is desirable because protein is constantly being lost in the urine. Salt is restricted during periods of massive edema, and a diet with no added salt may be recommended after remission to assist in decreasing the salt appetite. Normal amounts of water are given unless otherwise ordered.

The patient's appetite is generally poor. Serve small quantities of food, attractively arranged on brightly colored dishes. Colored straws may also be used. Serve favorite foods if they are nutritious. Sit with the child during the feeding whenever possible. Relax and allow plenty of time. Encourage self-feeding.

Fluid Balance. The patient's urine must be carefully measured. This is difficult with the child who is not toilet-trained or who has had a regression in urinary habits. Diapers or pull-ups can be weighed on a gram scale before applying and after removal (1 g of weight = 1 mL of fluid). The character, odor, and color of the urine are also important. Careful monitoring of intake and output is advised.

Care of the Skin. Good skin care is especially important during periods of marked edema. Special attention is given to the neck, underarms, groin, and other moist areas of the body. The male genitals may become edematous; supportive clothing may be necessary. Cotton or clothing may be used to separate the skin surfaces to prevent a rash from forming.

Positioning. The child is repositioned frequently to prevent respiratory infection. A pressure-equalizing mattress reduces the risk for skin breakdown. A pillow placed between the knees when the patient is lying on the side prevents pressure on edematous organs. The child's head is elevated during the day to reduce edema of the eyelids and to make the patient more comfortable. Children with mild edema can participate in usual activities with frequent periods of rest.

Infection Prevention. Because steroids mask the signs of infection, the child must be watched closely for more subtle symptoms of illness. Examine the child's skin at sites of punctures, wounds, pierced ears, catheters, and so on. Watch for temperature variations, increased BP, and changes in behavior. Report suspicions promptly because septicemia is life threatening. Prompt antibacterial therapy is begun when an acute infection is recognized.

Nurses make every effort to protect the patients from exposure to upper respiratory tract infections. Handwashing is crucial. Children should be separated from other infectious patients. **No vaccinations or immunizations should be administered while the disease is active and during immunosuppressive therapy.**

Emotional Support. The nursing care of the patient with nephrosis is of the greatest significance because this disease requires long-term therapy. The child might be hospitalized periodically and becomes a familiar personality to hospital personnel. Parental guidance and support should be given by all members of the nursing team. Family education about weighing, measuring abdominal girth, and determining urine specific gravity and urinary albumin is necessary. The parents should be encouraged to remain with the child as much as possible.

Whenever possible, the child is treated at home and brought to the hospital for special therapy only. Parents are instructed to keep a daily record of the child's weight, urinary proteins, and medications. Signs of infection, such as abnormal weight gain, and increased protein in the urine must be reported promptly. The child is allowed to be up and about after the acute stage of the illness subsides to participate in normal childhood activities.

The child with nephrosis is kept under close medical supervision over an extended period. The prognosis is considered favorable but depends on the patient's response to drug therapy (Nursing Care Plan 12-1).

SPECIAL TOPICS

COMMUNICABLE DISEASES

Prevention and control are key factors in limiting the spread of communicable diseases. Prevention is obtained mainly through immunization. Control is through the early identification and isolation of cases.

When a communicable disease is suspected, a thorough history must be obtained. The nurse asks whether the child has recently been exposed to a communicable disease, has been immunized, or has had the disease. The nurse may inquire whether the patient has experienced any of the prodromal symptoms (symptoms indicating the onset of a disease).

Most communicable diseases can be treated at home unless the child is immunosuppressed or complications occur. The child may be given tepid baths or have lotions (calamine) applied to relieve itching. Nails should be kept short, and mittens may be worn by younger children who persist in scratching. Benadryl may be given if the child cannot be soothed. Care should be taken when applying certain over-the-counter lotions, however, because some of these may also contain Benadryl. Acetaminophen or ibuprofen is given for an elevated temperature. Aspirin should be avoided because of its connection with Reye syndrome. Older children may gargle with saline rinses or use lozenges for sore throat relief. Anorexia is common, but children tend to increase their intake if they are limited to liquids and bland foods. Quiet activities should be provided to allow for rest and provide diversion.

Table 12-7 summarizes the nursing care of several common communicable diseases. Sections on anthrax and smallpox have been added to familiarize the student with information on these diseases in the event of bioterrorism. Box 12-2 on p. 270 differentiates chickenpox from smallpox. Figure 12-11 on p. 270 further illustrates the differences between these two diseases.

Community Cue

The Centers for Disease Control and Prevention (CDC) play an active role in researching diseases, including those that could result from bioterrorism. All health care providers should be aware of their educational resources *(http://www. cdc.gov/)*. Information is also available in Spanish.

DEVELOPMENTAL DISABILITY
Description

A developmental disability is any mentally or physically disabling condition that begins during childhood and is expected to continue throughout life. This includes children with mental retardation, sensory deficits (speech, hearing, vision), orthopedic problems, and other conditions including autism and cerebral palsy (McKinney et al., 2005). Autism is classified as a *pervasive developmental disorder* (PDD) and is discussed

NURSING CARE PLAN 12-1

The Child with Nephrotic Syndrome

NURSING DIAGNOSIS *Excess fluid volume related to fluid shift from intravascular to interstitial spaces, as a result of glomerular damage*

Goals/Outcome Criteria	Nursing Interventions	Rationales
Child begins to lose accumulated interstitial fluid as evidenced by: • Increased urinary output • Decreased edema • Weight loss	Administer medications as prescribed; liquid medication is more appropriate for children.	Steroids act on the glomeruli by suppressing the immune response; diuretics may be indicated.
	Test urine daily for protein.	Trace amounts or absence of urine protein indicates the disease is in remission.
	Weigh daily with the same scale and at the same time of day.	Monitors fluid gain or loss.
	Measure abdominal girth.	Monitors fluid accumulation in abdominal area.
Child maintains normal intravascular fluid volume as evidenced by: • Moist mucous membranes • Good skin turgor • Stable vital signs	Strictly measure intake and output: • Place input and output sign on bedside. • Instruct all visitors to keep track. • Weigh diapers or pull-ups before and after (1 g weight = 1 mL of fluid). • Use toilet "hat" for urine output measurement. • Measure intake amount in "sippy cup" if used. • Provide sufficient amounts of the child's favorite fluids—fluids should neither be restricted nor encouraged.	Provides data about fluid balance. Caretakers need to have understanding of importance of keeping accurate record.
	Monitor vital signs.	Decreasing BP, increasing pulse can indicate hypovolemic shock.
	Allow child to participate in usual activities as tolerated, but provide sufficient rest.	Excess fluid volume can deplete energy.

NURSING DIAGNOSIS *Imbalanced nutrition: less than body requirements related to decreased appetite*

Goals/Outcome Criteria	Nursing Interventions	Rationales
Child eats sufficient amounts to maintain usual growth	Provide a well-balanced diet; adequate protein and no added salt is recommended during acute phase.	A well-balanced diet is essential for growth and energy.
	Serve small quantities of favorite nutritious foods on brightly colored dishes; use colored straws.	Small quantities are not too overwhelming to a preschool child; interesting plates can often entice a reluctant child to eat.
	Encourage the child to eat with others.	Eating is a social process.
	Allow the child to choose foods with parent's help.	Encourages child's autonomy.

NURSING DIAGNOSIS *Risk for infection related to altered immunity*

Goals/Outcome Criteria	Nursing Interventions	Rationales
Child remains free of infection as evidenced by: • Normal body temperature • Intact skin with no redness or exudate • Normal respiratory function	Use meticulous handwashing.	Prevents spread of infectious organisms.
	Reduce contact with others who are ill.	Reduces opportunities to acquire an infection.
	Monitor vital signs.	Fever can indicate an underlying infectious process in the absence of other signs.
	Examine the skin at sites of punctures: wounds, IV, catheters.	Local redness, swelling can suggest infectious process.

Continued

NURSING CARE PLAN 12-1—cont'd

The Child with Nephrotic Syndrome—cont'd

Goals/Outcome Criteria	Nursing Interventions	Rationales
	Teach parent how to recognize and report signs of infection.	Many children with nephrosis are treated at home; parents need knowledge.
	Administer antibiotics as directed and for the entire period prescribed.	Used to treat infections.

NURSING DIAGNOSIS *Risk for impaired skin integrity related to pressure from edema.*

Goals/Outcome Criteria	Nursing Interventions	Rationales
Child's skin remains intact with no areas of redness or evidence of abnormal pressure	Bathe daily and clean diaper area as needed.	Reduces surface microorganisms, reduces action of acidic urine or feces on skin.
	Dry meticulously, particularly in skin folds; separate skin surfaces with cotton or clothing.	Moist areas are prime mediums for organism growth.
	Support edematous scrotal area with pad and t-binder.	Helps reduce pressure in the area.
	Turn and reposition frequently if child is on bed rest; use a pressure-equalizing mattress.	Prevents undue pressure in the same areas.
	Advise parent to avoid dressing the child in tight clothing.	Prevents chafing and skin irritation.

NURSING DIAGNOSIS *Ineffective coping related to stress of long-term remissions and relapses*

Goals/Outcome Criteria	Nursing Interventions	Rationales
Child and family describe adaptation to usual lifestyle.	Teach parents what to expect about the course of the illness.	Knowing what to expect increases control and decreases stress.
Child and family show stress-reducing strategies.	Teach management strategies, such as urine testing, monitoring for infection, skin care, daily weights, medication administration.	Participation in management increases coping.
Family promptly reports changes in the child's condition and complies with illness regimen.	Refer to social services or appropriate agency for financial help if needed.	Coping with illness is facilitated if financial worries are decreased.
	Allow family members to express concerns.	Listening and providing emotional support reduces stress.

? CRITICAL THINKING QUESTION

■ The mother of a 6-year-old with nephrotic syndrome is asking why her child is "so puffy." She also wants to know why her child is on prednisone and how long this needs to continue. How do you explain all of this to her? What discharge instructions need to be given to this mother?

---

in Chapter 10. The Centers for Disease Control and Prevention (2005) state that mental retardation is "characterized both by a significantly below-average score on a test of mental ability or intelligence and by limitations in the ability to function in areas of daily life, such as communication, self-care, and getting along in social situations and school activities." It requires a multidimensional approach; with appropriate support, the life of the person with mental retardation generally improves.

Mental retardation affects 2% to 3% of the population. According to Behrman et al. (2004), there are two overlapping populations of retarded children. There are those with mild mental retardation (approximately 85% of the population), which is associated with environmental influences, and those with severe mental retardation, which is associated more with biological causes. Some persons have a congenital malformation of the brain; others have had damage to the brain at a critical period in prenatal or postnatal development. Conditions that can develop during the prenatal period include PKU, Down syndrome, fetal alcohol syndrome, malformations of the brain (such as microcephaly, hydrocephalus, craniosynostosis), maternal infections,

Text continued on p. 270.

Table 12-7 *Communicable Diseases*

DISEASE	COMMUNICABILITY PERIOD AND ROUTE	CLINICAL MANIFESTATIONS	TREATMENT AND NURSING CARE	COMPLICATIONS
Anthrax *Incubation period:* Generally less than 2 wk for all forms; can be several months if *inhalational* anthrax *Causative agent:* *Bacillus anthracis* (an aerobic, gram-positive, encapsulated, spore-forming, nonmotile rod) Note: The anthrax vaccine is recommended for people at risk for repeated exposures to *B. anthracis* spores only and is not licensed for use in children.	No person-to-person transmission *Route:* Cutaneous (skin contact with spores or spore-contaminated materials), inhalational (inhalation of spores), and gastrointestinal (ingestion of contaminated meat)	Cutaneous: Pruritic papule or vesicle enlarges and ulcerates in 1-2 days, with subsequent formation of a central black eschar. Lesion is painless, with surrounding edema, hyperemia, and regional lymphadenopathy. Patients may have fever, malaise, and headache. Inhalational: Prodrome of fever, chills, nonproductive cough, chest pain, headache, myalgias, and malaise may occur initially; 2-5 days later, patients have hemorrhagic mediastinal lymphadenitis, hemorrhagic pleural effusion, bacteremia, and toxemia resulting in severe dyspnea, hypoxia, and septic shock. Radiograph shows widened mediastinum. Gastrointestinal: Intestinal form presents with nausea, anorexia, vomiting, fever, severe abdominal pain, massive ascites, hematemesis, and bloody diarrhea. Oropharyngeal form presents with oropharyngeal ulcers, neck swelling, sepsis. Can result in hemorrhagic meningitis.	Ciprofloxacin or doxycycline for all three forms initially; may combine with rifampin, vancomycin, imipenem, penicillin, ampicillin, clindamycin, chloramphenicol, and clarithromycin. Treatment should continue for at least 60 days. Ciprofloxacin or tetracycline are not routinely used to treat children but may be used for life-threatening infections. Standard precautions are used for hospitalized patients. Supportive care is used depending on the type of anthrax. Inhalational anthrax may require drainage of pleural effusions and is managed in the intensive care unit.	Fatality rates with treated cutaneous anthrax are less than 1%; however, mortality can exceed 50% with inhalational or gastrointestinal disease.
Chickenpox (varicella) *Incubation period:* 10-21 days *Causative agent:* Varicella-zoster virus	5 days after onset of rash and until all lesions are crusted *Route:* Airborne: droplet infection Direct or indirect contact Dry scabs are not infectious	General malaise, slight fever, anorexia, headache. Successive crops of macules, papules, vesicles, crusts. These may all be present at the same time. Itching of the skin. Generalized lymphadenopathy.	Oral acyclovir should be considered for otherwise healthy people at increased risk, such as people older than 12 yr of age, pulmonary disorders, etc. IV antiviral therapy is recommended for immunocompromised patients. Symptomatic. Prevent child from scratching. Keep fingernails short and clean. Sedation may be necessary. Use soothing lotions to allay itching. If secondary infections occur, antibiotics may be given. *Do not give aspirin* because of high risk for Reye syndrome. Salicylate therapy should be stopped in a child who is exposed to varicella.	Bacterial superinfection; thrombocytopenia, arthritis, encephalitis, nephritis, Reye syndrome (with aspirin use). See Box 12-2 for comparison of chickenpox and smallpox.

Continued

Table 12-7 Communicable Diseases—cont'd

DISEASE	COMMUNICABILITY PERIOD AND ROUTE	CLINICAL MANIFESTATIONS	TREATMENT AND NURSING CARE	COMPLICATIONS
Diphtheria *Incubation period:* 2-7 days or longer *Causative agent:* Corynebacterium diphtheriae	In untreated people, organisms can be present in discharges from the nose and throat and from eye and skin lesions for 2-6 wk after infection *Route:* Droplets from respiratory tract of infected person or carrier Contact with discharges from skin lesions	Local and systemic manifestations. Membrane over tissue in nose or throat at site of bacterial invasion. Hoarse, brassy cough with stridor. Toxin from organisms produces malaise and fever. Toxin has affinity for renal, nervous, and cardiac tissue.	A single dose (IV preferred) of equine antitoxin should be administered on the basis of clinical diagnosis, even before culture results are available (test for sensitivity to horse serum). Antimicrobial therapy with erythromycin or penicillin G procaine is given for 14 days in addition to antitoxin. Strict bed rest. Prevent exertion. Cleansing throat gargles may be ordered. Liquid or soft diet. Gavage or parenteral administration of fluids may become necessary. Observe for respiratory obstruction. Equipment for suctioning should be available. Oxygen and emergency tracheostomy may be necessary. Isolate.	Local infections: low grade fever with gradual onset. Serious complications include severe neck swelling (bull neck), upper airway obstruction, myocarditis, and peripheral neuropathies.
Epidemic influenza *Incubation period:* 1-4 days *Causative agent:* Virus	Not known, possibly during febrile stages *Route:* Airborne droplet infection, direct contact	Manifestations in respiratory tract. Sudden onset with chills, fever, muscle pains, cough. If infection is severe and spreads to lower respiratory tract, air hunger may develop.	Symptomatic. Provide bed rest and increased fluid intake. Antibiotics and sulfonamides may prevent secondary infection. Acetaminophen (antipyretic), drugs to control cough, and analgesics for pain may be given. *Do not give aspirin* because of high risk for Reye syndrome. Amantadine (antiviral medication) is approved for treatment in children 1 yr of age and older.	In severe cases, pulmonary edema and cardiac failure. Secondary invaders may produce bacterial infections of respiratory tract.
Erythema infectiosum (fifth disease) *Incubation period:* 4-14 days or longer *Causative agent:* Parvovirus B19	Uncertain *Route:* Infected persons	Three-stage rash: Erythema on face, mostly on cheeks (disappears in 1-4 days). 1 day after face rash, maculopapular red spots appear on upper and lower extremities, progressing proximal to distal; lacy appearance. Rash subsides but reappears if skin is irritated (sun, heat, cold); may last 1-3 wk. Child not contagious after rash appears.	Reinforce benign nature of the condition to parents. No treatment indicated. Exposed pregnant women should notify obstetrician. Avoid exposing children with sickle cell disease and immunosuppressed children.	Aplastic crisis in children with sickle cell anemia.

Disease / Incubation / Causative agent / Route	Clinical Manifestations	Therapeutic Management / Nursing	Comments / Complications
Exanthema subitum (roseola) Incubation period: 5-15 days Causative agent: Human herpesvirus type 6 Route: Unknown, primarily affects children less than 2 yr old	Persistent high fever for 3-4 days in child who appears well. Precipitous drop in fever to normal with appearance of rash. Rash: discrete rose-pink macules appearing first on trunk, then spreading to neck, face, and extremities. Nonpruritic, fades on pressure, lasts 1-2 days.	Antipyretics to control fever. Anticonvulsants for child who has history of febrile seizures. Teach parents measures for combating high temperature. Reinforce benign nature of illness.	Febrile seizures.
Hepatitis type A Incubation period: 15-50 days (average 30 days) Causative agent: Hepatitis A virus (HAV) Route: Few days before to 1 mo or more after onset. Oral contamination by intestinal excretions. Contaminated food, milk, or water. Hepatitis A is a major potential health problem in daycare centers	Manifestations occur rapidly and vary from mild to severe, from mild fever, anorexia, generalized malaise, nausea, vomiting, unpleasant taste in mouth, abdominal discomfort, and nonexistent or mild jaundice to severe jaundice, coma, and death. Early leukopenia is seen. Bile may be detected in urine; bowel movements are clay-colored. Liver function tests are useful for diagnosis.	Symptomatic. No specific therapy for uncomplicated HAV infection. Enteric precautions are necessary for 1 wk after onset of jaundice. Persons caring for those who are not toilet-trained, have diarrhea, or are incontinent should use disposable gloves when carrying fecal waste. Prevention: In daycare centers, thorough washing of hands after changing diapers and before preparing and serving food. Because HAV may survive on objects in the environment for weeks (e.g., infant changing tables), adequate environmental hygiene is essential. Children should be immunized at 1 yr (12-23 mo) of age. Administer immunoglobulin to contacts of affected child under 1 yr in a daycare setting.	Usually benign in children. Liver damage, recurrence of symptoms. May be a source of chromosomal damage.
Hepatitis type B Incubation period: 45-160 days (average 90 days) Causative agent: Hepatitis B virus (HBV) Route: Few days before to 1 mo or more after onset. Person-to-person by percutaneous introduction of blood, direct contact with secretions or blood contaminated with HBV; routine preexposure immunization recommended for all infants; appropriate immunoprophylaxis of infants born to HBsAg-positive women and infants born to women with unknown HBsAg status; some risk in children on hemodialysis, children receiving blood or blood products (including those with hemophilia), and IV drug users	Manifestations occur slowly. See hepatitis A for clinical manifestations.	Symptomatic. The child should be allowed to regulate own activity. Diet should be high-protein, high-calorie, high-carbohydrate, and low-fat. Food should be served in small, attractive, frequent feedings. Chief reasons for hospitalization are persistent vomiting and toxicity. Fluids may be given parenterally. Prevention: Universal immunization of infants and preteen children not immunized during infancy. Careful handling of blood and secretions; universal precautions.	Acute fulminating hepatitis characterized by rapidly rising bilirubin, encephalopathy, edema, ascites, and hepatic coma. Chronic HBV infected are at risk for serious liver disease including primary hepatocellular carcinoma (HCC) with advancing age.

Continued

Table 12-7 *Communicable Diseases—cont'd*

DISEASE	COMMUNICABILITY PERIOD AND ROUTE	CLINICAL MANIFESTATIONS	TREATMENT AND NURSING CARE	COMPLICATIONS
Hepatitis type B— cont'd			No specific therapy for acute HBV infection is available. HBIG and corticosteroids are not effective.	
Lyme disease *Incubation period:* 1-55 days *Causative agent:* *Borrelia burgdorferi*	Not communicable from person to person; patients with active disease should not donate blood *Route:* Spread by ticks; most common hosts are white-tailed deer and white-footed mice	Begins with a skin lesion at the site of a recent tick bite. The red macule expands to form a large papule with a raised border and a clear center. Systemic manifestations include malaise, lethargy, fever, headache, arthralgias, stiff neck, myalgias, and lymphadenopathy. Late manifestations involve the joints and the cardiac and neurological systems. Often first appears as single joint redness, swelling, and limitation.	Early treatment is doxycycline for children 8 yr and older. All ages: amoxicillin or cefuroxime. Later-stage disease is treated with high-dose IV ceftriaxone or penicillin. Prevention by teaching parents to observe for signs of disease during tick season. Protective clothing should be worn in areas where tick exposure is likely. Ticks should be removed.	Neurological complications, carditis, and chronic arthritis may develop. Transplacental infection has resulted in fetal death, prematurity, and congenital anomalies.
Measles (rubeola) *Incubation period:* 8-12 days *Causative agent:* Virus	From 4 days before to 5 days after rash appears *Route:* Direct contact Airborne by droplets and contaminated dust	Coryza, conjunctivitis, and photophobia are present before rash. Koplik spots in mouth, hacking cough, high fever, rash, and enlarged lymph nodes. Rash consists of small reddish brown or pink macules changing to papules; fades on pressure. Rash begins behind ears, on forehead or cheeks, progresses to extremities, and lasts about 5 days.	Symptomatic. Keep child in bed until fever and cough subside. Light in room should be dimmed. Keep hands from eyes. Irrigate eyes with physiologic saline solution to relieve itching. Tepid baths and soothing lotion relieve itching of skin. Encourage fluids during fever. Humidify the child's room. Antibacterial therapy given for complications. Vitamin A supplementation is recommended. Immunoglobulin can help prevent or modify measles within 6 days of exposure.	Vary with severity of disease: otitis media, pneumonia, tracheobronchitis, nephritis. Encephalitis may occur. Subacute sclerosing panencephalitis (SSPE), a rare degenerative central nervous system (CNS) disease, may occur. The mean incubation period is 7 yr after measles illness.
Measles, German (rubella) *Incubation period:* 14-23 days *Causative agent:* Virus	During prodromal period and for 5 days after appearance of rash *Route:* Direct contact with secretions of nose and throat of infected person Airborne by contaminated dust particles	Fetus may contract rubella in utero if mother has the disease; slight fever, mild coryza. Rash consists of small pink or pale red macules closely grouped to appear as scarlet blush that fades on pressure. Rash fades in 3 days. Swelling of posterior cervical and occipital lymph nodes. No Koplik spots or photophobia as in measles.	Symptomatic. Bed rest until fever subsides. Children should be excluded from school or daycare for 7 days after onset of rash. Infants with congenital rubella should be considered contagious until 1 yr old unless cultures are repeatedly negative.	Chief danger of disease is damage to fetus if mother contracts infection during first trimester of pregnancy. Neonate may have *congenital rubella syndrome* with permanent defects (cataracts, cardiovascular anomalies, deafness, microcephaly,

Disease / Causative agent	Transmission	Signs and symptoms	Treatment / Nursing care	Complications
Mumps (infectious parotitis) *Incubation period:* 16-18 days *Causative agent:* Virus	1-6 days before symptoms appear until swelling disappears *Route:* Direct or indirect contact with salivary secretions of infected person	Salivary glands are chiefly affected. Parotid, sublingual, and submaxillary glands may be involved. Swelling and pain occur in these glands either unilaterally or bilaterally. Child may have difficulty in swallowing, headache, fever, and malaise.	Local application of heat or cold to salivary glands to reduce discomfort. Liquids or soft foods are given. Foods containing acid may increase pain. Bed rest until swelling subsides. Children are excluded from school or daycare for 9 days from onset of parotid gland swelling. Mumps vaccine should be l given at east 2 wk before or 3 mo after administration of IG or blood transfusion.	mental retardation, etc.). Virus can be isolated from blood, urine, throat, cerebrospinal fluid, lens, and other involved organs. Infants may shed virus for 12-18 mo. Severe complications rare. Encephalitis may occur. Complications are less frequent in children than in adults. Meningoencephalitis, inflammation of ovaries or testes, or deafness may occur.
Pertussis (whooping cough) *Incubation period:* 7-10 days *Causative agent:* *Bordetella pertussis*	4-6 wk from onset *Route:* Direct contact Airborne by droplet spread from infected person	Begins with symptoms of upper respiratory tract infection. Coryza, dry cough, which is worse at night. Cough occurs in paroxysms of several sharp coughs in one expiration, then a rapid deep inspiration, followed by a whoop. Dyspnea and fever may be present. Vomiting may occur after coughing. Lymphocytosis occurs.	Symptomatic. Azithromycin is the drug of choice for treatment or prophylaxis of pertussis in infants younger than 1 mo of age. Erythromycin may limit communicability. Protect child from secondary infection. Erythromycin to household and daycare contacts. Primary or booster vaccination of exposed children under 7 yr. Provide mental and physical rest to prevent paroxysms of coughing. Provide warm, humid air. Oxygen may be necessary. Avoid chilling. Offer small, frequent feedings to maintain nutritional status. Refeed if child vomits. Small amounts of sedatives may be given to quiet the child. Most infants under 6 mo are hospitalized; intensive care may be required.	Very serious disease during infancy because of complication of bronchopneumonia. Otitis media, marasmus, bronchiectasis, and atelectasis may occur. Hemorrhage may occur during paroxysms of coughing. Encephalitis may occur.

Continued

Table 12-7 *Communicable Diseases—cont'd*

DISEASE	COMMUNICABILITY PERIOD AND ROUTE	CLINICAL MANIFESTATIONS	TREATMENT AND NURSING CARE	COMPLICATIONS
Poliovirus infection (poliomyelitis) *Incubation period:* 3-6 days *Causative agent:* Enteroviruses	During period of infection, latter part of incubation period, and first wk of acute illness *Route:* Oral contamination by pharyngeal and intestinal excretions	Acute illness. Initial symptoms of upper respiratory tract infection, headache, fever, vomiting. *Nonparalytic:* Previous symptoms plus sore or stiff muscles of neck, trunk, and extremities. Nuchal rigidity. *Paralytic:* Includes muscular paralysis. Clinical manifestations may vary from mild to very severe following symptomless period after initial symptoms.	Both parents and child need support and reassurance, for they are fearful of the term *polio.* Treatment and nursing care are symptomatic. Because oral polio vaccine is no longer available in the United States, the chance for exposure to vaccine-type polio is remote.	Emotional disturbances, gastric dilation, melena, hypertension or transitory paralysis of bladder may occur. Severe complications of paralytic polio include respiratory failure and permanent muscle deficits.
Rocky Mountain spotted fever *Incubation period:* 2-14 days *Causative agent:* *Rickettsia rickettsii*	Not communicable from person to person *Route:* Spreads by wood ticks or dog ticks from animals to humans (if tick is found, it should be removed without crushing)	Sudden onset of nonspecific symptoms: headache, fever, restlessness, anorexia. 1-5 days after onset, pale, discrete, rose-red macules or maculopapules appear mainly on distal extremities, including palms and soles.	Doxycycline is the drug of choice. Chloramphenicol or fluoroquinolone are also prescribed. The usual duration of therapy is 7-10 days. Avoidance of tick-infested areas is the best prevention.	CNS symptoms, electrolyte disturbances, peripheral circulatory collapse, and pneumonia may occur.
Smallpox (Variola) *Incubation period:* 7-17 days *Causative agent:* Virus (*variola*) NOTE: A smallpox vaccination plan has been implemented in the United States; however, the plan does not currently include immunization of children.	Patients are not infectious during the incubation period or febrile prodrome but become infectious with the onset of mucosal lesions, which occur within hours of the rash; the first week of rash illness is the most infectious period, although patients remain infectious until all scabs have separated *Route:* Droplets (from the oropharynx of infected individuals); may be transmitted from aerosol and direct contact with infected lesions, clothing, or bedding	Severe prodromal illness with high fever (generally 102° F-104° F [38.9° C-40.0° C]), malaise, severe headache, backache, abdominal pain, and prostration *(exhaustion),* lasting for 2-5 days. May include vomiting and seizures. The prodromal period is followed by lesions on the mucosa of the mouth or pharynx that last less than 24 hr before the onset of rash. The patient is considered infectious once the lesions appear. The rash begins on the face and spreads rapidly to the forearms, trunk, and legs in a centrifugal distribution. Many have lesions on the palms and soles (see Box 12-2). After 8-10 days, lesions begin to crust. Once all the lesions have separated (3-4 wk), the patient is no longer infectious.	Treatment is supportive. VIG (Vaccinia Immune Globulin) is used for certain complications of immunizations and has no role in treatment of smallpox. The vaccination may provide some protection against the disease if administered within 3-4 days of exposure. Patients are isolated in a private, airborne infection isolation room with negative pressure ventilation. *Anyone* entering the room must wear an N95 or higher-quality respirator, gloves, and gown even if there is a history of recent successful immunization. If the patient leaves the room, he or she should wear a mask and be covered with sheets or gowns to decrease the risk for possible transmission. Cidofovir has been suggested as having a role in smallpox therapy but no data are available.	Fatality rates reached 30% in the past; death occurred during the second week of illness from overwhelming viremia. The potential for modern supportive therapy in improving outcome is not known.

Streptococcal infection, group A betahemolytic (streptococcal sore throat, scarlet fever, scarlatina) Incubation period: 2-5 days Causative agent: Betahemolytic streptococci, Group A strains	Onset to recovery Route: Droplet infection Direct and indirect transmission may occur	Initial symptoms of streptococcal sore throat are seen in pharynx. The source of this organism may also be in a burn or wound. Toxin from site of infection is absorbed into bloodstream. The typical symptoms of scarlet fever are headache, fever, rapid pulse, rash, thirst, vomiting, lymphadenitis, and delirium. Throat is injected, and cellulitis of throat occurs. White tongue coating desquamates, and red strawberry tongue results. Other manifestations may include otitis media, mastoiditis, and meningitis.	Penicillin G is the drug of choice. Erythromycin is used for penicillin-sensitive individuals. Adequate fluid intake, bed rest, pain-relieving drugs, and mouth care are important. Diet should be given as the child wishes: liquid, soft, or regular. Warm saline throat irrigations may be given to the older child. Increased humidity for severe infection of upper respiratory tract. Cold or hot applications to painful cervical lymph nodes.	Complications are caused by toxins, the streptococci, or secondary infection. Complications of pneumonia, glomerulonephritis, or rheumatic fever may occur.

Modified from Marlow, D., & Redding, B. (1998). *Textbook of pediatric nursing.* Philadelphia: Saunders. Data from the American Academy of Pediatrics. (2006). *Red book.* Retrieved from *www.aapredbook.org.*

and anoxia. Birth injuries or anoxia during or shortly after delivery can also cause retardation. Diseases such as meningitis, lead poisoning, neoplasms, and encephalitis can cause mental retardation in a child or adult at any age. Other causes of retardation include near-drowning and traumatic brain injury. Heredity is a factor in mental retardation. It is also possible for children to live in such a physically and emotionally deprived environment that they become mentally retarded.

The American Association of Mental Retardation emphasizes both intelligence and behavior as criteria. Tests to measure intelligence are numerous. Intelligence is represented by intelligent quotient (IQ) scores obtained from standardized tests given by trained professionals. The IQ test score is generally 70 or below when the diagnosis of mental retardation is made. The IQ test is only one aspect in diagnosing mental retardation; significant limitations in adaptive behavior skills and evidence that the disability was present before age 18 years are two additional elements that are critical in determining the diagnosis (AAMR, 2002).

One test that is frequently given to children and adolescents is the Stanford-Binet Intelligence Scale. Intelligence tests differ somewhat, depending on the age of the subject. Intelligence testing of children is difficult to evaluate and is best done on an individual basis. Personality tests such as picture story tests, ink blot tests, drawing tests, and sentence-completion tests may also be administered. All such tests have their limitations and are subject to the abilities of the person interpreting them. Nonetheless, the tests are of value when used in conjunction with a thorough study of the child's physical, mental, emotional, and social development.

Signs and Symptoms

The diagnosis is determined after a thorough study by a team of experts, including a pediatrician, psychologist, psychiatrist, nurse, and social worker. Conditions such as epilepsy, cerebral palsy, severe malnutrition, emotional disturbances, blindness, deafness, and speech disorders must be ruled out.

Severe mental retardation might be noticeable at birth (see Data Cues), and the nursery nurse must be alert to cues. Early recognition in certain cases can lessen the disability. For example, routine testing of newborns for conditions such as PKU and congenital hypothyroidism allows for early treatment and facilitates normal intelligence.

Other symptoms are associated with landmarks of the growth process. A child who does not smile, sit,

---

Box 12-2 | *Differentiating Chickenpox from Smallpox*

Chickenpox (varicella) is the most likely condition to be confused with smallpox. In chickenpox:

- Lesions are superficial vesicles (smallpox has deep-seated, hard/firm vesicles or pustules)
- Lesions appear in crops; on any one part of the body there are lesions in different stages (papules, vesicles, crusts; smallpox has lesions that evolve from macules to papules to pustules over days, with each stage lasting 1 to 2 days)
- Greatest concentration of lesions on the trunk; fewest on distal extremities (smallpox lesions are greatest on face and distal extremities)
- First lesions appear on the face or trunk (smallpox lesions first appear on oral mucosa, face, forearms)
- Palms and soles rarely involved (smallpox lesions are on palms and soles)
- No fever or mild fever before rash (smallpox has fever exceeding 101° F (38.3° C) 1 to 4 days before rash, with headache, backache, chills, vomiting, or severe abdominal pain)
- Patient lacks history of varicella or varicella vaccination

Data from Department of Health and Human Services, Centers for Disease Control and Prevention. Atlanta, GA (2002).

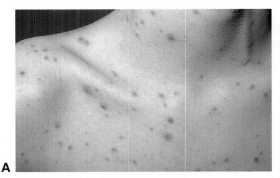
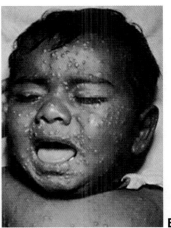

FIGURE **12-11** **A,** Lesions of chickenpox. **B,** Lesions of smallpox.

climb stairs, stand, or walk within the usual age limits might be retarded, although these signs can be caused by other problems. A child may also be slow in speech, in learning self-care, or in toilet training. Unusual clumsiness and failure to respond to stimuli are early indications. Sometimes this disability is not discovered until the child enters school.

Even though children with mental retardation are often categorized by IQ levels, each child must be frequently reevaluated according to individual progress. Many children who have received early intervention beginning in infancy outperform all expectations. A plan for each child should be devised to maximize the child's potential.

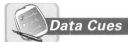

Data Cues

Signs Suggesting Cognitive Disability in Newborns and Infants

- Failure to suck
- Feeding difficulties
- Spasticity
- Convulsions
- Listlessness, irritability
- Floppy, hypotonic muscles
- Decreased alertness
- Unresponsive to eye contact
- Unusual clumsiness
- Jaundice
- Unusual-looking stools
- Unusual odor to urine
- Enlarged tongue
- Asian appearance in white infants
- Stubby fingers or toes
- Failure to achieve developmental milestones (smiling, rolling over, sitting, etc.)

Treatment and Nursing Care

Developmentally disabled infants should be started in infant stimulation programs as soon as possible. Nurses need to recognize that the pace of development is slower than that for the child without a disability. These children also lack the ability to think abstractly, so they have difficulty transferring learning from one situation to another. They learn by habit formation, which involves routine, repetition, and relaxation. Nurses working with these children must have a good understanding of the growth and developmental process. It is important that the child show a **readiness** for the task, whether it is toilet training, feeding self, or dressing. The atmosphere should be one of friendliness, and directions should be kept simple.

The nurse caring for developmentally disabled children in the hospital needs to know each child's stage of maturation and abilities. A detailed history, including a habit and care sheet, is completed. Self-help activities are documented.

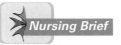

Nursing Brief

A list of words, sounds, and gestures, along with their meanings, posted on the developmentally disabled child's bed aids personnel in communicating with the patient.

Communicating with the patient may be difficult. It is important to follow home routines as closely as possible. The progress the child has made should not be allowed to slip during hospitalization. Good communication between parents and nurse helps make the transition from home to hospital as smooth as possible for the child.

Communication Alert

In obtaining information about the child from the parents, a positive approach is recommended. A request such as "Tell me about Gina's eating habits" is preferable to "Does Gina feed herself?" and is likely to yield more helpful information.

Developmentally disabled children are referred for early intervention as soon as possible after diagnosis. The American Association on Mental Retardation (AAMR) *supports* approach evaluates the specific needs of the individual and focuses on strategies and services that optimize individual functioning. *Supports* are defined as the resources and individual strategies necessary to promote individual development of the person with mental retardation. Support areas include home living, education, human development, community living, employment, health and safety, behavior, social, and protection and advocacy (AAMR, 2002).

The current trend in dealing with developmentally disabled children is to "mainstream" them into public schools and society with the support system described previously. In 1975, the U.S. Congress passed the Education for All Handicapped Children Act (PL 94-142), which guarantees the right of developmentally disabled persons and other disabled persons to receive appropriate education at public expense. Developmentally disabled children who are being educated in the public schools have individual educational plans that delineate services and specific educational adaptations to meet their needs. Many communities also have sheltered workshops in which developmentally disabled adults can work. These centers provide an opportunity for individuals to be more independent and increase their self-esteem. All children benefit from having developmentally disabled children interacting with them on a daily basis.

Like other children, developmentally disabled children must have limits set on behavior. The adult must be firm and consistent. Correction must directly follow any offense. Love, liberal praise, respect, and infinite patience are essential in helping developmentally disabled children to develop to fullest capacity.

The parents of a developmentally disabled child need support, compassion, and understanding, not pity. For nurses to work effectively with the child and the family, they must face their own feelings and develop a positive attitude. Sharing ideas and feelings with experienced professionals who work with developmentally disabled individuals helps nurses acquire enthusiasm for what these children and families can accomplish.

The problems confronting the parents usually become more complicated as the child develops physically and chronologically but still requires constant supervision. Puberty can be a particularly difficult period. Some parents make the decision that they are no longer able to care for their child adequately at home. The decision to institutionalize the child is a difficult one. Many things must be taken into consideration, such as the health of the parents, the effect on other children in the family, the community services available, and the financial status of the family. Even when the decision is made, there are long waiting lists in many places. Facilities are overcrowded, and the tendency is to take those who are most severely developmentally disabled first.

It is important that nurses be familiar with the resources in their communities so that they can direct the family to them. The local chapter of the National Association for Retarded Citizens (ARC of the United States) can provide information and support. The child guidance clinic or the psychological services of a nearby college or hospital may be tapped. The visits of the public health nurse are invaluable in many cases. Patients also may be eligible to obtain help from their local vocational and rehabilitation agency. Respite care workers afford needed rest and increased mobility for parents. In some communities, parent groups meet to discuss mutual problems. Arrangements for proper dental health must be made.

Developmentally disabled children can participate readily in recreational programs with supervision. The Special Olympics program, for example, facilitates participation in various individual and team sports. The enthusiasm of the children and volunteers in this program is overwhelming.

Community Cue

Nurses play a primary role in preventing mental retardation through educating the community about environmental dangers, teaching pregnant women about appropriate nutrition and prenatal care, and educating parents and children about injury prevention.

Key Points

- Minor burns can usually be handled at home. Major burns need to be handled by a hospital burn unit.

- Children with amblyopia or strabismus should be recognized early. Correction is necessary to prevent potential loss of vision.
- Support groups such as the Ronald McDonald House can aid the family of the child with leukemia face significant family stressors.
- The focus of care for the child with hemophilia has shifted toward home care. Many children are treated for bleeding episodes at home by their family or with self-administration of clotting factors.
- Bleeding after a tonsillectomy can be identified by frequent swallowing, restlessness, fast thready pulse, and vomiting of bright red blood.
- Celiac disease is managed through dietary restrictions. All gluten is to be removed from the diet.
- Maintaining activity and mobility for as long as possible is an essential nursing goal for children with Duchenne muscular dystrophy.
- Encephalitis is an inflammation of the brain tissue. The child may be at risk for residual neurological problems such as seizures.
- Education of parents with children having recurrent seizures involves understanding appropriate interventions during a seizure, proper medication administration, and family coping mechanisms.
- Several factors contribute to the incidence of UTIs in children; one of the most common is VUR.
- Acute poststreptococcal glomerulonephritis is caused by an untreated strep infection.
- Management of nephrotic syndrome includes reducing loss of proteins in the urine, decreasing edema, and preventing infection.
- Nursing interventions in the treatment of communicable diseases are focused on identification, prevention of transmission, providing comfort, and prevention of complications.
- Nurses today need to be aware of indications of bioterrorism, including signs and symptoms of anthrax and smallpox.
- Early intervention using infant stimulation programs is essential in the care of children who are developmentally disabled.

 Go to your Companion CD-ROM for an Audio Glossary, video clips, and more.

evolve Be sure to visit the companion Evolve site at http://evolve.elsevier.com/Price/pediatric/ for WebLinks and additional resources.

ONLINE RESOURCES

American Association on Mental Retardation: http://www.aamr.org

American Burn Association: http://www.ameriburn.org/

Centers for Disease Control and Prevention: http://www.cdc.gov/

Hemophilia One is a patient resource website: http://www.hemophiliaone.com/

National Association for Retarded Citizens (ARC of the United States): http://www.thearc.org/

evolve http://evolve.elsevier.com/Price/pediatric/

Upon completion of this chapter, the student will be able to:

1. Define the vocabulary terms listed
2. Describe the physical and psychosocial development of children from 6 to 12 years, listing, where appropriate, age-specific events and types of guidance
3. Discuss how to assist parents in preparing a child for school entry
4. List two ways in which school life influences the growing child
5. Identify the positive and negative aspects of television viewing and playing video games
6. Discuss safety issues related to the school-age child
7. Plan a diet that provides adequate nutrition for the school-age child

Key Terms

Be sure to check out the bonus material on the Companion CD-ROM, including selected audio presentations.

latchkey children (p. 284)
latency
myelinization (MĪ-ĕ-lĭ-nĭ-ZĀ-shŭn; p. 273)
sibling rivalry (p. 273)

GENERAL CHARACTERISTICS AND DEVELOPMENT

School-age children, from ages 6 to 12 years, differ from preschool children in that they are more engrossed in fact than fantasy. They have an ardent thirst for knowledge and accomplishment. They admire teachers and adult companions whom they consider wise. They attempt to use the skills and the knowledge that they obtain to master activities that they enjoy—music, sports, art, and so on. Children in school learn that they must cooperate with others. Participation in group activities increases. Acceptance becomes paramount. The type of acceptance these children receive at home and at school affects the attitudes that they develop about themselves and their roles in life.

Children at this age are aware that their parents are only human and can make mistakes. Conflicts may arise, particularly if what the child learns in school differs from what is practiced at home. Between the ages of 6 and 12 years, children prefer friends of their own gender. They also prefer the company of their friends to that of their brothers and sisters. They find outward displays of affection by adults embarrassing. Sibling rivalry, intense feelings that can develop when a child feels he or she is competing for parental attention, can develop when a new infant sibling joins the family unit.

PHYSICAL GROWTH

Growth is slow until the spurt, which occurs directly before puberty. Weight gains are more rapid than increases in height. The average gain in weight per year is about $5\frac{1}{2}$ to 7 pounds, or 2.5 to 3.2 kg. The average yearly increase in height is approximately 2 inches, or 5.5 cm. Head circumference increases only 2 to 3 cm throughout this entire period. This reflects slowed brain growth with complete brain growth occurring at 10 years of age. Myelinization, the growth process of the myelin sheath around the nerve fiber, is complete by 7 years of age and results in the refinement of fine motor coordination (Behrman et al., 2004).

Muscular coordination is improved, and the lymphatic tissues become highly developed. The skeletal bones continue to ossify. The body is supple, and sometimes skeletal growth is more rapid than the growth of muscles and ligaments. The child may appear gangling. There is a noticeable change in facial structure as the jaw lengthens. The sinuses are frequently sites of infection. Sinus headaches may occur. The 6-year molars (the first permanent teeth) erupt. The gastrointestinal tract is more mature. The heart grows slowly and is now smaller in proportion to body size than compared with any other point in time.

The shape of the eye also changes with growth. The exact age at which 20/20 vision occurs is subject to discussion. Before research done in the 1970s, it was generally thought that visual acuity did not reach an adult level until age 7 years or later. The best evidence that is currently available indicates that 20/30 vision is achieved by age 3 years and 20/20 vision by age 4 years (Behrman et al., 2004). This rather drastic revision is a result of new and improved techniques regarding measurement. The capabilities of the child's sense organs, including hearing, have an important bearing on learning abilities.

The vital signs of the school-age child are similar to those of the adult. Temperature is 98.6° F (37° C), pulse is 85 to 100 per minute, and the respiratory rate is 18 to 24 per minute. The systolic blood pressure ranges from 96 to 107 mm Hg, and the diastolic from 57 to 66 mm Hg. (Refer to Chapter 3 for additional information on vital signs.) Boys are slightly taller and somewhat heavier than girls until changes indicating puberty appear. The differences among children are greater at the end of middle childhood than at the beginning.

Language skills continue to develop. School-age children speak in full sentences. They continually add new words to their vocabulary. School-age children may swear to try and impress other children or to express anger. They also delight in the newly found use of humor. In the early school-age years, they delight their parents by telling "knock-knock" jokes.

In evaluating language development, the parent and the nurse should discuss the child's ability to comprehend and use both written and spoken language.

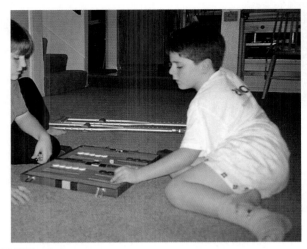

FIGURE **13-1** Competition can be common in the school years. Games can also assist in sharpening a child's cognitive skills.

energy is directed toward cognitive and physical skills. This, however, does not imply a complete lack of sexual activity at this age.

DEVELOPMENTAL THEORIES

According to Piaget (cognitive development), the school-age child thinks and reasons in concrete terms, progressing from inductive to deductive logic. Children at this age learn to comprehend the ideas of conservation and reversibility. Conservation is the ability to recognize two equal quantities regardless of their form. For example, although the same amount of water appears less in a tall glass than in a short glass, the school-age child can determine that it is the same amount of water. Reversibility is the ability to think in either direction. School-age children can take a result and reverse it so as to determine whether it is correct or not. This concept is used in addition and subtraction.

According to Erik Erikson's theories of psychosocial development, the school-age child is in the stage of industry versus inferiority. The child is a worker and producer and wants to accomplish tasks. Competitiveness is common (Figure 13-1). The school-age child's social world is continually expanding, and he or she achieves new competencies. However, without success in this area, they feel inferior. Parents and teachers need to support children in achieving success and developing self-esteem.

Kohlberg (moral development) describes the school-age child as being at the "conventional level." Rules are the basis for moral judgments, and they must be followed to please others. The school-age child begins to understand what is right and what is wrong. As a result, the child develops a conscience.

Freud believes that at this stage romantic love for the parent of the opposite gender diminishes and that the children start to identify with the parent of the same gender. This is also a period of **latency** when the child's

BIOLOGICAL AND PSYCHOSOCIAL DEVELOPMENT

Table 13-1 summarizes growth and development for the various school-age groups.

THE 6-YEAR-OLD

Six-year-old children are bursting with energy and are always on the go. They soon become overtired, and it is necessary to set limits to their activities. Although they like to start tasks, they do not always finish them because their attention span is fairly brief. They tend to be bossy and sometimes rude, but they are sensitive to criticism. Sex investigations begun in earlier years may persist. Their conscience is active, and they find it difficult to make decisions.

One of the most obvious physical changes at this age is the loss of the temporary teeth. The important 6-year molars also erupt. Six-year-old children can jump rope, throw and catch a ball, and tie shoelaces. They perform numerous other feats that require muscle coordination. Their language differs from that of the preschool child. These children use language for a purpose rather than for the pure joy of talking. Their vocabulary consists of about 2500 words. They need 11 to 13 hours of sleep a night.

Although 6-year-old children begin to show a preference for associating with children of the same gender, boys and girls do still play together at this age. Certain activities, such as imaginative play, are common to both genders. Most children enjoy collecting objects that catch their fancy, such as leaves, stones, and shells. Play at this time usually reflects events that occur in the immediate environment.

Table 13-1 | *Growth and Development During School-Age*

AGE (YR)	PHYSICAL AND MOTOR	MENTAL	ADAPTIVE	PERSONAL-SOCIAL
6	Growth and weight gain continues slowly Weight: 16 to 23.6 kg (35.5 to 53 lb); height: 106.6 to 123.5 cm (42 to 48 in) Central mandibular incisors erupt Loses first tooth Gradual increase in dexterity Active age; constant activity Often returns to finger feeding More aware of hand as a tool Likes to draw, print, and color Vision reaches maturity	Develops concept of numbers Counts 13 pennies Knows whether it is morning or afternoon Defines common objects such as fork and chair in terms of their use Obeys triple commands in succession Knows right and left hands Says which is pretty and which is ugly in a series of drawings of faces Describes objects in a picture rather than simply enumerating them Attends first grade	At table, uses knife to spread butter or jam on bread At play, cuts, folds, pastes paper toys, sews crudely if needle is threaded Takes bath without supervision; performs bedtime activities alone Reads from memory; enjoys oral spelling game Likes table games, checkers, simple card games Giggles a lot Sometimes steals money or attractive items Has difficulty owning up to misdeeds Tries out own abilities	Can share and cooperate better Has great need for children of own age Cheats to win Often engages in rough play Often jealous of younger brother or sister Does what adults are seen doing May have occasional temper tantrums Is a boaster Is more independent, probably influence of school Has own way of doing things Increases socialization
7	Begins to grow at least 5 cm (2 in) a yr Weight: 17.7-30 kg (39-66½ lb); height: 111.8-129.7 cm (44-51 in) Maxillary central incisors and lateral mandibular incisors erupt More cautious in approaches to new performances Repeats performances to master them Jaw begins to expand to accommodate permanent teeth	Notices that certain parts are missing from pictures Can copy a diamond Repeats three numbers backward Develops concept of time; reads ordinary clock or watch correctly to nearest quarter hour; uses clock for practical purposes Attends the second grade More mechanical in reading; often does not stop at the end of a sentence, skips words such as "it," "the," and "he"	Uses table knife for cutting meat; may need help with tough or difficult pieces Brushes and combs hair acceptably without help May steal Likes to help and have a choice Is less resistant and stubborn	Is becoming a real member of the family group Takes part in group play Boys prefer playing with boys; girls prefer playing with girls Spends a lot of time alone; does not require a lot of companionship
8-9	Continues to grow at 5 cm (2 in) a yr Weight: 19.6-39.6 kg (43-87 lb); height: 117-141.8 cm (46-56 in) Lateral incisors (maxillary) and mandibular cuspids erupt Movement fluid; often graceful and poised Always on the go; jumps, chases, skips Increased smoothness and speed in fine motor control; uses cursive writing Dresses self completely Likes to overdo; hard to quiet down after recess	Gives similarities and differences between two things from memory Counts backward from 20 to 1; understands concept of reversibility Repeats days of the week and months in order; knows the date Describes common objects in detail, not merely their use	Makes use of common tools such as hammer, saw, or screwdriver Uses household and sewing utensils Helps with routine household tasks such as dusting, sweeping Assumes responsibility for share of household chores Looks after all of own needs at table Buys useful articles; exercises some choice in making purchases	Is easy to get along with at home Likes the reward system Dramatizes Is more sociable Is better behaved Is interested in boy-girl relationships but does not admit it Goes about home and community freely, alone or with friends Likes to compete and play games Shows preference in friends and groups Plays mostly with groups of own gender but is beginning to mix

Continued

Table 13-1	*Growth and Development During School-Age—cont'd*			
AGE (YR)	**PHYSICAL AND MOTOR**	**MENTAL**	**ADAPTIVE**	**PERSONAL-SOCIAL**
8-9 cont'd	More limber; bones grow faster than ligaments	Makes change out of a quarter Attends third and fourth grades Reads more; may plan to wake up early just to read Reads classic books but also enjoys comics More aware of time; can be relied on to get to school on time Can grasp concepts of parts and whole (fractions) Understands concepts of space, cause and effect Classifies objects by more than one quality; has collections Produces simple paintings or drawings	Runs useful errands Likes pictorial magazines Likes school, wants to answer all the questions Is afraid of failing a grade; is ashamed of bad grades Is more critical of self Takes music and sport lessons	Develops modesty Compares self with others Enjoys Scouts, group sports
10-12	Weight: 24.3-58 kg (54-128 lb); height: 127.5-162.3 cm (50-64 in) Posture is more similar to an adult's; overcomes lordosis Boys: Slow growth in height and rapid weight gain; may become obese in this period Girls: Pubescent changes may begin to appear; body lines soften and round out Remainder of teeth erupt and tend toward full development (except wisdom teeth)	Writes brief stories Attends fifth to seventh grades Writes occasional short letters to friends or relatives on own initiative Uses telephone for practical purposes Responds to magazine, radio, or other advertising Reads for practical information or own enjoyment (stories or library books of adventure or romance or animal stories)	Makes useful articles or does easy repair work Cooks or sews in small way Raises pets Washes and dries own hair Is responsible for a thorough job of cleaning hair, but may need reminding to do so Is sometimes left alone at home for an hour or so Is successful in looking after own needs or those of other children left in his or her care	Loves friends; talks about them constantly Chooses friends more selectively; may have a "best friend" Enjoys conversation Develops beginning interest in opposite gender Is more diplomatic Likes family; family really has meaning Likes mother and wants to please her in many ways Demonstrates affection Likes father who is adored and idolized Respects parents

From Hockenberry, M.J., & Wilson, D. (2007). *Wong's nursing care of infants and children* (8th ed.). St. Louis: Mosby.

Six-year-old children need time and support to help them adjust to school. If they have nursery school or kindergarten experience, the transition may be more comfortable. Most children go to school expecting the same atmosphere they are accustomed to at home. For example, if parents are critical or overly protective, children automatically assume that the teacher will be too. When the experience at school differs markedly from their expectations, they feel insecure and may be hostile toward the teacher. Parents need to observe children for signs of fatigue and stress. Although they have reached the appropriate age, not all children are ready for school. Children who are ready for school still need time and support from parents and teachers before they can settle down and become completely comfortable in the classroom. At school, the child is also exposed more frequently to infection. Preschool immunizations and a physical examination are indicated.

THE 7-YEAR-OLD

Children at 7 years are generally less of a problem than they were at 6 years. It is a quieter age, and the child does not go looking for trouble. Some educators have noted that second graders are the easiest to teach. They

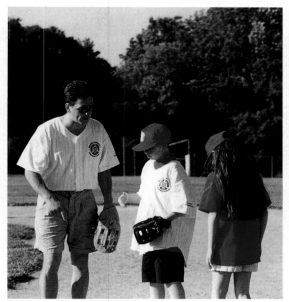

FIGURE **13-2** Organized activities provide both genders with physical and emotional outlets.

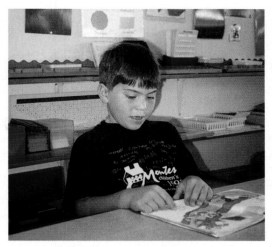

FIGURE **13-3** Reading can become an enjoyable activity. It should be encouraged.

set high standards for themselves and for their family, have a good sense of humor, tend to enjoy teasing (wiggle loose teeth to annoy adults), and are a little more modest than they were at an earlier age. They enjoy being active but can also appreciate periods of rest. The second grader may acquire a "crush" on a friend of the opposite gender.

These children know the months and seasons of the year. They also begin to tell time. They have a beginning concept of arithmetic, can count by twos and fives, and know that money is valuable. Their hands are steadier. Interest in God and heaven is heightened.

Active play is still important to both genders (Figure 13-2). The boys are more apt to tease the girls than to participate in such games as jump rope or tag. Both genders enjoy bike riding and table games. Realistic toys, such as dolls that can be bathed and fed or trains that back up and whistle, appeal to the 7-year-old. Comic books are also popular (Figure 13-3). Becoming increasingly independent, these children imagine themselves accomplishing feats more adventurous than those of their parents. They cannot understand why Mom and Dad lead such dull lives.

Stealing

Stealing is one problem that may arise during this age. This is generally a sign that some need of the child is not being met. It may be actual or perceived. In many cases, the child steals only to distribute the loot to neighborhood friends. This may in actuality be an attempt to buy friendship. The children's independence has separated them to a degree from their parents. As a result, if they cannot establish good relationships with their friends, they may feel left out. When children steal something, parents should

tell them that they are aware of the fact and should insist on some form of restitution. They should not humiliate the child, but they must make it clear that such actions are not permitted. As always, accept the child but not the deed. Afterward, try to understand the circumstances that are causing such behavior.

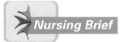
Nursing Brief

Before the age of 3 years, small children frequently take things that do not belong to them. This is not stealing because the child does not know any better.

THE 8–YEAR-OLD

The 8-year-old wants to do everything and can play alone for longer periods than a 7-year-old. Work is usually creative. Group activities such as Brownies and Cub Scouts are enjoyed, and companions of the same gender are preferred. Group fads begin to appear. Eight-year-olds like to be considered important, particularly by adults. They may behave better for company than for the family. Hero worship is evident.

The arms and hands of the 8-year-old seem to grow faster than the rest of the body. The large and small muscles are better developed, and movements are smoother and more graceful. The child can write rather than only print. The child also understands that a certain number of days must pass before special events, such as Christmas, birthdays, or discharge from the hospital, can occur.

Competitive sports are enjoyed, but the child is generally a poor loser. Long involved arguments occur over decisions made by referees. Wrestling is frequent, and dramatic play is popular. Most children like to be the hero or heroine of their favorite program. Neighborhood secret clubs are organized, and all members must pay strict attention to the rules.

THE 9-YEAR-OLD

The 9-year-old is dependable and is not as restless as the 8-year-old child. More interest is shown in family activities, and more responsibility is assumed for personal belongings and for younger brothers and sisters. Tasks are also more likely to be completed. Children resist adult authority if it does not coincide with their opinions or ideals. They are, however, more able to accept criticism regarding their actions. Individual differences are pronounced.

Worries and mild compulsions are common. Children avoid cracks in the pavement: "Step on a crack, break your mother's back." They realize that these actions are senseless but still feel obliged to repeat them. Nervous habits may also appear and may widely vary; nail biting is one example. The child should not be scolded for such actions because they are caused primarily by tension. The nervous habits usually disappear once home and social life become more relaxed.

Hand-eye coordination is well developed and manual activities are managed with skill. The child works and plays hard and often becomes overtired. About 10 hours of sleep a night are needed. The permanent teeth are still erupting.

Competitive sports, reading, listening to music, and watching television and movies are popular. Contact sports should be limited to minimize permanent growth-related injuries (Figure 13-4). The child begins to develop interests such as music and may desire to take lessons. Children know the date, can repeat months of the year in order, can multiply, and do simple division. They take care of their bodily needs, and by now table manners have considerably improved.

THE 10-YEAR-OLD

This marks the beginning of the preadolescent years. Girls are more physically mature than boys. The child begins to show self-direction, is courteous to adults, and thinks quite clearly about social problems and prejudices. Although 10-year-olds want to be independent and resent being told what to do, they are receptive to suggestion. The ideas of the group are more important than individual ideas. Interest in sex and sex investigations continue.

Girls are often more poised than boys. Both genders are fairly reliable about household duties. Slang terms are used. The 10-year-old can write for a relatively long period of time and maintains a good writing speed. The child uses fractions and knows numbers over 100. Boys and girls begin to identify themselves with skills that pertain to their particular gender role. There is an intolerance of the opposite gender. The play enjoyed by the 10-year-old is similar to that enjoyed by the 9-year-old. In addition, the child takes more interest in appearance.

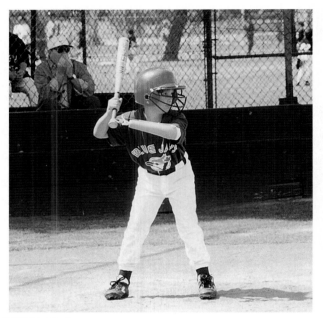

FIGURE **13-4** The child should be allowed to explore and participate in a variety of activities.

THE 11- TO 12-YEAR-OLD PERIOD

Adjectives that describe this age group include intense, observant, all-knowing, energetic, meddlesome, and argumentative. This period before the onset of puberty is one of complete disorganization. It may begin earlier in some children than others because the onset and rate of physical maturity greatly vary. Before the end of this period, the hormones of the body begin to influence physical growth. Posture is poor. There are 24 to 26 permanent teeth.

The child has an overabundance of energy and is constantly on the go. Girls become "tomboyish" in their actions. Table manners are a thing of the past, and the refrigerator is constantly emptied. Children this age are less concerned with appearance. They seem to be preoccupied a great deal of the time. This, along with physical activities and numerous anxieties, partially accounts for the decline in school grades. Ability to concentrate decreases, and parents complain that the children "never hear anything." When asked to do a new task, they moan and groan.

Groups of friends are still important (Figure 13-5). They are not ready to stand alone, but they cannot bear the thought of depending on their parents. They insist that they must overcome their problems without parental help. Their attitude implies, "Can't you see that I'm not a child anymore?"

The older school-age child also begins to see and understand other points of view. Morals and religious ideals become stronger. They begin to play with abstract ideas and become interested in the "whys" of health measures. They understand human reproduction. During prepuberty, they are very much interested in the body and watch for signs of

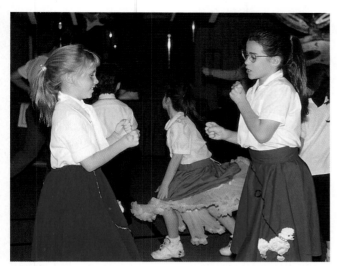

FIGURE **13-5** The school-age child relies on friends for advice. They are not always ready to ask parents to help with problem solving.

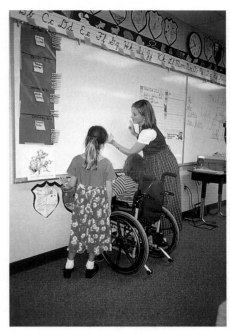

FIGURE **13-6** The school environment can provide the child with the opportunity to interact with children who have different backgrounds. For the child with a chronic condition, school can provide the opportunity to develop social and cognitive skills.

growing up. Girls look forward to menstruation and wearing their first bra. Boys and girls tend to ignore those of the opposite gender, but in reality they are much aware of them. There is a tendency to tease one another. Their descriptions of each other are far from complimentary: "stupid," "crazy," "nerd." Both genders enjoy earning money by doing odd jobs. Preadolescents often seek an adult friend of the same gender to idolize.

Guiding preadolescents is not easy. The primary task of the middle years of childhood is developing social competence. Parents and authority figures need to help children learn how to get along with peers and how to follow group rules. They need to set limits and establish consequences for unacceptable behavior. They also need to monitor television shows, video games, and music lyrics. Parents need to encourage self-discipline and teach young children to respect authority figures. School-age children need freedom within limits and recognition that they are no longer babies. They should know why parents make a decision. They should not be expected to blindly follow household rules. Their conscience enables them to understand and accept reasonable discipline. Constant verbal nagging is ignored. These children should be provided with constructive opportunities that enable them to get rid of pent-up emotions and energies. Their irritating behavior is more easily accepted once one realizes that a good deal of it is indeed "just a phase."

Community Cue

Anticipatory guidance at the school-age well checkup includes topics such as sex education, nutrition, physical activity, and injury prevention.

ENVIRONMENTAL INFLUENCES

SCHOOL

Schools have a profound influence on the socialization of children. Children bring to school what they have learned and experienced in the home. Although some children come from healthy intact families that are financially secure, many do not. Children themselves may be physically disabled, developmentally disabled, or abused; others may have a chronic illness (Figure 13-6). Parents may be unemployed or abusers of alcohol or other drugs or may have numerous other physical or stress-related conditions. In addition, children may be unable to verbalize their needs; therefore caretakers must become particularly astute in their observations. Even though children may seem similar, what each one is able to absorb intellectually is directly related to their emotional health and, more often than not, to the emotional health of the family. Schools reflect the social values and the economic standing of the community that supports them. If a community has various ethnic and economic groups, conflicts may appear in the schools. School-age children are exposed to many adults and peers whose values and expectations may be different from what they have experienced. In addition, children can no longer be protected from prejudices regarding beliefs, color, or ethnic background. The teacher becomes an important role model for the child. The child is influenced by the teacher and by fellow students. The sensitive nurse can assist parents by affirming the individuality of children. The nurse should encourage parents to tell their children how proud they are of their academic progress.

School can be stressful for children, especially when they are first starting school or are changing schools. In these situations, parents and teachers need to be supportive of the child. It is also important that parents take an active role in their child's education by getting to know the child's teachers, volunteering in the school, and informing the teachers if there are unusual or sudden stressors in the child's life. Children who are starting school should be introduced to the crossing guard if they walk to school or to the bus driver if they ride the bus. Initially, they should also be supervised at the bus stop. School-age children should know their home phone number and address.

By the time a child reaches middle school, anticipatory guidance includes dealing with sex education, peer abuse, organization of time, and the increased hazards of substance abuse. The nurse can assess patterns of communication between the parents and the child and can assist with specific behavioral problems. Parents may have a problem letting go. The nurse can be supportive of their endeavors as long as they are in accordance with the child's maturity. The transition to junior high/middle school generally means multiple classrooms, a series of teachers, and a change of buildings. The child is developing adult characteristics and has new feelings about the body, parents, teachers, and peers. Anticipatory guidance includes a review of normal physiology and how it changes with puberty. Information concerning sexuality is reviewed, and the child is encouraged to ask questions whenever they arise. A warm, ongoing relationship between parents and child helps to provide a safe atmosphere of caring. Adults should develop a heightened awareness for such things as school attendance problems, tardiness, and signs of loneliness or depression. Parents should continue to encourage their children to discuss any school problems and worries with them. It is important to foster the child's ability to communicate with teachers, parents, and other authoritative figures. School-age children need to learn to understand what is right and what is wrong. They also need to learn how to manage anger and resolve conflicts without violence. It is important that parents and children set realistic goals. Adults should periodically ask themselves, "When was the last time this child had a success?" Homework should be the child's responsibility, with minimum assistance from parents.

Gender

Children may face other problems in school. Research has identified that boys receive more praise than girls. Boys tend to get negative feedback concerning the quality of work such as neatness or spelling. On the other hand, girls get negative feedback about the content of their work. This causes boys to feel that their lack of success is from a lack of effort, and girls

feel that their failure is from a lack of ability. Teachers, therefore, need to be more aware of possible biases. They also need to focus their attention on efforts, not gender.

BULLYING

Bullying is a problem for a staggering number of children in elementary and middle school. A reported 5 million children have been victimized by this behavior. Bullying not only can result in long-term health and mental problems but also can have violent consequences. The U.S. Department of Education has been investigating school shootings, such as the one at Columbine. Although they did not define a "profile" for a school shooter, they did note that the shooters reported being victims of chronic bullying (Vossekuil et al., 2002).

By being aware of the warning signs, the school nurse may be able to identify a child who is a victim of bullying (see the Data Cues box). School officials should be involved because bullying usually occurs at school or on the way to and from school. The school environment should be safe for children, and additional adult supervision may be necessary. Both the victim and the bully need help. Victims and their families should be given tools that help them to deal with this problem. Bullies and their families also need to be given tools to help the bully achieve a socially acceptable behavior. Children who display aggressive behavior and start bullying at a young age are at high risk for more serious social problems.

Teasing and bullying are serious problems. They need to be recognized, and action must be taken. School officials, health care providers, and parents need to work together to encourage acceptable behavior and healthy socialization. Parents and school officials can find guidelines for dealing with these problems online (*www.bullyproofing.com* and *www.sopriswest.com*).

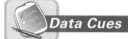 **Data Cues**

Warning Behaviors That a Child Is Being Bullied

Somatic	Serious problems
Stomach	School failure
Insomnia	Drug and alcohol abuse
New-onset enuresis	Violence
Behavior changes	Self-mutilation
Irritability	
Poor concentration	
Refusal to attend school	

From Scott, J.U., Hague-Armstrong, K., & Downes, K.L. (2003). Teasing and bullying: What can pediatricians do? *Contemp Pediatr, 20*(4), 105-120. Copyright © 2003, Advanstar Medical Economics Health Care, Inc. Reproduced with permission.

TELEVISION

Television has a powerful influence on children. The amount of time children spend watching television

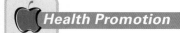 **Health Promotion**

Guidelines for Parents for Bullying and Teasing

VICTIM

Do not overreact; use calm manner
Listen to the child's perception of the problem
Use open-ended question to allow child to tell in his or her own words
Use drawing if child has difficulty communicating
Discuss what makes children be bullies
Review different options such as conflict resolution using forgiveness, shaking hands
Older children can ignore the teasing event and seek other company
Use role playing for practice
Encourage other friendships or organized activities such as clubs or teams
Praise child who faces up to fears
Reinforce to the child that the parent will protect him or her
Parents can talk to witnesses for further information
Parents can try to resolve conflict by involving the teaser's/bully's parents
Parents should involve any caregivers responsible for the teaser/bully
Parents should approach school officials for incidents that occur on school grounds or function
Consider group meeting of all involved individuals to resolve problem
Parents can involve law enforcement
Support school-sponsored programs that discourage teasing and bullying

BULLY

Parents must be aware of the seriousness of the behavior
Determine the reason for the child's behavior
Use expression of disappointment rather than anger when dealing with child
Encourage child's participation in organized, supervised activities
Observe child in play settings
Enforce the philosophy that the parent will not tolerate behavior that hurts other people
Respond to incidents of bullying with negative consequences
Encourage discussion of bullying incidents with other individuals who may be involved, such as school officials
Teach alternative approaches including negotiating skills
Notice and reward good play behavior
Consider mental health counselor if child does not respond or needs further understanding

Adapted from Scott, J.U., Hague-Armstrong, K., & Downes, K.L. (2003). Teasing and bullying: What can pediatricians do? *Contemp Pediatr, 20*(4), 105-120. Copyright © 2003, Advanstar Medical Economics Health Care, Inc. Reproduced with permission.

has declined since 1980. However, this is misleading because it does not include the time children spend playing video games. Television has been called the "great babysitter" of our time. Some complaints regarding children watching television are that (1) it does not challenge the imagination, (2) it interferes with solitude and play, and (3) it promotes materialism and passivity. Also, people portrayed on television are frequently stereotyped.

The American Academy of Pediatrics (AAP, 2001) recommends that parents should not only encourage the careful selection of programs but also watch and discuss the content with their children and adolescents. Parents should also create an "electronic media-free" environment in their children's rooms.

VIDEO GAMES

Video games have become the second favorite pastime of children (Figure 13-7). The advantages of video games include the development of eye-hand coordination, visual perception, attention to details, and the interactive component. Children are always using various strategies to win the game.

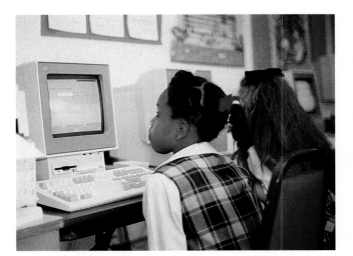

FIGURE **13-7** Children spend several hours a week both at home and school using a computer. Any computer games should be monitored by parents and school officials.

As the video game industry has grown, the amount of time children spend playing and the level of graphic violence have also increased. Violence in video games can either be fantasy based or human based. This means the characters are either imaginary (elves,

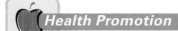

Health Promotion

Consequences of Excessive Television

- Displaces active types of recreation
- Interferes with conversation and discussion time
- Discourages reading
- Leads to poorer school performance (if more than 4 hours of television watching per day)
- Discourages exercise
- Affects how a child feels toward life and other people if television shows are violent
- Promotes and encourages material possessions

Parental Guidelines for Positive Television Viewing

- Encourage active recreation.
- Read to children.
- Limit television to 2 hours per day or less (1/2 hour if child is doing poorly in school).
- Do not allow television to be used as a distraction or babysitter for preschool children.
- Turn off television during meals.
- Teach critical viewing.
- Teach children to turn off the television at the end of a show.
- Encourage children to watch educational television shows.
- Forbid violent television shows; discuss reality of violence.
- Discuss purpose of commercials.
- Discuss reality and make-believe.
- Set a good example.

Schmitt, B.D. (2005). Patient Handouts. *Television: Reducing the negative impact.* MD Consult; *http://home.mdconsult.com.*

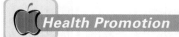

Health Promotion

Consequences of Excessive Video Game Playing

- Dominates leisure and study time
- Promotes solitary activity, reducing social interaction with family and friends
- Encourages acceptance of violent behavior in real life
- Leads to fallen grades, inadequate sleep, decrease in outdoor play, and social isolation

Parental Guidelines for Video Game Playing

- Limit to 2 hours or less per day.
- Encourage games without excessive violence.
- Provide educational games.
- Encourage alternative activities such as physical games, reading.

Schmitt, B.D. (2005). Patient Handouts. *Video games.* MD Consult; http://home. mdconsult.com.

monsters, aliens) or realistic (people or animals). Many of these games allow the player to assume the role of a shooter and award points for the number of people shot. Other games involve cars running over people and again award points for running over individuals. Many of these games continue to have improved graphics, which allows the violence to become more realistic.

Parents should monitor the rating of video games. The Entertainment Software Rating Board (ESRB) rates games for computers and home video systems. Parents can find ratings for specific software at their website (*www.esrb.org*).

PEERS

Peer relationships that form during the school-age years can greatly affect the socialization of the school-age child. Peers can positively and negatively influence school-age children. At this age, children can also be influenced through joining informal "clubs" that have official rules and secret passwords or joining formalized, cooperative groups such as scouts. Older school-age children, especially if they have limited family interaction or cohesiveness, can be affected by formal gang activity. Gang membership is strongly tied to drug use, sexual activity, violence, and crime. Children need to be taught to walk away if any gang member approaches them. Avoidance is the best policy. Education is crucial in preventing children from becoming involved in gangs.

School-age children need to be wary of peers or other persons offering illegal substances to them. Educational programs such as DARE (Drug Abuse Resistance Education) are taught to school-age children across the country. There have been questions as to the effectiveness versus the cost of the DARE program. There are new programs such as ALERT, LST (Lifeskills Training Program), and SFP (Strengthening Family Program). The goal of these programs is for children and families to gain life skills necessary to becoming responsible citizens.

GUIDANCE

Children who are in school continuously need the understanding of people who are concerned with their care. The types of relationships they have had are reflected in their behavior. They must know that they are wanted and loved. They need to know that their parents are proud of them and of their accomplishments, both in and out of school (Figure 13-8). They need approval, recognition for tasks well done, and a minimum of criticism. They need assistance in recognizing and keeping in touch with their feelings. At this age, they are quite critical of themselves. They need help with self-acceptance. Their judgment improves with age. Their decision-making capabilities need encouragement. For example, a parent can say, "I feel you can make that

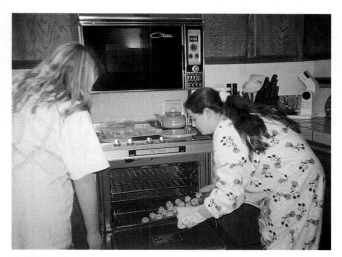

FIGURE **13-8** Learning to cook can be an enjoyable activity for the school-aged child. These activities can provide positive accomplishments.

decision yourself." Some of their decisions reflect their immaturity. If these are life-threatening or may cause injury, it may be necessary for parents to intervene. However, children learn from making minor mistakes. Parents and nurses who empathize with school-age children are able to better understand their views.

Preadolescents want to be accepted by their group; they imitate the group's speech, manner of dress, and actions. Interest in organizations is at its peak. Children enjoy scouting programs and young people's groups affiliated with their religious organization. Parents should encourage such group activities because they are both physically and morally strengthening.

School-age children need time and a place to study. They should have a desk of their own or at least a private area of the house where they are able to concentrate. Furniture should be of the proper size; lighting should be adequate. They must learn to take responsibility for their assignments and school supplies and to keep their room orderly. Parents can encourage them by showing an interest in what they are learning, joining parent-teacher organizations, and visiting the teacher periodically. They must also vote on civic matters that benefit the school system in their community.

At this age, an allowance or at least a means of earning money provides children with opportunities to learn the value of money. It takes time and encouragement for them to learn to spend money wisely. These experiences aid in making the school-age child a more responsible person.

SEX EDUCATION

Sexuality refers to the physical, psychological, social, emotional, and spiritual makeup of an individual. Young school-age children are curious about their bodies. This is sometimes evident in their play (doctor or nurse). As children grow and develop, so does their desire for knowledge about male and female roles. Adults can no longer answer questions in three or four words.

Sex education is a lifelong process. Parents convey their attitudes and feelings about all aspects of life, including sexuality, to the growing child. Teaching is not so much a matter of talking or providing formal instruction as it is a matter of reflecting the whole climate of the home, particularly the respect shown to each family member. Sexuality is only one of the child's capacities and should not be portrayed as a fearful, isolated, episodic kind of experience.

Children's questions about sex should be answered simply and at their level of understanding. It is helpful to have age-appropriate books in the home that help in answering questions. Correct names should be used to describe the genitals. The hospitalized child who says "My penis hurts" is understood by all. Private masturbation is normal and is practiced by both genders at various times throughout their lives. It does not cause acne, blindness, insanity, or impotence. The young boy needs to be prepared for erections and nocturnal emissions ("wet dreams"), which are to be expected and are not necessarily the result of masturbation. The young girl should be prepared for menarche and provided with the necessary articles in anticipation of this event. This is of particular importance to the early maturer because an elementary school may not provide sanitary napkin machines in the restrooms. Both genders are concerned during the school years with the disproportion of their bodies and they may be self-conscious when undressing. They may compare themselves with their friends. They need reassurance about their feelings concerning their awakening sexuality, which affects their thoughts and behavior.

Sex education programs in the schools are still subject to various group and community pressures. Most are fragmented and provide only basic information about anatomy and physiology with a general discussion of hygiene. If this is the case and if school-age children realize that their parents are uncomfortable with the subject, they turn to their peers, who often supply erroneous and distorted information. Some school programs emphasize that with each new freedom comes a responsibility. In addition, decision-making skills are taught. Children should be taught that when they do not make a decision, they have made a decision.

Regardless of their practice setting, nurses can aid in the sex education of parents and children through careful listening and anticipatory guidance. When it is appropriate, they should review normal developmental behavior and provide age-specific information, such as information about masturbation. They can provide families with useful written information that stresses sexuality as a healthy rather than an illness-related concept. Cultural differences should be taken into account during counseling.

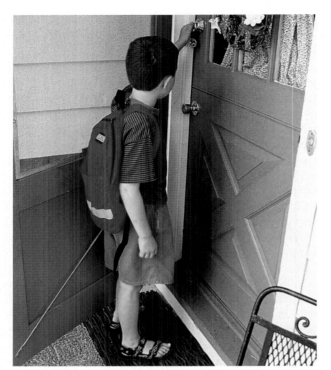

FIGURE **13-9** A child unlocks the door to let himself into his home after school.

Teenagers frequently share their concerns; the nurse must be prepared to assess their level of knowledge and assist in solving problems. An unexpected pregnancy in adolescence, although often traumatic, can also serve as framework for continued sex education.

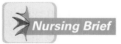

When discussing sexuality with the school-age child, it is necessary to identify slang or street terms. Most children hear the terms but may be confused about their meanings.

LATCHKEY CHILDREN

The number of latchkey children is growing, children left unsupervised after school (Figure 13-9). Many are asked to assume responsibilities that they are not ready to perform. Several factors contribute to this trend, most of which revolve around the changing nature of the family. There has been an increase in single-parent families that are predominantly headed by women and whose income is at or near the poverty level. In addition, the high cost of living may make it necessary for both parents to work to make ends meet. The nuclear family also is often separated geographically from the extended family; therefore relatives are not available for child care.

Latchkey children are at increased risk for accidents because of mischief or immature judgment. They may get into trouble more often than those children who are supervised after school. Studies show that these children are more likely to use alcohol and other illegal drugs. They may also show heightened feelings of fear and loneliness. They have fewer opportunities to socialize with friends because they may be instructed to remain alone in the house. It is important that children know where to go and whom to call, such as a neighbor or relative, in case of an emergency.

The Home Care Tip box shows parental and child guidance for latchkey children. Nurses should be aware of services in their community that are designed to meet the needs of latchkey children. They should provide this information to families. Hotlines have been established in various communities that provide telephone check-in for children and reassurance programs. Nurses can also investigate community after-school services and other programs.

🏠 Home Care Tip

Safety Tips for Latchkey Children

1. Establish a routine that includes a phone call when the child gets home. The child may call a "telephone friend" if the community offers this service. Incorporate special things into the routine such as a prearranged trip to a friend's house. Be sure the routine includes such things as snack ideas, homework responsibilities, caring for the family pet, or simple household chores to be done. Include allowed activities and those that are not allowed.
2. Teach the child phone numbers, especially his or her own. Include numbers for parents at work, grandparents, neighbors, and emergency numbers. Be sure these are posted. A good location is the refrigerator. Ensure that the child knows his or her address and the correct spellings of parents' names and own name.
3. Be sure the child knows to keep doors locked and *never* open the door to anyone (unless the child has called the grandparents, neighbor, or emergency number for help).
4. Post and review safety rules and basic first aid (see Health Promotion box for safety tips).
5. Instruct child *never* to enter the home if the door is ajar or a window is open or broken. Have the child call for help from a neighbor's house.
6. Teach child to tell phone callers that the parent or caregiver is busy; *never* say the parent or caregiver is not at home.
7. Teach child how to exit the home in case of a fire and to *never* reenter a burning building. Be sure the child knows what to do for other emergencies, including earthquakes.
8. Discuss with the child the importance of not telling others (including peers) they come home alone after school. Do not display household key in public.
9. Teach child what to do in storms, power outages, etc.
10. Be considerate of the child. Parents should always call if they will be late. Praise the child for acting responsibly.

CHILD ABDUCTION

One of parents' greatest fears in raising children is child abduction. There are several categories for missing children, but abduction by a nonfamily member can be the most frightening. Although the number of children abducted by a nonfamily member is smaller than the number taken by a noncustodial family member, the risk for death is higher with a nonfamily member. In the past children have been taught not to talk to strangers, not to take candy from a stranger, and not to go with a stranger, but perpetrators are finding ways to blur the "stranger" distinction. They can be the child's coach or neighbor. The Internet has provided an additional mode of contact for the perpetrator, who can establish a relationship over a period of time. The topic of strangers should be discussed with the child, and the child should learn to deal with strangers with confidence rather than with fear and avoidance.

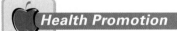

Health Promotion

Parental Guidelines for Preventing Abductions

- Don't let your child go out alone; use the buddy system.
- Always know where your child is and what his or her plans are.
- Teach your child to always say no if feeling uncomfortable.
- Teach your child to know his or her name, address, phone number with area code, and your work number.
- Teach child how to use a pay phone or cell phone and how to contact emergency number.
- Don't have jackets or T-shirts with your child's name in view.
- Be aware of anyone who pays a great deal of attention to your child.
- Have current ID kit done on your child (www.pollyklaas.org).

There are commercial devices that parents can use to track their children, such as Ionkids monitors or Wherify watch. These devices can have GPS (global positioning systems), which can identify the location of the child. Cell phones are available that allow the child to contact the parent using a push-button.

DIVORCE

Divorce is a concern for children of all ages, not just the school-age child. However, unless a divorce is handled carefully, the impact on this particular age group can have serious consequences.

Parents can use the many books available to assist with discussions about divorce. Although younger school-age children may openly show their grief, older school-age children may keep their feelings inside while experiencing deterioration in school performance and peer relationships. Children need to be allowed to express their emotions, and counseling may help them work through their feelings.

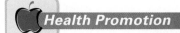

Health Promotion

Guidelines for Coping with Divorce

- Provide reassurance that both parents love the child.
- Keep constant as many aspects of the child's world as possible.
- Provide reassurance that the noncustodial parent will visit.
- Find substitutes if the noncustodial parent becomes uninvolved.
- Provide opportunities for the child to discuss painful feelings.
- Clarify that the divorce is final and that the child is not responsible.
- Try to protect the child's positive feelings about both parents.
- Maintain normal discipline in both households.
- Do not argue with the ex-spouse about the child in the child's presence.
- Try to avoid custody disputes.

Schmitt, B.D. (2005). Patient Handouts. *Divorce: Helping children cope.* MD Consult; *http://home.mdconsult.com*

SAFETY

As children become more mobile, the scope of possible injuries increases. This age group tends to have a high incidence of cuts, abrasions, fractures, strains, and sprains. In addition, although school-age children seek more independence, they often do not have the judgment necessary to ensure safety. They may not be able to judge their own bicycle speed or that of an oncoming car; they may be coerced into playing with matches or a handgun. School-age children (especially boys) enjoy skateboarding and riding various motorized vehicles. Both boys and girls of this age enjoy in-line skating and bicycle riding. Precautions need to be taken with these activities. With skateboarding and in-line skating, protective gear must be worn. On a skateboard, the child needs a helmet, protective padding, and wrist guards. Children must be taught to *never* ride in or near traffic. They also need to learn that ramps can be especially dangerous.

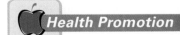

Health Promotion

Guidelines for In-Line Skating

- Always wear protective gear.
- Skate under control and leave plenty of room to stop.
- Always skate on the right side of paths and sidewalks; pass on the left.
- Avoid uneven pavement and heavy traffic areas.
- Observe traffic regulations and yield to pedestrians.

Motorized vehicles (tractors, personal watercraft, mopeds, mini-bikes, all-terrain vehicles, and snow mobiles) are both tempting and dangerous for school-

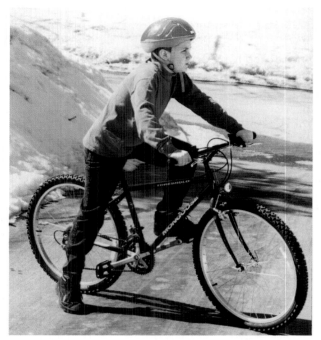

FIGURE **13-10** The right-size bike is important; the child should be able to sit on the bike and place the balls of both feet on the ground. Wearing a protective helmet is mandatory for safe cycling. The helmet should sit on top of the head in a level position with a secure strap. It should not rock side to side or front to back.

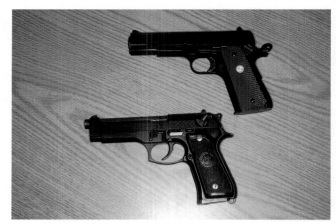

FIGURE **13-11** A child can easily mistake a real handgun for a very realistic looking toy gun, with possible tragic results. Can you identify the real gun? (It is the one on the bottom.)

age children. These children often lack the coordination and judgment to avoid crashes. These vehicles achieve high speeds yet provide little protection. The AAP recommends that children not operate these vehicles (AAP, 2000).

Bicycle safety includes the use of a helmet (the same helmet can be used for in-line skating and skateboarding) that meets the American National Standards Institute (ANSI) or Snell Memorial Foundation (Snell-approved). Bicycle helmets can absorb most of the impact of a crash, thus protecting the head from serious injury (Figure 13-10). Other precautions to take when bicycle riding include obeying all traffic lights and signs, avoiding tricks and double-riding, riding in the same direction as traffic, not wearing headphones when riding, using caution near driveways and alleys, and carrying objects in a backpack or basket. *Never* wear clothing that could become caught in the bicycle chain, *never* ride at night, be sure the child's feet touch the ground when sitting on the seat, and always keep the bike in good repair.

Another safety-related area of concern with school-age children is the use of guns. Firearm violence has become a crisis in the United States. School-age children are curious about and attracted to gun use. They may see it as a symbol of power or superiority. Every 2 hours, someone's child is killed with a gun, either in a homicide, suicide, or unintentional injury (Schor, 1999). A large number of children are also seriously injured by guns. The AAP supports gun control legislation. They

believe handguns, deadly air guns, and assault weapons should be banned. Until then, handgun ammunition should be regulated, restrictions should be placed on handgun ownership, and the number of privately owned handguns should be reduced (AAP, 2004). **Never allow a child access to a gun.** Loaded guns must never be kept in the house or car, ammunition must be locked away in a separate location, and guns should be equipped with trigger locks. Children need to learn that if they ever see a gun in a friend's house, they should not touch it and they should tell their parents. If they ever see a gun at school, they should report it to a teacher or a principal immediately. Children should never use a toy gun that looks so realistic that an adult would not be able to distinguish it from a distance (Figure 13-11).

The Health Promotion box presents a guide for preventing additional injuries and accidents in school-age children.

HEALTH PROMOTION AND MAINTENANCE

HEALTH EXAMINATIONS

The yearly preschool physical examination is given in the spring preceding admission. This allows time for correcting any problems that are found. Booster immunizations are given as needed (see Appendix A). Blood pressure, height, and weight must all be evaluated. Ensuring that the child regularly visits the dentist is also part of the examination. Blood cholesterol may be evaluated, especially if the child is at risk (e.g., from heredity).

School-age children need to be evaluated for the amount of exercise they receive. Exercise should be done daily. It can range from bicycle riding to organized team sports. If this is not encouraged, obesity may result as a preteen problem.

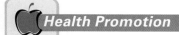

Health Promotion

Injury Prevention During School-Age Years

DEVELOPMENTAL ABILITIES RELATED TO RISK FOR INJURY

Is increasingly involved in activities away from home
Is excited by speed and motion
Is easily distracted by environment
Can be reasoned with

Is apt to overdo
May work hard to perfect a skill
Has cautious, but not fearful, gross motor actions
Likes swimming

Has increasing independence
Is adventuresome
Enjoys trying new things

Adheres to group rules
May be easily influenced by peers
Has strong allegiance to friends

Has increased physical skills
Needs strenuous physical activity
Is interested in acquiring new skills and perfecting attained skills
Is daring and adventurous, especially with peers
Frequently plays in hazardous places
Confidence often exceeds physical capacity

INJURY PREVENTION

Motor Vehicles

Educate child regarding proper use of seat belts as a passenger in a vehicle.
   Maintain discipline as a passenger in a vehicle (e.g., keep arms inside, do not lean against doors or interfere with driver).
Remind parents and children that no one should ride in the bed of a pickup truck.
Emphasize safe pedestrian behavior.
Insist on use of safety apparel (e.g., helmet) where applicable, such as when riding a bicycle, motorcycle, moped, or all-terrain vehicle.

Drowning

Teach child to swim.
Teach basic rules of water safety.
Select safe and supervised places to swim.
Check sufficient water depth for diving.
Have child swim with a companion.
Use an approved flotation device in water or boat.
Advocate for legislation requiring fencing around pools.
Learn CPR.

Burns

Make sure smoke detectors are in homes.
Set hot water temperatures (120° F-130° F) to avoid scald burns.
Instruct child in behavior in areas involving contact with potential burn hazards (e.g., gasoline, matches, bonfires or barbecues, lighter fluid, firecrackers, cigarette lighters, cooking utensils, chemistry sets); avoid climbing or flying kites around high-tension wires.
Instruct child in proper behavior in the event of fire (e.g., fire drills at home and school).
Teach child safe cooking (use low heat; avoid any frying; be careful of steam burns, scalds, or exploding foods, especially from microwaving).

Poisoning

Educate child regarding hazards of taking nonprescription drugs and chemicals, including aspirin and alcohol.
Teach child to say "no" if offered illegal or dangerous drugs or alcohol.
Keep potentially dangerous products in properly labeled receptacles, preferably locked and out of reach.

Bodily Damage

Help provide facilities for supervised activities.
Encourage playing in safe places.
Keep firearms safely locked up except during adult supervision.
Teach proper care of, use of, and respect for devices with potential danger (power tools, firecrackers).
Teach children not to tease or surprise dogs, invade their territory, take dogs' toys, or interfere with dogs' feeding.
Stress eye, ear, or mouth protection when using potentially hazardous objects or devices or when engaged in potentially hazardous sports (e.g., baseball).

Continued

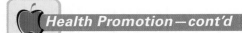

Health Promotion—cont'd

Injury Prevention During School-Age Years—cont'd

DEVELOPMENTAL ABILITIES RELATED TO RISK FOR INJURY	INJURY PREVENTION
Desires group loyalty and has strong need for friends' approval	**Bodily Damage—cont'd**
Attempts hazardous feats	Teach safety regarding use of corrective devices (glasses); if child wears contact lenses, monitor duration of wear to prevent corneal damage.
Accompanies friends to potentially hazardous facilities	Stress careful selection, use, and maintenance of sports and recreation equipment such as skateboards and in-line skates.
Delights in physical activity	Emphasize proper conditioning, safe practices, and use of safety equipment for sports or recreational activities.
Is likely to overdo	Caution against engaging in hazardous sports, such as those involving trampolines.
Growth in height exceeds muscular growth and coordination	Use safety glass and decals on large glassed areas, such as sliding glass doors.
	Use window guards to prevent falls.
	Teach name, address, phone number and to ask for help from appropriate people (cashier, security guard, policeman) if lost; have identification on child (sewn in clothes, inside shoe).
	Teach stranger safety:
	Avoid personalized clothing in public places.
	Caution child to never go with a stranger.
	Have child tell parents if anyone makes child feel uncomfortable in any way.
	Always listen to child's concerns regarding others' behavior.
	Teach child to say "no" when confronted with uncomfortable situations.

From Hockenberry, M.J., & Wilson, D. (2007). *Wong's nursing care of infants and children* (8th ed.). St. Louis: Mosby.

School health programs aimed at maintaining and promoting health are provided by most school systems. Nurses and other professionals who take part in such programs can play an important role in counseling parents. They also can help in meeting the needs of disabled children who are enrolled in their schools. A carefully taken health history provides the nurse with much-needed information (Figure 13-12).

Audiograms are done as part of the school health program, as are vision and scoliosis screenings. Deviations from normal in any of these areas require further assessment by the child's physician.

DAILY CARE

School-age children generally provide their own daily care. Teeth should be brushed at least twice daily with a pea-sized amount of fluoridated toothpaste. Drinking water should also contain fluoride. Twice-yearly dental visits should continue. The dentist may evaluate for application of dental sealants.

Children are so active during the day, both physically and mentally, that they soon become exhausted. Chil-dren from 6 to 8 years average approximately 11 to 13 hours of sleep a night. As they grow older, a little less is necessary. The 9- to 12-year-old averages about 10 hours per night. Parents can judge the amount of sleep children need by their behavior. If a child is eating and playing well and keeping up with schoolwork, chances are that the amount of sleep is sufficient.

PLAY

Play is still very much a part of the school-age child's life. It simply takes on a new dimension. During the beginning of this period, play occurs in groups, which are mostly of the same gender. These children still enjoy dolls, cars, and trucks. They ride bicycles and enjoy active games such as hide-and-seek, tag, jump rope, and roller skating. They become involved in sports. Team play has rules and goals. They also enjoy quiet activities and often start collections, play board games or card games, and read books. They enjoy being creative and learning new things. As they get older, school-age children become more independent and peer relationships (discussed earlier in the chapter) become more important.

I. GENERAL INFORMATION
Name _____ Date _____
Age and birth date _____ Language _____
Grade _____ Informant _____
Sex _____ Parents' home and business
Religion _____ phones _____

II. FAMILY PROFILE (health history of family members)
Mother _____
Father _____
Siblings _____
Paternal grandparents _____
Maternal grandparents _____
Life change events: death, divorce, new baby, moves of family, illness, separation, etc.
_____
_____

III. CHILD PROFILE
Newborn status: Did baby leave hospital with you? _____
Birth defects _____
Developmental history: Age for crawling _____ sitting _____
  walking _____ speech _____ toilet training _____
Immunizations _____
Habits, general behavior in school _____ Home _____
Sleeping patterns _____ Fears _____
Exercise _____ Friends _____
Interests _____ Special skills _____
_____
Previous illness or accidents _____
Is child taking any medications? _____
Hearing aid _____ Glasses _____
Dental care _____ Allergies_____
Typical foods consumed:
  breakfast _____
  lunch _____
  supper _____
  snacks _____
Eating problems _____ Elimination _____
Menses _____ Sexual maturation _____
Sex education _____ Personal hygiene _____
Review of systems _____
_____

IV. NURSE'S OBSERVATIONS AND COMMENTS
General physical description _____
_____
Results of screening procedures: vision _____ audiometer _____
Scoliosis _____ Other _____
Individual health education and guidance _____
_____
Problem-solving plan _____
_____

  Interviewer _____

FIGURE **13-12** Health assessment summary of the school-age child.

NUTRITION

The eating habits of school-age children are usually not a problem as long as a variety of nutritious foods are offered. Review the discussion about MyPyramid in Chapter 9 (see Figure 9-5) for the recommended food intake for school-age children. A good breakfast is important. The chief breakfast foods necessary are fruit, cereal, and milk. Eggs add variety. Older school-age children need to have the importance of breakfast stressed because they may decide that breakfast is no longer important or they may feel too rushed in the mornings. Peers may also influence this behavior. Menus centered on nutritional foods are more substantial than those consisting of doughnuts or sweet rolls. Nutritious snacks are also important to provide energy for after-school activities and homework. Good nutrition also prevents problems of obesity that can occur with school-age children.

Depending on individual activity levels, a 7-year-old girl needs approximately 1200-1800 calories per day, and boys of the same age need about 1400-1800 calories per day. The 12-year-old girl needs 1600-2200 calories, whereas 12-year-old boys require about

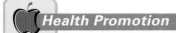
Health Promotion

Guidelines for Portions of Food Groups for School-Age Children

GROUP	1200 CALORIES	1800 CALORIES	2400 CALORIES
Fruits	1 cup	1.5 cups	2 cups
Vegetables	1.5 cups	2.5 cups	3 cups
Grains	4 ounces	6 ounces	8 ounces
Meats/beans	4 ounces	5.5 ounces	6.5 ounces
Milk	2 cups	3 cups	3 cups
Oils	4 teaspoons	5 teaspoons	7 teaspoons

U.S. Department of Agriculture. Center for Nutrition Policy and Promotion. Retrieved from *http://www.MyPyramid.gov* .

1800-2400 calories, again depending on activity level. The U.S. Department of Agriculture has developed new dietary guidelines, which are available online (*www.mypyrimid.gov*). This site provides information for parents, kids, and school officials.

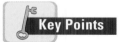
Community Cue

The school nurse can work with teachers to provide nutrition instruction in the classroom. Children can participate in learning activities that focus on nutrition education to encourage good habits.

The federal government has established the School Breakfast Program in many areas. The National School Lunch Program has been ongoing. Summer lunch programs are also available in some communities. These lunches must meet certain nutritional standards (the goal is to provide one third of the recommended daily allowance of foods).

Key Points

- School-age children are more engrossed in fact than fantasy; they begin to master activities they enjoy and learn they must cooperate with others.
- Growth is slow until just before puberty. Muscular coordination is improved, and vital signs are near those of an adult. Language continues to develop, and school-age children build an impressive vocabulary.
- The school-age child thinks in concrete terms and is in the stage of industry versus inferiority. He or she begins to understand right and wrong and develops a conscience.
- Each age brings out individual differences and personalities. Parents need to understand these differences as their child matures.
- School is an important influence in children's lives. Teachers, parents, and other caregivers need to instill values and help school-age children develop social competencies.

- Teasing and bullying can lead to long-term mental problems. Both the victim and the bully need assistance in handling these situations.
- Television and video game play should be limited. Both can have a detrimental effect on children.
- Peers are also a strong influence on children. Gangs and drugs are real temptations in children's lives; parents, teachers, and other caregivers must educate children to deter these activities.
- Sex education is discussed with the school-age child. Simple, straightforward answers at the child's level of understanding are the best advice for parents.
- Latchkey children need reminders and reassurance to keep them safe after school.
- Child abduction prevention guidelines should be discussed with children based on developmental age.
- Divorce is a problem for school-age children and children of other ages. When divorce occurs, parents need to be honest and provide reassurance to children.
- Safety is also a priority for school-age children. Although they have different types of injuries than do toddlers and preschoolers, school-age children still need supervision and education to prevent injuries.
- Good nutrition based on MyPyramid is important at this age. Children are growing slowly but steadily, and healthy eating habits formed at this age are important later on in life.

 Go to your Companion CD-ROM for an Audio Glossary, video clips, and more.

evolve Be sure to visit the companion Evolve site at http://evolve.elsevier.com/Price/pediatric/ for WebLinks and additional online resources.

ONLINE RESOURCES

American Academy of Pediatrics: www.aap.org

Bright Futures: www.brightfutures.org

Entertainment Software Rating Board: www.esrb.org

National Resource for Safe Schools: www.safetyzone.org

Missing Children: www.pollyklaas.org

U.S. Department of Agriculture: www.usda.gov

U.S. Department of Agriculture—MyPyramid: www.mypryamid.gov

Objectives

Upon completion of this chapter, the student will be able to:

1. Define the vocabulary terms listed
2. Differentiate between insulin-dependent and non–insulin-dependent diabetes mellitus
3. Outline the educational needs of the child with diabetes and of the parents in the following areas: nutrition and meal planning, glucose monitoring, insulin administration, and exercise
4. Describe the nursing care of the school-age child with asthma, including monitoring of respiratory status, respiratory treatments and medications, and the psychosocial implications of the condition
5. List three major and two minor manifestations of acute rheumatic fever as determined by the modified Jones criteria
6. List the symptoms of appendicitis and discuss what modifications in treatment and postoperative nursing care are necessary if a school-age child has a ruptured appendix
7. Identify the pathophysiology of Legg-Calvé-Perthes disease and the management approach
8. Devise a nursing care plan for a 12-year-old girl with juvenile rheumatoid arthritis, including teaching about home management
9. Discuss two ways in which the nurse can help an 8-year-old boy with a brain tumor address body image concerns
10. Relate the symptoms of a child with attention deficit/hyperactivity disorder with corresponding social, educational, and emotional difficulties and describe strategies to help the child and family cope with the condition

Key Terms

Be sure to check out the bonus material on the Companion CD-ROM, including selected audio pronunciations.

DSM-IV-TR (p. 321)
iridocyclitis (Ĭ-rĭd-ō-sĭ-KLĪ-tĭs; p. 315)
Jones criteria (p. 308)
latent period (LĀ-těnt; p. 308)
nystagmus (nĭ-STĂG-măs; p. 319)
papilledema (pă-pĭl-ă-DĒ-mă; p. 319)
peak expiratory flow rate (PEFR; ĕks-PĪ-răh-TŌ-rē; p. 304)

School-age children are slowly but steadily maturing. They may have health issues that cover a wide variety of areas. They spend most of their time in school and continue to be exposed to infectious illnesses. They can also have issues and health problems that may have a long-lasting effect on their lives.

SKIN

PEDICULOSIS

The infestation of humans by lice is known as *pediculosis*. The three types of pediculosis are pediculosis capitis, or head lice; pediculosis corporis, or body lice; and pediculosis pubis, or crab or pubic lice. The various types usually remain in the part of the body designated by their name. They are transmitted from person to person or from contaminated articles. Their survival depends on the blood they extract from the infected person. Severe itching in the affected area is the main symptom. Treatment in all cases is aimed at ridding the patient of the parasite, treating the excoriated skin, and preventing the infestation of others. The most common form seen in children is head lice. The child or parents may be embarrassed by the presence of lice, but infestations spread quickly in schools and do not reflect on the hygiene of the families.

Description

Head lice affect the scalp and hair. The adult attaches numerous eggs, known as *nits*, to the hair shafts approximately $1/8$ inch from the scalp (Figure 14-1). Nits hatch within 3 or 4 days. Head lice are more common in girls than in boys because of hair length. The parasite may be acquired from hats, combs, or hairbrushes. It is easily transferred from one child to another and is seen most frequently in the school-age child and in preschool children who attend daycare centers.

Signs and Symptoms

The child has severe itching of the scalp. Scratching of the head can cause further irritation. The hair may become matted. Occasionally pustules and excoriations are seen about the face. Nurses who admit patients to

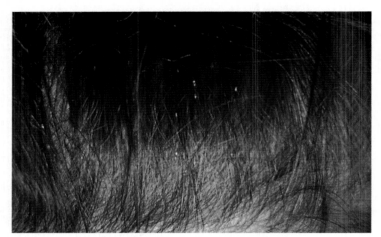

FIGURE **14-1** Head lice nits appear as tiny white dots along the hair shaft. Typically they are firmly attached to the hair around and behind the ears.

pediatric units should be on the alert for head lice. In particular, inspect the hairline at the back of the neck and about the ears. Crusts, nits, and dirt may cause matting of the hair and a foul odor.

Treatment and Nursing Care

Management is directed toward killing the adult lice, getting rid of the nits, and treating any infections of the face and scalp. Family members and playmates of the child should be examined and treated as necessary. The drug of choice is permethrin (Nix), which is available in cream rinse form to apply after shampooing. This drug has a high kill rate for both nits and lice. The manufacturer's directions should be followed carefully. Watch for an allergic response, particularly in children with a history of skin problems. Nonprescription pyrethrin shampoos (A-200, RID) are also commonly used. Lindane (Kwell) has also been used; however, it has more reported side effects and should not be used to treat head lice in children. If the eyebrows and eyelashes are involved, a thick coating of petrolatum (Vaseline) is applied, followed by removal of remaining nits. Nits on the head are removed by combing the hair with a fine-tooth comb.

Charting includes date and time, condition of scalp and hair before treatment, odor (if noticeable), type of shampoo used, how the procedure was tolerated, and the amount of relief obtained. Any signs of systemic infection should also be documented.

Clothing or bedding is laundered in hot water. Mattresses may be sprayed with a disinfectant. Wool clothing requires dry cleaning or can be placed dry into a clothes dryer set on hot cycle for at least 20 minutes. Children should be cautioned against swapping caps, headscarves, and combs. Parents are instructed to inspect the child's head regularly. Encourage parents to report infestations to the school nurse because widespread outbreaks are encountered periodically.

Cutting the child's hair is discouraged because it can be a source of stress to the child, who is already being singled out as "the child with lice." Oral Benadryl may be given for pruritus. Parents should be cautioned to watch for symptoms of secondary infection caused by breaks in the skin from scratching.

Recent studies of dry-on, suffocation-based pedicalicide lotion that does not require use of neurotoxins, nit removal, or household cleaning have shown promising results with a 96% cure rate. This approach should be considered since there is growing resistance with permethrin and lindane. The pedicalicide lotion is applied once a week with up to three applications. The lotion is applied; then after 2 minutes, it is combed out of the hair. The hair is dried using a heated hair dryer and can be shampooed after 8 hours (Pearlman, 2004).

ENDOCRINE SYSTEM

DIABETES MELLITUS (TYPE 1)
Description

Diabetes mellitus (DM) is a chronic metabolic condition in which the body is unable to metabolize and use carbohydrates, fats, and proteins properly because of a deficiency of insulin, an internal secretion of the pancreas. Insulin deficiency leads to impaired glucose transport (sugar cannot pass into the cells; Figure 14-2) and accelerated metabolism of stored fats for energy.

Insulin-dependent DM (IDDM; type 1) is the most common endocrine/metabolic disorder of childhood. The condition is found worldwide, affects multiple body organs, and is unique in that it requires a great deal of self-management by the person affected. Patient and family education and compliance are extremely important to the successful management of the condition and the prevention of complications. Morbidity and mortality are associated with chronic complications that affect small and large blood vessels, resulting in retinopathy, nephropathy, neuropathy, ischemic heart disease, and obstruction of large vessels.

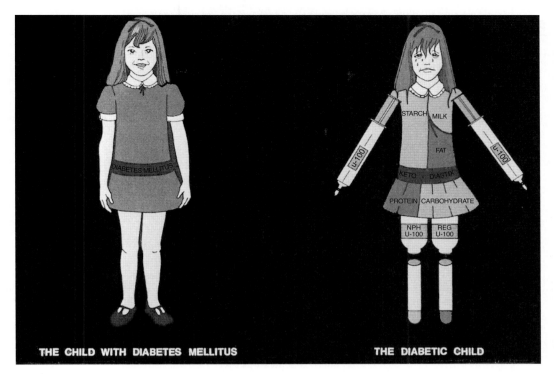

THE CHILD WITH DIABETES MELLITUS   THE DIABETIC CHILD

FIGURE **14-2** This illustration originally designed by Dr. L.B. Travis in 1968 is relevant today. The child with diabetes *(left)* represents our perception of what children with diabetes should look like and how they should view themselves. However, when professionals use the adjective "diabetic" to describe these children, there is small wonder that many children see themselves as a composite of what they feel is the disease itself *(right)*. (From Travis, L.B., Brouhard, B., & Schreiner, B. (1987). *Diabetes in children and adolescents.* Philadelphia: WB Saunders.)

Classification. Diabetes is not a single entity but several different disorders. These disorders differ in cause, pathophysiology, and genetic predisposition. All result in disturbed glucose metabolism. Previously, DM was classified by treatment. The old classification was IDDM (type 1) and non–insulin-dependent DM (NIDDM, or type 2). The American Diabetes Association has recommended a new classification system that includes type 1 and type 2 (Table 14-1). For the purposes of this discussion, only type 1 DM will be addressed in detail.

Type 1 DM was formerly known as juvenile-onset diabetes or brittle diabetes. It is characterized by partial or complete insulin deficiency. Although some insulin production may be seen during certain phases of the disease, patients eventually become completely insulin deficient. Type 1 DM is considered to be caused by an autoimmune process in which the body destroys the insulin-producing islet cells in the pancreas of those who are genetically vulnerable. Environmental and genetic factors are strongly implicated. Apparently, type 1 DM is sometimes set off by seemingly harmless viruses believed to provoke the immune system into mistakenly destroying its own islet cells. The presence of islet cell antibodies (ICAs) and the evidence that associates type 1 DM with other autoimmune conditions appear to support an autoimmune etiology.

Incidence. In the United States, surveys indicate the prevalence of type 1 DM to be 14.9 per 100,000 (Behrman et al., 2004). The frequency increases with age. Symptoms of type 1 DM may occur at any time in childhood, but the rate of occurrence of new cases is highest among 5- to 7-year-old children and children entering puberty. In the former, the stress of school and the increased exposure to infectious diseases, particularly viral illness, may be responsible. During puberty, increased growth, increased emotional stress, and the effects of growth and sex hormones on insulin action may be implicated.

Type 1 DM occurs equally in boys and girls. Socioeconomic correlations have not been seen. The risk of type 1 DM is higher in families, particularly in the siblings and children of individuals with diabetes. The risk is highest in twins of those affected. Pancreatic ICAs are found in up to 85% of patients with newly diagnosed diabetes, which supports an autoimmune component. Other contributing factors may include cow's milk fed to children under the age of 2 years, increasing incidence of obesity, and viral infections as triggers. Research has focused on prevention of diabetes in at-risk patients. This includes antibody testing and measurement of insulin response. Testing of low-dosage insulin administration to at-risk patients to delay or prevent the onset of diabetes did not provide evidence for disease prevention (Behrman et al., 2004).

The disease is more severe in childhood because the patients are growing, they expend a great deal of energy, their nutritional needs vary, and they have to face a lifetime of diabetic management. Children with type 1 DM often do not have the typical textbook picture of the disorder; therefore the nurse must be particularly astute with subjective and objective observations.

Table 14-1	*Classification of Types of Diabetes Mellitus*			
TYPE	**ONSET**	**CLINICAL FEATURES**	**OTHER COMMENTS**	
Type 1 DM	Primarily in childhood but can occur at any age	Polydipsia, polyuria, polyphagia, weight loss occurring for usually less than 1 mo Hyperglycemia: random plasma glucose above 200 mg/dL with symptoms or fasting blood glucose above 126 mg/dL and 2-hr postprandial blood glucose above 200 mg/dL with no symptoms Glycosuria, ketonuria Vaginal monilial infections in adolescent girls Elevation of antiislet or antiinsulin antibodies and presence of other indicators of immune connection	Child requires insulin to maintain life Type 1 can be diagnosed in children before symptoms appear and in family members at risk Type 1 appears to have both genetic and environmental components	
Type 2 DM	Usually after age 40 yr but can occur at any age	Hyperglycemia: fasting blood glucose above 126 mg/dL and 2-hr glucose tolerance test result above 200 mg/dL on more than one occasion without precipitating factors Patient is usually obese Serum insulin level can be normal or less than normal	Condition has some genetic basis Some affected children need insulin on occasion (e.g., during severe stress or illness)	

Recently, physicians have noted type 2 DM increasing in incidence in children. The condition accounts for approximately one third to one half of all newly diagnosed individuals under 18 years of age. The diabetes appears to affect mostly children who are obese and who have Native American, African-American, or Hispanic origins. Causative factors appear to be sedentary lifestyle (increased hours in front of the television and decreased physical activity) and poor dietary habits with increased sugar consumption. Children who have a BMI greater than 95% are at risk for developing type 2.

Signs and Symptoms

Children with type 1 DM have a classic triad of symptoms: **polyuria** (excretion of large amounts of urine), **polydipsia** (excessive thirst), and **polyphagia** (constant hunger). Despite the hunger and increased food intake, the child loses weight.

The symptoms can appear insidiously, with fatigue, anorexia, nausea, lethargy, and weakness. The skin becomes dry. Vaginal yeast infections may be seen in the adolescent girl. Often the symptoms of concern in the young child are bedwetting or urine accidents during play periods in a previously trained child.

Laboratory findings indicate **hyperglycemia** (excess sugar in the blood). Glucose may be found in the urine (**glycosuria** or **glucosuria**), which occurs after the blood glucose level reaches 180 mg/dL. Other laboratory tests might include insulin levels and antibody studies. Type

1 DM can also occur abruptly, usually during a viral infection or time of stress. Children with abrupt onset often become very ill with symptoms of **ketoacidosis** (severe hyperglycemia, ketones in the blood and urine, and acidosis). Diabetic ketoacidosis (DKA) is also referred to as diabetic coma, although a person may have DKA with or without a coma (Figure 14-3).

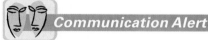 **Communication Alert**

When parents dominate a conversation and the child is not given an opportunity to answer a question, the nurse directs the conversation to the child. For example, during an admission interview of a child admitted for DKA, the nurse can say to the child, "Can you tell me what happened yesterday before your mother found you in your bedroom?"

Diabetic ketoacidosis can be triggered by conditions that increase insulin demand (fever, stress, infection). DKA may also affect the child with diabetes who has skipped one or more insulin doses, sometimes deliberately. The symptoms range from mild to severe and occur in hours to days. The skin is dry, and the face flushed. Patients appear dehydrated. They are thirsty but may vomit if fluids are offered. They perspire and are restless. There may be generalized pain in the abdomen and throughout the body. A characteristic fruity odor of the breath is apparent because the patient expels acetone from the respiratory system. Blood pressure and pulse

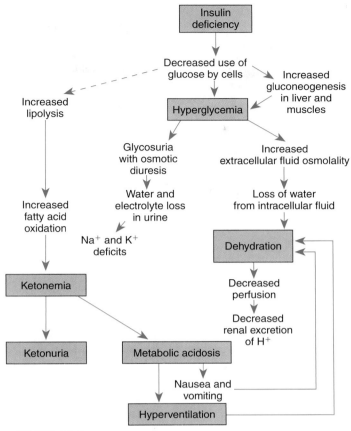

FIGURE **14-3** Pathophysiology of acidosis in diabetes mellitus.

increase. As the condition worsens, the child becomes weak and drowsy. Breathing patterns are peculiar in that they are rapid and deep and there is no normal period of rest between inspiration and expiration; this is termed **Kussmaul breathing.** The patient becomes unconscious. Death results unless insulin, fluids, and electrolytes are administered.

Treatment and Nursing Care

Diabetic Ketoacidosis. The correction of depleted fluids, frequent checking of vital signs, hourly blood glucose tests, regular blood chemistry measurements, and close observation of consciousness are necessary. Baseline studies include venous blood glucose, serum acetone, pH, total carbon dioxide (TCO_2), blood urea nitrogen, electrolytes, calcium, phosphate, white blood cell count, urinalysis, and appropriate cultures. Glucose levels in the blood and urine, electrolyte counts, and any other abnormal laboratory values are continuously monitored until the child's condition stabilizes. Low doses of regular insulin are administered intravenously or subcutaneously, and the patient is observed. A cardiac monitor is helpful in determination of cardiac effects of changing potassium levels. If the patient has an infection, the infection is treated. Cerebral edema, although rare, can be life threatening. Careful monitoring of neurological status is essential. A diabetic flowchart at the bedside is used to register all pertinent information. Response to treatment is gradual, occurring over a period of hours.

Long-Term Management: Physical Aspects. The aims of treatment of juvenile diabetes are (1) to promote normal growth and development through metabolic control, (2) to enable the child to have a happy and active childhood, and (3) to prevent complications. Ideally, teaching begins when the diagnosis is confirmed. A planned educational program is necessary to provide a consistent body of information, which can then be individualized. The patient's age and financial, educational, cultural, and religious background must be considered.

The patient and the family are instructed about the location of the pancreas and its normal function. The nurse explains the relationship of insulin to the pancreas, differentiating between type 1 and type 2 DM. All information is given gradually and at the level of understanding of the child and the family. Audiovisual aids and pamphlets are incorporated into the session. Most patients with newly diagnosed diabetes are hospitalized for varying periods of time for intense instruction; many hospitals hold group clinics for patients and their relatives. These sessions are conducted by various professionals such as the physician, dietitian, and nurse. Patients who are living with the disease provide encouragement and help by sharing concerns. Health professionals become directly involved with the patient's progress and can offer necessary feedback and support. Continuous follow-up is extremely important.

Since the release of results from the Diabetes Control and Complication Trial (DCCT), the focus of management of diabetes is intense insulin therapy to normalize blood glucose levels. Intense therapy includes multiple insulin injections, frequent blood glucose monitoring, strict dietary intake, and exercise. The importance of glycemic control (tight blood sugars) in decreasing the incidence of symptoms and complications of the disease has been established. The goal is to maintain blood glucose levels (Box 14-1).

Insulin Administration. Insulin is used principally to control DM. Insulin is a specially prepared extract obtained from the pancreas of cattle or pigs. Human insulin, developed with recombinant DNA technique, is the most frequently used because it is associated with a lesser incidence of allergies. When injected into the patient with diabetes, insulin enables the body to burn and store sugar. Insulin is given routinely with subcutaneous injection. Insulin pumps are being used in carefully selected children. More highly purified insulins are being developed to reduce complications.

The dosage of insulin is measured in units, and special syringes are used in its administration. A 100-unit (U-100) insulin is the standard form in the United States. Each marking on the 1-mL (U-100) syringe represents *two* units of insulin. The 50-unit disposable syringe is intended for small doses. All vials of U-100 insulin have color-coded caps, and all labels use black print on a white background. Bold letters indicate type: "R" for regular, "N" for neutral protamine Hagedorn (NPH), "L" for lente, "U" for ultralente, and "S" for semilente.

The various types of insulin and their actions are listed in Table 14-2. The main difference is in the amount of time necessary for effect and the length of coverage provided. The values listed are only guidelines. The response of each child with diabetes to any given insulin dose is highly individual and depends on many factors, such as site of injection, local destruction of insulin by tissue enzymes, and insulin antibodies.

Regular rapid-acting insulins are clear. Both NPH, an intermediate type, and ultralente, a long-lasting insulin, have had small amounts of chemicals added to prolong their action and to make them more stable. They offer protection over a period of hours, enabling the patient to do without repeated injections of unmodified insulin. These insulins are cloudy and require mixing before extraction from the vials (Skill 14-1), which is done by rolling the bottle gently between the palms of the hands. Insulin should not be used if it is discolored. Premixed insulin preparations are now available if the family has difficulty with the insulin-mixing technique, but because they are available only in standard doses, they may not be useful for children with doses that need to be altered frequently. Three new insulin medications are lispro, aspart, and glargine. Lispro and aspart are both rapid-acting. Glargine is a basal insulin that most clearly imitates the human insulin as it is absorbed equally throughout the 24-hour period.

Box 14-1   *Blood Glucose Control Levels for Type 1 and/or Type 2 Diabetes Mellitus*

	BEFORE MEALS	BEDTIME
Toddlers and preschoolers under 6 years	100-180	110-200
School age (6-12 years)	90-180	100-180
Adolescent (13-19 years)	90-130	90-150

From National Diabetes Education Program (2006). Overview of diabetes in children and adolescents. Retrieved July 12, 2006, from *http://www.ndep.nih.gov/diabetes/youth/htm*

Table 14-2   *Types of Insulin and Their Effects*

INSULIN TYPE	BRAND NAMES	HYPOGLYCEMIC EFFECT		
		ONSET	PEAK (HR)	DURATION (HR)
RAPID-ACTING				
Lispro	Humalog	5-15 min	1-2	4-6
Aspart	Novolog	5-15 min	1-2	4-6
Regular insulin	Humulin R, Novolin R, Velosulin	0.5-1 hr	—	6-8
Semilente insulin	Semilente	1-1.5 hr	5-10	12-16
INTERMEDIATE-ACTING				
Lente insulin	Humulin L, Novolin L	1-2.5 hr	7-15	24
NPH insulin	Humulin N, Insulatard, Novolin N	1-1.5 hr	4-12	24
LONG-ACTING				
Ultralente insulin	Humulin U Ultralente	2-4 hr	10-16	24
Glargine analog	Lantus	1-2 hr	Flat	24

Skill 14-1 Mixing Insulin

1. Verify insulin label and have insulin at room temperature to assist in decreasing painful injection.
2. Wash hands and clean injection site.
3. Gently rotate insulin bottle or pen.
4. Draw back the amount of air into the syringe that equals the total dose.
5. Inject the amount of air into the long-acting (NPH) vial that equals the NPH dose. Remove the syringe from the vial.

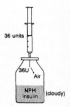

6. Inject the amount of air into the regular-acting insulin vial that equals the regular-acting dose.

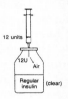

7. Invert the regular-acting insulin vial and withdraw the regular-acting insulin dose amount. Observe for any bubbles and remove.

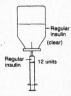

8. Without adding more air to the NPH vial, carefully withdraw the NPH dose.

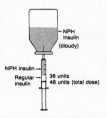

By following these steps, problems can be avoided with contamination of regular insulin with intermediate-acting or long-acting insulin. Should the regular insulin be contaminated, the action time would be affected and the insulin would not be effective in an acute situation such as DKA (American Diabetes Association, 2003).

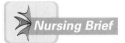

Nursing Brief

Glargine is a clear formula unlike other long-acting insulins and cannot be mixed with any other type of insulin.

Conventional insulin therapy is a one- or two-dose schedule that combines intermediate-acting and rapid-acting insulin. The combination is given before breakfast and dinner. Insulin doses are regulated according to blood glucose measurements. A more intense regimen of more frequent injections according to premeal and early morning (3 AM) glucose levels provides better control and reduces some long-term complications but is difficult to achieve in children and increases the number of hypoglycemic episodes.

Insulin is administered **subcutaneously.** Parents and children must be taught why it is necessary to take the hormone and how to administer it by injection. A child can generally be taught to give self-injections after the age of 7 years. The earlier this is learned, the better. Proper instruction of the patient is one of the most important aspects of the treatment of diabetes. The physician prescribes the type and amount of insulin and specifies the time of administration. The site of the injection is rotated to prevent poor absorption and injury to tissues (Figure 14-4). Injection model forms made from construction paper and site rotation patterns are useful. One suggested site rotation is to use one area for a week. Move to a different site within that area for each injection. The injection sites should be about 1 inch apart. The young child can use a doll for practice. Parents usually find the experience of injecting their own child difficult. One mother stated that for the first few months she gave the injection in the child's hips so that her daughter could not see the expression on her face. Commercially available devices may be used for insulin administration, such as syringe-loaded injectors or pen injectors.

Allergic responses to insulin can be divided into those that occur locally at the injection site, the rare systemic sensitivity (true insulin allergy), and immunological reactions. Lipoatrophy (loss of fat) and lipohypertrophy (increased fat) refer to changes in the subcutaneous tissue at the injection site. Proper rotation of sites and the availability of the newer purified insulins have helped eliminate these conditions. The child is taught to feel for lumps every week and to avoid using any sites that are suspicious. The nurse should ascertain what brand of insulin the patient is using. In general, switching brands of insulin (e.g., Eli Lilly,

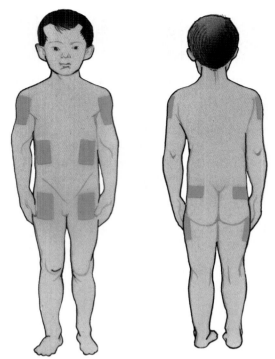

FIGURE **14-4** Sites of injection of insulin. The site of injection should be changed daily to prevent poor absorption and injury to tissues. Rotation should occur both within and among body areas.

Squibb) is not wise because they may be made slightly differently. Questions should be directed to the hospital pharmacist. Refrigeration of insulin to prevent deterioration is no longer necessary. Avoid extremes in temperature and check expiration dates.

Frequently, the doctor orders a combination of a short-acting insulin and an intermediate-acting one; for example, "Give 10 units of NPH insulin and 5 units of regular insulin at 7:30 AM." This offers the patient immediate and longer-lasting insulin coverage. A two-dose schedule has also been used with success. Occasionally, the two-dose schedule results in middle-of-the-night hypoglycemia. In such instances, evening intermediate-acting insulin dose reduction or altered timing of the doses according to physician recommendation can help. Long-acting insulin is seldom given to children because of the danger of hypoglycemia during sleep.

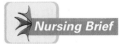

The only oral medication approved for children with type 2 DM is metformin.

Hypoglycemia. **Hypoglycemia** (low blood glucose), also known as insulin shock, occurs when the blood glucose level becomes abnormally low (below 70 mg/dL). This condition is caused by an excess of insulin in the body. Factors that may account for this imbalance include poorly planned or excessive exercise, insufficient food,

inappropriate insulin dose, or errors made because of improper knowledge of insulin and the insulin syringe. Children are more prone to insulin reactions than adults because (1) the condition itself is more unstable in young people, (2) they are growing, and (3) their activities are more irregular. Mild episodes of hypoglycemia are not unusual in the child with diabetes.

The symptoms of an insulin reaction, which range from mild to severe, are generally noticed and treated in the early stages. They appear *suddenly* in the *otherwise well* person. Examination of the blood reveals a lowered blood glucose level. The child becomes irritable and may behave poorly, is pale, and may feel hungry, cold, and weak. Sweating occurs (see Data Cues). Symptoms related to disorders of the nervous system arise because glucose is vital to the proper functioning of nerves. The child may become mentally confused and giddy and may have a headache; muscular coordination is affected. If insulin shock is left untreated, coma and convulsions can occur.

The immediate treatment consists of administering sugar in some form, such as orange juice, cola beverages, ginger ale, hard candy, or a commercial product such as Glutose. If the child begins to feel better within a few minutes and the blood glucose level exceeds 70 mg/dL, the child may eat a small amount of protein or starch (sandwich, milk, cheese) to prevent another reaction.

Glucagon, a hormone that raises the blood glucose level by causing a rapid breakdown of glycogen into glucose in the liver, is recommended for the treatment of severe hypoglycemia. Glucagon acts quickly to restore the child to consciousness in an emergency situation; the child is then able to consume some form of sugar. Glucagon is a hormone produced by the pancreatic islets that also produce insulin. Normally a fall in blood glucose makes the body release this substance. Because the islet cells are destroyed in children with type 1 DM, glucagon is not adequately released. Commercial glucagon is packaged in individual dose units that are stable in powdered form. When it is diluted, glucagon can be given subcutaneously, intramuscularly, or intravenously. Families of patients on insulin therapy can be instructed to administer it subcutaneously or intramuscularly. If the child does not respond rapidly to glucagon administration, the physician should be contacted. When patients are unconscious, they should be kept warm by covering with a blanket. Do not give anything by mouth; get medical attention.

Blood Glucose Self-Monitoring. Blood glucose self-monitoring has dramatically changed the approach to diabetes. Previously, blood tests for glucose could be carried out only in a doctor's office or laboratory. The patient had to rely on urine tests, which often gave a confusing picture, particularly when the urine had been in the bladder for several hours (glucose could appear in the urine when the patient's blood glucose

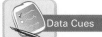Data Cues

Hypoglycemia	Hyperglycemia	Ketoacidosis
Caused by insulin excess	Caused by inadequate insulin	Caused by insulin deficiency
Excessive activity without extra carbohydrate intake	Little or no activity	
Missed or delayed meal	Excessive food	
Sudden onset in healthy child	Slowly	Appears over hours or days
Blood glucose <70 mg/dL	Blood glucose >240 mg/dL	Blood glucose >240 mg/dL
		Urine ketones positive
Initial symptoms of sweating, tremor, feeling cold, anxiety, hunger	Initial symptoms of polyuria, polydipsia, polyphagia, fatigue, weight loss, blurred vision	Initial symptoms include those seen in hyperglycemia with abdominal pain, flushed, restless, fruity breath odor, dry skin
Late symptoms of confusion, weakness, dizziness, nausea and vomiting, headache, stupor, convulsions		Late symptoms of acidosis, dehydration, Kussmaul breathing, coma, death
Give oral carbohydrates, glucagon, intravenous glucose	Give insulin, exercise, increase oral fluids	Give insulin (intravenously), intravenous fluids, electrolyte replacement

level was actually low). Only a blood check can show the actual amount of sugar in the blood at the time of the test. Technology has made it possible for patients to test their own blood glucose in the home. Although still under the supervision and consultation of the physician, the patient can nonetheless make rational changes in insulin dosage, nutritional requirements, and daily exercise. This is of great psychological value to the child, teenager, and parents because it reduces feelings of helplessness and complete dependence on medical personnel.

Home glucose monitoring should be taught to all young patients or their caretakers (Figure 14-5). It is important that the patient not only be skilled in the techniques but also understand the results and how to incorporate them into the daily regimen. This means involvement of the entire health care team in ongoing supervision, demonstration, and support. Although instructions come with the various products, it is highly recommended that patients receive individual training.

The obtaining of blood specimens has been simplified with the use of capillary blood-letting devices such as the Autolet. This device automatically controls the depth of penetration of the lancet into the skin. Other brands include the Hemalet, Autoclix, and Monojector. The sides of the fingertips are recommended because there are fewer nerve endings and more capillary beds in these areas. The best fingers to use are the middle, ring, or little fingers on either hand. If the child washes the hands in warm water for about 30 seconds, the finger bleeds more easily. To perform the test, a drop of blood is put on a chemically treated reagent strip (Chemstrip bG or Dextrostix). Meters are available for reading blood glucose determinations. The test

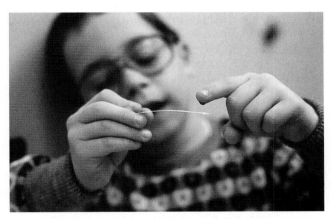

FIGURE **14-5** The school-age child can perform blood glucose monitoring at home.

strip with a drop of blood is inserted, and the reading appears.

Cost, convenience, and lability of the disease are factors to consider in selection of devices. Most products can be obtained at the local pharmacy. Newer and more precise instruments are being developed constantly. Frequency of use is determined by the physician.

Nutritional Management. The advent of blood glucose self-monitoring has enabled more flexible nutritional plans, and yet **consistency** (amount of food and time of feeding) remains the cornerstone of appropriate nutritional management. Contrary to popular belief, no scientific evidence shows that persons with diabetes need special foods. In fact, what is good for the person with diabetes is good for the entire family. The nutrient needs of children with diabetes are essentially no different from those of children without diabetes, with the exception of the elimination of concentrated carbohydrates (simple sugars) and refined sugars. These cause a marked increase in blood glucose and generally should be avoided.

The goals of nutritional management in children are to ensure normal growth and development, to distribute food intake so that it aids metabolic control, and to individualize the diet in accordance with the child's ethnic background, age, gender, weight, activity, family economics, and food preferences. Once a diet order is received from the physician, the dietitian calculates the distribution of carbohydrates, protein, and fat. Portion size is shown with food models and measuring cups and spoons. Regularly spaced meals and snacks are emphasized, and the family is taught how to read labels and the differences between carbohydrates, protein, and fat.

The two major approaches to nutritional management include the use of exchange lists and the constant carbohydrate diet. Exchange lists consist of foods separated into several food categories (fruit, milk, meat, bread, vegetables, fats). A food plan is developed that prescribes the amount or portion size of allowed food in each category. The child is given a choice from any number of foods in an individual category to meet the prescribed amount. In this way, the plan is flexible and according to the child's preferences.

The constant carbohydrate diet is a fairly new approach to meal planning. The goal is to maintain a consistent amount of carbohydrate at each meal and snack. Regularity of meals is stressed. The amount of carbohydrate may, and usually does, vary between meals. The initial carbohydrate pattern is determined by the individual's current food intake. To calculate the number of grams of carbohydrate in food, exchange lists that divide foods according to carbohydrate content are used. This food plan appeals to young patients with diabetes because of its ease in use and flexibility.

The importance of fiber in diets is well documented. In the patient with diabetes, fiber has been shown to reduce blood glucose and serum cholesterol levels. Fiber appears to slow the rate of absorption of sugar by the digestive tract. Raw fruits and vegetables and whole grain breads and cereals are good sources of fiber.

Because persons with diabetes have an increased risk for heart disease, the reduction of serum cholesterol is another concern. These persons (like most of the general public) need to reduce their intake of animal fats or substitute vegetable fat for animal fat. The use of polyunsaturated fats in cooking is advised.

The form of the food is also important. An apple, apple juice, or applesauce may precipitate different blood glucose responses. Portions, the type of processing, cooking, and combinations of foods have also been shown to have a bearing on these responses.

Aspartame (Nutra-Sweet) was approved by the U.S. Food and Drug Administration in 1981. It is used in items that do not require cooking. Aspartame is made of two amino acids. Both contain insignificant amounts of carbohydrate. One granulation form is called *Equal*. Sucralose (Splenda) is the newest low-calorie sweetener on the market. Sucralose can be used anywhere sugar can be used, such as in beverages, baked goods, and processed foods. Other artificial sweeteners are not recommended for children.

Exercise. Exercise is important for the child with diabetes because it causes the body to use sugar and promotes good circulation. It lowers the blood glucose and in this respect acts more like insulin. The patient with diabetes who has planned vigorous exercise should carry extra sugar to avoid insulin reactions. The patient should also carry money for candy or a drink or for a telephone call. The blood glucose level is high directly after meals, so active sports can be participated in at such times. Less active games should be enjoyed directly before meals. The child with diabetes should be able to participate in almost all active sports. Poorly planned exercise, however, can lead to difficulties. Like any other child, the child with diabetes should not swim unsupervised.

Skin Care. The patient should be instructed to bathe daily and dry well. Cleansing of the inguinal area, axillae, and perineum area is especially important because yeast and fungal infections tend to occur there. Inspect skin for cuts, rashes, abrasions, bruises, cysts, or boils. Treat promptly. If the skin is very dry, oil such as Alpha-Keri may be used in the bath water. Adolescents are taught to use electric razors. Avoid exposing the skin to extremes in temperatures. Inspect injection sites for lumps.

Foot Care. Although circulatory problems of the feet are less common in children, proper foot hygiene habits need to be established. Instruct the patient to wash and dry the feet well each day. Inspect for interdigital cracking, and check the condition of the toenails. Trim the nails straight across. Do not use corn remedies, iodine, or alcohol. Change socks daily, and avoid tight socks or large ones that bunch. Replace shoes often as the child grows. Wear boots only for short periods to minimize sweating. The patient should not go barefoot. If problems arise, consult a physician or podiatrist.

Infections. Obtain immunizations against communicable diseases. Cystitis, subcutaneous nodules, and monilial vulvitis occur with greater frequency in patients with diabetes. During late adolescence female patients should see a gynecologist yearly.

Urine Checks. Routine urine checks for sugar are being replaced by the more accurate glucose blood monitoring. However, this procedure does not test for acetone, which the patient may need to determine, particularly when the blood glucose level is high and during illness. Daily checks may also be advocated for some patients. The term *urine check* rather than test is less confusing to young children. During hospitalization, urine testing may be ordered. The two-drop method, with a second voided specimen, is frequently used. A second specimen is not always possible to obtain from a child; therefore it may be prudent to test the first one. If this occurs, record as first or second voiding. The nurse reads the manufacturer's directions and reviews the directions with the child. Regardless of which method is used, *exact timing* is important. The dipstick method is used more frequently than tablets because it is convenient and simple. Clinitest tablets are poison and must be kept away from children and confused adults. Test results may be affected by large doses of aspirin, antibiotics, and other medications. Check expiration dates on the carton or bottle. Instruct the child to wash hands before and after the procedure. Record results. Quantitative urine collection is sometimes ordered. All voided specimens over a period of time are collected in a receptacle. The results show how many grams of glucose are eliminated during the time allocated (generally 24 hours).

Glucose-Insulin Imbalances. The patient is taught to recognize the signs of insulin shock and ketoacidosis. Early attention to change and daily record keeping are stressed. Many excellent teaching films and brochures are available. The child should wear a Medic-Alert bracelet. Wallet cards are also available. Teachers, athletic coaches, and guidance officers should be informed about the disease and should have the phone numbers of the patient's parents and physician.

Psychosocial Aspects. Children newly diagnosed with type 1 DM often go through a transitional or "honeymoon" stage. Because the body still releases small amounts of insulin until complete destruction of islet cells occurs, initial dosage requirements of insulin may decrease temporarily. This does not mean that the condition is resolving. Parents need to understand that insulin doses vary but that the child continues to need lifelong insulin administration.

Because children with diabetes are growing, additional dimensions of the disorder and its treatment become evident. Growth is not steady but occurs in spurts and plateaus that have a bearing on treatment. Infants and toddlers may have hydration problems, especially during illness. Preschool children have irregular activity and eating patterns. School-age children may grieve over the diagnosis and ask, "Why me?" They may use the illness to gain attention or to avoid responsibilities. The onset of puberty may require adjustments in insulin as a result of growth and the antagonistic effect of the growth and sex hormones on insulin. Adolescents often resent this condition, which deviates from their concept of the body ideal. They have more difficulty in resolving the conflict between dependence and independence. This may lead to rebellion against the parents and the treatment regimen.

The impact of the disease on the rest of the family must also be considered. One mother commented, "I was so scared. I felt very strongly that whether my child lived or died depended on me. It was overwhelming. I couldn't allow myself mistakes. This was reinforced by all the do's and don'ts of the instructions." Parents may also feel guilty for having passed on the disease. Siblings may feel jealous of the patient. The sharing of responsibility by parents is ideal but is not necessarily a reality. In fact the successful management of the condition greatly depends on parent involvement and family organization skills. Everyone may have difficulty accepting the diagnosis and the more regimented lifestyle it imposes. Each family member must cope with a personal reaction to the stress of the illness.

It is important that the child assume responsibility for care gradually, according to cognitive and developmental readiness, and with a minimum of pressure. Overprotection can be as detrimental as neglect. Parents who have received satisfaction from their child's dependence on them may need help letting go. An experience at a camp for children with diabetes is helpful in this respect.

Emotional upsets can be as disturbing to the patient as an infection and may require food or insulin adjustments. Early detection of and intervention in deteriorating personal relationships and rebellion against diabetic management decreases the severity of the effects on the child. The nurse should be attuned to little problems that are frequently veiled requests for help. Family therapy and other forms of psychotherapeutic help may be necessary. Support by caretakers helps with preventing difficulties. Table 14-3 summarizes some stresses experienced by the child with diabetes and possible nursing interventions.

Other Issues. With planning, children can enjoy travel with their families, and older adolescents can travel alone. Before traveling, the child should be seen by the physician for a checkup and prescriptions for supplies. A written statement and a card identifying the child as having diabetes should be carried. Realize that crossing time zones may affect relative mealtimes. Keep additional supplies of insulin, sugar, and food with the child. *Never* check these with luggage, especially on an airplane. If foreign travel is planned, parents need to become familiar with the food in the area so that dietary requirements can be met. Local chapters of the American Diabetes Association or the Juvenile Diabetes Foundation can help vacationing families in an emergency.

The person with diabetes usually tolerates surgery well. Insulin may be given before or after the operation. If the patient is restricted to NPO (nothing by mouth), calories may be supplied with intravenous glucose. Details vary according to the procedure and the child's diabetes treatment. Careful review of the patient's history helps in formulating nursing care plans and provides a basis for teaching. The goal is to prevent hypoglycemia during the perioperative NPO period because the body is stressed from the surgery.

Table 14-3 | *Summary of Predictable Stress on Children with Type 1 Diabetes and Their Families*

ISSUE	NURSING INTERVENTION
INFANT	
Trust versus mistrust	Stress consistency in need fulfillment
Onset and diagnosis particularly difficult during infancy; anxiety can be transmitted to baby	Involve both parents in education
	Avoid information overload
	Instill hope and confidence
	Focus on child rather than disease
	Review normal growth and development of infancy
	Assist in problem solving (babysitters, difficulty in obtaining specimens, baby food exchange lists, etc.)
TODDLER	
Autonomy versus shame and doubt	Prepare child for procedures or separations
	Encourage exploration of environment
	Stress limit setting as a form of love
Is this a temper tantrum or high or low blood glucose?	Admit it is difficult to distinguish temper tantrums from symptoms
	If worsens or is prolonged or physical symptoms appear, check blood glucose; tight monitoring of blood glucose is highly recommended
	Provide 24-hr telephone number
PRESCHOOL CHILD	
Initiative versus guilt	Foster sense of competence
May view injections as punishment	Educate parents to provide consistent warmth, reassurance, and love
May view denial of sweets as lack of love	Educate parents to provide consistent warmth, reassurance, and love
	Discuss feelings about personal life and diabetes
	Avoid negative connotation by words (e.g., "bad blood test," "cheating")
	Help parents sort out child's fantasies
"Picky eater"	Plan favorite party dishes on occasion
	Invite a playmate for lunch
	Suggest alternative nutritious snacks
ELEMENTARY SCHOOL PUPIL	
Industry versus inferiority	Assist child in how to respond to teasing from peers ("Ick, needles!")
May feel hospitalization will be cure	Explain "honeymoon" stage of disease
Grief over lack of cure	Accept child's disappointment
Rebellion over treatment regimen	Gradually have child assume self-management of insulin and specimen tests; this increases feelings of mastery and control
Rebellion over food plan	Provide lists of fast-food exchanges
Anxiety about disclosure of condition to friends	Group-related education with peers who have diabetes
Embarrassed about reactions in school, missed days	Open dialogue between health personnel and teachers, school nurse, fellow students
Unpredictable effects of exercise	Continual reinforcement of treatment principles with specific regard to hypoglycemia or hyperglycemia and emergencies
AT PUBERTY	
Bouncing blood glucose levels may make child feel out of control	Explain that growth and sex hormones affect blood glucose levels
	Girls, in particular, have difficulties about the time of menstruation
	Adjustments in insulin and food are common for most children with diabetes at this stage
Anger at the disease ("Why must I be different?")	Assist patient in acceptable ways of expressing anger; discuss anger with parents, since they are often the target of it
More frequent hospitalizations	Provide encouragement and support; be alert to marital stress and sibling deprivation
TEENAGER	
Threatens sexual identity and body image	Encourage teenager to meet other adolescents with diabetes (camps, support groups, if not tried earlier); this helps decrease isolation
Surge toward independence, risk taking, or greater than usual need for security	Provide consistency with limit setting, avoid overcontrol—listen, listen, listen
Worries about health, prospects for marriage and family	Adolescents need to have full instruction regarding pregnancy risk or male potency; provide a safe environment for discussion; make appropriate referrals
Alcohol and drug abuse	Encourage patient's interest in diabetic research
	Share concerns and dangers with teenager

The child needs to see the physician regularly and have a physical examination every 3 to 4 months. The patient should also be taught to visit the dentist regularly for cleaning of teeth and gums; appointments should be scheduled for right after meals. Brushing and flossing daily are important. Eyes should be examined regularly; blurry vision must not be disregarded. Magazines such as *Diabetes Forecast* and *Diabetes in the News* offer excellent suggestions and guidance.

Role of the Nurse. Nursing responsibilities begin with preparing the child for meals. Blood glucose is usually checked before meals and at bedtime and may need to be checked in the early morning hours if there is a problem with hypoglycemia during sleep. Because of the importance of food intake for the child with diabetes, distracting toys are removed during mealtimes. The child's meals and snacks are served **on time**. Children who receive regular insulin before meals may have an insulin reaction if food is not taken within 20 minutes. If nurses are scheduled for lunch when diet meals are served, they should notify the team leader and should not assume that others will feed the child. No foods or liquids, with the exception of water, are given between meals unless authorized by the physician or dietitian. Be sure that the tray is served to the **correct patient**. A mistake can occur, particularly if several children are on special diets. This can happen more easily on the pediatric unit, where many patients roam about freely. Foods the child especially enjoys or dislikes are noted.

When the child has finished, the nurse observes the types and amounts of foods that the patient refused and charts them in the nurses' notes. These are brought to the attention of the dietitian, who determines the number of calories that need to be made up and orders a between-meal snack such as orange juice to compensate. Anorexia or vomiting is reported promptly. After the meal, the nurse washes the child's hands and face and returns the toys.

Education of the patient is an ongoing process. Too much information given at one time may be overwhelming to parents and discouraging to the child. Well-informed nurses can do much in the way of reinforcement and support. They can clarify such terms *as dietetic, sugar-free, juice-packed, water-packed,* and *unsweetened*. Meal trays in the hospital provide an excellent opportunity for teaching. Children should bring their own lunch to school. The nurse reinforces the interaction between nutrition, insulin requirements, and exercise and answers questions from the child or family.

Teenagers need to be advised that alcohol lowers the blood sugar. It suppresses gluconeogenesis and is high in calories. Most cocktail mixes contain sugar; however, water, sugar-free pop, club soda, and tomato juice do not. Although the consumption of alcohol is to be discouraged, if a young person of drinking age wishes to drink, it is better to drink *after* dinner or to consume the beverage with some type of food.

The Future of Research on Diabetes. Diabetic research is being conducted on many fronts. Geneticists are helping determine how diabetes is inherited so that someday they will be able to predict who will inherit the disease. If a virus is involved, a vaccine may help in its prevention. Pancreas transplantation has been performed, and the success rate is improving. β cells have been transplanted in animals, with the result that the animals have been cured. Another possibility is that of an artificial pancreas. Its precursors might be the insulin pumps being refined today. Administration of insulin via inhalation is being researched. The laser beam has aided in the treatment of complicated eye conditions. Such advances hold promise for the hope of resolving or eradicating the dilemma of diabetes.

RESPIRATORY SYSTEM

ASTHMA
Description
Asthma is the most common chronic illness in childhood. It is also the leading cause of emergency department visits, hospital admissions, and school absenteeism (Kliegman et al., 2006). Eighty percent of cases of asthma occur before the age of 5 years. Asthma is more frequently seen in poor children, partly because they often live in old homes with high concentrations of precipitating allergens. School nurses are seeing an increasing number of children with asthma on a daily basis and require a good understanding of the course of treatment for asthma. Nurses are giving inhalation treatments in school; such treatments can help the child manage the condition on a day-to-day basis.

Asthma is a reversible obstruction of the large and small airways caused by mucosal edema, smooth muscle constriction, and thick tenacious mucus. Also known as **reactive airway disease,** asthma may be precipitated by allergens such as pollens, foods, dust mites, and animal dander, which irritate the airways and initiate bronchoconstriction and the inflammatory process. Asthma may also be triggered by temperature changes, cold air, viral infections, and exercise. One of the major triggers of asthma is exposure to cigarette smoke.

Stress can precipitate an asthma attack or exacerbate the condition. Because asthma is a chronic disease of childhood, the stress on the child and family is important to consider.

A family history of allergies is often seen, although the child may have different manifestations. Careful management of asthma in children improves the prognosis, and most children do well. Children with severe asthma usually continue to have asthma in adulthood (Behrman et al., 2004). **Status asthmaticus** is defined as an episode of asthma that does not respond

---

Box 14-2 | *Classification of Asthma*

MILD INTERMITTENT
Symptoms less than twice a week
Asymptomatic between exacerbations
Exacerbations are brief
Nighttime symptoms less than twice a month
Normal PEFR between exacerbations
PEFR is greater than 80% of predicted value

MILD PERSISTENT
Symptoms more than twice a week but less than 1 time
  a day
Exacerbations may affect activity
Nighttime symptoms are more than twice a month
PEFR is greater than 80% of predicted value

MODERATE PERSISTENT
Daily symptoms
Daily use of inhaled short-acting β_2-agonist
Exacerbations occur more than twice a week
Exacerbations may last for days
Exacerbation affect activity
Nighttime symptoms are more than once a week
PEFR is greater than 60% to less than 80% of predicted
  value

SEVERE PERSISTENT
Continual symptoms
Frequent exacerbations
Limited physical activity
Frequent nighttime exacerbations
PEFR is less than 60% of predicted value

Adapted from National Asthma Education and Prevention Program Expert Panel Report 2. (April 1997). *Guidelines for the diagnosis and management of asthma.* Bethesda, MD: National Institutes of Health/National Heart, Lung, and Blood Institute.

to ordinary therapeutic measures. Hospitalization is necessary, perhaps in the intensive care unit (ICU).

Signs and Symptoms

Symptoms can occur abruptly (e.g., after sudden exposure to cold air or cigarette smoke) or over a period of days (precipitated by upper respiratory infection or mild exposure to an allergen). Initially the child has a tight nonproductive cough. Wheezing, particularly expiratory wheezing, may be audible or heard through a stethoscope. Depending on the severity of the problem, the child can have signs of increasing respiratory distress develop (tachycardia, dyspnea, tachypnea, retractions, pallor). The child appears tired and might have difficulty talking.

Asthma is categorized into four classifications (Box 14-2). Appropriate management of asthma depends on the child's symptoms and includes a baseline measurement of the peak expiratory flow rate (PEFR), or the force of expiration from maximum lung inflation. This is done with a special meter, which most children over the age of 5 years can be taught to use successfully. Children determine their personal best PEFR on their

meter and when replaced the child needs to reestablish a new personal best with the new meter (Hockenberry & Wilson, 2007). Thereafter, daily (or more frequent) monitoring of PEFR and comparison with the child's personal best can indicate how well the asthma is being controlled.

Oxygen saturation monitoring can help determine the severity of an episode. The child may exhibit elevated eosinophils in a complete blood count (CBC) and elevated immunoglobulin E (IgE) levels. Allergy skin tests may reveal precipitating allergens. Chest radiographs can show underlying respiratory infection.

Some school-age children and adolescents have exercise-induced bronchospasm, which often does not indicate underlying asthma. Wheezing, shortness of breath, and chest tightness appear after vigorous exercise. There is bronchoconstriction without underlying inflammation. Treatment of exercise-induced bronchospasm consists of taking an inhaled β-agonist 15 minutes before exercise. Also effective is the use of leukotriene receptor antagonists with exercise-induced asthma. These drugs are more attractive because of the oral route and decreased dependency. The child should avoid exercising in the cold because cold air can precipitate the condition.

Treatment and Nursing Care

The goal of treatment is to manage the condition appropriately so that the child can maintain optimal lifestyle and development. The treatment is focused on reducing episodes, minimizing the inflammatory process, decreasing the number of hospitalizations, avoiding precipitating factors, and facilitating normal growth and development.

The physician should obtain the child's history in detail. Skin tests may be administered to determine whether allergy is a cause. If so, it is necessary to eliminate the offender, whether it is an environmental agent or a food. Special measures should include the reduction of dust mites, mold, animal dander, cockroach allergens, and tobacco smoke in the home.

Medications are classified into two categories: long-term medications (**controllers**) and short-acting (**rescuer**) medications. Table 14-4 lists the common medications in both categories. The preferred route of administration of many of these medications is inhalation because it allows the medications to act directly on the airways. Inhalation treatments can be given via nebulizer, in which the medication is mixed with normal saline solution and aerosolized, **metered-dose inhaler** (MDI), or **dry powder inhaler** (DPI). Even young infants can benefit from nebulizer treatments (Figure 14-6). Bronchodilators can also be given via MDI if the child is able to follow the instructions (Skill 14-2). Most children over 5 years of age can manage an MDI. Some younger children can use an MDI with an attached spacer device,

Table 14-4 | *Asthma Medications*

CONTROLLER	TRADE NAME	DOSE FORM	SIDE EFFECTS
CORTICOSTEROIDS **Inhaled**			
Beclomethasone dipropionate	Beconase, QVAR	MDT, intranasal	Growth retardation, nasal irritation, unpleasant taste, headache; not recommended for children <6 years
Budesonide	Rhinocort, Pulmicort	MDI, intranasal	Growth retardation, nasal irritation, dry mouth; avoid chickenpox exposure
Flunisolide	Aerobid, Nasalide	MDI, intranasal	Growth retardation, gastrointestinal upset, unpleasant taste; not recommended for children <6 years
Fluticasone propionate	Flovent, Flonase	MDI, intranasal	Nausea, vomiting, dizziness, dental problems
Triamcinolone acetonide	Azmacort, Aristocort	MDI, oral, intranasal	Growth retardation, nausea, fatigue, lethargy, dizziness; not recommended for children <6 years
Systemic			
Methylprednisolone	Medrol, Solu-Medrol	Oral	Mask infection, growth retardation, cushingoid signs
Prednisolone	Prelone, Orapred, Pedipred	Oral	Insomnia, nervousness, mood swings, facial flushing
Prednisone	Sterapred	Oral	Insomnia, heartburn, nervousness, appetite changes, mood swings, nausea, vomiting
Antiinflammatory Agents			
Cromolyn sodium	Intal, Crolom, Nasalcrom	MDI, intranasal, oral	Fatigue, unpleasant taste, tachycardia, headache, rash, nasal congestion
Nedocromil	Tilade	MDI	Headache, unpleasant taste, cough, nausea
Leukotriene Modifiers			
Zafirlukast	Accolate	Oral, chewable tablet	Headache, nausea, vomiting, dizziness
Montelukast	Singulair	Oral	Headache, flu-like symptoms, abdominal pain
Long-Acting β_2-Agonists			
Salmeterol	Serevent	MDI, diskhaler	Tachycardia, tremor, nervousness, headache
Theophylline	Slo-bid, Theo-dur	Oral Not used as much	CNS hyperstimulation, seizures
Formoterol	Foradil	MDI	Tremors, dizziness, dysphonia
RESCUE **Short-Acting β_2-Agonist**			
Albuterol	Proventil, Ventolin	MDI, syrup, Neb	Tremors, anxiety, insomnia, tachycardia, heartburn, vomiting
Terbutaline	Brethine, Brethaire	MDI, Inject	Tremors, anxiety, insomnia, tachycardia, heartburn, vomiting
Levalbuterol	Xopenex	Neb	Tachycardia, tremor, insomnia, nausea, headache
Corticosteroids—Systemic			
Methylprednisolone	Medrol	Oral	Mask infection, growth retardation, cushingoid signs
Prednisolone	Prelone	Oral	Insomnia, nervousness, mood swings, facial flushing
Prednisone	Orasone, Deltasone, Meticorten	Oral	Insomnia, heartburn, nervousness, increased appetite
Anticholinergics			
Ipratropium bromide	Atrovent	MDI	Tachycardia, eye pain, cough, nervousness
Anti-IgE Antibodies			
Omalizumab	Xolair	SubQ	Headache

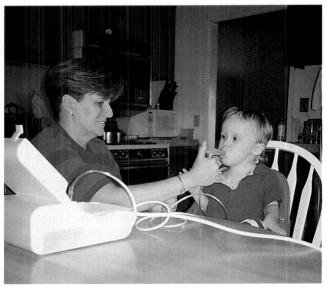

FIGURE **14-6** Appropriate use of a nebulizer involves placing the mouthpiece directly in the mouth. The child is encouraged to breathe normally.

which directs the medication more precisely and has excellent outcomes.

A new class of drugs is oral antileukotrienes (e.g., Singulair and Accolate). They have been useful for the prevention of asthma attacks. They are used in conjunction with corticosteroids and can reduce the level of need for corticosteroids. Singulair is given daily, and Accolate is given twice a day. Another new medication is omalizumab, an anti-IgE antibody that is administered by subcutaneous injection and has demonstrated positive results with moderate to severe allergy-related asthma in children 12 years or older (Kinane & Scirica, 2006).

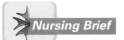

Nursing Brief

The key to chronic asthma management is long-term control of airway inflammation. Education is the key to reducing underappreciation of the disease, failure to follow treatment guidelines, nonadherence, and difficulty with inhalation devices.

Skill 14-2 Use of a Metered-Dose Inhaler

1. Remove cap from MDI and hold canister upright.
2. Shake the inhaler canister three or four times.
3. Tilt head back slightly and exhale normally.
4. Position the inhaler in one of the following ways:
   - Close lips around mouthpiece of inhaler.
   - Open mouth and hold mouthpiece two fingerbreadths from mouth.
   - Use a spacer.

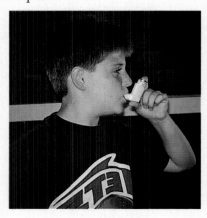

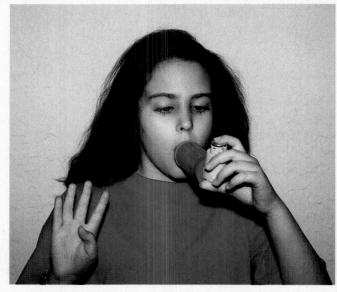

5. Start to breathe in slowly and press down on the inhaler to release the medication as you are inhaling.
6. Continue inhaling slowly and deeply (3 to 5 seconds).
7. Hold breath for a count of 10 (5 to 10 seconds) to allow the medicine to reach the lungs and then exhale.
8. Wait 1 to 2 minutes and repeat the puff.
9. Rinse out the mouth with water and spit out especially when taking an inhaled corticosteroid.

Children with acute exacerbations of asthma, which require a visit to the doctor's office or emergency room, usually are treated with nebulized albuterol every 20 minutes for 1 hour with oxygen. If the symptoms improve, the child is placed on a daily routine of bronchodilators and short-term oral steroids (3-day to 5-day course). If the child's condition does not resolve and the oxygen saturation is less than 90%, the child should be admitted to the hospital.

On admission, an intravenous solution is started and oxygen is given with nasal prongs, hood, or mask. Nebulized albuterol is continued either continuously or intermittently. Anticholinergic drugs, such as ipratropium bromide, may be added to assist in additional bronchodilation. Currently, aminophylline does not appear to provide additional benefits and is not usually administered. For severe airway obstruction that does not respond to treatment, aminophylline may be administered. Because aminophylline can cause cardiac dysrhythmias, children receiving aminophylline intravenously should be placed on a cardiac monitor during the course of therapy. Intravenous steroids, such as methylprednisolone, are administered to control the inflammatory response. Before discharge, the treatment is changed to oral medication.

Facilitating Optimal Gas Exchange. Place the child in a high Fowler's position. Some children may prefer to have a pillow placed on the over-bed table and to extend their arms over it. This allows maximal use of the accessory muscles of breathing. The child may receive humidified oxygen with mask or cannula. Infants and young children often do better with nasal prongs because they do not feel as though they are suffocating, as they might with a mask. An oxygen mask should not be used if it causes the child anxiety.

The nurse should organize care to provide for periods of uninterrupted rest. Cuddling and rocking the younger child often reduces distress and promotes sleep. Older children can be distracted with quiet music or games.

Vital signs, breath sounds, and a respiratory assessment, which includes oxygen saturation measurement, are done at least every 2 to 4 hours. Children in acute distress are monitored more frequently.

The child may be apprehensive because of the respiratory distress. The nurse should display a calm manner and remain with the child during periods of distress. Often, encouraging the child to breathe slowly, or to breathe along with you as you breathe slowly, decreases the child's anxiety and allows for maximum air exchange.

Maintaining Hydration. The child who is hospitalized with asthma should have an intravenous infusion started. If the child is not in acute respiratory distress, clear oral fluids should also be offered. The child's need for fluids is increased because of fluid loss through dyspnea and diaphoresis. The fluids offered should

Skill 14-3 Use and Interpretation of Peak Flow Meter

Use

1. Move slide marker to zero.
2. Standing upright with no gum or food in mouth, hold meter horizontal.
3. Relax, taking a few slow deep breaths.
4. Close mouth around mouthpiece and keep tongue away from mouthpiece.
5. Blow out hard and as fast as possible.
6. Note the marker number and repeat the previous steps for a total of three times, waiting at least 30 seconds between each time.
7. Record the highest of the three tries.
8. The peak flow meter reading should be done close to the same time each day. Readings should be done at least once a day, preferably in the morning.
9. A chart or record should be maintained.

Interpretation

1. Green zone (80% to 100% of personal best): no symptoms are present and routine treatment plan can be followed.
2. Yellow zone (50% to 79% of personal best): indicates caution. An acute episode may be present. Medication may need to be increased.
3. Red zone (<50% of personal best): indicates airway narrowing. Short-acting bronchodilator should be administered. If peak flow meter does not return immediately and stay in yellow or green zone, medical attention should be sought.

not be cold because these may cause bronchospasm. The child's intake and output are measured.

Encouraging Self-Care and Asthma Management Skills. Before discharge, the older child and parent are taught self-care. The patient is taught to recognize early signs of difficulties and personal triggers that can serve as forewarnings of an attack. The importance of following directions in the administration of medications is stressed, as is awareness of side effects. The use of nebulizers or aerosol devices is also taught.

Review the procedure for measuring PEFR (Skill 14-3). Some peak flow meters are colored like traffic lights. These zones should be individualized by the physician for each child. Remind the child to measure PEFR at the same times each day, usually morning and evening. If the child does the measurement after taking routine medications, the measurement should be done 15 minutes after the medication.

Specific information about how often and when to use a particular inhaler is also emphasized. The child

Table 14-5 | *Symptoms of Acute Rheumatic Fever*

SYMPTOMS	DESCRIPTION
Carditis	Involves the myocardium (heart muscle), the pericardium, and endocardium, but particularly the *mitral valve*, located between the left atrium and left ventricle. Inflammation causes dysfunction of the valve initially; later, scarring leads to mitral stenosis. Myocardial lesions called *Aschoff bodies* are also characteristic of the disease. Murmurs can be heard, and ECG alterations are present. The burden on the heart is great because it has to pump harder to circulate the blood. As a result, it may become enlarged and fail.
Polyarthritis	Painful, tender, warm, red, and swollen joints, especially the knees, elbows, ankles, wrists, and shoulders. Symptoms in one joint may disappear, only to appear in another joint (migratory arthritis). This pattern may continue for a few weeks without treatment with antiinflammatory medications. There is no permanent joint damage.
Erythema marginatum	Small red circles and wavy lines on the trunk and extremities that appear and disappear rapidly. The rash may come and go for several months.
Sydenham chorea	Characterized by involuntary, purposeless movements of the muscles. Begins as clumsiness, which is often noted by teachers. The child may stumble and spill things and may have difficulty buttoning clothes and writing. When the facial muscles are involved, grimacing occurs. The child may laugh and cry inappropriately. In severe cases, the patient may become completely incapacitated and deterioration in speech may be noticeable. Symptoms decrease when the child is at rest. Chorea is self-limiting, and full recovery is expected. It can last as little as 2 weeks or more than a year.
Subcutaneous nodules	Hard, painless swellings that occur most frequently over bony prominences (scalp, spine, joints).

needs to be seen regularly by the physician to evaluate progress and adjust medications. Review signs of respiratory infection: where, when, and whom to call for help. The child and family should be aware of early signs of an asthma attack and methods of limiting such an attack.

Regular exercise is stressed. Swimming is an excellent sport for children with asthma, although they can participate in many other sports as well. If the child with asthma also has exercise-induced bronchospasm, use of an inhaler before exercising is important.

Listen to and provide support for the patient, parents, and siblings. Review stress reduction strategies with the child. These often can avert an impending attack. Parents should be encouraged to allow the child to live a normal life within the limits of a chronic condition. Refer the family to social services for additional support and to the Asthma and Allergy Foundation of America or the American Lung Association. Be certain that all children discharged from the hospital have appropriate inhalation equipment for the home management of their condition (Nursing Care Plan 14-1).

CARDIOVASCULAR SYSTEM

ACUTE RHEUMATIC FEVER
Description
Acute rheumatic fever is a systemic disease that involves the joints, heart, central nervous system (CNS), skin, and subcutaneous tissues. It follows an infection with certain strains of group A β-hemolytic streptococci (GABHS). The condition is uncommon in the United States, but there have been outbreaks. Its peak incidence rate occurs between the ages of 5 and 15 years (Behrman et al., 2004). Rheumatic fever has a high family incidence

and is more common worldwide in lower income groups and in overcrowded conditions. It is more prevalent in fall, winter, and spring because carrier rates among schoolchildren are believed to increase during these seasons. Genetic factors also have been implicated. The incidence of rheumatic fever fell dramatically with the widespread use of antibiotics in the 1960s and 1970s. The disease remains a concern, however, because of its potential to cause permanent cardiac problems.

Rheumatic fever is considered an autoimmune inflammatory response of connective tissue to untreated GABHS. Rheumatic fever typically follows an upper respiratory tract infection (tonsillitis, pharyngitis). Throat cultures done at the time of diagnosis of rheumatic fever are not always positive for streptococci because there is a latent period of 1 to 3 weeks between the streptococcal infection and the onset of rheumatic fever. It is thought that during this period the body becomes sensitized to the organism and develops an immune response to it. This immune response affects the particular body tissues described previously. The disease is self-limiting.

Signs and Symptoms
Symptoms range from mild to severe and may not occur for several weeks after a streptococcal infection. The classic symptoms are outlined in Table 14-5. The diagnosis of rheumatic fever is difficult, and for this reason, the revised Jones criteria have been developed and modified over the years (Figure 14-7). The presence of two major criteria, or of one major and two minor criteria, along with evidence of recent streptococcal infection, indicates a high probability of rheumatic fever (Figure 14-8). The diagnosis of Sydenham chorea or carditis without any other known cause is sufficient alone to suggest rheumatic fever (Behrman et al., 2004).

NURSING CARE PLAN 14-1

The Child with Asthma

NURSING DIAGNOSIS *Gas exchange, impaired, related to increasing airway obstruction from inflammation and mucus*

Goals/Outcome Criteria	Nursing Interventions	Rationales
Child shows adequate gas exchange, as evidenced by: • Pink skin color • Normal respiratory rate and rhythm • Ability to talk and sleep comfortably • Absence of wheezing, cough	Provide inhaled bronchodilators and other medications as ordered; monitor for effects and side effects.	Relax bronchial tissue and open up the airway. Cromolyn prevents late allergic response; steroids reduce inflammation.
	Monitor vital signs and oxygen saturation closely (at least every 2-4 hr) for signs of increased respiratory distress. Maintain oxygen saturation between 92% and 95%.	Close monitoring allows rapid recognition of respiratory distress.
	Place child on a cardiac monitor according to hospital protocol if receiving aminophylline; carefully monitor theophylline levels.	Theophylline can cause cardiac rhythm abnormalities.
	Provide humidified oxygen as ordered via least stressful route.	Facilitates adequate oxygenation in the lung.
	Place child in upright position.	Facilitates lung expansion.
	Organize care to provide maximum rest periods.	Decreased energy expenditure decreases need for oxygen.
	Encourage relaxation strategies such as slow, deep, breathing; listening to quiet music or stories. Rock the infant or young child.	Relaxation decreases stress and respiratory effort.

NURSING DIAGNOSIS *Fluid volume, risk for deficient, related to fluid loss from increased expirations and diaphoresis*

Goals/Outcome Criteria	Nursing Interventions	Rationales
Child maintains adequate hydration, as evidenced by: • Good skin turgor • Adequate urination • Absence of thirst • Moist mucous membranes	Provide intravenous fluids as ordered.	Maintains fluid balance while the child may be unable to take oral fluids.
	Give clear oral fluids when respiratory effort decreases; give fluids child likes.	Providing fluids child likes increases child's interest in taking them.
	Avoid cold fluids.	Can cause bronchospasm.
	Give small, frequent sips rather than larger amounts; use straws, "sippy" cups, or other devices that interest the child.	Giving large volumes of fluid can result in vomiting when the child coughs; large volumes also cause distention, which limits diaphragm movement.
	Monitor intake and output.	Provides data on hydration status.

NURSING DIAGNOSIS *Coping, ineffective, related to stress of acute and chronic illness*

Goals/Outcome Criteria	Nursing Interventions	Rationales
Child has decreased stress: • Appears calm and in control • Shows stress-reducing measures	Encourage regular participation in exercise.	Exercise releases hormones that facilitate a feeling of well-being.
	Advise the child to participate in exercise or sports that require short periods of energy (sprints, baseball, gymnastics) or in swimming.	Short bursts of energy allow the child to recover in between; swimming provides external source of moisture for airways.
	Advise child to find enjoyable activities that reduce stress (e.g., bike riding, talking to friends, playing games).	Reducing stress helps the child cope with daily living.
	Advise parents to encourage child to participate in normal developmental activities.	Overprotection increases stress by decreasing the child's self-esteem.

Continued

NURSING CARE PLAN 14-1—cont'd

The Child with Asthma—cont'd

NURSING DIAGNOSIS *Deficient knowledge about home management, related to inexperience with equipment, medications, and principles of disease management*

Goals/Outcome Criteria	Nursing Interventions	Rationales
Parent and older child appropriately manage condition at home: • Demonstrate equipment • Describe signs indicating condition is worse • Intervene appropriately • Describe principles of infection prevention	Review teaching about MDI, nebulizer equipment, and PEFR measurements. Have child and parent demonstrate use of equipment. Review medications and when to use them. Provide a list of criteria for when it is necessary to adjust medications or call the doctor. Help parents with environmental control measures (e.g., allergy-proofing the home, installing air purification systems or dehumidifiers to reduce mites and molds). Teach prevention of respiratory infections, avoiding exposure to colds, meticulous cleaning of inhalation equipment, yearly influenza vaccine.	Review reinforces teaching. Return demonstration allows for evaluation of learning. Reinforces teaching. Reducing home allergens can reduce episodes in children with allergic asthma. Preventing respiratory infection reduces exacerbations of asthma.

NURSING DIAGNOSIS *Interrupted family processes, related to chronic condition and frequent exacerbations*

Goals/Outcome Criteria	Nursing Interventions	Rationales
Family adjusts to child's chronic illness, as evidenced by: • Appropriate intervention during acute episodes • Child's normal development • Absence of inappropriate anxiety	Encourage the parent to participate in the child's care during exacerbations. Keep parent informed about changes in condition. Maintain child's usual routine and usual treatment regimen if possible. Encourage close communication between family and the school nurse. Listen to family concerns. Refer for financial or psychological help if indicated.	Involving the parent decreases parental and child stress. Parents know more about how their child reacts to situations than the health care personnel. Decreases stress associated with hospitalization and increases coping. Appropriate communication increases consistency in care. Listening provides a basis for planning. Stress adversely affects family relationships and coping.

CRITICAL THINKING
SNAPSHOT

■ A 12-year-old comes to the community health clinic with his mother. He is wheezing and short of breath; his chest is tight, and he is coughing. He is lethargic and sitting in a tripod position. His color is pale, and his skin is cool and clammy. As the nurse, what is your initial assessment of this child? What are your initial interventions? What changes in his breath sounds would concern you?

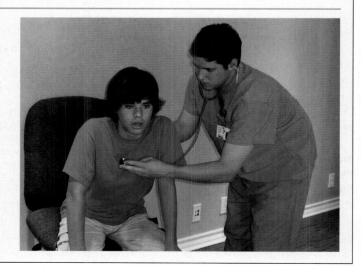

MAJOR CRITERIA   MINOR CRITERIA

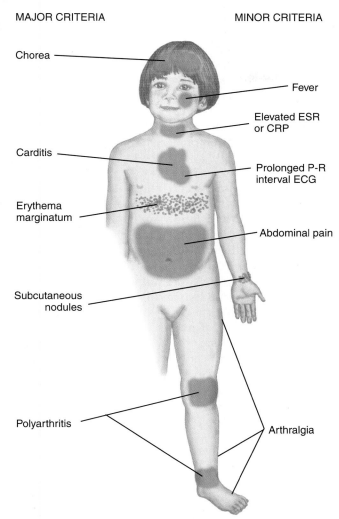

FIGURE **14-7** Major and minor criteria for the diagnosis of acute rheumatic fever.

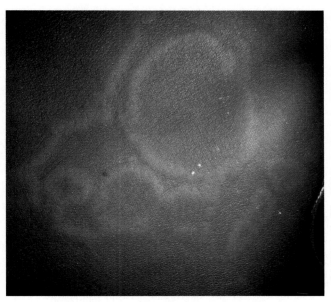

FIGURE **14-8** Erythema marginatum with complete rings that have flat centers and raised erythematous margins.

Abdominal pain, often mistaken for appendicitis, sometimes occurs. Fever varies from slight to very high. Pallor, fatigue, anorexia, and unexplained nosebleeds may be seen.

A careful history and physical examination are done. Certain blood tests are helpful. The erythrocyte sedimentation rate (ESR) is elevated. Abnormal proteins, such as C-reactive protein (CRP), may also be evident in the serum. Leukocytosis may occur but is not regularly present.

Culture demonstration of streptococcal infection may not be possible. In that event, antibodies against the streptococci (measured with antistreptolysin-O titer) confirm recent streptococcal infection. Additional studies may include chest radiography.

The electrocardiogram (ECG), a graphic record of the electrical changes caused by the beating of the heart, is useful. Changes in conductivity, particularly a prolonged P-R interval (first-degree heart block), may indicate carditis. Tests are repeated throughout the course of the disease so that the doctor may determine

when the active stage has subsided. Rheumatic fever has a tendency to recur, and each attack carries the threat of further damage to the heart. The recurrences are most frequent during the first 5 years after the initial attack and decline rapidly thereafter.

Treatment and Nursing Care

Treatment is aimed at preventing permanent damage to the heart, relieving uncomfortable symptoms, and preventing recurrence of rheumatic fever. All children should be treated for streptococcal infection at diagnosis.

Elimination of the initial infection is followed by long-term **chemoprophylaxis** (prevention of disease by drugs). Intramuscular penicillin G benzathine (Bicillin), given as an intramuscular injection every 28 days, is the drug of choice to prevent recurrence for patients with a history of rheumatic fever or evidence of rheumatic heart disease (Kliegman et al., 2006). Oral penicillin does not have the same reliability but may be considered for patients with minimal involvement whose reliability about medications can be ascertained. The duration of therapy varies from 5 years to the lifetime of the patient, depending on individual and environmental factors. Sulfadiazine is recommended for long-term therapy for patients who cannot tolerate penicillin.

Antiinflammatory drugs (salicylates or nonsteroidal antiinflammatory drugs [NSAIDs]) are used to decrease pain and inflammation. Aspirin is the drug of choice for joint disease but should be withheld until the diagnosis has been confirmed because it can mask the migratory nature of the arthritis (Behrman et al., 2004). The use of steroids is controversial and is reserved for patients with severe carditis and congestive heart failure.

Important concerns during therapy include aspirin toxicity and the effect of aspirin therapy on clotting time. More severe reactions such as gastric ulcer, hypertension, overwhelming infection, and psychic disturbances should be guarded against.

Chorea may need to be treated with diazepam or haloperidol. Seizure precautions may be necessary. Chorea movements are aggravated by anxiety; therefore the nurse should suggest activities that do not require fine motor coordination of the hands, which may cause frustration. Good communication with school personnel when the child returns to school increases understanding of the child's behavior.

Activity Limitations. Bed rest during the initial attack is not necessary but is recommended if carditis is present. Usually some limitation is placed on activity until the ESR decreases to normal or the congestive heart failure has resolved. Because most children with rheumatic fever are treated at home, the nurse needs to verify that the parent and child understand any prescribed activity limitations. The child benefits from access to quiet games and other interesting activities during the acute phase. Suggested passive diversions include an aquarium, growing plants of various types, stories, and quiet music. As the condition improves, part of the time may be taken up with simple self-care tasks. Hobbies such as needlework or stamp collecting are interesting and fun to start. Boys and girls can be encouraged to follow sports or a popular series on television; this helps them keep up with peer interests. Most children resume moderate activity shortly after the febrile phase.

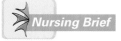
Nursing Brief

Nurses need to become skilled at providing quiet activities for the child who is ill. Provisions must be made for the child to carry out school work as the condition permits. If a long period of convalescence is indicated, a tutor is needed unless closed-circuit television or a school-to-home telephone is available.

Reducing Pain. The nurse instructs the parent to support painful joints with the hands when moving the child. Care includes special attention to the skin, especially over bony prominences.

Promoting Nutrition. During the initial stage of the disease, the child may have anorexia. Caution parents not to pressure the child at this time because it may lead to feeding problems during recovery. Offer small amounts of foods frequently. As the child's appetite improves, encourage nutritive essentials with occasional special treats. Consider ethnic food preferences. If the child has congestive heart failure, fluids need to be monitored.

Providing Emotional Support. Any disease that has the potential to permanently affect the heart produces anxiety in the child and parents. Keeping the parents informed about the child's condition helps them cope by relieving anxiety. It is important to emphasize that most children with rheumatic fever do well. The prognosis in rheumatic fever is favorable. Death from uncomplicated rheumatic fever is rare. Recurrent infections can cause damage to the heart, however, and although the nurse should be reassuring, infection prevention must be emphasized.

Prevention

Close medical supervision and follow-up care for children with rheumatic fever are essential. Preparation of the child and family for long-term antibiotic compliance is extremely important. Financial assistance is available to patients on long-term chemoprophylaxis. Local heart associations and disabled children's services, as well as state and municipal health departments, are among the sources of such aid.

Maintenance of healthy teeth and prevention of cavities are of special importance. The patient with rheumatic fever is susceptible to **subacute bacterial endocarditis,** which can occur as a complication of dental or other invasive procedures likely to cause bleeding or infection. High-dose antibiotic prophylaxis is indicated if the child is to undergo dental procedures or surgery, regardless of whether the child is receiving chemoprophylaxis for prevention of recurrent rheumatic fever (Hockenberry & Wilson, 2007).

The nurse is involved in prevention of rheumatic fever in the community by recognizing signs and symptoms of streptococcal infections, doing screening, and referring for treatment. Any child with symptoms who has been exposed to scarlet fever or to another person with a streptococcal infection needs investigation. Examination of family contacts is also important. Throat cultures are necessary in determining whether the organism is GABHS. The use of rapid antigen detection testing (RADT) has assisted physicians in detecting the organism quickly. There are reports of false-positive results in children, so that if a child has a negative RADT, a throat culture should be done to confirm the results. Once a diagnosis is established, the nurse stresses the importance of completing antibiotic therapy; parents sometimes neglect this once the child's symptoms disappear. The absence of acute signs and symptoms may inaccurately be associated with eradication of the organism.

GASTROINTESTINAL SYSTEM

APPENDICITIS
Description

Appendicitis occurs when the opening of the appendix into the cecum becomes obstructed. This may have a number of causes, among them fecaliths (blockage with fecal matter), infection, and allergy. Diet has also been implicated. Appendicitis is rare before age 2 years but is the most common cause of abdominal surgery during childhood. The incidence rate is higher in boys.

Signs and Symptoms

The symptoms in older children are similar to those in adults and include nausea, with or without vomiting; abdominal tenderness; fever; constipation or diarrhea; and an elevated white blood cell count. Pain, which is initially about the umbilicus, localizes in the right lower quadrant (RLQ) midway between the umbilicus and the iliac crest (McBurney's point).

The symptoms of appendicitis in the young child are more obscure. The patient has to be observed carefully over a period of time to determine the diagnosis. The child cries, is restless, and has a low-grade fever. Pain is more generalized and harder to pinpoint, and nausea and vomiting may occur. Because these symptoms accompany many childhood upsets, the diagnosis is more difficult to establish than in adolescents or adults. Having the child stand on the toes and then drop onto the heels often helps localize the pain in cooperative younger children. Pain, followed by a sudden absence of pain, can indicate rupture of the appendix. If the appendix ruptures, the infected contents spill into the abdominal cavity and a generalized infection called **peritonitis** results.

Absent or diminished bowel sounds, rigid abdomen, and rebound tenderness are also indicative of appendicitis. **Rebound tenderness** can occur when pressure placed on the RLQ is followed by quick release of pressure, resulting in severe pain. Rebound tenderness in the RLQ, although classic for appendicitis, is not reliable in children. Because it can be falsely negative or positive, eliciting it in the child can cause needless pain. Rectal examination elicits tenderness. Diarrhea may be present in retrocecal appendicitis.

A chest radiograph may be ordered to rule out lower lobe pneumonia, which sometimes mimics appendicitis. A careful history and physical examination are paramount. The presence of vomiting and the degree of change in the child's behavior are considered particularly significant. Children almost always refuse solids and liquids. The child may guard the abdomen or voluntarily lie down. **Guarding** is characterized by tightening or rigidity of the abdominal muscles when the abdomen is palpated. One position frequently seen in the child with appendicitis pain is lying on the side with the knees flexed toward the abdomen.

Treatment and Nursing Care

Appendicitis is treated with a surgical operation called an **appendectomy**. Surgery is performed immediately after diagnosis unless the patient is dehydrated and needs rehydration. Antibiotic therapy is instituted before surgery in the patient with a perforated appendix. **Heat is never applied because it might cause a rupture, leading to the possibility of peritonitis.**

Uncomplicated Appendicitis. Oral fluids and feedings are withheld pending surgery. As in other emergency situations, emotional support is given by the nurse and the patient's family. Cathartics are withheld when a patient has abdominal pain to prevent rupture of the appendix. The prognosis of uncomplicated appendicitis is good.

Temperature, pulse, respirations, and blood pressure are monitored. The dressing is observed for drainage. If an intravenous line is running, the type, amount, and rate are observed. The state of consciousness (e.g., alert, groggy), the presence of nausea or vomiting, the appearance of any drainage, and any other pertinent observations are noted.

The patient's position is changed frequently. Teach the patient to take deep breaths; an incentive spirometer can be used, as can bubbles for younger children. Wash the patient's hands and face and help with putting on a clean hospital gown. An accurate record of intake and output is kept. The first void should be noted. If the child has not voided by change of the shift, the nurse should report this. The physician's orders indicate whether or not the child with nausea can have sips of water or ice chips.

As soon as the child is able to take and retain water and other fluids by mouth, intravenous feedings are discontinued. Vital signs and bowel sounds are monitored as ordered or according to institutional policies. The patient is encouraged to move about in bed; reluctance to move and anorexia may be early signs of complications. Evidence of pain is reported, and analgesics are administered as ordered.

Pediatric patients recuperate quickly from uncomplicated surgery. Ambulation is generally not a problem. Children usually can return to school in 1 or 2 weeks, but specific instructions concerning restriction of activity should be reviewed before hospital discharge.

Ruptured Appendix. Early recognition of appendicitis decreases the danger of perforation. Because the diagnosis is difficult to make in younger children, the nurse may come in contact with more patients with a ruptured appendix on the pediatric unit than on adult divisions. In addition, the body systems of a child are less mature; thus the condition progresses rapidly. Parents may also be confused by the symptoms and hesitate to obtain medical attention. With a ruptured appendix, the child is acutely ill and the recovery period prolonged. After the appendix ruptures, the abdomen rapidly becomes rigid.

Medical management to prevent shock, dehydration, and infection is instigated before surgery. This usually includes intravenous administration of fluids and electrolytes, systemic antibiotics, nasogastric suctioning, and positioning in a low Fowler's position or on the right side to facilitate drainage into the pelvic area. The patient is given nothing by mouth. Intermittent suction is maintained at appropriate negative pressure, and irrigations are carried out as ordered to ensure patency of the nasogastric tube.

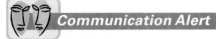

Communication Alert

The nurse can communicate to the school-age child the need to hold still during a procedure by saying, "You can help by holding your arm still. I will help you by putting my hand on your arm." After the procedure, the child should be praised for cooperation: "You were great. We could not have started that IV without your help."

Penrose drains are placed in the incision to drain exudate or abscess. Some surgeons prefer to leave the incision open and packed with Betadine or saline gauze. The nurse may do a wet-to-dry dressing change several times a day, removing the contaminated dressing and repacking the wound. Wound precautions are instigated according to hospital procedure. The area is kept clean and dry, and medication is applied if ordered. Administer analgesics for pain relief. Monitor intake, output, and bowel sounds. Supply nutritious foods as the diet is increased. Administer nursing care as described for the child with simple appendicitis, including appropriate modifications and interventions in nursing care plans. The child should be placed in a semi-Fowler's position to prevent spread of the infection. The child's hospital stay is increased, and intravenous antibiotic therapy is given.

MUSCULOSKELETAL SYSTEM

LEGG-CALVÉ-PERTHES DISEASE (COXA PLANA)
Description

This disease is one of a group of disorders called the **osteochondroses,** in which the blood supply to the **epiphysis,** or end of the bone, is disrupted. The tissue death that results from the inadequate blood supply is termed **avascular necrosis.** Legg-Calvé-Perthes disease affects the development of the head of the femur. Its cause and incidence are unknown. The disease is age related and is seen most commonly in boys between the ages of 4 and 8 years. It is more common in whites than in African Americans. This disease is unilateral in about 80% of cases. Healing occurs spontaneously over a period of 2 to 3 years; however, marked distortion of the head of the femur may lead to an imperfect joint or degenerative arthritis of the hip in later life.

Signs and Symptoms

The classic symptom is "painless" limping. Other symptoms include intermittent thigh pain that might be referred to the knee and limitation of motion. A number of cases are diagnosed in sports clinics. Legg-

Calvé-Perthes disease may or may not be preceded by trauma or infection. Radiographs confirm the diagnosis and show the extent of femoral head involvement.

Treatment and Nursing Care

The prognosis is more favorable with a young age of onset. Children who are older than 8 years of age may have degenerative arthritis develop. The goal in treatment is to prevent femoral head deformity. In recent years, extensive confinement of the child and weight-relieving methods have been replaced by allowing weight bearing and by keeping the femoral head deep in the hip socket while it heals. This is accomplished through the use of ambulation-abduction casts or braces that prevent dislocation of the femoral head and enable the acetabulum to mold the healing head in such a way that it does not become deformed. This treatment may be preceded by bed rest and traction to relieve muscle irritation. Newer surgical reconstruction and containment methods show promise in shortening the length of treatment. The prognosis in Legg-Calvé-Perthes disease depends on the age at onset, the stage of the disease at diagnosis, and the type of treatment initiated.

Nursing considerations depend on the age of the patient and the type of treatment. When immobilization of the child is necessary, the general principles of traction, cast, and brace care are used. Total or partial mobility is particularly trying for children and their families. Braces and casts hinder the patient's move toward independence and deprive him or her of many natural outlets for relieving stress. The natural inclination to compete physically is thwarted. It is important to emphasize safety principles when school-age children are in mobility braces.

Review brace care with the parent and child. Braces must be applied appropriately and preferably over light clothing. Observe the skin underneath the brace for signs of skin breakdown. Keep the skin clean and dry. Some practitioners recommend applying alcohol to the skin under friction areas. Check the brace regularly to be sure all parts are working properly.

If the child is admitted to the hospital for surgery, routine preoperative teaching is done. Postoperative care includes monitoring circulation, sensation, and motion, and other routine observations.

JUVENILE RHEUMATOID ARTHRITIS
Description

Juvenile rheumatoid arthritis (JRA) is the most common arthritic condition of childhood; it affects approximately 1 in 1000 children annually (Kliegman et al., 2006). Formerly considered to be one disease with several subtypes, it is now classified as several different syndromes. These inflammatory diseases involve the joints, connective tissues, and viscera. JRA is seen frequently in children. The exact cause is unknown,

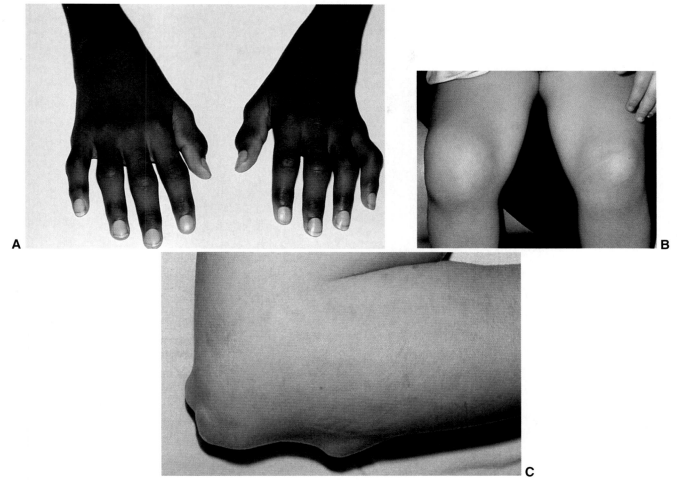

FIGURE **14-9 A,** Child's hands show swelling and inflammation of joints with polyarticular JRA. **B,** Swollen right knee of a toddler with pauciarticular JRA. **C,** Subcutaneous nodules over the pressure points of a child's elbow.

but infections and an autoimmune response have been implicated. The symptoms mimic many of those of nonrheumatic conditions, such as Lyme disease, septic arthritis, and osteomyelitis; these conditions need to be ruled out before a diagnosis of JRA is made.

Signs and Symptoms

The most common types of JRA are listed in Table 14-6. Symptoms vary from one patient to the next, and each type has a distinct method of onset: **systemic** (acute febrile), **polyarticular** (involving more than four joints), or **pauciarticular** (involving four joints or fewer). The course is chronic, with remissions and exacerbations. Some children who have disease of pauciarticular onset progress to a polyarticular course. Children rarely have permanent joint deformity, although many have some functional limitations. In systemic JRA, joint symptoms may be absent at onset but do develop in most patients.

Affected joints are swollen, warm, and stiff (Figure 14-9). Joint stiffness occurs mainly in the morning or after a period of inactivity (the "gel" phenomenon). Joint effusion and thickening synovial membrane

eventually erode cartilage and can cause joint destruction.

Children with pauciarticular disease are at risk for iridocyclitis, an inflammation of the iris and ciliary body of the eye. Symptoms include redness, pain, photophobia, decreased visual acuity, and nonreactive pupils. This condition occurs most frequently in young girls. Its course is unpredictable. All children with pauciarticular arthritis need slit-lamp eye examinations several times a year for at least the first 5 years after the diagnosis of JRA. Distortion of the pupil and cataracts may occur. The long-term visual prognosis is uncertain.

Bone mass increases most during adolescence, and the process is related to weight, amount of exercise, and diet. Because children with JRA are less mobile than others their age, are likely to experience anorexia and reduced nutritional intake, and are taking certain medications for their disease, they are more susceptible to **osteopenia** (low bone mass). If adequate bone mass is not attained during the teen years, osteoporosis in adulthood is more likely. The skeletal bone mass should be monitored closely.

Table 14-6 *Major Types of Juvenile Arthritis*

TYPE	INCIDENCE RATE	GENDER AFFECTED	AGE	JOINTS AFFECTED	OTHER MANIFESTATIONS	PROGNOSIS
Systemic	10%-20%	Both equally	Any	Few to multiple	High fever (especially in the evening), chills, rash on trunk and extremities, enlarged liver and lymph nodes, pericarditis/pleuritis, leukocytosis, abdominal pain, anemia, arthralgias before arthritis begins	Approximately 50% have chronic joint disease develop; prognosis depends on number of joints involved
Polyarticular, RF-positive	5%; may be familial	90% girls	>8 yr	Any or multiple large and small joints, upper and lower extremities, symmetrical pattern	Rapid, severe course; rheumatoid nodules (palpable near elbows); low fever; slight anemia	Early joint erosion, with many having permanent disability
Polyarticular, RF-negative	20%-30%	70%-75% girls	Early childhood School age	Multiple large and small joints	Arthritis persists, loss of bone mass, small percentage with iridocyclitis, growth disturbances, low fever, malaise, anorexia, anemia	Small percentage have joint damage
Pauciarticular	40%-55%; may be familial	*Girls:* 20%-35% have a polyarticular course develop after approximately 3 yr	Early childhood	Knees, ankles, elbows (<4 joints); asymmetric pattern	Chronic iridocyclitis with occasional loss of vision, malaise, low fever, slight anemia; slightly enlarged liver, spleen, and lymph nodes during active disease	More favorable prognosis regarding long-term joint function
		Boys: many have spondyloarthropathies develop	Late childhood	Large joints of lower extremities, hips, spine	Small percentage have acute iridocyclitis	

No specific tests exist for JRA. The duration of the symptoms is important, particularly when they last longer than 6 weeks. The diagnosis is determined from clinical manifestations, radiographs, laboratory test results (CBC, ESR, rheumatoid factor [RF] assay, antinuclear antibody [ANA] assay), and the exclusion of other disorders. Aspirated joint fluid is yellow to green and cloudy and has a low viscosity. The goals of therapy are to reduce pain and swelling, to promote mobility, to preserve joint function, to educate the patient and family, and to help the child and family adjust to living with a chronic disease.

Treatment and Nursing Care

Treatment is supportive. Drug therapy and exercise are the mainstays of therapy. First-line medications used to treat JRA are the NSAIDs, which include ibuprofen (Advil, Motrin), naproxen (Naprosyn; all available over the counter), and tolmetin. Ibuprofen now comes in liquid form, making it easier to give to small children. Aspirin is given less frequently than previously because of its association with Reye's syndrome. These agents do not change the course of the disease but reduce pain and stiffness.

If initial treatment with NSAIDs fails after adequate trial (at least 2 to 3 months of each medication chosen), other approaches are used. Corticosteroids used intraarticularly have been effective in preserving joints. Systemic corticosteroids are usually avoided unless extreme disease presents. Disease-modifying antirheumatic drugs have demonstrated effectiveness; these include methotrexate, sulfasalazine, and etanercept. Methotrexate can be safely given to children with careful monitoring of bone marrow and liver function.

Regular monitoring of all medications is imperative. NSAIDs are given with meals to avoid gastric irritation. Parents should be informed of the side effects, which include tinnitus, lethargy, hyperventilation, dizziness, headaches, nausea, and vomiting.

Physical and occupational therapy are included in the treatment of JRA. The purpose is to maintain and reduce function and reduce pain.

The nurse functions as a member of a team that includes the pediatrician, rheumatologist, social worker, physical therapist, occupational therapist, psychologist, ophthalmologist, and school and community nurses. The child may be hospitalized during an acute episode or for an unrelated illness. Treatment consists of medications, warm tub baths, joint exercises, and rest. The physical therapist oversees the type and amount of exercise performed. Daily range-of-motion exercises and play activities that incorporate specific routines help preserve function, maintain muscle strength, and prevent deformities. Morning tub baths and the application of moist hot packs help lessen stiffness. Resting splints may be ordered to prevent flexion contractures and preserve functional alignment. Proper body alignment with a regular change to the prone position (unless contraindicated) facilitates comfort. Either no pillow or a small flat pillow is advocated. Measures to alleviate boredom should be undertaken.

Home Care. The child is given instructions for home care. These are reviewed with the family to determine the level of understanding. A firm mattress or bed board is necessary to prevent joints from sagging. Age-appropriate tricycles and pedal cars promote mobility and exercise. Modifications in daily living, such as elevation of toilet seats, installation of hand rails, Velcro fasteners, and so on, may be necessary. Swimming is an excellent form of exercise. Assist parents in planning nutritional meals with adequate calcium and vitamin D. Weight gain is to be avoided because it places further stress on the joints. Emphasize the importance of regular eye examinations. Unnecessary physical restrictions should be avoided because these can lead to rebellion.

Facilitating School Attendance. Encourage school attendance. Excess absence from school, particularly for nonspecific symptoms, might suggest that the child is depressed or excessively preoccupied with the illness. In such cases, the meaning of the illness to the child and family and its effect on daily life need to be explored. Careful communication with the school nurse is essential for the child to have a successful school experience without interruptions in learning. The child should allow adequate preparation time in the morning to work out stiffness before arriving at school. There should be planned rest periods during the day, especially during disease flare-ups. Unobtrusive access to the school health office is important for these children so that they do not feel different from their peers.

Meeting Emotional Needs. Parents need assistance with establishing limits. Consistent negative behavior in social situations can present more problems than the actual disability. Overindulgence and preferential treatment often compromise the child's potential for happiness and independence. Siblings of chronically ill children may resent the special attention received by the patient. They may also be torn between loyalty to the brother or sister and their own need to be with others. Parents need ongoing counseling and the services of various community resources. One resource is the Arthritis Foundation. The child may benefit from association with other children who have arthritis.

This disease is characterized by periods of remission and exacerbations. There is no known cure for JRA. Parents need assistance in understanding the chronic nature of the disease and the potential for recurrence of signs and symptoms. Nurses can serve as advocates for the child by recognizing the impact of the disease and by openly communicating with the child, the family, and other members of the health care team.

| Table 14-7 | *Clinical Staging of Reye's Syndrome* |

GRADE	SYMPTOMS AT TIME OF ADMISSION
I	Usually quiet, **lethargic** and sleepy, vomiting, laboratory evidence of liver dysfunction
II	Deep lethargy, **confusion**, delirium, combative, hyperventilation, hyperreflexic
III	Obtunded, **light coma**, with or without seizures, decorticate rigidity, intact pupillary light reaction
IV	Seizures, deepening coma, **decerebrate rigidity**, loss of oculocephalic reflexes, fixed pupils
V	Coma, loss of deep tendon reflexes, respiratory arrest, fixed dilated pupils, **flaccidity/decerebrate** (intermittent); isoelectric EEG

From Behrman, R.E., Kliegman, R.M., & Jenson, H.B. (2004). *Nelson's textbook of pediatrics* (17th ed.). Philadelphia: Saunders.

NERVOUS SYSTEM

REYE'S SYNDROME
Description

Reye's syndrome is a pediatric disease characterized by a nonspecific encephalopathy with fatty degeneration of the viscera and altered ammonia metabolism. It mainly affects the liver and brain. The cause is unknown, although it is probably a mitochondrial disease. *Mitochondria* are structures within the cytoplasm of cells. Damage to these structures impairs enzyme activity. This leads to hyperammonemia and fatty acidemia, which along with other factors, are believed to cause the brain swelling seen in this disease. The disease is triggered by a virus, particularly influenza or varicella. Other controversial causes include genetic makeup, environmental factors, and the use of salicylates and phenothiazines. **The American Academy of Pediatrics does not advise giving aspirin to children with influenza or varicella because this drug appears to be linked to Reye's syndrome.** The incidence rate of this disorder has decreased markedly since pediatricians began advising parents not to treat children with aspirin for viral infections. Reye's syndrome affects children under 18 years of age; most cases occur between the ages of 4 and 12 years, with a peak incidence at 8 years. The younger the child, the higher the morbidity and fatality rates. Early diagnosis is crucial because of the rapid, life-threatening course of the disease.

Signs and Symptoms

The clinical picture is typical in that the child is recovering from an upper respiratory infection or chickenpox. The recuperation is interrupted by general malaise; then there is the sudden onset of persistent vomiting, which may continue for 24 hours, and lethargy (Table 14-7). Metabolic acidosis and respiratory alkalosis can occur.

The diagnosis is based on the patient's history, symptoms, and laboratory data. Examples of the latter include elevated findings on liver function tests (serum glutamate oxaloacetate transaminase [SGOT], serum glutamate pyruvate transaminase [SGPT], lactate dehydrogenase [LDH]) and serum ammonia levels, possibly decreased blood glucose levels, and elevated prothrombin times. Liver biopsy may be done if the diagnosis is questionable. Computed tomography (CT) may be ordered to rule out a brain tumor. The prognosis depends on the severity of the illness, with full recovery if patient does not have progression beyond stage III. Most survivors recover completely; however, some have complications of neurological sequelae.

Treatment and Nursing Care

The patient is admitted to the ICU. Treatment is supportive. Of particular priority is prevention of brain insult because the disease process in most other organs is reversible. Fluid management in conjunction with treatment of increased intracranial pressure (ICP) is crucial. Electroencephalography (EEG) is performed until stabilization is seen. Medications include osmotic diuretics (such as mannitol), sedatives, and barbiturates. Appropriate therapy for secondary infection is also instituted. Treatment programs are currently focused on monitoring and treatment for increased ICP. The nursing care is similar to any child with increased ICP. In addition, the nurse should evaluate the child's respiratory status frequently. Be on the alert for drug incompatibilities and avoid overhydration. Observe the patient for bleeding. A hypothermia pad may be used to prevent temperature elevations, which increase the demand for cerebral oxygen.

The rapid course of this disease is extremely frightening. Parents need information and reassurance. There is usually guilt. Family members may blame themselves for not recognizing the seriousness of the infection. Other children in the home may also be ill. Address parental concerns and prepare them for how the child looks, particularly if procedures with additional equipment have been introduced since their last visit. Assess family coping skills and refer family members to a chaplain, social service, Reye's Foundation, and so on. When patients awaken, they may be reserved, disoriented, and fearful of their environment. They may not recall any of the events surrounding hospitalization.

BRAIN TUMORS
Description

Brain tumors are the second most common type of neoplasm in children (the first is leukemia). Most childhood tumors occur in the area of the brain below the cerebellum. The cause of these tumors is unknown. They occur most commonly in school-age children.

| Table 14-8 | *Most Frequently Seen Childhood Brain Tumors* |

TUMOR	PEAK AGE (YR)	CHARACTERISTICS
Cerebellar astrocytoma (52% of all brain tumors)	6-14	Slow-growing, cystic tumor; very high rate of cure with surgery (90%)
Medulloblastoma (21% of all brain tumors)	2-6	Rapidly growing, highly malignant, occurs more often in boys *Treatment:* Surgery, craniospinal irradiation, chemotherapy *Prognosis:* 5-yr survival rate at 80% to 90%
Glioma of brainstem (19% of all brain tumors)	6-10	Slow-growing, diffuse tumor; cannot be removed with surgery; focal tumors can be removed; affects cerebral pathways and cranial nerves *Treatment:* Site radiation to shrink tumor, surgery for focal tumor *Prognosis:* Poor, but better if focal tumor is removed; 5-yr survival rate at 20%
Ependymoma (9% of all brain tumors)	5-6	Tumors grow at various speeds; because of location, invades vital centers, obstructs flow of cerebrospinal fluid *Treatment:* Partial surgical removal, irradiation of entire cerebrospinal axis *Prognosis:* Improving but related to age, location, and grade of tumor; 5-yr survival rate at 50%

The diagnosis is difficult because of the tumor's insidious onset. Metastatic tumors of the brain are rare in children. A synopsis of brain tumors in children is given in Table 14-8.

Signs and Symptoms

The signs and symptoms are directly related to the location and size of the tumor. Most tumors create increased ICP, with the hallmark symptoms of headache, vomiting, drowsiness, and seizures. Early morning headache relieved by vomiting may indicate a brain tumor. Nystagmus (constant jerky movements of the eyeball), double vision, strabismus, and decreased vision may be evident. Papilledema (edema of the optic nerve) may be seen. Other symptoms include ataxia, clumsiness, head tilt, behavioral changes, and cerebral enlargement, particularly in infants. Disturbances in vital signs are noticeable when the tumor presses on the brainstem. The diagnosis is determined from clinical manifestations, laboratory tests, magnetic resonance imaging (MRI) and CT, and biopsy.

Treatment and Nursing Care

Treatment is multidisciplinary and includes surgery, radiation therapy, and in some cases, chemotherapy. It should take place at a hospital with appropriate support. About 60% of children with brain tumors can be successfully treated using radiation, chemotherapy, and surgery (Yock & Tarbell, 2006).

In general, nursing care occurs in several phases. These phases are diagnosis, preoperative care, postoperative care, radiation therapy and chemotherapy, and convalescence. The nursing objectives in each area of care are specific but also overlap. One pervading theme is ongoing emotional support for the child and family during this taxing ordeal. "Waiting periods" for test results, surgery, and prognosis increase the anxiety levels of the entire family.

Nursing care follows the phase of treatment. Before surgery, emphasis is placed on careful explanations of various procedures and on familiarizing the patient and family with the recovery room, ICU, and the hospital personnel. Of importance is that the patient's head will be shaved at the incision site. The nurse should anticipate anxiety and provide empathy and support. The size of the postoperative dressing should be carefully explained. Applying a similar dressing to a doll may be helpful.

The postoperative care is the same as that given to the critically ill child. Adjuncts to care may include the use of a hypothermia blanket or a mechanical respirator. Parents must be prepared for the appearance of the child after surgery. The patient may be unconscious for a while, or there may be facial edema.

In supporting the family, several common issues may need to be addressed. These are the fear of pain, truthfulness versus withholding facts, feelings of helplessness and guilt, and concerns about the future. In addition, the fear of loss is always present. Depending on the circumstances, supportive care for the terminally ill child and for the family may be necessary. Oncology support groups are particularly helpful. The families identify with one another and share common concerns.

Radiation Therapy. Radiation treatment requires preparation. The radiologist outlines the areas to be treated. These marks should not be washed off. Small doses of radiation are given over a period of weeks. Determine what the radiologist has told the patient. Provide support to the child, who may feel that he or she will be burned. Advise the child that he or she will be alone in the room but will retain voice contact. Tour the facility with the patient. Recognize physical symptoms of fear such as dry mouth, pupil dilation, trembling, and clinging. Tape or lotion should not be placed on the skin before or during radiation treatment in an attempt to help prevent burns. Untoward effects of treatment may begin about the end of the first week. Headaches, anorexia, nausea and vomiting, diarrhea, and general lethargy may ensue. More severe effects include leukopenia, a decreased platelet count, skin breakdown, and hair loss. Reassure the family that the hair grows back but that it may be a different color or texture. Medication may be prescribed to help alleviate symptoms. Nutritious foods in small quantities should be offered. Provide a pleasant environment, one that is free of odors, sounds, and sights that might induce nausea. Radiation has been shown to impair intellectual development, effect growth, and interfere with normal hormone function. New treatments with stereotactic radiosurgery, stereotactic radiotherapy, intensity-modulated radiotherapy (IMRT), and proton radiation are providing new approaches with less damage to the normal tissue. These approaches promise fewer complications from treatment than radiation (Yock & Tarbell, 2006).

Chemotherapy. Chemotherapy regimens vary somewhat. The child and family are prepared for the possible side effects of medications. This is done initially by the physician in charge of treatment. Ongoing education by nurses is important because distraught parents can assimilate only so many facts. The nurse stresses the importance of return visits to monitor bone marrow depression and other parameters. Children need to know that the medicine is designed to make them feel better but that they may feel worse at first. The nurse should observe the sleeping child who has had nausea and frequent vomiting. The patient should be positioned to avoid aspiration. Prolonged vomiting may be an indication that the medicine should be withheld or reduced. When therapy is being administered on an outpatient basis, careful instruction of parents or guardians is paramount.

The period of convalescence is punctuated by frequent clinic visits that are anxiety-provoking. "Will the blood tests be all right?" "He's lost so much weight." "I hope he won't have to go back on medication." Some parents have to commute long distances to medical facilities. These problems involve all aspects of care of the chronically ill child. Many nurses try to maintain contact with discharged patients by mail, reunions at the clinic, and involvement in cancer camps. The community health nurse and school nurse become significant persons on discharge. It is important that the child receive adequate nutrition and hydration. The child should be assisted in relating to a new body image. This may be augmented by the use of caps, wigs, or head scarves. Residual effects depend on the type and extent of the tumor.

It is not unusual for information such as the death of a loved child to filter back to persons who were directly involved with care. This always creates grief, which must be dealt with by the medical persons involved.

SPECIAL TOPICS

OVERVIEW OF EMOTIONAL AND BEHAVIORAL DISORDERS

Growing up can be painful even under the best circumstances. It is difficult for the child in the early school years

to live up to so many rapidly developing standards. Guilt and anxiety develop. Finger sucking, nail biting, excessive fears, stuttering, and conduct problems are reflections of nervous tension. Disorders that may or may not be traced to emotional problems include constipation, diarrhea, stomachaches, dermatitis, obesity, frequent urination, enuresis, school phobia, and the common cold. The current trend toward prevention with identification of risk factors and performance of interventions is a major goal of children's mental health services. The term **psychosomatic** has come to refer to the bodily dysfunctions that seem to have an emotional and an organic basis. Each person has a different potential for coping with life. Truancy, lying, stealing, failure in school, and a crisis such as death or divorce of parents are but a few of the difficulties that may require the services of the child guidance clinic.

The first psychiatric clinic for children in the United States was established in Chicago in 1909 to serve delinquents. The basic staff of the modern child guidance clinic is composed of a psychiatrist, a psychologist, and a social worker; frequently, a pediatrician is also a member of the staff. Usually the child guidance clinic provides both diagnostic and treatment services. It may be part of a hospital, a school, a court, or a public health or welfare service, or it may be an independent agency.

The various psychiatric specialties may be confusing to the average person. A **psychiatrist** is a medical doctor who has specialized in mental disorders. The **psychoanalyst** is usually a psychiatrist but may be a psychologist (lay analyst); all psychoanalysts have advanced training in psychoanalytic theory and practice. The **clinical psychologist** has a PhD degree in clinical psychology from a recognized university. Many work in the school system with children, teachers, and families in an attempt to prevent or resolve problems.

There are also emotionally disturbed children who require the type of care provided in residential treatment centers. Their home situations may be such that they can respond to therapy only with a complete change of environment. In both the areas of diagnosis and treatment, the total situation to which the child reacts needs to be treated rather than just the individual patient. Short-term residential care in a general hospital (preadolescent unit) is a newer adjunct to therapy. The length of stay varies from about 2 weeks to 2 months. Most of these children have not responded well to individual outpatient therapy.

For nurses to work effectively with children who have emotional problems, they must first understand the types of behavior considered normal because the two are intimately related. Nurses are valuable members of the health care team in that they work closely with the child both in and out of the hospital. They keep a careful record of behavior and note relationships with members of the family. Such notations are meaningful to the physician who should be as concerned with preventing problems as with treating them. Is 4-year-old Janice wetting the bed? What about Bobby, who continually bangs his head against the crib during naptime? What does Allan do in the playroom? Is he sitting alone in a corner? Does he hit the other children? Is he constantly in motion? Does Eric seem indifferent to your attempts to establish rapport with him? Is there a physical cause for his behavior? Each action in itself might be considered well within the normal limits of behavior, but when carried to extremes, such actions may interfere with the child's experience of and reaction to reality and should be investigated further. Nurses should bear in mind that behavior one might describe as "bratty" may be interpreted very differently by persons skilled in understanding deeper levels of personality. They should feel free to discuss the conduct problems of patients with other members of the staff and should not consider these problems a threat to their own abilities.

One might ask where else the nurse sees such children: wherever the children are—in the home, in nursery school, in residential institutions, at child health conferences, in special clinics, in the doctor's office. Everyday, everywhere, children are trying to cope with stress. Many succeed and grow stronger. Many do not.

When parents request direction from nurses, they should be encouraged to seek help from their family physician or pediatrician or from a community mental health center. If the child is in school, the services of the school psychologist may prove valuable. Some churches employ counselors who are available free of charge to parishioners. The nurse should support organizations concerned with mental health, vote on issues that are pertinent to the welfare of children in the community, and offer services when they are needed.

Attention Deficit/Hyperactivity Disorder

Description. The term **attention deficit/hyperactivity disorder (ADHD)** refers to specific patterns of behavior that include inattention and impulsivity and might or might not involve hyperactivity. Boys are affected more frequently than girls. There is increased incidence in families, suggesting a genetic etiology. Affected children usually are of normal or above-average intelligence. Boys exhibit more behavioral problems, whereas girls tend to experience more frequent academic underachievement. ADHD can lead to social, emotional, and learning problems and subsequent decreased self-esteem.

The cause of ADHD is not thoroughly understood. Proponents of a biochemical causation suggest that hyperactive children have a total lack or diminished amount of dopamine. Others attribute the problem to an alteration of the reticular activating system of the midbrain that causes the child to react to every stimulation in the environment rather than to selected ones. Newer evidence indicates that genetic factors may play an important role. These disorders have also been linked to fetal alcohol syndrome and lead toxicity.

Signs and Symptoms. The American Psychiatric Association's Diagnostic and Statistical Manual of Mental Disorders has repeatedly tried to precisely define and categorize symptoms of ADHD. In its most recent edition (*DSM-IV-TR*), the Association identifies three major patterns of the disorder: (1) ADHD, predominantly inattentive type; (2) ADHD, predominantly hyperactive-impulsive type; and (3) ADHD, combined American Psychiatric Association, 2000). In each of these categories, symptoms must be present for at least 6 months, must have appeared before the age of 7 years, must be identified in more than one setting (home, school), and must cause significant impairment in psychosocial or educational adjustment and functioning (American Psychiatric Association, 2000). In addition, other causes for the behavior must be ruled out before a diagnosis can be made.

The diagnosis is difficult to establish because sometimes symptoms are subtle, and the diagnosis has become a "catch-all" for children with behavioral problems that might be the result of other causes. The diagnosis is made primarily from the patient history and interviews with family and teachers. Several screening tests are available to help with data collection.

The following are some manifestations that suggest ADHD:

- Is inattentive to details, careless with schoolwork or other activities
- Has difficulty organizing tasks
- Is unable to sustain attention for periods of time that would be appropriate for age
- Does not listen, follow instructions, or complete tasks; interrupts frequently
- Avoids activities and games that require concentration
- Is easily distracted, fidgety; has difficulty remaining seated
- Is forgetful, loses things
- Appears to have excessive energy

More specific criteria can be found in the manual. A child with these characteristics may have difficulties in school and in social situations. Children with ADHD are a challenge for parents, family members, and school professionals.

Treatment and Nursing Care. Children with ADHD should be managed by a multidisciplinary team consisting of a nurse, physician, social worker, psychologist, and special education teacher. Parents need support and should be referred to support groups. Family counseling may be warranted. Parents should be aware that only a physician can prescribe medication.

The specific medications used for the treatment of behavior problems in ambulatory patients are listed in Table 14-9. They are believed to act directly on the reticular activating system or to stimulate the release

Table 14-9	*Medications for Children with Attention-Deficit Disorder*		
DRUG	**DAILY DOSAGE (MG)**	**SIDE EFFECTS**	
Dextroamphetamine (Dexedrine) 5-mg, 10-mg tablets (also long-acting tablets); (Adderall) 5-mg, 7.5-mg, 10-mg, 12.5-mg tablets (also long-acting tablets)	5-80	Anorexia, weight loss, insomnia, emotional lability or oversensitivity, tics, growth delays	
Methylphenidate* (Ritalin) 5-mg, 10-mg, 20-mg tablets; (Concerta) 18-mg, 36-mg, 54-mg tablets; (Focalin) 2.5-mg, 5-mg, 10-mg tablets	10-80	Similar to dextroamphetamine Concerta is given once a day	
Pemoline (Cylert) 18.75-mg, 37.5-mg, 75-mg chewable tablets	37.5-131.25	Insomnia, anorexia, abdominal pain, nausea, headache, dizziness, drowsiness, depression Associated with elevation of hepatic enzymes and liver failure (needs close monitoring)	
Atomoxetine (Strattera) 10-mg, 18-mg, 25-mg, 40-mg, 60-mg, 80-mg, 100-mg tablets	100	Decreased appetite, insomnia, sedation, depression, tremor, pruritus, palpations, tachycardia, headache, nausea, vomiting, abdominal pain, hepatotoxicity	

*Primarily used because of rapid and predictable onset and relatively few side effects.

of norepinephrine from the brainstem. Although the use of drugs to modify behavior in children is controversial, extensive experience has shown its effectiveness, particularly in children with disorders of attention, activity, and organization. There is no evidence that these drugs are addictive; abuse is unlikely because the effect on the patient is opposite to that produced in persons without the problem. More controversial therapies include dietary modification (particularly eliminating food additives, such as preservatives and artificial flavors and colors) and the use of megavitamins. Side effects for many of these medications include anorexia. This side effect should be addressed by the encouragement of high-calorie foods, small frequent meals, administration of medication after meals, taking medication only when needed (taking off during weekends, summers), and changing to a different medication (Greydanus et al., 2003).

In addition to medications, the American Academy of Pediatrics recommends the use of behavior therapy. Programs may use training sessions with a trained therapist in behavior modification. The goal of this approach is to assist the parents in understanding the child's behavior and learning specific techniques for altering behavior (Stein & Perrin, 2003).

Initially, a careful medical history and neurological examination are indicated. Intelligence and psychological testing may aid in determining the specific assets and liabilities of the child so that an individual learning plan can be outlined. Many schools today have special learning disability classes in which the children are helped to establish self-discipline by consistent controls, elimination of distractions, and recognition and appreciation of accomplishments. Many children with ADHD function well in the regular classroom with certain educational and behavioral modifications. These methods are reinforced by the thoughtful nurse when such a child is hospitalized.

A priority in the care of these patients is a careful nursing admission history, a most useful tool in dealing with children who have problems of this nature. Nurses observe the patient's behavior alone and in interaction with the family. They document what they see, but they do not analyze. For example, a nurse would write, "Eric threw four crayons on the floor," not "Eric appeared distraught and misbehaved this morning." Careful attention is given to the child's attitude toward school. Other responsibilities might include dietary counseling if ordered, education in parenting, and assisting with screening and psychological testing. Functions pertinent to the nurse's work setting might also include referral to appropriate agencies and assessment of the home and school environment.

Listening to the child and the parents and providing support are particularly important. If the child is hyperactive, opportunities for gross motor play and screaming to externalize feelings, which can be encouraged at home, are limited in the hospital. The use of puppets, finger paints, and singing may be used to offset this imbalance. One nurse each shift is assigned to a particular child to provide continuity of care. Nursing care plans should include both short and long-term goals.

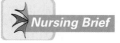
Nursing Brief

Parents should be aware that medications will not cure ADHD

When medications are necessary, the child and the family must understand the reasons for their use and their possible side effects. Periodic evaluation by the physician is essential. It is helpful if a behavior chart is kept and is submitted to the doctor before prescriptions are renewed. The child with a learning disability should not become a "sacrificial lamb" to the educational process, and the emphasis on education should not be disproportionate to the child's innate capabilities. Personal growth and self-esteem should be emphasized. Parents should be aware that other opportunities exist that can be adjusted to the child's abilities.

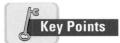

Key Points

- Head lice do not jump from individual to individual but are transferred by direct contact.
- The most frequently occurring pancreatic disorder is type 1 DM, which occurs with destruction of insulin-producing islet cells. Therapy is a combination of insulin, diet, and exercise.
- The goal of diabetes management is tight glucose level management. The child should be gaining self-management skills as age appropriate.
- Type 2 DM incidence rate is increasing in children.
- Asthma is the most common chronic childhood disease. The goal is to help the child manage the disease and to prevent hospitalization.
- Rheumatic fever is an autoimmune disease that occurs after a GABHS infection. The primary goal of treatment is to prevent cardiac complications, such as problems with the mitral valve.
- Appendicitis is difficult to diagnose in the young child because the child's vague symptoms may resemble other gastrointestinal problems.

- Juvenile rheumatoid arthritis therapy consists of administration of medications, such as NSAIDs, methotrexate, or aspirin, along with exercise, heat application, and support of joints.
- Aspirin is not given to children with influenza or chickenpox because of increased risk for Reye's syndrome.
- Attention deficit/hyperactivity disorder is difficult to establish and many times becomes a "catch-all" diagnosis for children with behavioral problems. Treatment requires a multidisciplinary team approach.

 Go to your Companion CD-ROM for an Audio Glossary, video clips, and more.

evolve   Be sure to visit the Companion Evolve site at http://evolve.elsevier.com/Price/pediatric/ for WebLinks and additional online resources.

ONLINE RESOURCES

American Diabetes Association: http://www.diabetes.org/home.jsp

Arthritis Foundation: http://www.arthritis.org/conditions/DiseaseCenter/jra.asp

Children and Adults with Attention Deficit Disorder: http://www.chadd.org//AM/Template.cfm?Section=Home

National Attention Deficit Disorder Association: http://www.add.org/

Objectives

Upon completion of this chapter, the student will be able to:

1. Define the key terms listed
2. Identify two major developmental tasks of adolescence
3. Discuss three ways in which youth can help prevent violence
4. Discuss anticipatory guidance for a 15-year-old girl just beginning to date
5. Describe three ways an adolescent can be given responsibility
6. Describe at least five ways a home health care worker can assist in caring for a disabled child
7. Explain three ways parents can be assisted in the skills of parenting adolescents
8. Discuss how health care workers can assist adolescents in making informed decisions regarding body piercing and tattoos
9. Summarize the nutritional requirements of the adolescent and cite two factors that may contribute to dietary deficiencies in this age group
10. Discuss the three leading causes of accidents in adolescence and suggest methods of prevention for each

Key Terms

Be sure to check out the bonus material on the Companion CD-ROM, including selected audio pronunciations.

adolescence (ĂD-ō-LĔS-ĕns; p. 324)
androgens (ĂN-drō-jĕnz; p. 325)
asynchrony (ā-SĬN-krō-nē; p. 325)
emancipated minor (ē-MĂN-sĭ-PĀ-tĕd; p. 333)
estrogens (ĔS-trō-jĕnz; p. 325)
identity (p. 324)
intimacy stage (p. 324)
mature minor doctrine (p. 333)
menarche (mĕ-NĂR-kē; p. 325)
puberty (PŪ-bĕr-tē; p. 325)
respite care (p. 331)
thelarche (thĕ-LĂR-kē; p. 325)

GENERAL CHARACTERISTICS AND DEVELOPMENT

Adolescence is the period of life that begins with the appearance of secondary sex characteristics and ends with cessation of growth and achievement of emotional maturity. The term comes from the word *adolescere*, meaning "to grow up." For purposes of clarification, adolescence is often divided into early, middle, and late periods. This is because a 13-year-old teenager is very different from an 18-year-old one. Middle adolescence appears to be the time of greatest turmoil for most families. Perhaps one of the most characteristic features of adolescence is its uncertainty. In our culture, it is a period of life that lasts a comparatively long time and involves a great number of adjustments.

Life is never dull with adolescents in the family. The adolescents' surge toward independence becomes more and more pronounced. This makes it practically impossible for them to get along with their parents, who represent authority. When adolescents submit to their parents' wishes, they feel humiliated and childish. If they revolt, conflicts arise within the family. Parents and teenagers have to weather this storm together and must try to come up with solutions that are more or less acceptable to everyone.

Numerous other factors also account for the restlessness of youth. Adolescents' bodies are rapidly changing, and they experience intense sexual drives. They want to be accepted by society but are not sure how to go about it. Adolescents question life and search to find what psychologists term as their sense of identity: "Who am I?" "What do I want?" Gaining an understanding of self-concept is an important aspect of adolescence. According to Orr (1998), when asked to respond to the question "Who am I?" early adolescents responded with lists of physical features and things they liked. The middle adolescent included some abstract categories ("I am friendly" or "I am nice"). The late adolescent answered with global, abstract categories ("I am a good person" or "I am ambitious"). This sense of identity is followed by the intimacy stage, in which teenagers must learn to avoid emotional isolation. Through shared activities such as sports, close friendships, and sexual experiences, they must face their fear of rejection. The older adolescent thinks about the future and is generally idealistic. This age also brings about an increased sophistication in moral reasoning. Thinking also has evolved to abstract reasoning.

Although these facts sound complicated in themselves, they are intensified by a constantly changing world. Even adults are confused by the rapid pace of living and the many technological advances. The feminist movement has challenged the traditional roles of men and women in society. In some households, gender roles are becoming less well defined. This is likely to change the ways in which parents act as models for their children. Many adolescents are living in single-parent homes or with working relatives, and little if any supervision is available. The Carnegie Council of Adolescent Development (1995) reports that "the demands and expectations as well as the risks and opportunities facing adolescents are both more numerous and more complicated than they were even a generation ago." The study found that adolescents are not receiving the guidance they need from parents and adults. In addition, they are pressured into drugs and sex at early ages. Many engage in antisocial activities and violence. Neighborhoods and schools are often unsafe. The report also indicates that "many have not learned how to handle conflict without resorting to violence." Because of adolescent turmoil, many teenagers show indications of psychiatric distress.

There is no one perfect way to guide adolescents. Most children come through the period of adolescence with flying colors and relatively few scars. Perhaps this is because each generation learns to live with the insecurities of its era, never having known any other. However, recognizing adolescents' needs is an important first step. Adolescents' reactions are individual; one must realize that, in contrast to the stereotyped descriptions, adolescence takes many forms in a free society. A great deal depends on the culture and the experience of a particular adolescent. All experts in teenage guidance agree on the importance of keeping the lines of communication open in the family. They also agree that it is important to listen and to watch for verbal and nonverbal cues that indicate an adolescent's need for help. Adolescents need to learn to develop problem-solving skills. They also must learn to deescalate conflicts. They need to refrain from teasing, bullying, and intimidating peers. Encourage them to participate in sports, school, and community activities. These types of programs help adolescents to get along with one another and often build self-esteem. Nurses can actively participate in speakers' bureaus and discuss youth violence. Initiatives such as *Kids Count*, sponsored by the American Nurses Association, need to be advocated in today's society to help reduce youth violence. Schools, parents, health care workers, and communities must continue to seek programs and policies that make schools safer. The challenge exists for nurses to assist in the prevention of injury and death from violence. School nurses and those in clinics and physician offices can and must promote violence-free communities and schools for our children (Scott et al., 2003).

BIOLOGICAL DEVELOPMENT

Preadolescence is a short period that immediately precedes adolescence. In girls, it comprises the years 10 to 13 and is marked by rapid changes in the structure and function of various parts of the body. It is distinguished by **puberty**, the stage at which the reproductive organs become functional and secondary sex characteristics develop. Both genders produce male hormones, **androgens**, and female hormones, **estrogens**, in comparatively equal amounts during childhood. At puberty, the hypothalamus of the brain signals the pituitary gland to stimulate other endocrine glands—the adrenals and the ovaries or testes—to secrete their hormones directly into the bloodstream in differing proportions (more androgens in boys and more estrogens in girls).

The age at which puberty takes place varies and is about 2 years earlier in girls than in boys. In both genders, it is preceded by spurts in height and weight. Overall, girls stop growing sooner and have smaller increases in height and weight than boys. During the pubertal growth spurt, weight increases 50%; this varies according to pubertal maturation, degree of adiposity, and size of muscle mass. During puberty, the growth spurt results in a 15% to 20% increase in height. The adolescent's general appearance tends to be awkward—long-legged and gangling. This growth characteristic is termed **asynchrony** because different body parts mature at different rates. The sweat glands are very active, and greasy skin and acne are common. Both genders mature earlier, grow taller, and are heavier than adolescents in past generations.

In most girls, changes in the breast with the development of a small bud of breast tissue (**thelarche**) signals the earliest sign of puberty. The average age is 11 years. **Menarche** (onset of menstrual periods) occurs approximately 2 years afterwards. Menarche can range from $10\frac{1}{2}$ to 15 years and still be within normal guidelines. According to Hockenberry & Wilson (2007), girls' peak height velocity occurs at about 12 years of age (6 to 12 months before menarche); girls gain 2 to 8 inches in height and 15 to 55 pounds during adolescence. In addition to secondary sex characteristics becoming more apparent before menarche, fat is deposited in the hips and thighs, causing them to enlarge. Hair grows in the pubic area and underarms. The body reaches its adult measurements about 3 years after the onset of puberty. At this time, the ends of the long bones knit securely to their shafts and further growth can no longer take place.

Although breast cancer is rare in adolescents, this is a time when girls are aware of their bodies and breast self-examination should be introduced. The American Cancer Society believes that breast self-examination should be routinely performed after age 20 years. The American Cancer Society provides various informational pamphlets describing the procedure.

The first sign of puberty in boys is usually the enlargement of the testes, which begins between ages 9½ and 14 years. Ejaculation and the appearance of pubic hair occur approximately 1 year after this. The production of sperm begins between ages 13½ and 14½ years. Complete fertility is not present at this time, but impregnation is possible. According to Hockenberry & Wilson (2007), boys' peak height velocity occurs around 14 years of age, followed by growth of the testes and penis. The penis elongates and widens, testes enlarge, and scrotum pigment becomes evident. Both axillary and facial hair increase, along with body odor. Voice changes are also noticeable. By late adolescence (17 to 21 years), adult genitalia is attained. The male voice deepens, and most linear growth is achieved. Overall, boys gain 4 to 12 inches in height; weight gain is from 15 to 65 pounds during adolescence.

The American Cancer Society recommends that boys examine their testes during or after a hot bath or shower. Each testicle is examined with the index and middle fingers of both hands on the underside of the testicle and the thumbs on the top of the testicle. It is normal for one testicle to be larger than the other. The testicles are gently rolled between the thumb and fingers. Testicular self-examinations are performed once a month. If a lump is discovered, it should be reported immediately. Males also need to report an abnormal enlargement of a testicle or a heavy feeling in the scrotum. In addition, they should report any pain or discomfort in a testicle or in the scrotum, especially if symptoms last as long as 2 weeks.

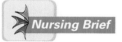
Nursing Brief

Although young girls are often taught breast self-examination, young boys are seldom instructed in the examination of the testes. Boys should also be taught to report enlargement or tenderness of their breasts because males, too, can develop breast cancer.

DEVELOPMENTAL THEORIES

Adolescents are in a period of transition from childhood to adulthood (Table 15-1). Erik Erikson identified the major task of this group as identity versus role confusion. At this time, children must determine who they are, where they are going, and how they are getting there. This should not imply that adolescents wait until this stage to develop individuation. During the toddler period, the child is first challenged with issues of autonomy that, if accomplished, make the adolescent task less of a challenge.

Adolescents want to be people in their own right, and they try out different roles (Figure 15-1). Self-concept (one's view of oneself) fluctuates during this time and is molded by the demands of parents, peers,

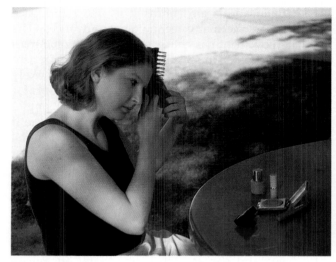
FIGURE **15-1** The adolescent is very concerned about personal appearance. A teenager's self-esteem is influenced by how far body image deviates from the mythical "body ideal."

teachers, and so on. Although gaining a self-concept is an ongoing process, adolescence can be a time that particularly challenges the child's view of self.

As adolescents move toward independence, they begin to separate from the family. Peer influences dominate decisions that relate to style of dress, but parents still hold sway over moral decisions and setting limits. Parents are often ambivalent about letting go. Disagreements with parents often revolve around dating, use of the family car, money, chores, school grades, choice of friends, smoking, sex, and the social use of drugs. Parental values and morals are questioned, especially if parents do not practice what they preach. Adults who associate with teenagers should try to create an atmosphere of interest and understanding. A caring environment that sets limits is essential. Adolescence is a little like being on a roller coaster. Parents, nurses, and other adults who interact with adolescents should be reminded that they should remain objective, calm, understanding, and loving.

According to Piaget's theory of cognitive development, development is systematic, sequential, and orderly. Early adolescents are still in the concrete phase of thinking. They take things literally. For instance, assume the nurse asks a young teenager girl, "Have you ever slept with anyone?" The teenager may not perceive this to have anything to do with a vaginal infection or sex. By middle adolescence, the ability to think in abstract terms has increased. Piaget calls this the stage of formal operations. Older adolescents can see a situation from many viewpoints and can imagine or organize unseen or unexperienced possibilities. The failure to develop formal thoughts is cited by some as connected to the failure to develop a high level of moral reasoning. Adolescents who have developed both are most likely to demonstrate a high degree of morality and consistency in their behavior.

Table 15-1 | *Growth and Development During Adolescence*

EARLY ADOLESCENCE (11-14 YR)	MIDDLE ADOLESCENCE (14-17 YR)	LATE ADOLESCENCE (17-20 YR)
GROWTH Rapidly accelerating growth Reaches peak velocity Secondary sex characteristics appear	Growth decelerating in girls Stature reaches 95% of adult height Secondary sex characteristics well-advanced	Physically mature Structure and reproductive growth almost complete
COGNITION Explores newfound ability for limited abstract thought Clumsy groping for new values and energies Comparison of "normality" with peers of same gender	Developing capacity for abstract thinking Enjoys intellectual powers, often in idealistic terms Concern with philosophic, political, and social problems	Abstract thought established Can perceive and act on long-range operations Able to view problems comprehensively Intellectual and functional identity established
IDENTITY Preoccupied with rapid body changes Trying out various roles Measurement of attractiveness by acceptance or rejection of peers Conformity to group norms	Modifies body image Very self-centered; increased narcissism Tendency toward inner experience and self-discovery Has a rich fantasy life Idealistic Able to perceive future implications of current behavior and decisions; variable application	Body image and gender-role definition nearly secured Mature sexual identity Phase of consolidation of identity Stability of self-esteem Comfortable with physical growth Social roles defined and articulated
RELATIONSHIPS WITH PARENTS Defining independence-dependence boundaries Strong desire to remain dependent on parents while trying to detach No major conflicts over parental control	Major conflicts over independence and control Low point in parent-child relationship Greatest push for emancipation; disengagement Final and irreversible emotional detachment from parents; mourning	Emotional and physical separation from parents completed Independence from family with less conflict Emancipation nearly secured
RELATIONSHIPS WITH PEERS Seeks peer affiliations to counter instability generated by rapid change Upsurge of close, idealized friendships with members of the same gender Struggle for mastery takes place within peer group	Strong need for identity to affirm self-image Behavioral standards set by peer group Acceptance by peers extremely important—fear of rejection Exploration of ability to attract the opposite gender	Peer group recedes in importance in favor of individual friendship Testing of male-female relationships against possibility of permanent alliance Relationships characterized by giving and sharing
SEXUALITY Self-exploration and evaluation Limited dating, usually group Limited intimacy	Multiple plural relationships Decisive turn toward heterosexuality (or, if homosexual, knows by this time) Exploration of "self-appeal" Feeling of "being in love" Tentative establishment of relationships	Forms stable relationships and attachment to another Growing capacity for mutuality and reciprocity Dating as a male-female pair Intimacy involves commitment rather than exploration and romanticism
PSYCHOLOGICAL HEALTH Wide mood swings Intense daydreaming Anger outwardly expressed with moodiness, temper outbursts, and verbal insults and name-calling	Tendency toward inner experiences; more introspective Tendency to withdraw when upset or feelings are hurt Vacillation of emotions in time and range Feelings of inadequacy common; difficulty in asking for help	More constancy of emotion Anger more apt to be concealed

Hockenberry, M.J., & Wilson, D. (2007). *Wong's nursing care of infants and children* (8th ed.). St. Louis: Mosby.

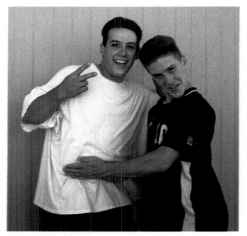

FIGURE **15-2** The peer group is often the adolescent's "safety net" in the search for independence and identity.

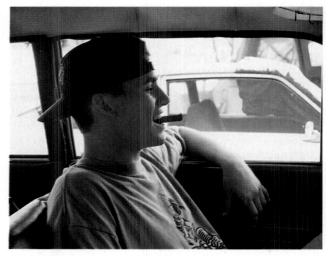

FIGURE **15-3** Peer pressure heavily influences an adolescent's decision to try tobacco, alcohol, and drugs.

Lawrence Kohlberg posited adolescence at a post-conventional morality stage, in which the person "focuses on individual rights and principles of conscience" (James et al., 2002). Older adolescents consider others' points of view and consider what rights and values are the best for everyone. They are able to do this because they can engage in abstract thinking. Social responsibility is recognized, and moral decisions can be made.

From the perspective of Sigmund Freud, adolescence is the "genital stage." The adolescent begins to love others and peers. Parents also provide a love that helps set a realistic direction for the teenager. In adolescence, theorists believe, a maturity has developed that sets the stage for adult development. Through support and guidance, nurses can assist children and adolescents through the stages of development necessary to reach that maturity.

SPECIAL NEEDS

PEER RELATIONSHIPS

Adolescent peer groups vary in number, interests, social background, and structure. They may consist of small groups of the same gender or of both genders. In late adolescence, peer groups may be small groups of couples. The young person may belong to one or several groups. The peer group serves as a mirror for "normality" and helps to determine where one fits in. Belonging to a peer group is vitally important to helping the adolescent define the self. Acceptance by one's friends helps decrease the loneliness and the sense of loss that many teenagers experience on the road to adulthood (Figure 15-2).

On the other hand, the social norms and pressures exerted by the group may cause problems (Figure 15-3). The selection of friends and adolescents'

allegiance to them may bring about conflicts within the family. Parents need help in understanding that teenagers' exaggerated conformity is a necessary step in moving away from dependence and in obtaining approval from people outside the nuclear family. Failure to develop social competence may produce feelings of inadequacy and low self-esteem.

Nurses can assist the parents through supporting and educating them in the dynamics of this age group. They can direct families to groups such as peer helpers (for the adolescent) and to community educational programs sponsored by various agencies. Organizations such as Parents Without Partners might be another avenue. Nurses must also remember that teenagers who do not belong to the dominant system, such as those from different cultural, social, or economic backgrounds, may see themselves as being quite different from their friends. In such cases, the use of family networks may prove helpful.

CAREER PLANS

Some adolescents enter high school with a definite idea of what they would like to do. Many, however, are unsure of what type of career they want to pursue. To choose a career that he or she is best suited for, the teenager must first know the self and understand what choices are available. What particularly interests him? What is she good at? What are the shortcomings?

By this time, the adolescent has already taken some rather definite steps toward a goal. On completing high school, the choice of high school curriculum and the types of grades received determine eligibility for entrance into college or preparation for a specific vocation (Figure 15-4). Parents should observe the interests of their children and encourage them to take advantage of their particular talents. Whenever possible, a teenager should investigate various fields by talking to people who are involved in them. Valuable information can also be

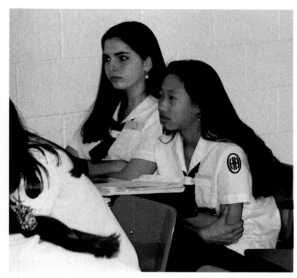

FIGURE **15-4** School is an important part of the adolescent's life.

obtained by career exploration, which is available at most colleges and with pamphlets from professional organizations, the government, and other sources. School guidance counselors administer aptitude tests that serve as an additional guide. They also can work with teenagers to expose them to as wide a selection of careers as possible. The final decision must be made by the adolescent. If people are to be happy with their work, they must choose it of their own free will and not because of parental expectations.

Many types of work are open to young women. Although they may choose to marry, many girls are selecting careers that support an independent lifestyle. Women also make up a large proportion of the work force and are being introduced into more nontraditional jobs. Nevertheless, teenagers face more unemployment than adults. They need to be creative, assertive, and well groomed when seeking employment.

The job market today is extremely competitive—and almost nonexistent for those without skills or education. Unemployment is high among minority groups and in some geographic locales. Although there are numerous causes for this, the individual unable to find a fulfilling job often experiences feelings of hopelessness and decreased self-esteem. Productive employment of young people needs to fit into their total framework of life. It also needs to offer an opportunity for personal growth. Some constructive aspects of employment include building self-esteem, promoting responsibility, testing new skills, constructively channeling energies, providing money for increased independence, engaging young persons in interactions with adults, and allowing them to assume an active rather than a passive role. In contrast, when adolescents are forced to take a job because of economic or personal pressures, they may have to drop out of school. With few skills and no experience, they may remain locked in low-level employment. This is often perpetuated from one generation to the next.

RESPONSIBILITY

Young people look forward to challenges. Parents must watch for ways that they may free their children to take on new responsibilities. Even routine jobs can be made more inspiring if youths are taught to see them in relation to their overall objective. Astronauts have a certain amount of dull routine to their jobs; so do doctors, nurses, and scientists. They are able to accept routine tasks because they contribute to the effectiveness of the entire project. Young adolescents must also be taught the value of money. An allowance helps them to learn management. If money is simply handed out as requested, it is more difficult for the adolescent to develop a sense of responsibility regarding finances. Allowances should be increased from time to time to comply with the age and needs of the teenager.

Middle and older adolescents who have jobs can be taught the use of a checkbook and a savings account. Many find satisfaction in being able to purchase their own clothes. If a boy or girl buys a car, he or she soon discovers that it takes money to run and repair it. Experiences such as these provide valuable lessons in finance. A common way of earning money among younger teenagers is babysitting. Many boys and girls begin to baby sit at about 12 or 13 years of age. Babysitting courses are valuable because these young people need to be prepared for this important responsibility. Courses are regularly taught by the American Red Cross, Campfire Boys and Girls, and local hospitals. Safe Sitter is an international organization that promotes babysitting skills. Safe Sitter has teaching sites established in all 50 states, as well as in England and Canada.

EMOTIONAL NEEDS

Teenagers worry frequently. They are able to talk about fears that are not too intimate, such as school examinations, how they will look with this or that type of haircut, and so on. They need assistance, however, in getting in touch with their feelings and in sorting out confused feelings. Adults must provide a confidential accepting atmosphere to foster quality communication. One of the more difficult aspects of communicating with adolescents is their fluctuating attitude. They may vary from being unconcerned about deadlines to being in a state of panic. They may wish to please but may be overly critical of themselves and their own performance. They may try to control others by being overly talkative. This may come from a desire to demonstrate their competence. Physical symptoms such as stomachaches, headaches, and insomnia surface and disappear periodically. Anxiety over future events, relationships with peers, and meeting others' expectations is also prevalent. Teenagers often experience their parents' pain and feel tremendously responsible for the family's burdens and failures. For many, the image of what a

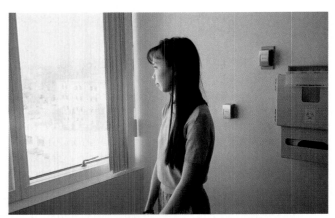

FIGURE **15-5** Adolescents can spend time daydreaming as a normal outlet.

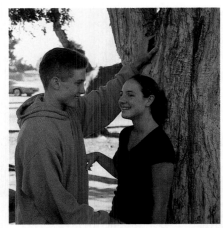

FIGURE **15-6** During adolescence, emerging sexuality is expressed in the development of intimate relationships. Many young couples date on a regular basis and prefer dating only one other person.

family should be is derived from television. Adolescents who have lifetime handicaps, alcoholic parents, physical or mental illness, or other serious problems such as poverty need the support of the medical community and other community resources. Bizarre behavior may be a signal for long overdue help.

DAYDREAMS

Adolescents spend a lot of time daydreaming, in the solitude of their rooms or during a biology lecture. Most of this is normal and natural for this age group (Figure 15-5). Daydreaming is usually considered harmless if the young person continues usual active pursuits. It also serves several purposes. Adolescence is a lonely, in-between age; daydreaming helps fill the void. Acting out imaginatively what will be said or done in various situations prepares teenagers to deal with others, so when confronted with real scenarios, they are better able to handle and cope with the situation. Daydreams are also a valuable safety valve that allows the expression of strong feelings.

HETEROSEXUAL RELATIONSHIPS

During adolescence, romantic friendships emerge. Special talents and interests influence selection of activities. Social outings to the mall or beach are heavily influenced by the desire to meet members of the opposite gender. Participation in group and individual activities enhances social stature. All adolescents enjoy parties, movies, athletic competitions, and sports. Teen nightclubs and rock concerts are, however, generally reserved for later adolescence.

Adolescents need to meet and become acquainted with members of the opposite gender. Adolescents may start by first admiring from a distance. This is accompanied by daydreams. Gradually, the young person attempts to attract the attention of the person in whom he or she is interested. Competition and rivalry may be keen. A person may date a number of people or merely one. Dates may be frequent or sporadic (Figure 15-6).

The adolescent's cultural background has an influence on patterns of dating. Conflict often arises when the teenager from a different cultural background wants to be independent and quickly adopts American norms of dating while parents insist on strict traditional values. This is particularly noticeable with daughters.

Dating represents one of the early social decision points of growing up. As such, it may become a battleground in the struggle for independence. Parental opposition is often based on unspoken fears of rejection and the adolescent's increased sexual experience or the possibility of pregnancy. Parents may respond by imposing strict restrictions in regard to curfews, chaperones, use of the car, and so on. When these problems are not discussed openly with the young person, the adolescent may react by rebelling, by sexual acting out, or by other means. Often these means are designed to test injunctions of control rather than out of a desire for the sexual act itself.

Date Rape

Teens need to be educated on "date rape." Unfortunately, this can occur simply because boys believe girls want to have sex, even when they say "no." When a girl says "no," her wishes are to be respected. If her date does not take "no" for an answer, teenage girls should be taught to shout, scream, fight back, or run away to protect themselves. In addition, teens need to be aware of the effects of Rohypnol, the "date rape drug." Rohypnol is illegally imported into the United States at an alarming rate. The effect of this drug is 10 times stronger than that of Valium. Teens need to learn not only about the effects of this drug but also how to avoid places and situations where it could be used.

CHRONIC ILLNESS/DISABILITY

Chronic illness during adolescence runs counter to developmental needs. Specific programs that foster

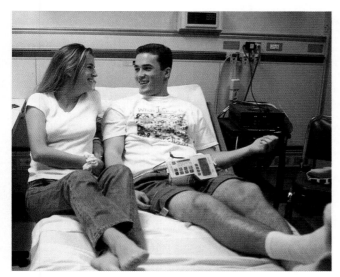

FIGURE **15-7** The chronically ill adolescent can develop strong intimate relationships that can provide a source of support and companionship during hospitalization. This should be encouraged by the hospital staff.

feelings of security and independence within the limits of the situation are essential. Behavioral problems are lessened when patients can verbalize specific concerns with people who are sensitive to their problems. If they feel rejected by and different from peers, they may become depressed. To be in school and to be considered one of the group is important. Hospital school programs for adolescents with long-term hospitalization enable teenagers to keep pace with their classmates and to achieve their educational goals. Recreational programs are also helpful in combating boredom and providing outlets for tension. Peers should be encouraged to spend time with the adolescent who requires long-term hospitalization (Figure 15-7). Nurses need to help patients cope with body image concerns. They must develop an awareness of the teenager's particular fears of forced dependence, bodily invasion, mutilation, rejection, and humiliation, especially within the peer group. The nurse should anticipate a certain amount of reluctance to adhere to hospital regulations, which reflects the adolescent's need for self-determination. Recognizing this as an asset rather than a liability enables the nurse to respond in a constructive manner.

Adolescents who have a developmental disability that affects the intellect or the ability to cope face some unique difficulties. They are often overprotected, unable to break away from supervision, and deprived of necessary peer relationships. The pubertal process with its emerging sexuality becomes a worrisome concern for parents and may precipitate a family crisis. It is becoming more common for hospitals to provide an interdisciplinary team that works to meet the needs of adolescents and their families.

Many adolescents with chronic illnesses or developmental disabilities are assisted at home through home health. Home health agencies, public school districts, and community agencies work together to meet the physical and psychosocial needs of the patient. **Respite care** for parents enables a helper to come into the home to relieve parents of the responsibility of caring for the child for brief periods of time. This enables the parents to shop, transact business affairs, or simply take a much-needed break or vacation.

One mother whose 13-year-old daughter had a severe developmental disability (cerebral palsy, blindness, mental retardation) offered these suggestions for the health care worker assisting in the home:

- Observe how the parents interact with the child.
- Do not wait for the child to cry out for attention because the youngster may be unable to communicate in this way.
- Watch for facial expression and body language.
- Post signs above the bed denoting special considerations, such as "Never position on the left side," "Do not feed with plastic spoon," and so on.
- Listen to the parents and observe how they attend to the physical needs of the youngster.
- Do not be afraid to ask questions or discuss apprehensions you may feel concerning your ability to care for the child.
- Be attuned to the needs of other children in the home.
- Be creative in exploring avenues for socialization because these teenagers are seldom invited to birthday parties, slumber parties, or other social activities available to most adolescents.
- Explore community facilities and support groups that might be of benefit to the family.

HEALTH PROMOTION AND MAINTENANCE

PARENTING A TEENAGER

At times, parents have difficulty coping with adolescents. The shift that has occurred in parenting philosophy, from the rigid rules of discipline to permissiveness to the current middle-of-the-road position, causes confusion. Some parents are unsure of their own opinions and may hesitate to exert authority. Others refuse to change any of their beliefs to accommodate youth. The teenager, who is the subject of a heavy concentration of parental attention, can become overanxious. Mothers have a particular problem because they have to find substitute satisfactions for the loss of a dependent child. However, as adolescents mature, they become more secure and are able to develop a new and more satisfactory relationship with their parents.

Adolescence may be one of the greatest parenting challenges. Raising children to be independent and responsible is the goal of all parents. Children should understand that there are house rules and consequences.

| Table 15-2 | *Summary of Findings from "Youth Risk Behavior Surveillance—2005"* |

AREAS	FINDINGS
Physical activity and fitness	Youth participation in physical activity remained the same; more young people are taking part in daily physical education classes (36%)
Nutrition	The number of youth at risk of being overweight increased (15.7%)
Tobacco	Decrease in adolescents reporting smoking (23%); smokeless tobacco rates reduced significantly (8%)
Alcohol and other drugs	74% lifetime alcohol use; 43% have current alcohol use; marijuana use has decreased slightly (38%); steroid use has decreased (4%)
Mental health and mental disorders	Suicide attempt rates among young people are leveling (16.9%)
Violent and abusive behavior	Number of rapes is 7.5%; homicide rates are increasing; student reporting of weapon carrying at school is leveling (18.5%), but physical fighting has increased (35.9%)
Unintentional injuries	The reported number of youths not wearing seat belts is leveling (10.2%) Youths not wearing bicycle helmets (94.6%)

From Centers for Disease Control and Prevention. (2006). Youth risk behavior surveillance USA—2005. *MMWR, 55*(SS05), 1-108.

Children need to understand society's rules and consequences, which will teach responsibility for actions committed outside of the home. Both of these ideas encourage teens to become responsible adults while allowing them to make mistakes and assume the responsibility for their actions.

Parents need to be reassured that all parents make mistakes with their children. This may be an excellent time for parents to role-model for their children the ability to say "I'm sorry" or "I made a bad decision." Parents should be encouraged to know their children's friends and parents, become involved in their school and activities, and keep the lines of communication open. They also need to provide their teenager with privacy. Parents need to wait until teenagers are ready and then give them the opportunity to discuss their problems. However, teenagers often end up discussing problems with friends instead. Parents who are experiencing difficulties in parenting may be referred to professional help.

HEALTH EXAMINATIONS

The prevention of illness in this age group, as in all others, is of primary importance. Yearly physical examinations are recommended for healthy adolescents. Immunizations need to be reviewed and updated (see Appendix A). A menstrual history and gynecological examination should be a routine part of the assessment of the adolescent girl. With sexually active teenagers, school nurses and other health care practitioners must take an active role in teaching about the prevention of sexually transmitted diseases. They also might need to refer the teenager for treatment.

Adolescents are often reluctant to seek health care. This reluctance can be influenced by factors such as perceived availability of confidential services, characteristics of health care providers, geographic access, and financial limitations (Hockenberry et al., 2003). They also feel nothing will or can go wrong with

them and often feel they are invincible. Multiple resources may be the most effective adolescent health promotion effort. School-based clinics and school-linked clinics and physician offices and community clinics can offer services the adolescent needs for health promotion. It is important that nurses and physicians make adolescents feel comfortable in the waiting room and in the examining room. The physician-patient relationship can be enhanced when a good rapport is established. When facing the issues of the teenage years, adolescents need to be able to turn to a supportive nurse or physician.

The media can also have an impact on the health of the adolescent. The media can offer health promotion messages such as antismoking, antiviolence, and antidrug campaigns. Through these messages, today's youth can make informed decisions and help maintain good health habits.

Healthy Youth 2010 is a document that outlines the adolescent component of the *Healthy People 2010* objectives (*Healthy People 2010* was discussed in Chapter 1). An interim report, "Youth Risk Behavior Surveillance USA—2005," summarizes some of the findings (Table 15-2). This summary stresses the importance of health promotion among our youth. Nutrition, tobacco, alcohol use, and suicide remain areas that require the attention and educational efforts of health care workers and the community.

CONFIDENTIALITY

Respecting a teenager's right to confidentiality is essential to establishing trust. In general, the nurse does not divulge or share information without the patient's consent. Many problems can be avoided if the confidentiality of the relationship is clearly defined during initial meetings. At this time, nurses explain to teenagers that there are certain situations that must be reported: plans to harm themselves or harm others or any abuse that may have occurred. Patient records must be carefully monitored to avoid loss or access by unauthorized personnel. The nurse should not give any private information about the teenager to telephone callers or visitors.

The term emancipated minor generally refers to adolescents less than 18 years of age who are no longer under their parents' authority. Married minors or minors in the military are automatically considered emancipated and may give consent for medical treatment for themselves and their children. The mature minor doctrine recognizes that individuals mature at different rates. In most parts of the United States, the young adolescent may receive medical assistance for certain conditions such as sexually transmitted diseases, contraception, pregnancy, abortion, and drug abuse without parental awareness. These laws are designed to afford the young person immediate medical help without fear of reprisal. However, they are subject to controversy. All states allow minors to obtain treatment in life-threatening situations when legal guardians are not available. Because laws vary from state to state, nurses must be continually informed about the policies and the legislation within their practice state. This information is usually available from the local medical or nursing association office.

SEXUALITY

Sexuality defines those characteristics that make each of us either female or male. A person's sexuality is affected by psychological, biological, and social factors. Because the adolescent is in a period of growth, the various factors of sexuality may be in conflict. The adolescent is not prepared for the responsibility of having a child and yet is biologically capable of reproduction. The number of teenagers giving birth has continued to decrease in adolescents ages 15 to 19 since the most recent peak in 1991. Sexual activity continues to increase. Adolescents are becoming sexually active at younger ages. Current statistics indicate that 46.8% of adolescents have engaged in intercourse, with girls having a higher rate (CDC, 2006).

During this period, the adolescent has an increased need to learn about sexuality. Values must be clarified, and decision-making skills evaluated. The adolescent may be told that not making a decision about sexual activity is indeed making a decision. Although parental involvement in sex education is encouraged, parents often wait until adolescence to talk with their children. In other cases, they might prefer giving others the responsibility of educating their children. Consequently, the adolescent receives information from peers, the media, and other sources that may be incorrect or biased.

If the adolescent receives incorrect information about the body, misconceptions should be identified and teaching should be done regarding menstruation, pregnancy, sexually transmitted diseases, and contraception. Most adolescents do not want to become pregnant, and yet many do not use contraceptives. Adolescents need to be informed about safe sex practices. Contraceptive information needs to be available to prevent pregnancy. Condom information needs to be available to protect against the transmission of HIV and other sexually transmitted diseases. Both boys and girls need to be knowledgeable about protective measures. The school nurse or clinic nurse can often provide this information to adolescents.

Adolescents have fears and concerns that are specific to their sexuality. The girl who is the tallest person in her class is often just as concerned as the boy who is the shortest. Adolescent girls are also concerned about when to wear a bra, when they will begin their menstrual period, and when they will take on the characteristics of a woman. Adolescent boys may be worried because they do not have the height and strength of their peers. There is a wide age range for the physical changes that take place during puberty, and the adolescent needs to be reassured that they are normal. An excellent time to teach normal growth and development to the developing adolescent is at the time of assessment. Nurses can talk about concerns as they examine each part of the child's body. Because there is such a wide variation in the age at which each child develops, nurses should point out to adolescents that they are exactly where they should be for their particular stage of sexual development.

Sex education in public schools tends to concentrate on the physiology of sex, on the reproductive systems, and on sexually transmitted disease. It is usually less informative about the psychological and value aspects of sexuality and the facts concerning contraception. Peers play a major role in providing information on sex. This is because few adolescents can talk freely to their parents about sex (particularly regarding their own sexual behavior and problems). However, sexual values, attitudes, and information are conveyed in less conscious ways by role modeling. In this way, parents serve as an initial source of sex role learning for their daughters and sons. In their sexuality and intimacy, adolescents reflect society's new openness about sexual matters and are inclined to see sexual behavior as a matter of personal choice rather than of morality or law. Parents need to provide factual information.

HOMOSEXUALITY

Homosexual experiences in adolescence are not uncommon. This experimentation is not necessarily a positive prediction of one's sexual preference as an adult. It may merely reflect a desire to explore alternative lifestyles or may arise from curiosity. Homosexuality, although no longer classified as a disease, is nonetheless subject to great controversy. Whether or not the adolescent is homosexual, unspoken suspicions during adolescence can create anxiety and turmoil for the young person and the family. Parents need to accept their child and be supportive. It is also important that nurses remain sensitive to these issues when interacting with homosexual adolescents. Nurses need to be aware of their personal biases to determine their potential effectiveness with this population. Refer adolescents to counseling when they question their sexual orientation and preference.

BODY PIERCINGS AND TATTOOS

Teens and other young people receive body piercing and tattoos because they want to make a "statement" or because they simply feel that it is fashionable and expressive. Ears, navels, tongues, eyebrows, lips, nostrils, nipples, and genitals are all sites used for piercing. Ideally, piercing and tattooing should be performed by an experienced licensed person. Unfortunately, no national regulations exist regarding the piercing or tattooing of minors. Generally, unlicensed uncertified "professionals" perform these procedures. At the very least, new disposable gloves and sterilized or disposable needles must be used to prevent HIV and hepatitis B. There is also a risk for tetanus. The skin at the site of the piercing is inspected regularly for signs of infection or allergic reaction. Jewelry should never be shared. Healing can take anywhere from 8 weeks to more than a year when a body part is pierced (Anderson & Martel, 2002). Self-inflicted or friend-inflicted piercing and tattoos are to be avoided because improper technique is often used.

It is important that health care workers examine their own feelings regarding these issues and not stereotype or pass judgment when caring for youth with piercing or tattoos. It is also up to health care workers to provide education regarding piercing and tattoos to today's youth and to assist them in making informed decisions.

NUTRITION

Adolescent girls have special nutritional needs. They have fewer caloric requirements than boys do. There is a concern with body image that may lead to anorexia or bulimia. The nurse should emphasize that skipping meals can lead to a decrease in essential nutrients. Encourage physical exercise to maintain body weight and eating nutritious foods that are low in calories such as skim milk and fruits. The adolescent should avoid high-calorie fast foods (Figure 15-8). Besides salad bars, many fast food chains have added grilled and high-fiber foods to their menus.

Many adolescent boys are concerned with their body image and body building. They should have a well-balanced diet with increased calories. Part of the dietary requirement is proper hydration without the use of supplements.

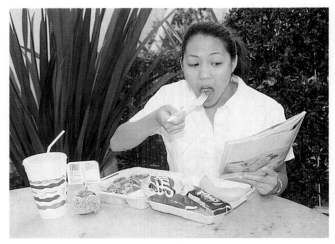

FIGURE **15-8** Snacking on empty calories is common among adolescents.

Overeating can lead to adult obesity. Adolescents who are obese need guidance in weight reduction. They should be instructed to:

- Eat a variety of foods low in calories and high in nutrients.
- Eat less fat and fewer fatty foods.
- Eat less sugar and sweets.
- Eat more fruits, vegetables, and whole grains.
- Increase physical activity.

Teenagers are growing rapidly, and they need foods that provide for the increase in height, body-cell mass, and maturation. Dietary deficiencies are more apt to occur at this age because of the acceleration in growth and increasingly irregular eating patterns. Depending on activity level, 13-year-old girls need approximately 1600-2200 calories per day and boys of the same age require 2000-2600 calories per day. The 18-year-old female needs 1800-2400 calories, whereas 18-year-old males need 2400-3200 calories, again depending on activity level. The U.S. Department of Agriculture has developed new food guidelines through the MyPyramid plan *(www. mypyramid.gov)*.

The most noticeable changes in the adolescent's eating habits are skipping meals, an increase in between-meal snacking, and an increase in eating out. Breakfast and lunch are often omitted. Part-time jobs, school activities, and socialization may result in the teenager's eating little or nothing during the day and then catching up in the evening. Fast food restaurants are inexpensive and quick for the busy adolescent. These foods tend to be high in calories, fat, protein, sugar, and sodium and low in fiber. Most fast food chains have added salad bars and other healthier foods. These appeal to the diet-conscious teenager and to vegetarians. Carbonated drinks often replace milk, resulting in low intakes of calcium, riboflavin, and vitamins A and D. The few fruits and vegetables eaten provide insufficient fiber.

Nutritional research on this age group is still meager, partly because studies must account not only for age but also for physical maturity. Minerals most apt to be inadequate in the adolescent diet are calcium and iron. Zinc is known to be essential for growth and sexual maturation and is therefore of great importance in adolescence. The retention of zinc increases, especially during the growth spurts, and leads to more efficient use of this nutrient's sources. Good sources of zinc include meat, liver, eggs, and seafood, particularly oysters. Sources for vegetarians include nuts, beans, wheat germ, and cheese. The importance of calcium lies in its key role in bone formation. In both boys and girls, the recommended dietary allowance (RDA) for calcium increases from 800 mg at age 10 years to 1500 mg during the growth spurt. The primary source of calcium is dairy products. The need for iron is increased in both genders at this time. This increased need is caused primarily by increases in muscle mass and blood volume in boys and to a lesser extent in girls. A menstruating woman loses 15 to 30 mg of iron per cycle. Iron absorption varies in individuals. Good sources of iron include liver, poultry, fish, dried beans, vegetables, egg yolk, and enriched breads. Protein needs are increased, particularly during pubertal changes in both genders and for developing muscle mass in boys. Calcium is important for the adolescent because during adolescence 40% to 60% of peak bone mass is developed. Bone mass has relevance for decreasing osteoporosis later in life. Girls need 44 to 46 g/day, whereas boys need 45 to 59 g/day. Finally, girls need about 2200 kcal/day; boys need 2500 to 3000 kcal/day.

SPORTS AND NUTRITION

The best training diet is one that contains foods from each of the basic food groups in sufficient quantities to meet energy demands and nutrient requirements. There is no evidence that eating large amounts of special foods or nutrients is beneficial in terms of athletic performance. Protein supplements are not necessary and could even be harmful. Sweat losses must be replaced by drinking plenty of fluids during the workout. Carbohydrates should not be used as the sole energy source because they are stored for relatively short spans in the body. Sodium and potassium replacement usually is met by eating a well-balanced diet. Caffeine and alcohol deplete body water and are to be avoided. Anabolic steroids, used by some athletes to gain weight and increase strength, are detrimental to bone growth. Iron is particularly necessary for female athletes who may be borderline or deficient in their intake of this mineral. On the day of the event, the athlete is advised to eliminate roughage, fats, and gas-forming foods.

PERSONAL CARE

SLEEP

Sleep requirements vary among individuals. Adolescents may obtain the 8 hours generally suggested but

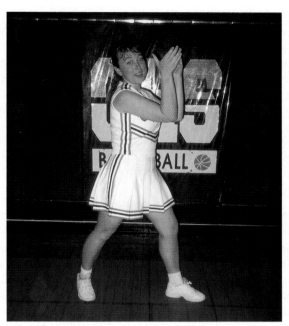

FIGURE **15-9** Cheerleading is an example of an activity that promotes physical fitness and helps the adolescent learn to work with others in a small group.

often at irregular hours. Many young people who are employed have to work very late hours, particularly in the summer months. This necessitates sleeping later in the morning. Another trend is for the young person who has worked long hours during the day to try to make up for lost time after work. It would seem that adolescents are either sleeping all the time or burning the candle at both ends! Complaints of fatigue are heard more often at home than elsewhere. The nurse should advise parents to become aware of the young person's sleep patterns. Crankiness, frustration, impatience, accident proneness, and other such behaviors may indicate lack of sleep. Finally, teenagers need to sleep on a bed with a firm mattress, preferably in their own room.

EXERCISE

Exercise has many benefits. Adolescents do not have to participate actively in sports; they can easily exercise by taking a brisk walk, riding a bike, or swimming. Although many teenagers are not athletes, they can benefit from a less sedentary lifestyle. These patterns, when carried over into adulthood, contribute to good health (Figure 15-9).

PERSONAL HYGIENE

Personal hygiene information is necessary at this time when the body changes of puberty require more frequent bathing and the use of deodorants. The nurse can help the adolescent figure out procedures and the various claims of reliability for products dealing with hair removal, menstrual hygiene, and cosmetics. Nurses need to stress the importance of not sharing razors with friends.

CLOTHING

Clothing is of great interest to the adolescent. Peer influence and the media have a major impact on fashion. How adolescents dress may indicate the peer group to which they belong. Dress varies from very contemporary to conservative, depending on the particular teenager's preferences. Much of this is just for fun and provides for good conversation. The power of television advertising in regard to clothes sales and other commercial messages may be explored.

DENTAL CARE

The prevalence of tooth decay has decreased substantially over the past few years. This is believed to be the result of the widespread use of fluorides, including community fluoridation and the use of dental products containing fluorides. Teenagers, nevertheless, are at risk for dental caries because of inadequate dental maintenance and frequent snacking on sucrose-containing candies and beverages. When dental hygiene is neglected, the period of greatest tooth decay in the permanent teeth is from ages 12 to 18 years. Poor oral hygiene (inadequate brushing, flossing, and rinsing, particularly after meals) fosters the accumulation of plaque and food debris. Missing, aching, or decayed teeth contribute to poor nutrition. Young people with unattractive teeth may have low self-esteem. According to the media, healthy white teeth are synonymous with popularity and sex appeal. A visit to the dentist twice a year is out of reach for many financially strapped young people. For others, it is a low family financial priority. There is a need for more school dental programs and other innovative measures to reach a major proportion of our young people.

SAFETY

The primary danger to the adolescent is the automobile. Road accidents kill and cripple teenagers at alarming rates. Many schools today offer driver training courses as an integral part of the educational program. In these courses, students learn the basic skills of driving, as well as the responsibilities that driving entails. Unfortunately, this does not ensure compliance. Preventing motor vehicle accidents is of utmost importance to every community. Seat belts must be worn every time an adolescent rides in a car (Figure 15-10). No one should ever drink and drive. Students Against Drunk Drivers (SADD) is an organization for youth against drinking and driving. Adolescents who ride motorcycles, motor scooters, or motorized bicycles should know the rules of the road and should wear special safety equipment, such

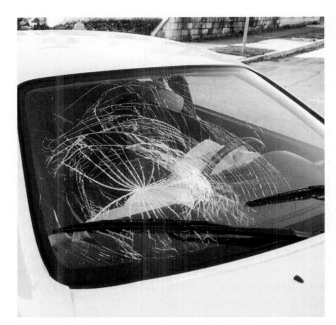

FIGURE **15-10** Accidents involving motor vehicles are a leading cause of injury and death in children and adolescents. Passengers need to have seat belts even if the car has an airbag.

as helmets, for protection. Adolescents must also be told that riding in the back of a pickup truck is dangerous—and possibly fatal.

Homicide is now the second leading cause of death among 15-year-olds to 24-year-olds. Most of these homicides involve firearms. The third leading cause of death among 15-year-olds to 24-year-olds is suicide, which has increased at alarming rates in adolescents over the past several years. Teenagers who do not achieve a sense of identity can experience self-doubt. Loss of relationships and depression can also leave the adolescent vulnerable to suicidal tendencies. It is important for parents and health care workers to be alert for signs of depression or isolation in the adolescent. It is also crucial to work on promoting self-esteem and identity.

Although most adolescents know how to swim, accidents that involve diving into unsafe areas and using alcohol or drugs while playing in the water are not uncommon.

Both accidental and deliberate morbidity and mortality caused by firearms continue to be a major concern during the adolescent period. Regarding handling firearms, this age group is characterized by the feeling of "it couldn't happen to me." Gang-related injuries and deaths often involve the use of firearms. Many adolescents are involved in serious crimes (Figure 15-11), some of which involve guns and violence. Gun control continues to be controversial. At the very least, control must be stringent for this age group. Those who do use firearms legally must be taught to respect the power of firearms and how to use them safely.

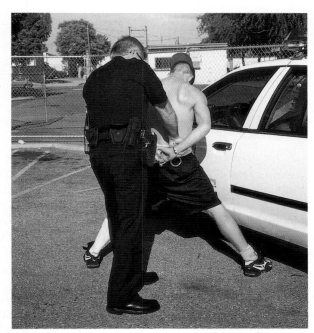

FIGURE **15-11** Increasing numbers of older children and adolescents are involved in serious crimes against persons and property.

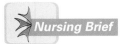

Boys and girls should both be taught sports injury prevention. Physical conditioning should be emphasized in relation to all intense physical activity (e.g., team sports).

INTERNET SOLICITATION

Children using the home computer is becoming the typical picture of family life. Children and adolescents are spending more time at the computer, for both educational and personal purposes. Internet access allows adolescents to explore topics such as pornography and gambling in the privacy of their home. Reports indicate that 1 million to 2 million adolescents engage in gambling, which can be difficult to monitor and can lead to hidden addictions (Verkler, 2005).

Online predators are able to access unsuspecting children by using chat rooms and instant messaging. With the increasing use of handheld devices, the home computer is not the only mode of contact. Parents need to have an understanding of computers, how to trace websites, and how to use filtering devices. Health care providers need to raise awareness of the potential dangers of Internet access for all ages. The AAP has partnered with Microsoft to offer a free web-based safety service (Windows Live Family Safety Setting), which will provide parents with a tool to control and track Internet access. The service hopes to encourage dialogue between parents and children regarding websites (AAP, 2006).

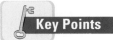

Guidelines for Internet Safety

- Never share personal information
- Never meet with an online contact
- Discuss with a parent or adult about relationships developed over the Internet
- Never send an message over the Internet that you would not say in person

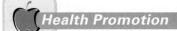

- Adolescence begins with the appearance of secondary sex characteristics and ends with cessation of growth and the achievement of emotional maturation.
- Adolescents question life and search for their sense of identity. They seek to understand who they are, where they are going, and how they are getting there.
- It is important in today's society that adolescents learn to develop problem-solving skills and learn to de-escalate conflicts.
- Early adolescents are in the concrete phase of thinking; older adolescents develop abstract formal thinking.
- Peer relationships are important in helping adolescents define themselves.
- With increasing maturity comes increasing responsibility. Adolescents need to learn to understand financial management.
- Dating represents one of the early social decision points of growing up.
- Parents need to clarify house rules and consequences; society's rules and consequences teach responsibility outside of the home.
- Annual health examinations are equally important to the adolescent; anticipatory guidance includes nutrition, exercise, and safety.
- Adolescents must come to terms with their own sexuality; this is affected by psychological, biological, and social factors.
- Parents should have an open dialogue with adolescents regarding Internet usage and safety.

 Go to your Companion CD-ROM for an Audio Glossary, video clips, and more.

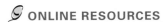 Be sure to visit the companion Evolve site at http://evolve.elsevier.com/Price/pediatric/ for WebLinks and additional online resources.

ONLINE RESOURCES

American Academy of Pediatrics: www.aap.org

Bright Futures: www.brightfutures.org

Safe Sitter: http://www.safesitter.org

Teen gambling: www.nati.org

CHAPTER 16

Disorders of the Adolescent

Objectives

Upon completion of this chapter, the student will be able to:

1. List and describe the more common disorders of adolescents
2. Contrast the clinical presentation and nursing care of the teenager with anorexia nervosa with that of the teenager with bulimia
3. Formulate a nursing care plan for the adolescent confined in a brace for the treatment of scoliosis
4. Describe several measures designed to prevent sports injuries
5. Detail the special needs of teenagers with sexually transmitted diseases
6. List four risk factors that might indicate an adolescent is contemplating suicide
7. Identify health issues for substance abuse drugs

Key Terms

Be sure to check out the bonus material on the Companion CD-ROM, including selected audio pronunciations.

anorexia nervosa (ăn-ŏ-RĔK-sē-ă nĕr-VŌ-să; p. 343)
asymmetry (ā-SĬM-ĕ-trē; p. 349)
bulimia (bū-LĒ-mē-ă; p. 345)
comedo (KŎM-ĕ-dō; p. 338)
dysmenorrhea (dĭs-mĕn-ō-RĒ-ă; p. 352)
mittelschmerz (MĬT-ĕl-shmārts; p. 352)
premenstrual syndrome (PMS; prē-MĔN-strū-ăl; p. 352)
sebum (SĒ-bŭm; p. 338)

Adolescents are marching toward adulthood. As these children grow physically into young adults, they leave behind many of the illnesses that are typical of younger children. New illnesses that occur during this time span are related to physical growth, self-image, experimentation, and access. Adolescents' health issues involve behavior choices that can have later ramifications.

SKIN

ACNE VULGARIS
Description

Acne is an inflammation of the sebaceous glands and hair follicles in the skin. At puberty, because of hormonal influence, the sebaceous follicles enlarge and secrete increased amounts of a fatty substance called sebum. Genetic factors and stress are also thought to play a part. The course of acne may be brief or prolonged (lasting 10 or more years). Premenstrual acne in girls is not uncommon. The principal lesions include comedones, papules, and nodulocystic growths.

Signs and Symptoms

A comedo (plural, *comedones*) is a plug of keratin, sebum, and bacteria. Keratin is a protein substance that is the main constituent of epidermis and hair. There are two types of comedones, open and closed. In the open comedo, or blackhead, the surface is darkened by melanin. Closed comedones, or whiteheads, are responsible for the inflammatory process of acne. With continued build-up, the walls of the follicle rupture, releasing their irritating content into the surrounding skin. A pustule may appear when this develops near the exterior (Figure 16-1). This process occurs no matter how carefully the teenager washes because surface bacteria are not involved in the pathogenesis. Acne is usually seen on the chin, cheeks, and forehead. It can also develop on the chest, upper back, and shoulders. It is usually more severe in winter.

Treatment and Nursing Care

The basic treatment of acne has changed considerably over the past few years. It is no longer thought that certain foods trigger the condition; therefore chocolate, peanuts, and cola drinks are not restricted unless the patient is convinced of a correlation between a specific item and the condition. A regular well-balanced diet is encouraged. Patients who are not taking tetracycline or vitamin A benefit from sunshine. General hygienic measures of cleanliness, rest, and avoidance of emotional stress may help prevent exacerbations.

Cleansing with mild soap and water removes surface oil, although excessive cleansing should be avoided because it leaves the skin dry and irritated. Lipid-free cleansers, synthetic detergent bars, astringents, and exfoliants can be used to clean the skin. Squeezing pimples increases local inflammation. Use of a flesh-colored topical preparation over active lesions can improve appearance while lesions are resolving.

If topical preparations are needed, over-the-counter benzoyl peroxide lotions or prescription-strength gels

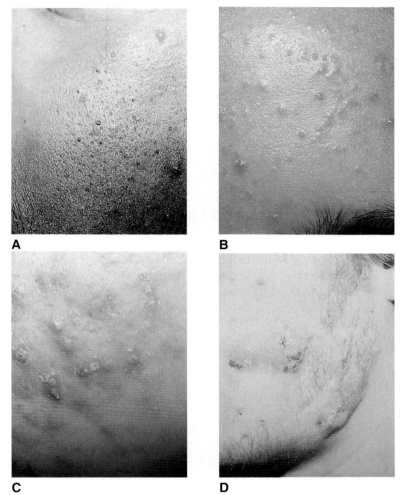

FIGURE **16-1**   Acne. **A,** Comedonal acne with blackheads. **B,** Comedonal acne with whiteheads. **C,** Papulopustular acne with inflamed papules and pustules. **D,** Cystic acne with deep cysts and marked erythema that can cause future scarring.

act to dry and peel the skin and suppress fatty acid growth. Topical retinoic acid derivative (Retin-A) aids in the elimination of keratinous plugs. It is applied daily, beginning with the lowest strength and increasing the strength until acne is controlled without excessive peeling or irritation. Vitamin A acid can increase sensitivity to the sun, so precautions should be taken when it is used. Antibiotic topical preparations, such as erythromycin solution in easy-to-use pads, minimize surface bacteria. They can be used in conjunction with benzoyl peroxide.

For adolescents with severe acne that does not respond to topical treatment, systemic medications may be indicated. Tetracycline, doxycycline, or erythromycin may be given in conjunction with topical medications in more serious cases. Monilial vaginitis is a secondary complication sometimes seen with the use of these drugs and should be explained to the unsuspecting female teenager. Tetracycline can interfere with the action of certain birth control pills, so the adolescent girl needs to be sure to tell the dermatologist if she is using oral contraceptives.

Accutane (13-*cis*-retinoic acid) is now being used for patients with severe pustulocystic acne who have not benefited from other types of treatment. It has many side effects, including conjunctivitis, hypertriglyceridemia, elevated blood cholesterol serum, blood dyscrasia, elevated liver enzymes, dry mucous membranes, photosensitivity, and pruritus. The patient requires careful monitoring and the physician needs to be registered in the manufacturer's System to Manage Accutane-Related Teratogenicity (SMART) program to prescribe the medication (Feldman et al., 2004). **Because of its highly teratogenic effects, Accutane is not prescribed during pregnancy or to those at any risk for pregnancy because of the possibilities of fetal deformity.** Many physicians prescribe oral contraceptives in conjunction with Accutane. The long-term effects of this medication have not been established. There have been concerns regarding depression and suicide with the use of Accutane; however, at present there is not an established correlation. **Dermabrasion** (planing of the skin to minimize scarring) is done selectively because it is not always successful.

Acne is very distressing to the adolescent, particularly when the face is extensively involved. Sometimes even a minimal problem is seen as disastrous when it happens before an important event. The self-conscious young person feels different and embarrassed. The nurse who is attuned to the feelings of individuals can provide understanding support. Although the teenager is educated to assume responsibility for his or her regimen, inclusion of the parents helps prevent conflict surrounding it.

HEMATOLOGIC SYSTEM

INFECTIOUS MONONUCLEOSIS
Description

Infectious mononucleosis is a global disease caused by a herpes-type Epstein-Barr virus (EBV). It occurs chiefly in older children and adults; its peak incidence is in persons between 17 and 25 years of age or earlier in low socioeconomic groups. Studies suggest that the organism is transmitted by contact with saliva, either directly or on contaminated eating utensils; however, its communicability is considered low. The incubation period is from 1 to 2 months.

Signs and Symptoms

Symptoms vary from mild to moderately severe and may last for several weeks. They include low-grade fever, sore throat, headache, fatigue, skin rash, and general malaise. The lymph glands enlarge. Splenomegaly develops in approximately half the patients. Liver involvement with mild jaundice occurs in a small number of persons and requires bed rest until liver function returns to normal.

The diagnosis is confirmed with the examination of peripheral blood. Lymphocytosis and the presence of atypical lymphocytes are seen. A rising titer of antibody to EBV is also indicative; the **MonoSpot** test is rapid, can detect the infection earlier than the heterophile antibody test, and is now widely used. Complications, although uncommon, include rupture of the spleen, secondary pneumonia, neurological manifestations, and heart involvement.

Treatment and Nursing Care

Treatment is supportive because the disease is self-limiting. Acetaminophen, aspirin, or nonsteroidal anti-inflammatory medication such as ibuprofen is given as needed. An antipyretic is given to reduce fever and discomfort. An initial period of rest or restricted activities is usually needed, and returning to usual activities is based on the child's energy level. Gargling with warm saline solution and sucking on throat lozenges can be helpful for pharyngitis. Adequate fluid intake is necessary, in particular bland, cool liquids that are not irritating to the throat. Smoking should be discouraged. There is no special diet. Isolation is not necessary. The patient is alerted to signs of secondary infection. Activities are increased as the fever and fatigue diminish. The patient with an enlarged spleen is cautioned to avoid heavy lifting, trauma to the abdomen, and vigorous athletics until the splenomegaly subsides. For the athlete with an enlarged spleen, contact or collision activities should be restricted for at least 3 to 4 weeks. Severe abdominal pain is unusual, except in the presence of splenic rupture, which requires immediate attention.

The teenager with mononucleosis may be discouraged and depressed. The teenager worries about job, schoolwork, and the ability to continue extracurricular activities of importance. Open communication with school officials and classmates helps alleviate some of the anxieties. The prognosis in mononucleosis is good. It is no longer considered a prolonged, debilitating disease. Many cases go unrecognized. Two vaccines are currently ready for trials for the EBV virus (Macsween, 2003).

LYMPHATIC SYSTEM

HODGKIN'S DISEASE
Description

Hodgkin's disease is a malignant disease of the lymph system that primarily involves the lymph nodes. It may metastasize to the spleen, liver, bone marrow, lungs, or other parts of the body. The Reed-Sternberg cell, which can be seen on microscopic examination of lymph node tissue, contains two nuclei and is diagnostic of the disease. Hodgkin's disease is rare before 10 years of age, but the incidence rate increases during adolescence and early adulthood. It is twice as common in boys as in girls. There are four subtypes, each with a different age at onset, clinical findings, and prognostic factors.

Signs and Symptoms

The presenting symptom is generally a painless lump in the cervical area or other lymph node site (supraclavicular, axillary, inguinal). Characteristically, there are few other manifestations. The swelling is generally first noted by the patient or the parents. In more advanced cases, there may be high spiking fever, anorexia, weight loss, night sweats, general malaise, rash, and itching of the skin. Because this condition affects immune cells, the affected adolescent can be more prone to infection.

Infectious causes of enlarged lymph glands should be ruled out (e.g., infectious mononucleosis is common among adolescents). Blood counts may show changes in white blood cell differentials. A chest radiograph may show mediastinal involvement. The diagnosis is confirmed with a lymph node biopsy, which reveals Reed-Sternberg cells.

Determining the stage of the disease is necessary for prescribing a treatment regimen. Initially, computed

Table 16-1 | *Interventions for Adolescents Undergoing Cancer Chemotherapy*

PROBLEM	INTERVENTION
Infection risk	Explain the function of the immune system and how chemotherapeutic medications affect it
	Use visual aids whenever applicable
	Review methods to prevent infection—meticulous handwashing, avoiding exposure to colds or illness, importance of routine checkups and immunizations
Bleeding	Advise cautious physical activity and avoid contact sports if platelet count is low
	Review management of nosebleeds
	Help the adolescent plan for low-risk social activities
Stomatitis, nausea, vomiting	Use a local anesthetic on ulcerated oral lesions before meals
	Advise using a soft toothbrush, WaterPik, and mouthwash
	Give ordered antiemetic before chemotherapy treatment; practice relaxation techniques
	Provide frequent small meals; discuss altered taste and foods that will appeal
Fatigue	Encourage frequent rest periods
	Coordinate in-school rest periods with the school nurse
	Explore quiet areas of interest
Body image changes	Encourage the adolescent to express feelings about changes in skin and hair and activity level
	Use wigs, scarves, hats, eyebrow pencils, false eyelashes, and other cosmetic devices to minimize appearance of hair loss; remind the adolescent that the hair loss is temporary
	Suggest clothing that minimizes body changes and enhances appearance
Enforced dependence during treatment	Involve the adolescent in decision making
	Advise parent not to be overprotective but to allow autonomy within treatment limits
	Encourage peers to visit or phone; provide opportunities for "rap" sessions with peers
Fear	Refer the adolescent to a peer support group
	Allow to express any fears, concerns, or doubts
	Refer patient and family for spiritual support
	Clarify information about the disease, procedures, or treatments
	Refer to a camp for children with cancer if the adolescent is interested

tomography or magnetic resonance imaging can help determine the extent of the disease. Lymphangiography can assess lower abdominal lymph node involvement. In some cases, a laparotomy may be performed to determine the stage of the disease. At this time, the spleen may be removed and biopsies of the liver, accessible nodes, and bone marrow are performed. The stages in Hodgkin's disease are defined as follows:

Stage I: Disease restricted to a single, non-lymph node site or localized in a single group of lymph nodes. Asymptomatic.

Stage II: Two or more affected lymph node areas on the same side of the diaphragm, or one affected non-lymph node area and one or more affected lymph node regions on the same side of the diaphragm.

Stage III: Involvement of lymph node regions on both sides of the diaphragm; involvement of adjacent organ or spleen.

Stage IV: Diffuse disease; least favorable prognosis.

Further clarification of disease extent depends on the presence or absence of systemic symptoms of fever or weight loss (Kliegman et al., 2006).

Treatment

Well-established treatment regimens are now available to combat Hodgkin's disease. Both low-dose radiation therapy and chemotherapy are used in accordance with the clinical stage of the disease. The prognosis for remission is favorable. Cure is primarily related to the stage of the disease at diagnosis.

Nursing care is mainly directed toward the symptomatic relief of the side effects of radiation therapy and chemotherapy (see Chapter 12 for management of side effects and Table 16-1 for interventions adapted for adolescents). Education of the patient and family is paramount because most patients are cared for in the home.

A common side effect of irradiation is malaise. The teenager tires easily and may be irritable and anorexic. The skin in the treated area may be sensitive and should be protected against exposure to sunlight and irritation, particularly during treatment. After treatment, a sun-blocking agent containing PABA (para-aminobenzoic acid) should be used to prevent burning. The attending physician may prescribe an ointment to relieve itching of the skin. Nothing should be applied to the treatment area without the recommendation of the doctor. There may be diarrhea after abdominal radiation therapy. The patient **does not** become radioactive during or after therapy.

After splenectomy, the patient faces the long-term risk for serious infection. This is explained to the parents and teenager. Elevations in temperature need to be monitored carefully. There may also be infection with little or no fever as a result of masking by certain medications. In such cases, throat specimens may need to be taken for culture as should specimens of blood, urine, sputum, or stool. Instruct parents or the adolescent to feel free to call the clinic, particularly if there is a change in the condition or if they are apprehensive or confused about symptoms. Medication readjustments should not be attempted unless specifically advised by the physician.

Because adolescents are cognitively able to understand the implications of serious disease, emotional support is paramount. Nurses must be prepared in particular for periods of anger, which may be directed at them. Suitable exercise, such as the use of a punching bag, allows for safe direction of anger. Routine use helps prevent the unnecessary build-up of tension. Activity in general is regulated by the patient. The physician advises the patient if special precautions are necessary.

GASTROINTESTINAL SYSTEM

OBESITY

Description

Obesity, or **overnutrition,** is the accumulation of excess body fat. It is the most common nutritional disorder in Western society today, and its treatment record is dismal. Obesity has become an important issue with children. Statistics show that 15% of children ages 6 to 19 years have a BMI at or above 95%, labeling them as obese. Children of African-American and Mexican American descent have above a 20% obesity rate. Obesity has far-reaching implications. Heart disease and the incidence of type 2 diabetes are only two of the serious conditions that result from obesity. Obesity is difficult to define during adolescence because of height, age, and body structure variations within this age group. An increase in lean body mass and fat is characteristic of this age group; therefore one must know what stage of puberty teenagers are in and whether or not they have completed the growth spurt before calling them obese. The Centers for Disease Control and Prevention (CDC) has developed growth charts that use body mass index (BMI) for age to determine percentiles. Obesity in children is defined as having a BMI greater than the 95th percentile for age. Children with a BMI between the 85th and 95th percentile for age are defined as at risk for obesity.

Signs and Symptoms

Weight gain can occur at any age but appears most frequently in the first year of life, at 5 to 6 years of age, and during adolescence (Kliegman et al., 2006). Most children stay plump during puberty and then return to their normal size after growth is complete.

Obesity becomes particularly significant during adolescence, when feelings of inadequacy are pronounced. Obese adolescents are concerned about their appearance but are unable to conform to the standards of the group. They are often the subject of cruel ridicule. For instance, overweight males frequently appear to have developed breasts, white striae may appear on the abdomen, and the penis appears disproportionately small. Obese teenagers date less and may feel rejected, unattractive, and unloved. Accompanying the emotional anxieties

are the more obvious physical handicaps. Overweight teenagers may be unable to participate in sports or other school activities and are more accident-prone. Their choice of careers is more limited. Although some obese adolescents experience emotional consequences, many do not and become well-adjusted adults. However, the physical consequences of obesity can adversely affect adult health.

Causes

There are many theories concerning the causes of obesity. In reality, the etiology is complex, and researchers are only beginning to discover some of the underlying genetic and emotional contributing factors. The onset of obesity can be traced to excess food intake, reduced physical activity, or both. Contrary to popular belief, obesity due to abnormal function of the glands is rare. Genetic studies have shown an increased incidence of obesity in twins, even though they may have been raised in separate homes. Children born to obese parents are more likely to become obese. However, environmental factors such as ethnic diet, family eating practices, and psychological factors are also operating, making it difficult to isolate these from genetic factors.

The risk for obesity persisting into adulthood increases with a later onset (adolescence versus infancy) and the severity of the obesity. The longer the adolescent is overweight, the more difficult it is to overcome the problem. The only way to obtain a permanent solution to obesity is to decrease intake and increase the amount of energy used through activity.

Compulsive overeating is an eating disorder in which adolescents eat not because they are hungry but because they use food to satisfy emotional rather than physical needs. Compulsive overeating leads to obesity because persons who overeat are unable to tell when they are full. Many adolescents who compulsively overeat try fad diets, starvation, and other inappropriate methods for losing weight. In most cases, these methods are unsuccessful and increase the feeling of hopelessness these adolescents experience.

Treatment and Nursing Care

The optimal treatment of obesity usually includes a combination of diet modification and exercise. Often the goal is not to lose weight but to avoid gaining weight during puberty. The weight remains stable as the adolescent grows in height. Teaching the adolescent about good nutrition, proper food choices, and the importance of regular moderate exercise helps develop healthy patterns for the future.

If a diet is necessary, it must be carefully planned with a nutritionist or dietitian to ensure enough calories and nutrients for growth. Dieting is difficult and often unsuccessful. When obesity begins in early childhood, a person is faced with a lifetime of fighting calories. This is complicated by the fact that food is readily available in the United States and that advertisers bombard the public with tempting treats. Parents must be keenly interested in helping control their child's weight if a diet is to be successful. Changing methods of cooking and types of food prepared to create a healthy plan for the entire family is more successful than preparing different food for the dieting adolescent. Many specialized cookbooks and magazines help families prepare meals that are appealing yet not high in fat or calories. Adolescents should avoid cookies and cakes and should substitute fresh fruits for between-meal snacks. The nurse should emphasize that diets must be carefully planned and based on accurate nutrition information. Adolescents are apt to go on diets that they invent themselves and that are dangerous to their health. Whenever such a major satisfaction as eating is denied, it must be replaced by something equally satisfying and rewarding, such as new social activities, hobbies, friends, or sports.

Behavior modification techniques have shown success. This approach helps a person identify and control poor eating patterns. Such techniques include eating only at the table, using a smaller plate, eating only at specific times, recording food intake (food diary) and feelings at the time of eating, and so on. A point system or system of rewards is established on initiation of this technique. Groups such as Weight Watchers, Overeaters Anonymous, or diet workshops, although helpful, are frequented mostly by adults. A few parents accompany their teenagers and participate themselves.

Support groups specifically for adolescents are more acceptable. These are usually found in teenage clinics, schools, and specialized summer camps. Diet pills are not recommended. Their long-term effectiveness is minimal, and the potential for misuse by the teenager is high. Jejunoileal bypass, or lap banding, can have complications and is seldom advised unless the child is morbidly obese. The long-term consequences of this procedure have yet to be established.

The nurse interested in helping teenagers with weight reduction can play an important role. Many nurses are or have been personally involved with losing weight and know how frustrating this can be. Motivating the adolescent requires ingenuity and patience. A sense of hope must be instilled, and the adolescent must be involved in the treatment plan. Positive parental involvement seems to increase the chances of the teenager's success. Failure is almost certain if the parent is committed to weight reduction and the child is not. Nurses should approach the obese adolescent in a nonthreatening way. They should try to recognize achievements and increase the adolescent's self-esteem. The basic dignity of the individual should always be foremost. Family therapy may be necessary to alleviate tension and promote understanding; nurses can assist in the referral process. They can also be the source of contact for a registered dietitian.

Preventing obesity in children is important. The earlier in life this begins, the better. Identification of the infant or child at risk is necessary while the child is still under parental control and before eating and activity patterns are firmly established. Breastfeeding is desirable for infants, in that sufficient quantities of milk are obtained and there is less chance of overfeeding. Solid foods should be delayed until 6 months of age. Inform mothers that a baby's food requirements diminish greatly as growth slows at about the first year. Discourage overfeeding because fat babies are not necessarily healthy babies. Advise parents that a crying baby does not necessarily mean that the infant is hungry.

Parents should foster activities that promote freedom of movement and exercise during the first few years of life. If there are any questions concerning weight gain, these should be voiced during well-baby conferences.

During the school years, nutritious snacks rather than junk foods should be kept in the home. Television viewing and video games should be restricted to 2 hours per day, and walking and other exercise should be encouraged. Parents need to promote participation in a regular exercise program. Sound nutritional practices are of particular importance during puberty, when there is an increase in fat cells. Teenagers are capable of assuming responsibility for what they eat.

Helping the child's self-esteem through encouragement, praise, and support is essential. The depressed young person may turn to food as an outlet for emotions. Be generous and specific with your praise. Sprinkle your conversation with such comments as "I knew you could do it," "That's quite an improvement," "You made it look easy," "I couldn't have done better myself." This type of positive approach may help the child or young person feel better and decrease the need to overeat.

ANOREXIA NERVOSA
Description

The American Psychiatric Association, in the fourth edition of *Diagnostic and Statistical Manual of Mental Disorders* (*DSM-IV-TR*, 2000), defines anorexia nervosa as an eating disorder characterized by self-imposed starvation, extreme weight loss or failure to gain expected weight for growth (less than 85% of expected weight), and body image disturbance. Affected adolescents have a morbid fear of being or becoming fat. Amenorrhea (defined as the absence of three consecutive menstrual cycles) occurs in postpubertal adolescents.

The disorder occurs primarily in girls and affects about 1% to 5% of American teenage girls and 1% of teenage boys. The adolescent sees herself as being fat, even in the stages of advanced emaciation. The term *anorexia* is misleading, for many patients do not have a lack of appetite. Instead, they experience intense hunger, which they deny or satisfy by eating and purging binges. A combination of factors may cause the disease, including genetic or physiological

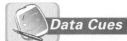
Data Cues

Anorexia Nervosa and Bulimia

DATA	ANOREXIA NERVOSA	BULIMIA
Age at onset	12-16 yr	15-20 yr
Weight	Markedly decreased below normal	Normal or slightly above normal
Body image	Distorted; person sees herself as fat even when emaciated	Realistic, but person feels eating behaviors are out of control
Underlying psychological problems	Perfectionist, unrealistic expectations of self and others, unmet needs for nurturance; desire for autonomy places the adolescent in frequent conflict with restrictive parents; decreased self-esteem	Anxiety, guilt, feelings of worthlessness and inadequacy, impulsiveness, decreased self-esteem, parents with too high expectations

predisposition, sociocultural influences, and impaired psychological development.

Some theorists believe that families of these young people are dysfunctional. They may exhibit such behaviors as overprotectiveness, rigidity, lack of privacy, and inability to resolve conflicts. Affected adolescents appear to be in conflict with their parents about achieving autonomy. In addition, the patient's illness may serve to maintain family balance because the parents focus on the needs of the child and thus avoid other internal conflicts.

Signs and Symptoms

Early signs and symptoms may be vague; often, in retrospect, the condition may seem to have begun with a diet or with some emotional trauma. The onset can often be pinpointed to the young girl's inability to wear some of her clothes or to life changes such as a move, parental divorce, or the death of a relative or close friend (see Data Cues).

Initial weight loss may be gradual or sudden, but as the patient's weight drops, her sense of being overweight rises. Despite lack of intake, the patient initially has a great deal of energy and may exercise strenuously to reduce more rapidly. Later, the adolescent loses the energy to participate even in activities of daily living. Adolescents with anorexia nervosa often have a preoccupation with food or with cooking for others and may exhibit bizarre eating behaviors. On physical examination, some of the following conditions become evident: emaciated appearance, dry skin, amenorrhea, lanugo hair over the back and extremities, cold intolerance, low blood pressure, low pulse, abdominal pain, and constipation. Electrolyte imbalance may be noticeable in the patient who induces vomiting or uses laxatives or diuretics. Elevated calcium levels indicate that osteoporosis is occurring.

Teenagers with anorexia have feelings of helplessness, lack of control, low self-esteem, and depression. Socialization with peers diminishes. Mealtime becomes a family battleground, increasing the conflict and power struggle. Some adolescents feel guilty and may go on an eating binge, which is followed by self-induced vomiting as the fear of gaining weight returns. The perception of body image becomes increasingly disturbed, and there is a lack of self-identity. The young person remains egocentric and unable to resolve normal adolescent tasks. The patient complains of bloating and abdominal pain after small amounts of food are ingested.

Treatment and Nursing Care

The treatment of anorexia is complex and involves several methods. A period of hospitalization may be necessary to correct electrolyte imbalance, establish minimal restoration of nutrients, and stabilize the patient's weight. In addition to fluid and electrolyte imbalance, criteria for hospitalization include severe loss of control or suicidal behavior, weight more than 25% lower than expected, too rapid weight loss, hypothermia, coexisting illness, and failure of outpatient treatment (Kliegman et al., 2006). Therapies include medical stabilization, psychotherapy, behavioral therapy, drug therapy, and family therapy. Nasogastric feedings and total parenteral nutrition are usually used only when other means have failed because they are only a temporary answer to a much larger problem. Such measures do not reflect normal eating patterns. Hospitalization is expensive and sometimes is not covered by insurance for the length of time necessary to effectively stabilize and treat the patient. The ongoing need for inpatient or outpatient therapy, or both, can lead to family financial stress.

The nurse can play an important role in ensuring that the atmosphere is relaxed and nonpunitive while maintaining clear behavioral limits. It is important for nurses to facilitate positive coping behaviors, gradually increasing autonomy and decision making and improved body image. Some hospitals now have units that specialize in eating disorders. Continued follow-up after discharge from the unit is essential.

Nurses working with adolescents in any capacity need to be alert to the symptoms of this disease because lack of recognition is one of the biggest obstacles to treatment. Making young people aware of the seriousness of this condition is an important nursing function. Because there is a higher incidence rate of anorexia nervosa in athletes (especially gymnasts, ballet dancers, and runners), it is important for coaches and parents to recognize early signs and symptoms. Educational materials, referral sources, and counseling are available from the National Association of Anorexia Nervosa and Associated Disorders. Encouragement and support from self-help groups are also valuable.

The prognosis for patients with anorexia nervosa is uncertain. Most patients gain weight in the hospital regardless of the type of therapy. This may not, however, predict future success. Success rate is about 70% (Behrman et al., 2004). Complications include gastritis, cardiac arrhythmia, inflammation of the intestine, kidney problems, and others. Deaths do occur, particularly in untreated persons.

BULIMIA
Description
Bulimia, or binge eating, is now recognized by *DSM-IV-TR* as a separate eating disorder from anorexia nervosa. It is characterized by the following behaviors: (1) regular, multiple episodes of binge eating (large amounts over a short period of time, occurring twice a week for at least 3 months) and feeling that the eating is out of control, (2) purging, or the use of methods to prevent weight gain from the binge eating (such as self-induced vomiting, laxatives, ipecac, diuretics, enemas), and (3) expressed dissatisfaction with body size or weight. It occurs more commonly in older adolescents and young women but can also be observed in males. Persons with bulimia binge periodically, usually on easily accessible high-calorie food items. These episodes are generally carried out in private. They may be followed by self-induced vomiting or the use of cathartics. Persistent vomiting can cause erosion of the enamel of the teeth, tooth decay, chronic esophagitis, chronic sore throat, inflammation, and parotitis. The person is aware that eating is out of control. Binging periods are preceded by anxiety and followed by feelings of dejection, guilt, and self-deprecation. (See previous Data Cues for a comparison summary of anorexia and bulimia.)

The treatment for bulimia is similar to that for anorexia but involves pharmacological management as well. Because depression and anxiety are underlying factors, the physician may try antidepressant or anti-anxiety agents. In addition to nursing management of physical consequences, the goals of nursing care are directed toward reducing anxiety by identifying alternative methods for dealing with it, increasing effective coping mechanisms, and facilitating appropriate family interaction.

MUSCULOSKELETAL SYSTEM

SCOLIOSIS
Description
Scoliosis refers to an S-shaped curvature of the spine. It is the most common nontraumatic skeletal condition in children. Not all scoliotic curves are progressive, and some may require only periodic evaluation. Untreated progressive scoliosis can lead to back pain, fatigue, disability, and heart and respiratory complications. Skeletal deterioration does not stop with maturity and may be aggravated by pregnancy.

Scoliosis affects children of both genders at any age, but it is most commonly seen in adolescents. Curvatures in adolescent girls seem to progress faster and require treatment more frequently than those in boys (Kliegman et al., 2006).

Scoliosis can be caused by several factors. It can be congenital, resulting from abnormal fetal vertebral development. Some neurological conditions that affect muscular strength, such as spina bifida, cerebral palsy, and muscular dystrophy, can cause scoliosis. Spinal tumors can also cause the condition.

The most common occurrence of scoliosis is idiopathic. The exact cause is unknown, but the incidence can affect children of both genders at any age. Most commonly affected is the adolescent. In many cases, scoliosis affects multiple family members, although the exact inheritance pattern has not been determined.

Signs and Symptoms
Often the first sign of scoliosis is an uneven hemline and difficulty fitting clothes. When viewed from the front, adolescents with scoliosis can have uneven shoulder levels, unequal arm-to-body spaces, or a protruding hip. One arm may appear longer than the other when the person bends forward. Sometimes the patient complains of a "crooked back." When viewed from the back, bent at the waist, the patient might have a protruding scapula, with one side of the back appearing higher than the other (Figure 16-2). A definitive diagnosis can be made from spinal radiographs, which show the severity and location of the curve.

Treatment and Nursing Care
Treatment is aimed at correcting the curvature and preventing further scoliosis. The course of treatment is determined by the child's age, the skeletal maturity, the degree and location of the curvature, and any underlying disease processes. Curves up to 20 degrees do not require treatment but are carefully followed, particularly if the adolescent is prepubertal. Follow-up examinations every 4 to 6 months can detect any progression of the curve.

Progressive curves between 20 and 40 degrees most often require bracing until the child's skeletal system is mature (Figure 16-3). The Milwaukee brace, a plastic and metal brace with a neck ring, was the type most

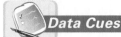

Data Cues

Scoliosis

CLASSIFICATION	SYMPTOMS	CAUSES
Functional (nonstructural)	Normal spine with temporary curvature, flexible	Underlying condition, such as difference in leg length, spasms, poor posture
Structural	Abnormal spinal structures, fixed	Birth defects, congenital defects, neuromuscular diseases, infections, tumors, metabolic diseases, connective tissue diseases
Idiopathic	Painless curve, neurologically normal	No known cause

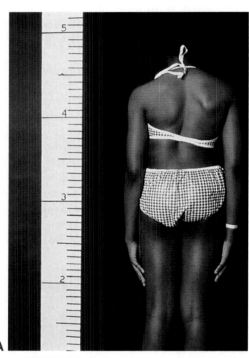

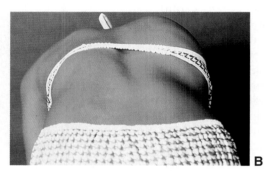

FIGURE **16-2** Idiopathic scoliosis. **A,** Scapular asymmetry is easily seen. Back bra strap can also assist in detecting asymmetry. **B,** Forward bending reveals a mild rib hump deformity.

commonly used for years; however, it is now used only rarely for scoliosis. Braces more commonly used are the Boston brace, which uses plastic shells, and the thoracolumbosacral orthosis (TLSO), a custom-molded jacket. For lower back curves, a plastic molded brace is used. Such a brace contributes to better compliance with the treatment program because it can be worn under clothing and is barely distinguishable (Nursing Care Plan 16-1). In addition to bracing, the child might also be involved in an active exercise program.

The child is usually required to wear the brace for 23 hours a day, although some experts believe the same effect can be obtained from wearing the brace for fewer hours. It is worn over a T-shirt. Because appearance is such a concern for adolescents, a brace is used only for curves whose apex is higher than the eighth thoracic vertebra.

Curvatures greater than 45 degrees most likely require surgical intervention in the form of a spinal fusion, with stabilization through the use of instrumentation (rods, wires, or both). There are many instrumentation systems available, such as Harrington rods, Dwyer instruments, Cotrel-Dubousset procedure (rods and wires), Zielke, and TSRH (Texas Scottish Rite Hospital). Depending on the procedure chosen, the surgical approach can be posterior or anterior. The anterior approach requires insertion of a chest tube. Some procedures are followed by bracing for several months.

Preoperative Care. The usual preoperative preparation of the patient is necessary for spinal fusion. It is important that the nurse evaluate and document the patient's neuromuscular status at this time so that it may be used as a basis for comparison after the procedure. All four extremities are observed for

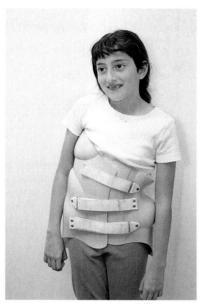

FIGURE **16-3** A brace can be custom designed to meet the child's specific needs.

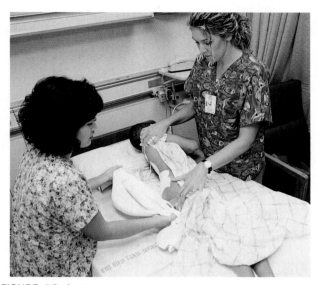

FIGURE **16-4** The log-rolling technique is used after back surgery to prevent a child from flexing the back while being turned from side to side in bed.

color, temperature, capillary filling, edema, sensation, and motion. The nurse explains to the patient that breathing exercises and frequent changes of position are necessary to prevent heart and lung complications. If postoperative log-rolling is anticipated, it can be practiced before surgery, or when possible, the patient may watch the procedure being done with another patient.

Postoperative Care. After surgery, adolescents can spend up to several days in the intensive care unit. When they return to the unit, they usually have a fairly extensive dressing, intravenous fluids, round-the-clock pain medications (often patient-controlled anesthesia), nasogastric tube, urinary catheter, wound drains, and a chest tube (if the anterior approach is used). The nurse can log-roll most patients to change their position in bed (Figure 16-4). Some patients can get out of bed with or without a brace after only a few days. The nurse encourages active and passive range-of-motion exercises for as long as the patient remains in bed. A physical therapist assists with ambulation when permitted.

In addition to routine postoperative management, the nurse carefully assesses the adolescent's vital signs and neurological, cardiovascular, and respiratory status frequently. Any changes in motion or sensation of the extremities must be reported immediately. Fever and abnormal wound drainage can indicate infection and should also be reported immediately because the danger of bone infection is great.

Adolescents often are reluctant to assume self-care after spinal surgery. In addition to being in pain, they are concerned about their safety. They express reluctance to move because of fear they will dislodge or break the fusion. Reassure patients that careful

movement does not harm the surgical site. The sooner adolescents participate in self-care, the faster they progress. Encourage the adolescent to shower as soon as is permitted. Some may need to use a shower chair initially.

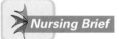
Nursing Brief

Insertion of a Harrington rod or other metal device delays a patient at an airport security scanner because the metal activates the alarm. A note can be obtained from the physician, which can be used as a clearance for air travel.

Begin home care instructions early in treatment. Demonstrate application of the brace to the parent and patient and be sure the parent can properly apply the brace before the adolescent is discharged. Give written instructions for any activity restrictions or necessary follow-up care.

Screening. An important nursing action for the management of scoliosis in the community is screening. This is done in school, preferably at the beginning of fourth grade. It should also be a part of every yearly physical given to prepubescent youngsters. Camp nurses also need to be aware of symptoms. Early recognition is of utmost importance in detecting mild cases amenable to nonsurgical treatment.

Screening in the school system is usually done by the school nurse or trained physical education teacher. Students are prepared for screening by the nurse or teacher explaining the purpose of the procedure and reassuring students that it merely entails observation of the back while standing and while bending forward. Tell the students that the screening is simple, quick,

NURSING CARE PLAN 16-1

The Adolescent with Scoliosis in a Brace

NURSING DIAGNOSIS *Risk for impaired skin integrity related to uneven pressure from the brace*

Goals/Outcome Criteria	Nursing Interventions	Rationales
The skin remains smooth without areas of redness or irritation or signs of skin breakdown	Advise the patient to wear a soft cotton T-shirt under the brace; be sure that the shirt is free from wrinkles.	Placing a thin layer of fabric between the brace and the skin reduces friction rubbing.
	Inspect areas under the brace daily after the adolescent showers.	Routine inspection allows for rapid identification of problem areas.
	Apply alcohol to areas of potential friction before reapplying the brace.	Alcohol helps keep the skin dry.
	Report persistent reddened areas to the brace fitter.	Brace modification can reduce friction areas.

NURSING DIAGNOSIS *Risk for injury related to altered body weight and function from bracing*

Goals/Outcome Criteria	Nursing Interventions	Rationales
The adolescent remains free from injury	Demonstrate and have the adolescent demonstrate alternative body movements used to accomplish activities of daily living: • Bending from the knees to pick something up • How to get out of bed by rolling to a side-lying position before pushing upright • Putting clothing on lower part of the body while sitting on the edge of a bed or chair	Demonstration helps the adolescent visualize changes that need to be made.
The adolescent adapts appropriately to altered body movements caused by the brace	Encourage the parent to be aware of and remove any potential hazards in the environment (e.g., slippery rugs, toys, other objects on the floor).	Alerting the parent to environmental hazards prevents injury.
	Advise the adolescent to be aware of hazards at school; make special arrangements for walking in corridors between classes if necessary.	Because schools are crowded, the injury potential is high and special arrangements may be necessary.
	Advise the adolescent to try activities slowly at first.	Helps patient adjust to altered body weight before resuming activity.

NURSING DIAGNOSIS *Disturbed body image related to the appearance of the brace*

Goals/Outcome Criteria	Nursing Interventions	Rationales
The adolescent adapts appropriately to any changes in appearance or function resulting from the brace, as evidenced by: • Ability to verbally express concerns • Participation in activities of interest • Continued contact with peers	Encourage the adolescent to discuss feelings about the appearance or limitations of the brace.	Facilitating expression of feelings helps the nurse identify and assist with concerns.
	Help the patient and family choose loose, stylish, colorful clothing to minimize the appearance of the brace and boost the adolescent's confidence.	Attractive clothing helps boost an adolescent's self-image and decreases feelings of being different from peers.
	Describe any activity restrictions (e.g., competitive sports) and help the adolescent explore alternate activities of interest (e.g., walking, slow jogging, moderate dancing); encourage the adolescent to be physically active.	Helps the adolescent identify areas of interest and activities that maintain physical fitness and promote socialization with peers.

Nursing Care Plan 16-1—cont'd

The Adolescent with Scoliosis in a Brace—cont'd

NURSING DIAGNOSIS *Ineffective therapeutic regimen management related to length of treatment time*

Goals/Outcome Criteria	Nursing Interventions	Rationales
The adolescent complies fully with the treatment, as evidenced by: • Wearing the brace the required amount of time • Stating the long-term benefits of the treatment	Reinforce the long-term positive outcome from the bracing. Be sure that the brace fits well and that the adolescent is comfortable; refer to the brace fitter if adjustments are needed. Allow the adolescent to express anger and frustration if needed.	Continued reinforcement helps validate the rationale for treatment and encourages compliance. Comfort increases compliance. Allowing expression of feelings prevents them from building up.

? CRITICAL THINKING QUESTION

■ An 11-year-old girl is admitted to the ICU after surgery for correction of scoliosis. She has an IV, a nasogastric tube to low suction, HemoVac, and a Foley catheter. She is NPO and on strict intake and output. She is repositioned by log-rolling every 2 hours. Her vital signs are as follows: temperature, 99.8° F; pulse, 96 beats per minute; respiration, 32 breaths per minute; and blood pressure, 135/78 mm Hg. She is moaning. What are the nurse's initial actions? What actions should be done first, and what needs continual evaluation?

---

and painless. Suggest that students wear clothing that is easy to remove, such as a pullover top, or that they wear a bathing suit. Boys disrobe to the waist, girls generally to the bathing suit top. No slip or undershirt should be worn. The procedure consists of examining the spine from the front, side, and back while the student stands erect and then observing the back as the student bends forward.

The examiner looks initially for general body alignment and asymmetry (one side of the body looking different from the other; Figure 16-5). Fourth grade boys are especially lordotic; therefore developmental patterns at various ages must be considered. Referrals are made as indicated. Because of familial tendencies in this condition, brothers and sisters of children with scoliosis should be examined. Community understanding of scoliosis benefits those who must obtain further treatment.

SPORTS INJURIES
Description

A high percentage of adolescents of both genders participate routinely in athletic activities. In the past 10 years, there has been an increase in the number of children participating in team and solo sports. Even children with such chronic conditions as asthma, diabetes mellitus, and seizures readily participate in sports. Athletic participation teaches valuable lessons about cooperation, achieving goals, persistence, and confidence building. Many states and school facilities require a preparticipation physical before the participation in the sport. The American Academy of Pediatrics (AAP) has devised a sport classification system with the following divisions: contact or collision sports, limited contact sports, and noncontact sports. Students should be evaluated for suitability for a particular sport. For example, a student with seizures should not participate in contact sports. The AAP provides an extensive list matching medical conditions with acceptable sports participation (American Academy of Pediatrics, 2001).

Many sports, however, have the potential for causing both minor injuries, such as strains and soft tissue injury, and catastrophic permanently disabling injuries. The injury potential of an individual sport depends on several factors, among them the amount and type of protective equipment required, rule enforcement and modification to prevent injury, correct assignment of athletes to teams based on developmental level and maturity, and adequate training of the coaching staff. Parents should be aware of the potential injuries. Overuse syndrome has increased in the pediatric population as the demand for excelling in sports is expected.

Signs and Symptoms

The symptoms of the most common sports injuries are presented in the Data Cues. In addition to those injuries described, athletes can sustain fractures and dislocations. Altered tissue blood flow, electrolyte deficiencies, or minor tissue injury can cause muscle cramps, which are experienced at one time or another by all athletes. Nurses need to be aware that some injuries can damage a skeletally immature child's growth plate, interfering with growth potential. Other injuries, such as anterior cruciate ligament tears, can be particularly

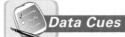

Frequently Seen Sports Injuries

INJURY	DESCRIPTION
Strain	Caused by stretch injury to soft tissue structures (muscle, tendon), often associated with overuse. Pain on movement, swelling (extent depends on severity of the injury).
Sprain	Ligament tear, most frequently seen in ankle, knee, shoulder, or elbow. Pain, "popping" feeling at time of injury, extensive swelling, bruising, joint instability, movement limitation.
Stress fracture	Fracture occurring at a bony insertion site, usually caused by overuse or from physical exercise without adequate training or preparation. Commonly seen in the lower extremities, depending on the sport involved (running, ballet, gymnastics, and so forth). Intermittent pain or limp that worsens with activity; local tenderness or swelling. Fracture is shown with radiography or more sensitive imaging studies.
Shin splints	Pain and discomfort in anterior lower leg from repeatedly running on a hard surface such as concrete.
"Stinger" or "burner"	Described as an "electric jolt" resulting from contact of an athlete's head with another athlete's body. Usually mild and disappears suddenly.
Concussion	Altered mental status caused by a blow to the head. Possible loss of consciousness, headache, vomiting.

severe, resulting in several months' loss of participation time and requiring extensive rehabilitation.

Sports injuries are diagnosed using radiography or other bone-imaging procedures. **Arthroscopy,** a surgical procedure designed to assess joint damage, is used to diagnose knee and shoulder injuries. Some tissue repair can be done with arthroscopy.

Treatment and Nursing Care

First aid treatment for most extremity injuries includes **RICE** (**r**est, **i**ce, **c**ompression, and **e**levation) during the first 72 hours (Figure 16-6). Immobilizing and elevating the injured limb at the scene prevents further injury until the adolescent can be evaluated. Crutches may be necessary for several days to keep the injured area rested. Compression of the injury with an elastic bandage helps minimize tissue bleeding and swelling.

For soft tissue injuries, such as strains and sprains, apply ice for 20 minutes three to four times a day for the first 48 hours. If using ice in a pack, protect the skin with a thin cloth before applying the pack.

Usually, the physician prescribes a rehabilitative physical therapy program for athletes with severe tissue injury. Muscle-strengthening exercises and weight work are usually necessary to stabilize the injured area before an athlete can return to the sport. Some severe injuries may require casting or surgical intervention. In these instances, nursing care is similar to that for any child undergoing surgery or casting.

Prevention

Several factors help prevent sports injuries. Some of these are an adequate warm-up and cool-down period; year-round conditioning; careful selection of activity according to physical maturity, size, and skill necessary; proper supervision by adults; safe, well-fitting equipment; and avoidance of participation when

in pain. Proper diet and fluids are also necessary. The nurse plays an important role in educating and directing parents to sources of accurate information to ensure that the physical, emotional, and maturational levels of the adolescent are appropriate for the activity. Parents are encouraged to inquire about the capabilities of personnel and the availability of emergency services before the beginning of the competition.

An often overlooked factor that contributes to sports injuries is emotional pressure. Many parents and coaches place undue pressure on the athlete to be the best or to win at all costs. Parents and coaches often argue with referees and umpires; they criticize their athletes if mistakes are made or if times are not good enough. Many athletes leave their sport because of intolerable pressure to succeed. This can cause decreased self-esteem at a time when positive self-esteem is developmentally important. Nurses need to reinforce to parents the value that participating on a team has for an adolescent and the dangers involved with too much pressure.

Authorities disagree about what constitutes a good sports physical examination; however, they are unanimous about the need for regular and pre-participation medical examinations. Most athletes are required to have a yearly sports physical for participation. Such examinations are updated with a questionnaire asking about any injury acquired between sports during a given year. The family history and an orthopedic screening are important in identifying risk factors. The problem with this approach is that adolescents who have yearly sports physicals often do not have regular comprehensive examinations. Because the physicals are specific for sports participation, other areas of health promotion—such as assessment of risk behaviors, diet, other illnesses that affect sports participation, and emotional health—are neglected. Recommendations

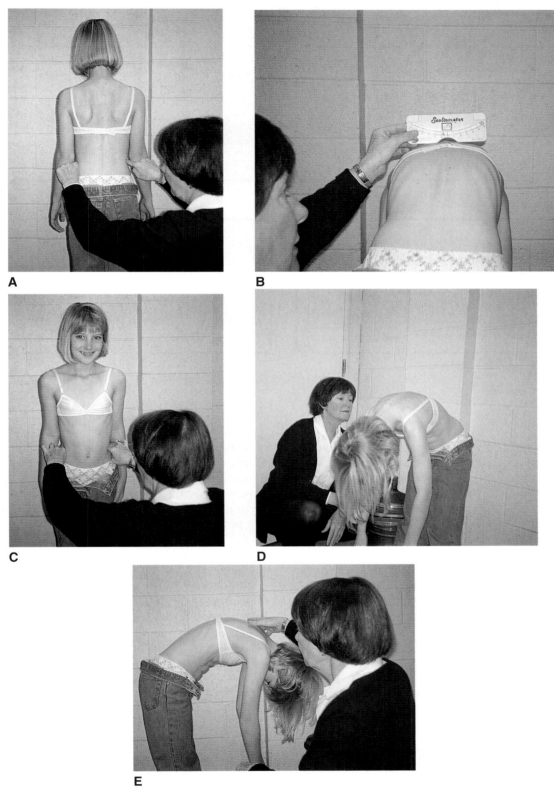

FIGURE **16-5**   Scoliosis screening is performed by the school nurse. **A,** The examiner begins by viewing the child from the back, looking for symmetry of the shoulders, scapulae, and waist creases. **B,** Next, the child is asked to place her hands together and bend forward. The examiner uses a scoliometer to obtain a rough estimate of the degree of spinal curvature. **C,** The examiner looks from the front for anterior chest deformity or asymmetry. **D,** When the child bends forward toward the examiner, particular curves may become more visible. **E,** Observing the child from the side allows the examiner to assess for kyphosis or lordosis.

RICE =

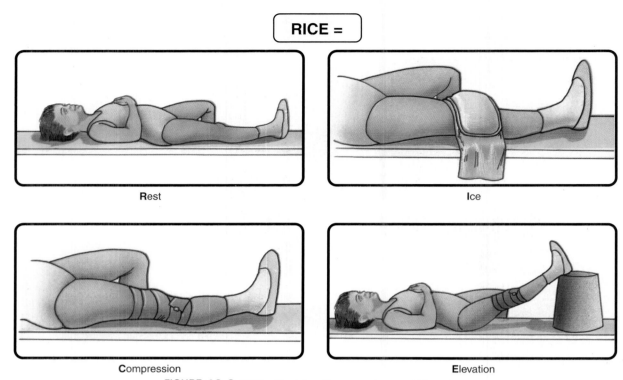

Rest

Ice

Compression

Elevation

FIGURE **16-6** RICE = Rest, Ice, Compression, and Elevation.

are that either sport physicals be expanded to include more thorough assessments of adolescents or that sports-specific assessments become a routine part of comprehensive physical examinations.

Considerations for Female Athletes

Irregular menses and **amenorrhea** (absence of menses) are relatively common with heavy exercise. This may be the result of a decrease in the percentage of body fat. Weight loss, thinness, and physical and emotional stress may also precipitate such irregularities. It is suggested that girls who stop menstruating for 2 months or more and those who menstruate irregularly be examined. Amenorrhea that is exercise induced can be confused with pregnancy by the teenager. Although breast injuries are not common, sports bras in several styles are available that provide protection and support.

GENITOURINARY SYSTEM

DYSMENORRHEA (PRIMARY)
Description

Primary dysmenorrhea, or painful menstruation, denotes pain associated with the menstrual cycle in the absence of organic pelvic disease. It is distinguished from **secondary dysmenorrhea,** in which the patient may have an underlying condition such as endometriosis, pelvic inflammatory disease, ovarian cysts, adhesions,

or congenital abnormalities. Mittelschmerz refers to midcycle pain during ovulation. For many years, dysmenorrhea was thought to be psychological. It is now recognized that painful menses result from myometrial stimulation by prostaglandins E_2 and F_{2a}, produced in the endometrium (Kliegman et al., 2006). The concentration of these prostaglandins is higher in women with dysmenorrhea than in control subjects.

About two thirds of postpubescent teenagers in the United States have some degree of dysmenorrhea. Approximately 10% are incapacitated from 1 to 3 days per month. Dysmenorrhea is the greatest single cause of lost school and work days in women. Its onset is usually before age 20 years.

Signs and Symptoms

Symptoms include cramping, abdominal discomfort, and leg aches, all of which begin at the onset of menses. Systemic symptoms such as nausea, vomiting, dizziness, diarrhea, backache, and headache can occur. Dysmenorrhea is graded from mild to severe. Primary dysmenorrhea occurs in the absence of organic disease. Secondary dysmenorrhea occurs as a result of organic disease.

Premenstrual syndrome (PMS) is more common in adults than in teenagers. Although the symptoms may overlap with those of dysmenorrhea, weight gain, breast tenderness, irritability, and insomnia before menstruation are also seen. The symptoms of

PMS resolve with the onset of menses. PMS does not generally occur before ovulatory cycles begin.

Treatment and Nursing Care

Painful menses should be evaluated to rule out any structural problem such as pelvic inflammatory disease, tumors, or endometriosis. Primary dysmenorrhea should be treated with NSAIDs which are prostaglandin inhibitors and assist in decreasing myometrial contractions. Ibuprofen or naproxen should be taken every 4 hours and usually requires 2 to 3 days of medications. These drugs should not be taken on an empty stomach and can cause fluid retention. Applying a warm heating pad to the lower abdomen may also decrease discomfort. When these measures fail, a thorough history and pelvic examination by a gynecologist should be performed to rule out organic disorders. Patients with dysmenorrhea who are also in need of contraception may be candidates for combination (estrogen-progesterone) oral contraceptives.

SEXUALLY TRANSMITTED DISEASES
Description

Sexually transmitted disease (STD) is the general name given to infections that are spread through direct sexual activity. This replaces the term *venereal disease*, which was used in the past. The two most common types of STDs are chlamydial infection and gonorrhea; however, more than 20 other diseases are now considered to be prevalent. Some of these are syphilis, genital warts, herpes progenitalis, cytomegalovirus infection, hepatitis B, and AIDS (acquired immunodeficiency syndrome). Other conditions, such as scabies and pediculosis pubis, can also be transmitted sexually. The effects of some untreated STDs can be debilitating and irreversible. More than one STD can be contracted at the same time. Many can be transmitted by a pregnant woman to her unborn child, causing serious problems in the fetus, such as blindness, birth defects, and death. The incidence of AIDS continues to increase, and public awareness of spread through sexual contact is a priority in prevention. Because persons with HIV infection may remain asymptomatic for many years, they may unknowingly spread the disease to others.

It was thought that with the advent of penicillin, STDs would be eradicated, but there has been a widespread resurgence. The reasons for this resurgence are many and include intertwining cultural, economic, social, and moral factors. Specific reasons include changing values and lifestyles in society; an increase in sexual contact, particularly in the middle and upper classes; an increase in the mobility of society and surges in the population; the reluctance of many persons to seek medical help (particularly adolescents); inadequate education about the diseases; increasing intravenous drug use; organism resistance to antibiotics; widespread apathy among professionals; social equality of the genders; and a change in

common methods of contraception. The occurrence of an STD in a prepubertal child should always prompt investigation into the possibility of sexual abuse.

The incidence of STDs among teenagers is high. Adolescent girls have some of the highest rates of STDs (Burstein & Murray, 2003). The reasons are physical and psychosocial. Today's adolescents are maturing earlier than previous generations, marrying later, engaging in sexual intercourse at younger ages, and having multiple sexual partners. Despite intense efforts to provide comprehensive sex education, adolescents continue to engage in risky behaviors. Alcohol and drug use contribute in large part to an increase in sexual activity among today's youth. Media images in popular music videos, commercials, and teen magazines are becoming an important source of inaccurate sex information for adolescents. Although misinformation contributes to the problem, adolescents are surprisingly well-informed about how to avoid risky behaviors. However, a discrepancy appears between what they know and what they actually do. Although the causes for this discrepancy are not fully understood, contributing factors include lack of appropriate adult role modeling; reacting in an emotional rather than intellectual manner in pressure situations (the heart ruling the head); lack of concrete practice with prevention techniques (putting on a condom, using a diaphragm or foam, and so forth); and low self-esteem.

Signs and Symptoms

Table 16-2 describes the clinical manifestations of the major STDs in the United States. Some additional information follows.

Chlamydia Infection. *Chlamydia trachomatis* infection has become the most common STD in the United States. The condition can persist for months or years and remain undiagnosed because it is often asymptomatic. The incubation period is approximately 1 week.

Should an infected woman give birth vaginally, the infant is at risk for development of neonatal conjunctivitis and pneumonia. Infants should be treated with oral erythromycin.

A positive culture for *Chlamydia trachomatis* from conjunctival, nasopharyngeal, vaginal, or rectal areas is diagnostic. Nonculture tests, such as immunoassays and fluorescent antibody tests, are available but should not be used if sexual abuse is suspected because of false-positive results.

Gonorrhea. The infectious agent that causes this highly communicable disease is *Neisseria gonorrhoeae*, an anaerobic bacterium that penetrates the mucous membrane surfaces lining the genital tract, rectum, and mouth. The bacteria thrive in warm, moist areas of the body and can also survive in the tissues around the eyes of the newborn infant and in the immature vulvar tissues of prepubescent girls. They quickly die outside the human body. The common names for this disease include GC, clap, a dose, strain, or the drip.

Text continued on p. 360.

Table 16-2 | *Sexually Transmitted Disease Summary*

DISEASE	CLINICAL PRESENTATION	THERAPY	COMPLICATIONS AND SEQUELAE	TEACHING
Chlamydia trachomatis	Asymptomatic infection to acute inflammatory symptoms. Males have urethritis and epididymitis. Females have urethritis, vaginitis, and cervicitis. Can be passed from mother to infant during delivery. Infants can have conjunctivitis and pneumonia develop.	Doxycycline, 200 mg twice daily (bid) for 7 days **or** Azithromycin, 1 g in a single oral dose **or** Ofloxacin, 600 mg in a single oral dose **or** Levofloxacin, 500 mg in a single oral dose **or** Erythromycin, 2 g/day is used for children under 6 mo and pregnant women.	In females, inflammation can progress to chronic pelvic inflammatory disease, which can cause infertility or ectopic pregnancy. Lymphogranuloma venereum (LVG) with genital lesions and regional lymphadenitis is a chronic consequence. Pneumonia in infected infants can be severe.	Identification and treatment during pregnancy can prevent infection in the neonate. Routine screening for *Chlamydia* during yearly pelvic examinations in sexually active adolescents aids in identification and treatment. Evaluate sexual contacts and treat if the last sexual contact was within 30 days of the first appearance of symptoms or within 60 days of diagnosis in an asymptomatic patient.
Gonorrhea	Asymptomatic. Men usually have dysuria, frequency, and purulent urethral discharge. Women may have abnormal vaginal discharge, abnormal menses, dysuria, or abdominal pain. Anorectal and pharyngeal infections may be symptomatic or asymptomatic.	Ceftriaxone, 125 mg intramuscularly (IM) once **or** Spectinomycin, 40 mg/kg IM once **plus** Azithromycin, 20 mg/kg orally once **or** Erythromycin, 50 mg/kg orally for 14 days.	Women with untreated gonorrhea may have pelvic inflammatory disease develop and are at risk for its sequelae. Men are at risk for urethral stricture, epididymitis, and infertility. Newborns born to women with untreated infection are at risk for scalp abscess at the site of fetal monitors, ophthalmia neonatorum, rhinitis, disseminated infection, or anorectal infections. Untreated persons are at risk for disseminated gonococcal infection (e.g., septicemia, arthritis, dermatitis, disseminated gonococcal infection [DG], meningitis, and endocarditis).	Understand how to take any prescribed oral medications. Return for evaluation if symptoms persist or recur after treatment. Refer sexual partner(s) for examination and treatment. Avoid sex until patient and partner(s) are cured. Use condoms to prevent future infections.

Gonorrhea distinguished by vulvar inflammation, edema, and purulent vaginal discharge.

Table 16-2 | *Sexually Transmitted Disease Summary—cont'd*

DISEASE	CLINICAL PRESENTATION	THERAPY	COMPLICATIONS AND SEQUELAE	TEACHING
Genital warts (human papillomavirus [HPV])	Present as single or multiple soft, fleshy, papillary or flat, painless growths around the anus, vulvovaginal area, penis, urethra, or perineum. Subclinical infection, particularly of the cervix, may occur and is best recognized with culdoscopy with application of 3% to 5% acetic acid (vinegar), which turns lesions white.	The goal of treatment is removal of warts and the amelioration of signs and symptoms, not the eradication of HPV. Treatment with podophyllin or trichloroacetic acid is helpful for adolescents, but safety is a concern in children. Other approaches include electrocautery, laser surgery, or surgical removal. *Note:* For women with cervical warts, dysplasia must be excluded before treatment is begun. Management should therefore be carried out in consultation with an expert.	Most anogenital warts are thought to be caused by HPV type 6 or 11. Other types (principally 16, 18, and 31) have been associated with genital dysplasia and carcinoma. The presence of genital warts in children suggests sexual abuse and requires follow-up. All women with anogenital warts should have an annual Pap smear, and atypical, pigmented, or persistent warts should be biopsied. Lesions may enlarge and produce tissue destruction. Giant condylomata may simulate carcinoma yet be histologically benign. In pregnancy, warts enlarge and are extremely vascular. Rarely, they may obstruct the birth canal, necessitating cesarean section. HPV can cause laryngeal papillomatosis in infants.	Return for weekly or biweekly treatment and follow-up until lesions have resolved. Women should have annual Pap smears. Partners should be examined for warts. Abstain from sex or use condoms during therapy. Using condoms may help prevent future infections.

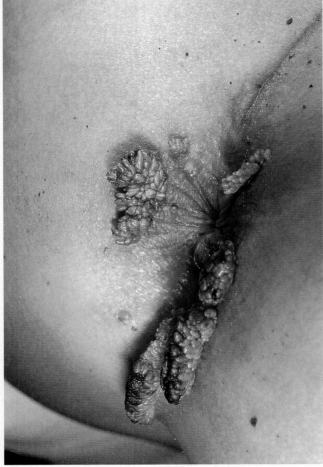

Genital warts in a 3-year-old.

Continued

Table 16-2 | *Sexually Transmitted Disease Summary—cont'd*

DISEASE	CLINICAL PRESENTATION	THERAPY	COMPLICATIONS AND SEQUELAE	TEACHING
Herpes genitalis	Single or multiple vesicles on the genitalia. Vesicles spontaneously rupture to form shallow ulcers that may be very painful. Because the vesicular phase may be missed, especially in women, genital ulcers may be the initial presentation. Lesions resolve spontaneously without scarring. The first occurrence is termed *initial infection* or *first clinical episode* (mean duration, 14-21 days). Subsequent, usually milder, occurrences are termed *recurrent infections* (mean duration of lesions, 8-12 days). The interval between clinical episodes is termed *latency.* Viral shedding may occur intermittently during latency.	No known cure exists. Systemic acyclovir treatment of acute disease may reduce symptoms and signs of herpes episodes and may accelerate healing but does not eradicate the infection nor affect subsequent recurrences. *First clinical episode (genital):* Acyclovir, 400 mg orally 3 times daily for 7-10 days or until clinical resolution occurs. *First clinical episode (Herpes proctitis):* Acyclovir, 400 mg orally 5 times daily for 10 days or until clinical resolution occurs. *Recurrent episodes:* Acyclovir, 400 mg orally 3 times daily for 5 days. *Suppression of recurrent genital herpes infection:* Continuous treatment reduces the frequency or severity of active disease in at least 70%-80% of patients with frequent (at least 6 per yr) recurrences. Acyclovir, 400 mg orally bid daily.	Aseptic meningitis may occur during the first clinical episode. Initial acquisition of HSV infection during pregnancy increases the likelihood of maternal-to-infant transmission; women with recurrent infection infrequently transmit the virus to the neonate during vaginal delivery. Neonatal herpes ranges in severity from clinically inapparent infection to local infections of the eyes, skin, or mucous membranes to severe disseminated infection that may involve the central nervous system.	Keep involved area clean and dry. Because both initial and recurrent lesions shed virus, patients should abstain from sex while symptomatic. An undetermined but presumably small risk for transmission also exists during asymptomatic intervals. Condoms may offer some protection. The risk for fetal infection should be explained to all patients. Nonpregnant women should be reassured that genital herpes does not affect their ability to have children and that, in the great majority of cases, delivery can be performed vaginally. Pregnant women should make their clinicians/obstetricians aware of any history of herpes. Genital herpes (and other diseases causing genital ulcers) has been associated with increased risk for acquiring HIV infection. Latex condoms can reduce risks.

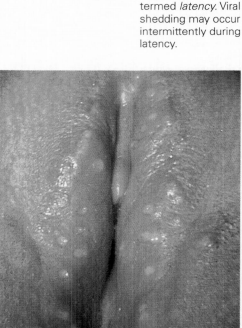

Herpes simplex with thick-walled vesicles and perineal pain.

Table 16-2 | *Sexually Transmitted Disease Summary—cont'd*

DISEASE	CLINICAL PRESENTATION	THERAPY	COMPLICATIONS AND SEQUELAE	TEACHING
Syphilis	*Primary:* The classic chancre is painless, indurated, and located at the site of exposure. *Secondary:* A highly variable skin rash, mucous patches, condylomata lata, lymphadenopathy, or other signs. *Latent:* Patients are without clinical signs, although they may intermittently have signs of secondary stage. *Neurosyphilis:* Neurosyphilis may be asymptomatic. If symptomatic, a variety of neurological symptoms and signs occur, including lightning pains, ataxia, bladder disturbances, confusion, and obtundation.	Primary, secondary, or early syphilis of less than 1 yr duration: Benzathine penicillin G, 2.4 million units IM, in 1 dose; 2-week course of oral tetracycline or doxycycline for patients with penicillin allergy. Syphilis of indeterminate length or of more than 1 yr duration: Benzathine penicillin G, 7.2 million units total, administered as 2.4 million units IM given 1 wk apart for 3 consecutive weeks. Neurosyphilis (inpatient therapy recommended): Aqueous crystalline penicillin G, 18-24 million units per day, administered as 3-4 million units every 4 hr intravenously (IV), for 10-14 days. May be followed by benzathine penicillin G, 2.4 million units IM weekly for 3 wk.	Both late syphilis and congenital syphilis are preventable complications on prompt diagnosis and treatment of early syphilis. Sequelae of late syphilis include neurosyphilis (although neurosyphilis may occur at any stage), cardiovascular syphilis (thoracic aortic aneurysm, aortic valve disease), and localized gumma formation. Congenital syphilis affects multiple organ systems. In addition to stillbirth and intrauterine growth retardation, sequelae of congenital syphilis may include mucocutaneous, skeletal, hematological, central nervous system, and ocular involvement.	Return for follow-up blood studies as indicated (usually 6 and 12 mo after therapy). Follow-up may be of longer duration or at more frequent intervals. Understand the importance of returning for follow-up treatment or taking oral medications correctly, if prescribed for evaluation and treatment. Avoid sexual activity until patient and partner(s) are cured. Use condoms to prevent future infections. Understand the risks associated with syphilis during pregnancy. Pregnant women should be screened early in pregnancy. Syphilis (and other diseases causing genital ulcers) has been associated with an increased risk for acquiring HIV infection. HIV-infected patients treated for syphilis should be followed clinically and serologically at 1, 2, 3, 6, 9, and 12 mo after treatment.

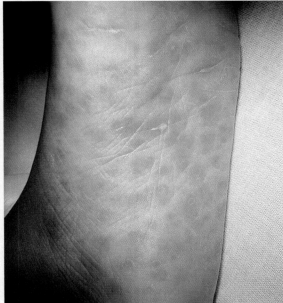

Skin rash of a child with secondary syphilis. Appears on palms of the hands and soles of the feet.

Continued

Table 16-2	*Sexually Transmitted Disease Summary—cont'd*			
DISEASE	**CLINICAL PRESENTATION**	**THERAPY**	**COMPLICATIONS AND SEQUELAE**	**TEACHING**
Hepatitis B	Clinical symptoms and signs are indistinguishable from other forms of hepatitis and may include various combinations of anorexia, malaise, nausea, vomiting, abdominal pain, dark urine, and jaundice. Skin rashes, arthralgias, and arthritis may also occur. Only 33% to 50% of acute infections are symptomatic. Acute infections may resolve, resulting in permanent immunity. In approximately 90% of infants who acquire the infection perinatally and 5% to 10% of acute cases in the older child, infection is persistent, resulting in a chronic carrier state, which can be asymptomatic.	No specific therapy is available for acute hepatitis B or for the chronic carrier state. Universal hepatitis B vaccine administration is recommended for all infants and for unimmunized children before they reach adolescence. Hepatitis B vaccine is also recommended for persons at risk for acquiring hepatitis B virus (HBV) infection. HIV coinfection reduces the humoral response to the hepatitis B vaccine. Infants born to infected (HBsAg-positive) mothers should receive both hepatitis B immune globulin (HBIG) at birth and hepatitis B vaccine at birth, at 1 mo, and at 6 mo. Sexual partners of persons with acute hepatitis B should receive the hepatitis B vaccine and should receive HBIG if seen within 14 days of the last exposure. Sexual partners of persons who are found to be chronic carriers of HBV should receive the hepatitis B vaccine. Before treatment, testing of sexual partners for susceptibility to HBV infection is recommended if it does not delay treatment beyond 14 days.	Long-term sequelae include chronic persistent and chronic active hepatitis, cirrhosis, hepatocellular carcinoma, hepatic failure, and death. Rarely, acute infection may be fulminant with hepatic failure, resulting in death. Infectious chronic carriers may be asymptomatic but are at increased risk for chronic liver disease or liver cancer later.	Long-term sequelae include chronic persistent and chronic active hepatitis, cirrhosis, hepatocellular carcinoma, hepatic failure, and death. Rarely, acute infection may be fulminant with hepatic failure, resulting in death. Infectious chronic carriers may be asymptomatic but are at increased risk for chronic liver disease or liver cancer later. Although often asymptomatic, hepatitis B can be life-threatening and can cause serious complications. Hepatitis B is presented by hepatitis B vaccine, which is both safe and highly effective. Persons at risk for exposure should be immunized with hepatitis B vaccine. Persons whose sexual partners have acute HBV infection should receive postexposure prophylaxis with hepatitis B vaccine and HBIG if seen within 14 days of the last exposure. Persons whose sexual partners are found to be chronic carriers of HBV should receive the hepatitis B vaccine. All pregnant women should be screened for HBsAg during pregnancy to ensure optimal management of the infant. Homosexually active men and parenteral drug users are at increased risk for both HBV and HIV infections. The frequency of clinical follow-up of persons with acute HBV infection is determined by symptomatology and the results of liver function tests. Use condoms to prevent sexual transmission to susceptible persons.

Table 16-2   Sexually Transmitted Disease Summary—cont'd

DISEASE	CLINICAL PRESENTATION	THERAPY	COMPLICATIONS AND SEQUELAE	TEACHING
HIV infection and AIDS	Initial symptoms in young children are failure to thrive and frequent episodes of oral *Monilia* infection. Other signs and symptoms include those specific to opportunistic diseases: shortness of breath and nonproductive cough resulting from *Pneumocystis carinii* pneumonia (PCP) and glossitis, dysphagia, and retrosternal pain associated with oral and esophageal candidiasis.	Although no vaccine or cure is available for HIV infection or AIDS, the development of treatment therapies, including antiretroviral agents, immunomodulators, and others, is progressing rapidly. For persons with HIV infection, zidovudine (ZDV, formerly called AZT), ddI, Epivir, d4T, and ddC may be effective in delaying the clinical conditions of HIV disease. Aerosol pentamidine and sulfamethoxazole / trimethoprim has been shown to be effective in preventing *Pneumocystis carinii* pneumonia. These drugs have serious side effects and require careful monitoring by knowledgeable clinicians. For persons diagnosed with AIDS, standard therapy consists of antiretroviral therapy, infection prophylaxis, and treatment of opportunistic diseases aggressively as they occur. Early treatment with ZDV (during pregnancy, at labor and delivery, and administration to newborns at birth) to HIV-positive pregnant women has decreased transmission to newborns to about 8%. Newborns of HIV-infected mothers are treated with ZDV for several weeks after birth.	Although most persons with HIV infection eventually have some symptoms develop related to their infection, some remain asymptomatic for 10 yr or more. About 30% of infants born to HIV-infected women are infected with HIV. The prognosis for these infants is poor, but therapeutic advances are being made.	Individuals initiating a sexual relationship should be counseled about sexual practices that reduce the risk for HIV transmission. Sexual partners should be informed of HIV seropositivity. Sexual practices should be limited to those that do not permit any exchange of blood, semen, or vaginal secretions. Condoms should be used consistently. Persons should not inject illicit drugs. Drug users should enroll or continue in a drug treatment program. If drug use practices continue, needles and syringes should *never* be shared. If sharing does occur, cleaning the "works" with bleach may decrease the risk for HIV transmission. Alcohol and other drugs that are not injected may result in carelessness in practicing safer sex. Women of childbearing age who may be at risk for HIV infection should be counseled about the risks for perinatal transmission and about contraception options. Pregnant women with known or suspected HIV infection should promptly notify their physicians to ensure optimal management of the pregnancy. STD causing genital ulcers has been associated with an increased risk for acquiring or transmitting HIV infection. Persons with HIV infection should be skin-tested for tuberculosis.

Symptoms in men appear within 2 to 7 days after sexual contact with an infected person (although some men are asymptomatic). The germs invade the urethral canal, causing a painful burning sensation during urination. Pus that gradually becomes thin and watery is discharged from the penis. Increased burning, urinary frequency, and urgency are signs of bladder infection. The disease may spread to the prostate gland, seminal vesicles, and testes. The scrotum, when inflamed, is hard, swollen, painful, and heavy.

Some 80% to 90% of women with gonorrhea are asymptomatic; therefore they may spread the infection without knowing it. Those who have symptoms experience mild burning or smarting in the genital area, with or without a light yellow discharge. There may be slight inflammation and swelling of the Bartholin glands, which makes sitting or walking painful. The patient may also have a feeling of pelvic heaviness and discomfort in the abdomen. Anal itching and urinary symptoms may prevail. After one or more menstrual periods, untreated disease may invade the reproductive organs, including the fallopian tubes and ovaries, or may spread to the pelvis, causing pelvic inflammatory disease. Scar tissue may cause sterility. The disease can be transmitted by homosexual practices in both male and female patients. Anal gonorrhea is increasing in prevalence and causes no symptoms. In both genders, arthritis, endocarditis, and death may occur if gonorrhea is untreated.

The diagnosis of gonorrhea is based on medical history, symptoms, and laboratory test results. In men, a smear of the discharge from the penis is taken with a cotton swab and transferred to a special culture plate or bottle, where the organisms are grown for identification. The physician may want to take separate cultures a week or two apart. In women, the doctor usually takes a specimen for culture from within the vagina. Fluorescent-tagged antibody methods are the most accurate laboratory tests in women but should not be used in young children because of the risk of false-positive results. Procedures are simple and painless, and the results are confidential. If the patient is a minor, he or she can still receive free, confidential treatment without parental consent from the city or state health department or most physicians. If the test results are positive, sexual contacts are traced so that they may be treated before complications arise.

Syphilis. Syphilis, also known as *lues,* causes destruction throughout the body. The disease is caused by the spirochete *Treponema pallidum*, a spiral organism that reproduces rapidly in warm, moist areas of the body and quickly invades other tissues and organs. The organisms enter the body during coitus or through cuts or other breaks in the skin and mucous membranes. The incubation period is usually 3 weeks but may be anywhere from 10 to 90 days.

The symptoms of syphilis occur in three stages: primary, secondary, and tertiary (third). The primary stage consists of the appearance of a painless sore called a **chancre** (pronounced "shanker"), which appears where the spirochete enters the body on genital, anal, or oral membranes. In women, the chancre may go unnoticed if it is located around the cervix or in the vagina. It disappears without treatment in about 6 weeks. During this time, the serological blood test results are negative, but the organism can be identified with examination of the scrapings from the sore under the dark-field microscope. Although the chancre disappears, the destructive work of the spirochete continues as it invades various body systems.

Secondary syphilis can begin from 4 weeks to 6 months after the infection. Symptoms subside and reappear intermittently. If left untreated, the disease enters a latent period in which there are no symptoms. The latent period may last for many years. The disease remains contagious during the first 2 years, after which it is generally not communicable. Serological test results are positive.

The tertiary stage occurs after the fourth year. The disease is noninfectious at this time but very serious. The spirochetes attack the heart, blood vessels, brain, and spinal cord, in any of which the infection can cause death. Insanity and blindness can result. Bone tissue is destroyed, and there is severe crippling or paralysis.

Because a mother who has syphilis can infect her unborn child, obstetricians perform a serological test (VDRL, for Venereal Disease Research Laboratories, or RPR, for rapid plasma reagin) at the first prenatal visit and just before delivery. This has been successful in preventing **congenital syphilis.** When the result is positive, the mother is treated with penicillin G, which effectively permeates the placenta regardless of the stage of pregnancy and protects the fetus. If the syphilitic mother is untreated, abortion, stillbirth, or congenital syphilis may result. Young unwed mothers and their babies are in jeopardy, particularly when early prenatal care is neglected. Case finding in adults is furthered by means of preemployment physicals, required by many companies, and by preinduction physicals by the uniformed services. The adolescent who has been raped and is at risk may need prophylactic treatment.

Genital Herpes. **Herpes simplex virus (HSV) type II** causes an STD of the genitalia. Its frequency among teenagers appears to be increasing. Genital herpes usually is caused by type II, but there is an increase of type I. The type I virus is isolated most frequently from lesions above the umbilicus, whereas the type II virus is generally isolated from genital lesions (American Academy of Pediatrics, 2006). The virus becomes latent after the initial infection, only to recur later. The incubation period is from 5 to 10 days, and the lesions may persist from 3 to 6 weeks. The infection can be extremely painful, especially if the urethra and bladder are involved. Sitz baths, heat lamps, and local compresses of Burow's solution can bring relief. Systemic symptoms include fever, headache, malaise, and anorexia. Tissue culture

Table 16-3	*Interventions for the Child or Adolescent with a Sexually Transmitted Disease*	
ISSUE	**GOALS**	**INTERVENTIONS**
Anticipatory guidance for children under 12 yr	To provide anticipatory guidance concerning sexuality at a level that the young person can comprehend throughout the developmental cycle	Encourage educational programs that explore sexuality issues according to developmental level Provide age-appropriate instruction concerning sexuality during well-child visits Teach children strategies to deal with inappropriate touching by others Emphasize the importance of telling an adult if anything inappropriate should occur
Anticipatory guidance for adolescents	To prevent infection through anticipatory guidance	Discuss sexuality risk factors at each well checkup (include information about the relationship between sexual activity and drug and alcohol use) Review structure and function of the reproductive system and personal hygiene Discuss values and decision making, possible sexual behavior and consequences, prevention of pregnancy and STDs Advocate for a comprehensive health education program in the schools
Suspicion of infection	To identify early symptoms and facilitate prompt treatment if infection occurs	Create a nonjudgmental atmosphere, listen, assess level of knowledge, observe nonverbal behavior, establish confidentiality Provide privacy when assisting with pelvic or genital examination; ensure proper draping of patient Inquire about sexual partners and direct them to treatment, if warranted; persons with multiple sexual partners, homosexuals, persons with new partners, and those with history of prior STD are at particular risk for infection Realize anger is often a mask for depression or grief; do not take it personally Suspect sexual abuse if the child is under age 12 yr; report to Department of Social Services if disease is confirmed or sexual abuse is suspected
Compliance with treatment	To ensure treatment plan is followed and to prevent infection of others	Advise to abstain during treatment and to use condoms if sexual activity continues Advise to take all of the prescribed medication; if the patient is taking tetracycline or doxycycline, advise to take it 1 hr before or 2 hr after meals (on an empty stomach) and to avoid dairy products, antacids, iron, and sunlight Tell patients taking tetracycline or doxycycline that these medications decrease the effectiveness of oral contraceptives so that other methods of birth control should be used during the treatment course
Preventing complications	To prevent reinfection and sequelae	Emphasize the importance of follow-up and routine Pap smears Discuss the possible complications of specific disorders, such as birth defects, infertility

isolates and identifies the virus. There is no known cure, although acyclovir administration can hasten healing and the course of the episode.

HSV type II, which can be fatal to the newborn infant, is acquired from the mother during passage through the birth canal. Overwhelming infection involving many of the body systems occurs. A cesarean section is performed on mothers known to have this virus.

Herpes is thought to be a predisposing factor in cancer of the cervix. Regular follow-up Pap smears detect early carcinoma.

Treatment and Nursing Care

Table 16-3 describes the treatment methods and public health approaches for the most frequently seen STDs. Regardless of how health care professionals may feel about the changes in society and sexual permissiveness, they must recognize that STDs exist and deal with them appropriately. For nurses to be of help to teenagers with an STD, they must create an environment in which the teenagers feel at ease. To support adolescents' self-esteem, nurses should listen carefully to concerns with a nonjudgmental attitude.

The nurse approaches the patient with sensitivity, recognizing that the teenager is embarrassed and in need of privacy, especially during examinations. Girls are often afraid of and always nervous about a pelvic examination. This is true even when their outward manner may seem otherwise. The nurse provides careful explanations of the procedure, indicates what the patient can do to relax, drapes the patient appropriately, and remains during the examination to provide reassurance. The findings are discussed with the patient, and questions are encouraged. Most teenagers need help in being drawn out and do not readily ask questions even when they do not understand.

The reporting of sexual contacts, required by law, is an emotionally charged topic that often prevents patients from seeking help. The person who is assured of confidentiality and who has been treated in a dignified manner is more apt to cooperate. Sexually active girls must take responsibility for their own health and should be encouraged to request a chlamydial and gonorrheal culture as a routine part of their physical examination.

The nurse needs to explain to adolescents of both genders that it is particularly important to seek immediate medical attention if they suspect that their partner has an STD. Menstruation should not interfere with gaining medical help. Advise young people that sex with only one partner does not eliminate the risk because this person may have had contact with others; the partner needs only one sexual experience with one infected person to transmit the disease.

Sexual experimentation, lack of education, and lack of caution make adolescents highly susceptible to STDs. The goals of care should include reducing the patient's fear, obtaining a thorough history, and developing a trusting relationship. If a therapeutic relationship develops between the adolescent and the nurse, then preventive teaching can take place.

The percentage of patients hospitalized with STDs is small because of adequate outpatient treatment measures. Diagnosed cases are isolated. Nevertheless, because of the insidious nature of these disorders, nurses must practice scrupulous techniques of hand-washing when assisting with vaginal and rectal examinations on new admissions and when handling equipment such as rectal thermometers and douche nozzles. Hands should be kept away from the face to prevent gonorrheal conjunctivitis.

An STD that affects the reproductive organs is a serious threat to self-image and creates a great deal of anxiety. The nurse needs to assess the person's level of knowledge and provide information at that level. Many young people have little knowledge of their bodies and their developing sexuality. Others have mild to deep-seated emotional problems that need to be addressed. They may be using sex as an escape from reality, to express hostility or rebellion, or to call attention to themselves. They may be involved in

relationships they no longer desire, so they need help in formulating positive attitudes toward themselves. They also need help understanding their behavior and that of others. In particular, adolescents need to learn that they are responsible for their own actions if they choose to be sexually active.

The prevention of STDs is everyone's concern and demands individual initiative and responsibility. Nurses must keep themselves informed about the latest techniques in diagnosis and treatment. Education of the public, particularly young people, is paramount. Nurses who work in settings frequented by teenagers can distribute some of the many excellent health pamphlets available. Structured courses in sex education should include presentations on STDs (there are also excellent audiovisual aids) and discussions on how to establish healthy sexual behavior patterns. The community health or school nurse is involved in case finding and referral. Delays because of fear of disclosure are tragic. Legislation has now been enacted in all 50 states that permit physicians to treat infected minors without first obtaining parental consent.

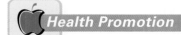

ABCs for STD Prevention

- Abstinence
- Be faithful (selective in choosing partner) for those who are sexually active
- Condoms
- Diagnosis (obtain screening and treatment)
- Education

Adapted from Polizzotto, M.J. (2005). Prevention of sexually transmitted diseases. *Clin Fam Pract, 7*(1), 127-137.

SPECIAL TOPICS

ADOLESCENT PREGNANCY

Approximately 1 million teenage girls give birth. Since 1991, there has been a 33% decrease in the adolescent pregnancy rate and a decline in the abortion rate for adolescent girls. Overall, 57% of teen pregnancies result in a birth, and less than 1% of infants are placed for adoption (Hillard, 2005). Teenage mothers are more likely to (1) drop out of school, (2) be unemployed because of limited education or lack of job skills, (3) be dependent on family or the welfare system, and (4) live in poverty.

During pregnancy, these young women are at risk for complications such as anemia, premature labor, high blood pressure, and placental problems. The use of tobacco, alcohol, drugs, and exposure to STDs can add additional problems to the pregnancy. Adolescents who are pregnant may be inconsistent with prenatal care, and their diet may be poor because of body image issues.

Health risks for the newborn whose mother is a teenager include low birth weight, prematurity, respiratory problems, and bleeding into the brain. Babies with low birth weight are 40 times more likely to die in the first month of life than are babies with normal weight. Children born to mothers who are 18 years of age or younger tend to have more difficulty in school and poorer health.

A girl who has a pregnancy in early adolescence is at risk for another pregnancy during her teenage years. Fathers of infants born to adolescent mothers are often older, many over the age of 20 years. Adolescent sexual activity and resulting pregnancy can be correlated with high-risk behaviors, such as alcohol and drug use.

First intercourse experiences among young people are typically characterized by the absence of effective contraception. For the pregnant girl, concerns of body image become blurred, education is interrupted, and she may be separated from sources of support, such as her peer group. The father's education may also be interrupted; he may become locked in low-paying employment and may face responsibilities for which he is ill prepared. Parenting classes, which provide guidance and support, and continuing education regarding the normal processes of child growth and development are vital for these young people and for the health and welfare of their children.

Growing evidence exists that comprehensive programs for the pregnant teenager and her baby, especially those that emphasize continued schooling, are associated with fewer repeat pregnancies. Many teenage fathers are included in prenatal education programs, allowed to participate in the birth, and allowed to visit the infants afterward; these fathers are more likely to remain in contact with their children as they grow.

Although school-based health education programs have had varying success in reducing the incidence of adolescent pregnancy, they remain an important source of accurate information for teens. Many teenagers prefer to postpone intercourse. It is important that they understand that a choice exists and that delay is acceptable. Sexually active adolescents need to receive information about contraception, although there may be no guarantee that the information will be put to use. Awareness of the responsibility of parenting, together with decision-making skills, can aid in lowering the number of teenage pregnancies.

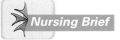

Nursing Brief

A major problem for teenagers is that they receive mixed messages from society about sexuality. In a society that is media focused, inappropriate messages linking sexuality and alcohol contribute to misinformation. It is important to help adolescents become media literate, increasing their skills to filter out information that is misleading.

DEPRESSION AND SUICIDE
Description

Suicide is one of the leading causes of death among persons between 15 and 19 years. It ranks second as a cause of death for adolescents and college students. The incidence rate increases during the spring. Completed suicide is more common among boys than girls, but girls make more attempts. Many adolescent suicides are not intended to be completed but are cries for help. The risk for death increases when there is a definite plan of action, the means are readily available (such as pills or guns), and the person has few resources for help and support. Firearms are the most common means. **Cluster suicide,** which is a situation where one suicide precipitates several others, is becoming more prevalent among adolescents and can be the result of the ideation of suicide.

Signs and Symptoms

Adolescents who do not have socially acceptable ways to express their frustrations may turn their anger and hostility inward. Their self-esteem is low and they feel trapped, rejected, and abandoned. Although each experience is individual, a group of teenagers who had attempted suicide had these common feelings: emptiness and loss, inability to experience pleasure, lack of concentration, confusion, inability to make decisions, and the sense that life lacked meaning and purpose. Physical problems revolved around eating and sleeping disturbances. They experienced lack of appetite and insomnia or the reverse, sleeping all day. Hyperactivity was yet another symptom. Behavioral problems surfaced; these included a drop in school grades, truancy, running away, promiscuity, and other forms of acting out. Alcoholism and substance abuse were significant contributing factors, as were the breakdown of family ties and the pressure to succeed. Some felt that their own expectations and those of others significant to them were too high.

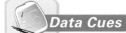

Data Cues

Risk Factors for Suicide

- Mood disorder
- Disruptive disorder (mostly males)
- Life stressors
- Low level of communication with family
- Maladaptive attribution and coping skills
- Substance abuse
- Family history of suicidal behavior
- Ideation of suicide
- Suicide threats

Previous suicide attempts (American Academy of Child and Adolescent Psychiatry, 2001)

More than half of suicide attempts are directly preceded by conflict with parents, ranging from misunderstandings to long-term, deep-seated problems.

Some teenagers are loners, isolated from their peers and family and unable to communicate their distress. Because the symptoms are difficult to distinguish from healthy adolescent reactions to stress, they may go unrecognized. However, if the manifestations are uncharacteristic and interfere with the person's ability to function on a daily basis, further investigation is imperative. In assessment of the situation, questions to the patient must be direct and specific. "Did you ever feel so upset that you wished you were not alive or wanted to die? Did you ever hurt yourself or try to hurt yourself? Are you planning to kill yourself? How? When?" Determine what coping skills the adolescent has used in the past to solve problems. If the person has made previous serious suicide attempts, the current suicidal situation should be considered more dangerous. **Never ignore an adolescent who threatens to commit suicide. Assume the adolescent is serious and act accordingly.**

Treatment and Nursing Care

Treatment is multidimensional. When possible, individual, group, and family therapy are provided in an outpatient setting such as a community mental health agency. Group therapy seems to be especially helpful for adolescents. The adolescent mental health or behavioral unit of a hospital provides a structured environment in which to associate with peers. It has the additional advantage of separating the adolescent from stressful surroundings and providing support and protection.

Depression is not always a negative experience. Often it is a reaction to a real or fancied loss. Although it is painful, it can lead to growth (Figure 16-7). The withdrawal accompanying depression is frustrating to those close to the young person, and they experience a feeling of helplessness. Nevertheless, it is futile to bombard the person with platitudes such as "Cheer up" and "Nothing can be that bad." Instead, the nurse should accept adolescents where they are and help them to look at and externalize their feelings. Ask them how you can help. Remain available to them. Activities that promote physical exercise can provide hostility outlets and are therapeutic. Some days nurses may feel ineffective and need to retreat. However, they should assure the young person that they will return. This helps lessen feelings of desertion. It is important that the nurse keep in touch with his or her feelings to avoid burnout. As teenagers begin to feel more secure, they reach out and progress at their own rate.

Adults are startled and disturbed when a 15-year-old boy or girl takes his or her life. Many adults view adolescence as a carefree time and forget the painful circumstances that surrounded their own young lives. Suicide is unacceptable in Judeo-Christian society, and many persons find it difficult to console the grieving family, which carries a heavy burden of guilt,

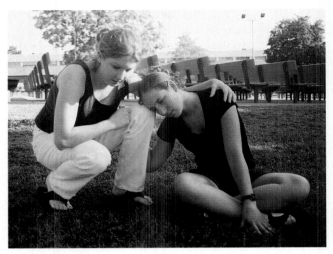

FIGURE **16-7** Adolescents are at risk for depression as they deal with the physical, emotional, and social changes that characterize this developmental stage.

anger, and sorrow. Self-help groups for survivors are available in most cities. The nurse needs assistance in identifying feelings toward the patient who expresses suicidal intentions.

It is usually better if the responsibility for a suicidal patient is shared by as many people as possible. A combined effort indicates to the young person that others care and are interested and ready to help. It is also beneficial for the team in that concerns can be discussed and grief can be shared in the event that the suicidal intent is carried out. In the hospital, the nurse is often the person most accessible and least threatening to the patient. Frequent, brief visits provide surveillance and also serve to break destructive thought patterns. The nurse must realize how sensitive the patient is to other people's reactions and should not add to the patient's guilt.

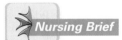
Nursing Brief

When a child asks for help or to talk about "a friend" who is talking about suicide, health care providers, parents, or teachers should be alert to the possibility that the child is indirectly talking about his or her own feelings.

Crisis intervention is necessary for acute and repeated episodes. Other voluntary services such as hot lines, drop-in centers, runaway houses, and free clinics focus on the immediate needs of the patient and are usually accepted by troubled youngsters. Unfortunately, there are not enough of these resources. Professionals need to be alert for warning signals of destructive behavior so that prompt intervention can be instigated; this might include earlier consideration of placement in a foster home. Community training courses for parenthood are becoming more popular and may provide another means of alleviating the complex problem of teenage suicide.

SUBSTANCE ABUSE
Description
The problem of substance abuse is serious and complex and of great magnitude. Government effort to control the supply and distribution of dangerous drugs has generally failed. Adult society, through its widespread acceptance of self-administered pills and alcohol, has compounded the problem; in particular, the drinking patterns of teenagers appear to directly reflect those of their parents and the community.

Numerous reasons have been cited concerning why adolescents resort to drug use. Possible reasons for increased use of drugs are a decrease in perceived risks, fewer school-based substance abuse programs, media that glamorizes tobacco and alcohol use, and lenient patterns of parenting (American Academy of Pediatrics, 2005). Other reasons cited are curiosity; peer pressure; rebellion; the need to escape from loneliness, boredom, or family problems; and the desire to become more sociable and to relax. Teenagers differ from adults in a preference for **polypharmacy** (the use of several drugs together), a sense of invulnerability, and a delay in psychosocial maturation with chronic drug use. Drug-seeking behavior may include stealing—shoplifting in particular—dealing in drugs, sexual promiscuity, and prostitution. In addition, a disproportionately high number of suicides are related to substance abuse. Gender-related differences have narrowed, particularly in the use of alcohol (more girls are experimenting with drugs and alcohol in their teens).

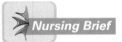

The use of tobacco and alcohol at an early age is a predictive factor for use of other drugs, use of greater variety of drugs, and use of more potent drugs (Figure 16-8).

Signs and Symptoms
The American Psychiatric Society has defined substance abuse as (1) a pattern of substance use that significantly interferes with normal activities of daily living, including fulfilling role obligations at home, school, or work, (2) use of substances when performing hazardous activities, (3) frequent substance-related legal difficulties, and (4) continued use despite the problems caused. Often adolescents begin by experimentation. However, there is a fine line separating use, dependence, and abuse.

Substances can cause **dependence,** an inappropriate reliance on the substance that persists despite efforts to cut down or control it. Dependence can be physiological, marked by **tolerance,** that is, an increasing need for greater amounts of the substance to produce the same effect, and **substance withdrawal,** physical withdrawal

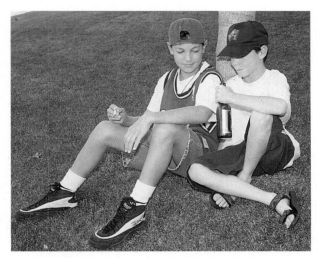

FIGURE **16-8** Cigarettes and beer are considered "gateway" substances that can lead to the use of other, illegal substances.

symptoms when the substance is reduced or stopped. Not all substances cause physiological dependence.

Table 16-4 summarizes the characteristics of some of the drugs more commonly abused by adolescents.

Treatment and Nursing Care
Treatment and nursing care for adolescents with substance abuse problems differ, depending on the drug involved. Prevention in the community and in schools through drug and alcohol education programs, identification and referral of students known to be users or at risk, and support for drug-free communities can reduce the incidence of substance use in teens.

The prevention of alcohol and other types of substance abuse begins by helping expectant parents develop good parenting skills. It is vitally important that children learn to feel good about themselves early in life. They need adults they can trust and who serve as good role models. As orderly development proceeds, the growing child learns to interact with others and develops a sense of identity. A positive self-image and feelings of self-worth help adolescents fine-tune their adaptive coping skills. In time, they can rely on their own problem-solving abilities and, it is hoped, will not need chemicals to deal with the complexities of life. Nurses in their various settings can contribute to this process. They can also educate their patients about the seriousness of substance abuse.

Although it is generally true that problem drinkers cannot be helped unless they want to be, more intervention is now being done. Most adolescents involved in substance abuse do not choose to enter treatment but are coerced by family members or the juvenile justice system. Although this is a controversial issue, clinical experience in substance abuse treatment settings has shown that many adolescents become interested in treatment and make behavioral changes after they have been required to enter a treatment program.

Table 16-4 *Long-Term Effects, Tolerance, Dependence, Adulteration, and Methods of Administration of Substances Adolescents Abuse*

SUBSTANCE	STREET NAME	EFFECTS	HEALTH ISSUES	METHOD OF ADMINISTRATION	TREATMENT	ISSUES
Alcohol	Booze	Sense of well-being, disinhibition, behavioral changes, impaired judgment, incoordination	Peptic ulcers, hepatitis, pancreatitis, fatty liver	Ingestion	Behavioral treatment with psychological and pharmacological aspects. Benzodiazepines (Valium, Librium) are used during first few days to help with withdrawal. Naltrexone (Revia) used in conjunction with counseling lessens cravings. Disulfiram (Antabuse) discourages drinking by causing nausea and vomiting when alcohol is used.	Family involvement with treatment is important. Alcoholics Anonymous (AA) for the alcoholic, Al-Anon for spouses or significant adults of alcoholics, Alateen for the children of alcoholics.
Tobacco, nicotine		Stimulates central nervous system (CNS), causing sudden release of glucose followed by depression and fatigue	Increase of chronic bronchitis, heart disease, cancer, increased number of stillbirths and prematurity for smoking pregnant women	Inhalation, ingestion (chewing)	Gradual cessation with psychological and pharmacological support. Nicotine replacement therapies include gum, transdermal patch, nasal spray, and inhalers. Drug Zyban has been approved for use (controls nicotine craving). Future vaccine being developed.	Heavily addictive with use, nicotine levels accumulate in body, tolerance occurs, leading to increased dependency. Leads to preventable cause of death in the United States and accounts for 7% of total U.S. health care costs. Easily available.
Methamphet-amine	Speed, meth, chalk, ice, crystal, glass	Releases increased level of dopamine, resulting in increased mood and body movement, wakefulness, increased physical activity, decreased appetite	Insomnia, confusion, tremors, memory loss, convulsions, anxiety and aggressive behavior; increases heart rate and blood pressure, leading to strokes; increased hyperthermia; extreme anorexia	Inhalation, snorting, injection, oral	No pharmacological treatments available at this time. Most effective treatment is cognitive behavioral interventions, which increase coping mechanisms. Recovery support groups used in adjunct can be effective.	

Continued

SUBSTANCE	STREET NAME	METHOD OF EFFECTS	HEALTH ISSUES	ADMINISTRATION	TREATMENT	ISSUES
Phencyclidine	Angel dust, ozone, wack, rocket fuel PCP combined with marijuana: killer joints and crystal supergrass	Feelings of strength and power, numbing effect on mind Distorts perception of sight and sound Violent behavior exhibited Muscle incoordination	Psychological effects producing violent or suicidal behavior; increased blood pressure and pulse with decrease in respirations; generalized numbness of extremities; high doses result in seizures, coma, and death; can mimic symptoms of schizophrenia	Inhalation, ingestion, snorting		Addictive, leading to psychological dependence, craving, and PCP-seeking behavior. Person should be kept in calm setting and not be left alone.
Lysergic acid diethylamide	Acid, boomers, yellow sunshine, blotter	Hallucinations, euphoria, rapid mood swings, panic, flashback	Dilated pupils, increased body temperature, increased heart rate and blood pressure, sweating, loss of appetite, sleeplessness, dry mouth, tremors	Ingestion		Effects are unpredictable and depend on amount taken, user's personality, mood, and expectations. Not considered addictive drug because does not produce drug-seeking behaviors.
3, 4 methylene-dioxymetham-phetamine	Ecstasy, Adam, XTC, X, clarity, lover's speed, love drug, hug, beans	Hallucinations, mental alertness; used to enable individuals to dance for extended periods of time	Confusion, depression, sleep problems, drug cravings, anxiety, paranoia, muscle tensions, nausea, sweating, increased heart rate and blood pressure; marked hyperthermia, cardiovascular failure, strokes, and seizures	Ingestion		Being used by young adults while attending clubs, raves (large, all-night dance parties), and rock concerts. Developing a rash after use may indicate future liver damage.

Table 16-4 *Long-Term Effects, Tolerance, Dependence, Adulteration, and Methods of Administration of Substances Adolescents Abuse—cont'd*

SUBSTANCE	STREET NAME	EFFECTS	HEALTH ISSUES	METHOD OF ADMINISTRATION	TREATMENT	ISSUES
Cocaine, crack	Coke, snow, blow, flake, C, nose candy, rock crank Cocaine or crack with heroin: speedball	Affects brain's key pleasure center by blocking removal of dopamine in synapse, causing a build-up of dopamine and results in pleasurable euphoric effects; feelings of energy, mental alertness, decreased need for sleep or food; bizarre, erratic, or violent behavior	Disturbances in heart rhythm, heart attacks, chest pain, respiratory failure, strokes, seizures and headaches, abdominal pain and nausea	Inhalation, injection, sniffing, snorting	Complex treatment including psychological, social, and pharmacological aspects. A combination of disulfiram, a medication used with alcoholism, and buprenorphine have been effective at reducing cocaine abuse. Antidepressants have shown some benefit. Behavior treatments have proven effective, with residential and outpatient facilities.	One of oldest drugs used. Two forms: hydrochloride salt (powdered form) and "freebase." Freebase is smokable, and powder is injected or taken intranasally.
Heroin	Smack, H, skag, junk, Mexican black tar	Euphoria with warm flushing of skin, dry mouth, and heavy extremities; followed by alternating wakeful and drowsy states; mental function becomes clouded with depression of CNS	Cardiac functions slow, respirations severely decrease, collapsed veins, bacterial infections, infection of heart lining and valves, arthritis, rheumatological problems, HIV	Injection, inhalation, sniffing, snorting	More effective with early intervention. Methadone (synthetic opiate that blocks the effects of heroin and eliminates withdrawal symptoms) has proved effective. LAAM (synthetic opiate) has longer duration of action, requiring dosing 3 times per week. Naloxone and naltrexone are effective as antidotes. Now available is buprenorphine, which does not produce the same level of dependence as methadone, makes discontinuing easier. Available through a physician's office.	Highly addictive. Street heroin is "cut" with other drugs or substances such as sugar, starch, powdered milk, or quinine. Can have strychnine or other poisons included. Strength of heroin or the contents makes overdose or death a high risk.

SUBSTANCE	STREET NAME	EFFECTS	HEALTH ISSUES	METHOD OF ADMINISTRATION	TREATMENT	ISSUES
Marijuana	Reefer, pot, weed, grass, boom, Mary Jane, gangster, chronic, ganga, widow, hash, herb, Bubblegum, Northern Lights, Fruity juice, Afghari #1	Euphoria, memory and learning problems, distorted perceptions, difficulty thinking or problem solving, increased appetite	Increased heart rate, panic attacks, respiratory problems such as bronchitis, chest colds, coughs, destruction of lung tissue, increases risk for cancer of head, neck and lungs	Inhalation, ingestion		Can be addicting. Most commonly used illicit drug in United States. Usually smoked as a cigarette (called a joint or nail) or in a pipe. Can be in a blunt (cigars emptied of tobacco and refilled with marijuana or in combination with crack).
Rohypnol	Rophies, roofies, roche, rope, "date rape" drug, forget-me pill	When combined with alcohol, produces a sedative hypnotic state with muscle relaxation and amnesia	Decreased blood pressure, drowsiness, visual disturbances, gastrointestinal disturbances, urinary retention	Ingestion		Can produce physical dependence on drug and cause withdrawal seizures.
Gamma hydroxy-butyrate	Liquid ecstasy, somatomax, scoop, grievous bodily harm, G, Georgia home boy	Euphoric, sedative effects, body-building effects; withdrawal effects of insomnia, anxiety, tremors, and sweating	Coma, seizures, especially when combined with use of metham-phetamine	Ingestion		Can be used as "date rape" drug in combination with alcohol. May be sold in fitness centers as synthetic steroid.

Continued

SUBSTANCE	STREET NAME	EFFECTS	HEALTH ISSUES	METHOD OF ADMINISTRATION	TREATMENT	ISSUES
Steroids (anabolic)	Arnolds, gym candy, juice, pumpers, stackers, weight trainers, roids	Performance-enhancing; designed to mimic the body building traits of testosterone but minimizes the masculine effects; reports of "feeling good", wide mood swings from violence to depression; paranoia, irritability, delusions, impaired judgement	Men: reduced sperm count, impotence, baldness, difficulty urinating, enlarged prostate, shrinking testicles, development of breasts Women: facial hair growth, menstrual changes, deepened voice, breast reduction Adolescents: premature growth halt Liver tumors and cancer	Ingestion, injection	Being developed as more is learned about long-term effects.	Long-term users experience addiction symptoms of craving, difficulty stopping use, and withdrawal symptoms. Easily obtained on black market.
Inhalants	Butyl nitrite: bolt, bullet, climax, locker room, rush Amyl nitrite: poppers, snappers Balloons with nitrous oxide: whippets Spray paint: Texas shoe shine	Quick excitement followed by drowsiness, disinhibition, staggering, agitation; body is depleted of oxygen and death can result; heart rate is rapid and erratic	Panic attacks, emotional instability, cardiac arrhythmia, CNS depression, brain damage, liver damage, respiratory arrest; "sudden sniffing death" can occur within minutes of a prolonged session	Inhalation, sniffing, snorting		Are readily available, cheap, and can be purchased legally. Three categories: volatile solvents, nitrites, and anesthetics.

Compiled from information from National Institute on Drug Abuse. (2006). *NIDA Infofax.* Retrieved July 10, 2006, from *www.drugabuse.gov.*

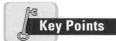

Key Points

- Acne is a common problem that can have serious psychological effects on the adolescent; severe acne can be successfully treated with Accutane.
- Hodgkin's disease is treated with radiation and chemotherapy.
- Obesity is an epidemic in children and adolescents and can lead to serious health problems.
- A multifocal approach that includes a family-centered focus with long-term lifestyle modifications is necessary for successful obesity treatment.
- Eating disorders can lead to weight loss and electrolyte imbalances if not recognized and treated.
- Childhood is a critical period for beginning obesity that has implications for future coronary heart disease.
- Children wearing body braces need to receive instructions in proper wearing techniques. Home instructions should be carefully discussed as should compliance issues.
- Overuse injuries are common in the adolescent population. Rest, ice, compression, and elevation are primary treatments.

- Alcohol use, potential drug abuse, and sexual relationships are important issues that should be explored with the adolescent.
- Substance abuse is a serious growing problem in the adolescent population. When counseling the adolescent, the health care worker should be supportive, understanding, and never judgmental.

 Go to your Companion CD-ROM for an Audio Glossary, video clips, and more.

evolve Be sure to visit the companion Evolve site at http://evolve.elsevier.com/Price/pediatric/ for WebLinks and additional online resources.

ONLINE RESOURCES

American Academy of Child and Adolescent Psychiatry: www.aacap.org

American Association of Suicidology: www.suicidology.org

American Foundation for Suicide Prevention: www.afsp.org

17 Pediatric Procedures

Objectives

Upon completion of this chapter, the student will be able to:

1. Discuss preparation techniques for the different developmental stages
2. Discuss safety precautions to take when bathing an infant
3. Describe the collection of various specimens from an infant or small child
4. Describe how to assist with a lumbar puncture
5. Contrast the administration of medicines to children and adults
6. Describe the preferred sites for intramuscular injections in infants and small children
7. Discuss precautions necessary when a child is receiving parenteral fluids and the rationale for each precaution
8. Discuss care of the child with a tracheostomy
9. Describe oxygen therapy related to children

Key Terms

Be sure to check out the bonus material on the Companion CD-ROM, including selected audio pronunciations.

alimentation (ĂL-ĕ-mĕn-TĀ-shŭn; p. 391)
lumbar puncture (p. 379)
nomogram (NŎM-ŏ-grăm; p. 380)
pulse oximeter (ŏk-SĬM-ĕ-tĕr; p. 396)
surface area (p. 389)
tracheostomy (trā-kē-OS-to-mē; p. 393)

PREPARATION FOR PROCEDURES

Preparation of the child for a procedure is one of the most important tasks of the health care worker. Children fear pain and bodily injury during hospitalization. Nurses must prepare the child with honest, age-appropriate explanations and carry out the procedure in the least stressful manner to the child. Hockenberry et al. (2005) refer to this as *atraumatic care*. Once nurses understand the stressors that affect hospitalized children, the effect of these stressors can be minimized with providing atraumatic care.

With infants, the parents are given the explanation and want to comfort the infant after the procedure. Toddlers can be given brief, simple explanations just before the procedure and may need to be restrained while the procedure is performed. Be sure the toddler does not view this as punishment. Parents may want to be there during the procedure to provide comfort but should not be viewed as the restrainer. An exception to this would be therapeutic holding done by the parent. Always provide comfort after the procedure. Preschoolers need simple explanations and should be allowed to touch and play with equipment if possible. Preschoolers engage in "magical thinking" and believe they have all-powerful thoughts. They may feel responsible for bad thoughts that coincide with events. They need to be reassured that their thoughts did not cause the event to occur. They also need to know that a procedure is not a punishment. They may need to be restrained as well. Always provide comfort (Band-Aids, stickers) after a procedure. The school-age child needs explanations through the use of drawings, pictures, and contact with equipment. Restrain only if needed. Praise cooperation and explain steps as you proceed. School-age children may be able to perform stress-reducing techniques such as visualization during the procedure. The adolescent generally needs no restraint, only clear explanations and praise for cooperation. Remember that child life therapists not only provide education before procedures, but often help children through procedures as well by providing distraction and other assistance. These therapists are helpful in the hospital and clinic setting.

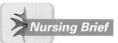
Nursing Brief

Always perform procedures in the treatment room.

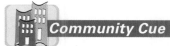
Community Cue

The Mayo Clinic website provides a slide show that demonstrates how parents can hold their child during procedures *(http://www.mayoclinic.com/health/childrens-health/CC00046)*. Refer parents to this when their child is in the hospital or clinic.

BASIC HYGIENE AND CARE

BATHING

Bathing not only promotes cleanliness and stimulates circulation to the skin, but also provides exercise and may help the child relax and feel more comfortable (Skill 17-1). Explain the procedure in appropriate terms. **Always remain with the child when bathing occurs.** Be sure to check any allergies the child may have. Always assess conditions that influence the type of bath given, such as a recent surgical incision, a cast, an intravenous (IV) line or Foley catheter in place, and so on. Examine the baby or child for skin abnormalities such as rashes, birthmarks, bruises, breaks in the skin, etc. *Never* use baby powder after the bath because the powder can cause breathing problems. Skill 17-1 can be taught to parents for home use.

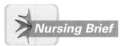

Always wash hands following *any* procedure performed.

SUCTIONING

A bulb syringe is used when it is necessary to provide an open airway by removing secretions from an infant's mouth and nose (Skill 17-2). Secretions may be the result of mucus or regurgitation of a feeding. Always assess the condition of the child after suctioning (Figure 17-1). There should be no sign of respiratory distress. Be sure parents know how to suction their baby's mouth and nose prior to discharge from the hospital.

FEVER AND SPONGE BATHING

Fever is defined as body temperature above 38° C (100.4° F) rectally. The physician may only recommend monitoring the fever, since it is the body's way of defending itself against illness and is part of the immune process. However, it is generally accepted that a fever of greater than 39° C (102.2° F) needs to be treated because children become more uncomfortable (Behrman et al., 2004). The child's metabolic rate also increases 10% for every 1° C increase. Antipyretic agents such as acetaminophen and ibuprofen are safe and effective in proper doses. Ibuprofen should only be used for children older than 6 months of age. Aspirin is not recommended because of the risk for Reye syndrome. Cooling the child by reducing the room temperature and removing blankets and clothing may be beneficial. In addition, tepid sponge bathing in warm water may be used to reduce hyperpyrexia (high fever) due to infection or hyperthermia resulting from external causes such as heatstroke (Behrman et al., 2004). Often, a tepid sponge bath is ordered if the child's temperature exceeds 40° C (104° F). When performed,

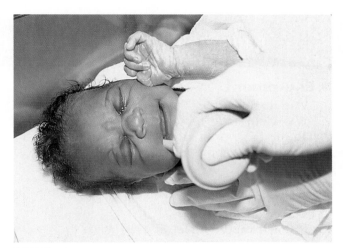

FIGURE **17-1** Suctioning secretions to clear the infant's airway. A bulb syringe can be used to clear most of the excessive secretions.

the sponge bath may be given in a tub or in the child's bed (Skill 17-3). The child should not be permitted to shiver because shivering produces heat, leading to a temperature increase. The bath is given for up to 20 to 30 minutes. **Alcohol should never be added to the water because it reduces the heat too rapidly and can be absorbed**. A table of Celsius (centigrade) and Fahrenheit temperature equivalents is provided in Appendix H.

COLLECTION OF SPECIMENS

COLLECTION OF URINE SPECIMENS

Urine specimens are often collected in doctors' offices and clinics, as well as in the hospital (Skill 17-4). All urine specimens need to be labeled and sent to the lab immediately because bacteria accumulate at room temperature. If there is a delay, the urine specimen is to be kept refrigerated or on ice. An example would be if the patient were taking a urine specimen to a laboratory that was obtained at home. Documentation of the procedure, including child's reactions, is also done. The physician may request that the specimen be collected with the **clean-catch** method, catheterization, or 24-hour collection.

The physician may also order a specimen so that the nurse can check certain lab results immediately, either in the clinic or the hospital. Examples of this may include specimens such as protein, albumen, glucose, ketones, or blood. These are checked with a urine dipstick without being sent to the lab. Results are recorded on the patient's chart.

Obtaining a Clean-Catch Specimen

Children who can voluntarily void can assist in obtaining a clean-catch specimen. Be sure to use familiar

Skill 17-1 Bathing an Infant or Small Child

■ Equipment

✓ Wash basin or tub
✓ Washcloth
✓ Towels
✓ Shampoo (as appropriate)
✓ Mild soap
✓ Cotton balls
✓ Clean clothing
✓ Diapers
✓ Lotion (as appropriate)

■ Safety Issues

- *Never* leave a child unattended around water.
- Prevent the child from slipping by placing a towel or rubber mat on the bottom of the tub or basin.
- Verify that the room temperature is warm enough and draft-free to prevent chilling.
- Only sponge bathe the baby until the cord has fallen off.
- Only sponge bathe the baby until the circumcision has healed.
- *Always* run cold water first to prevent burns.
- Hold on to infant securely, supporting the head while bathing.

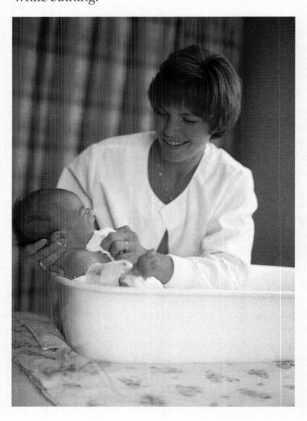

■ Method

1. Explain procedure.
2. Assemble equipment.
3. Wash hands. Use gloves if body fluid precautions are warranted.
4. Run water. Temperature should be 100° F (38° C). Check the temperature by submerging your wrist in the water or placing drops on the inside surface of your forearm. It should feel comfortably warm. (May use bath thermometer if available.)
5. Begin by removing secretions from the child's eyes with cotton ball immersed in plain water. Use a separate cotton ball for each eye.
6. Shampoo hair (if necessary); wash the scalp of an infant less than 1 year of age as necessary. Pour water over head. Apply shampoo and rinse. Avoid eyes. Dry head with towel when finished.
7. Bathe remainder of body. End with the perineal area. Remember to wash from front to back. Do not allow the child to chill. Wrap in towel when finished.
8. Apply lotion as needed.
9. Dress in clean clothing. Keep top edge of diaper below umbilicus site if not healed.
10. Teach hygiene practices to the parents as needed: frequency of bathing, shampooing hair, cleaning genitals, avoiding bubble bath (frequent occurrence of vaginal irritation), and so on.

■ Skills Checklist

✓ Prepare the child and family.
✓ Assemble equipment.
✓ Wash hands.
✓ Prepare basin, check temperature.
✓ Clean infant's eyes, wash hair and scalp.
✓ Bathe the rest of the child; prevent chilling.
✓ Dry. Apply lotion as needed.
✓ Teach as appropriate.
✓ Document the procedure. Be sure to note any abnormal skin conditions.

Skill 17-2   Suctioning with a Bulb Syringe

■ Equipment
✓ Bulb syringe
✓ Tissues
✓ Washcloth

■ Safety Issues
- Be sure infant shows no signs of respiratory distress after the procedure.
- Do not insert bulb straight to the back of the throat. This could result in a vagal response or gagging.
- Suction nares carefully so that tissue is not traumatized.

■ Method
1. Explain the procedure to the parent.
2. Gather equipment.
3. Wash hands; wear gloves.
4. Hold infant's head to one side.
5. Compress bulb.
6. Insert into mouth, along side of mouth.
7. Release bulb slowly.
8. Remove bulb syringe and empty by compressing several times as needed onto tissues or washcloth.
9. Suction nose carefully if necessary.
10. Discard tissues or place washcloth with soiled linen.

■ Skills Checklist
✓ Assess need for suctioning.
✓ Explain procedure.
✓ Wash hands; glove.
✓ Position infant.
✓ Compress bulb.
✓ Insert into mouth, release bulb.
✓ Suction nose if needed.
✓ Document procedure.

---

terms that the young child understands, such as "pee-pee" or "tinkle" when describing what the child is to do. Many children will be reluctant to void into a specimen container; have the parents assist as much as possible. Always wear protective equipment for Standard Precautions such as gloves when handling *any* specimen.

Special sterile containers are available for clean-catch specimens; follow the directions of the manufacturer. All require cleansing of the perineum or tip of the penis. When cleaning girls, cleanse the perineum with a soap or antiseptic agent, wiping from front to back. Repeat twice and follow with sterile water to prevent contamination of the specimen. After the urine stream has started, the midstream specimen should be caught in the sterile container, with care taken not to contaminate the container.

Infants and young children may have a sterile urine bag applied (see Skill 17-4). Check frequently under the diaper as leakage from the bag may occur. A slit may also be cut in the diaper to allow the bag to remain on the *outside* of the diaper where it is more visible.

Obtaining a Specimen with Catheterization
Obtaining a specimen with a catheter is the same as for adults, except that the size of the catheter is usually an 8 or 10 Foley (check institution policy). When necessary for surgical patients, the catheter may be inserted once the child has undergone anesthesia. This is less traumatic for children, who are usually frightened by this procedure.

Home Care Guidelines for Intermittent Catheterization Using a "Clean" Technique (CIC)
Some children require frequent catheterization. One example is the child with spina bifida. Parents can be taught how to catheterize their child at home. When children are old enough, they too can learn this procedure. A mirror is helpful for girls. Remember, repeated exposure to latex can cause latex allergies; therefore non-latex catheters are recommended. A clean technique is generally used. Always be sure the bladder is completely emptied to reduce the risk for urinary tract infections.
- Thoroughly clean the perineum or tip of penis with mild soap and water or povidone-iodine.
- Using the appropriate size lubricated catheter, insert until urine is obtained.
- Urine can flow freely into a clean container, urinal, bedpan, or toilet (if the child is old enough)
- Cleanse the area when finished.

If parents cannot afford a new catheter each time, catheters may be cleaned with soap and water, dried after use, and reused (for at least a week). Using this technique does not increase the chance of developing a urinary tract infection (American Urological Association Education and Research, 2002). Catheters may also be soaked in white vinegar solution once a week (to help with odor and mucus build-up). Additional cleaning techniques may be recommended by the physician.

Obtaining a 24-Hour Urine Specimen
At times, a 24-hour urine specimen may be requested to determine the rate of urine production and to measure the excretion of specific chemicals from the body. This

Skill 17-3 Sponge Bath to Reduce Fever

■ Equipment
✓ Basin of tepid (85° F to 90° F or 29° C to 32° C) water
✓ Three washcloths, towel(s)
✓ Two bath blankets
✓ Waterproof sheet

■ Safety Issues
• *Never* leave a child unattended around water.
• If the child shivers, stop the procedure.
• Assess color and pulse frequently.
• Record temperature before and 30 minutes after the procedure.
• *Never* add alcohol to water.

■ Method
1. Explain the procedure to the patient and family. Assemble the equipment at the bedside.
2. Wash hands. Screen the child. Take and record temperature, pulse, and respirations.
3. Cover the patient with a bath blanket or sheet. Fanfold bedclothes to the foot of the bed. Place a waterproof sheet and bath blanket beneath the patient.
4. Remove patient's gown.
5. Wash the patient's face and neck with tepid water.
6. Lift the corner of the bath blanket and bathe the child's body, part by part. Use long strokes. Expose one area of the body at a time.
7. Place moist, folded cloths over blood vessels that lie close to the skin (underarms and groin).
8. Turn the patient and repeat the procedure, beginning with the neck, then going to the shoulders, the back, and so forth.
9. Check color and pulse to be sure that the child is tolerating the procedure without adverse effects.
10. If the child begins to shiver, the procedure should be immediately stopped.
11. When the bath is completed, pat the skin dry and cover the patient with only a sheet.
12. Remove the waterproof sheet and blanket. Replace the hospital gown. An infant may be placed on a large towel, covered by a receiving blanket.
13. Arrange pillows and bedding for the patient's comfort.
14. Take the patient's temperature within 30 minutes of the time the procedure ended and record. If the temperature has not started to go down, check to see whether the procedure should be repeated. Note: The temperature is not expected to drop to normal but merely to a more reasonable level. Also record pulse and respirations.
15. *Chart:* Time procedure began, length of time administered, untoward reactions, patient's temperature before and after procedure.

■ Skills Checklist
✓ Prepare the child and the family.
✓ Assemble equipment.
✓ Wash hands.
✓ Record temperature, pulse, respirations.
✓ Drape patient.
✓ Remove gown.
✓ Wash face, neck, other body parts, one at a time.
✓ Place cloths; proceed to back of patient.
✓ Check color, pulse.
✓ Pat dry, regown.
✓ Assess comfort.
✓ Record temperature, pulse, respirations.
✓ Document procedure.

---

requires close supervision by the nurses on each shift to maintain accuracy of the test because lost specimens necessitate restarting the test. Problems can arise if the collection device does not adhere to the skin properly; therefore the nurse must be alert for this occurrence. Diversions suitable to the child's age are used. Certain tests require that chemicals be added to the bedside collection receptacle. It is important to clarify this before the procedure is begun. A sign is attached to the infant's crib to alert personnel to a 24-hour urine collection.

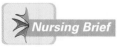
Nursing Brief

The rule of thumb for urine output is 0.5-2 mL/kg/hr.

COLLECTION OF STOOL SPECIMENS

Stool specimens from older children are obtained as for an adult (Skill 17-5). This is embarrassing for most children, who are turned off by the suggestion. The ambulatory child can use a collection device placed beneath a toilet seat. It is difficult for a child to tell the nurse that the sample has been collected. The nurse can acknowledge these feelings by giving the child permission to express them without being critical. The nurse might say, "I know this must be embarrassing for you. It is for grown-ups, too, but we need this because . . ."

COLLECTION OF BLOOD SPECIMENS

Blood specimens are generally collected by the laboratory technician or a specially trained nurse. Children

Skill 17-4 Obtaining a Specimen for Urinalysis

■ Equipment
✓ Sterile container
✓ Urine collection bag (infant)

■ Safety Issues
- Wear gloves because of contact with body fluids.
- Check urine collection bag frequently.
- Label specimen clearly.
- Deliver specimen immediately to the laboratory (bacteria may grow at room temperature).

■ Method
1. Explain the procedure.
2. Wash hands; wear gloves.
3. Use a sterile container or apply a urine collection device.
4. If a bag is used, secure the diaper over the bag or cut slit so that bag is outside the diaper.
5. Check bag every 20 to 30 minutes.
6. Label all specimens clearly and attach the proper laboratory slip. Collected specimens should be transported in a plastic bag (check institution policy).
7. Record in nurse's notes. Document color, amount, and any odor.

■ Skills Checklist
✓ Explain procedure.
✓ Obtain container/urine collection device (infant).
✓ Wash hands; glove.
✓ Apply urine collection device (infant) or have child void.
✓ Recover specimen.
✓ Label, send to laboratory.
✓ Document procedure.

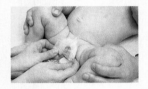
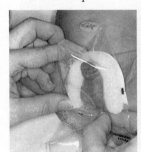

When applying newborn and pediatric urine collectors, there are two key points. 1, The skin must be clean and perfectly dry. Avoid oils, baby powders, and lotion soaps that may leave a residue on the skin and interfere with the ability of the adhesive to stick. 2, Application must begin on the tiny area of skin between the anus and genitals. The narrow "bridge" on the adhesive patch keeps feces from contaminating the specimen and helps position the collector correctly. With the child on his or her back, spread the legs and wash each skin fold in the genital area. A genital bath soap is best. Do not use a scrub soap solution; it may leave a residue that interferes with adhesion. Wash the anus last. Rinse and dry. For boys, wash the scrotum first, then the penis; wash the anus last. Allow a few moments for air drying. Remove protective paper from the bottom half of the adhesive patch. Most persons find it easier to keep the top half of the adhesive covered with paper until the bottom part has been applied to the skin. With a very active boy, you may want to keep all the paper in place until you have fitted the collector over the genitals. For girls, stretch the perineum to separate the skin folds and expose the vagina. When applying adhesive to the skin, be sure to start at the narrow bridge of skin separating the vagina from the anus. Work outward from this point. For boys, begin between the anus and the base of the scrotum. Press adhesive firmly against the skin and avoid wrinkles. When the bottom part is in place, remove paper from the upper portion of the adhesive patch. Work upward to complete application. (Courtesy Hollister Inc., Libertyville, IL.)

generally fear this procedure. EMLA cream can be used to lessen the pain. Remember, however, that the cream needs to be in place approximately 45 minutes before the blood sample is taken. If time permits, have the blood specimen obtained in the treatment room, keeping their bed a safe place. The antecubital fossa is a common site in children older than 2 years of age. The dorsum of the hand or foot can also be used (Figure 17-2). The heel is often used in infants (Figure 17-3). The heel needs to be warmed with a warmed washcloth or commercial warmer. This increases blood flow. Temperature should not exceed 42° C (107.6° F) to avoid burns. The external jugular vein can be used in infants when other sites have not worked. The femoral vein may be used when other sites have been exhausted. Jugular and femoral venipuncture are only done by the physician. If a child has a central venous catheter or port, specially trained nurses can obtain the blood specimen by following hospital procedure. Always use Standard Precautions when obtaining or assisting with blood specimens.

Positioning the Child
Positioning the pediatric patient for blood drawings is extremely important. The nurse is often asked to assist in these procedures. Figures 17-4 and 17-5 show

Skill 17-5 Obtaining a Stool Specimen

■ Equipment
✓ Clean container
✓ Tongue blade

Safety Issues
• Wash hands well. Wear gloves to obtain specimen.
• Label specimen appropriately.

■ Method
1. Explain procedure to child or parent.
2. Wash hands; wear gloves.
3. Obtain stool specimen directly from the diaper (if it has not been contaminated by urine) with the tongue blade, or use the tongue blade to retrieve the specimen from the collection device.

4. The specimen is labeled properly, and the laboratory slip is attached.
5. Some specimens must be sent to the laboratory while they are warm.
6. The nurse charts the time, color, amount, and consistency of the stool; the purpose for which it was collected (e.g., blood, ova, parasites, bacteria); and any related information.

■ Skills Checklist
✓ Explain procedure.
✓ Wash hands; glove.
✓ Obtain specimen.
✓ Label, send to laboratory.
✓ Document procedure.

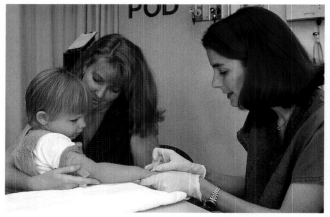

FIGURE **17-2** Using a parent to hold and comfort the child during a blood specimen procedure.

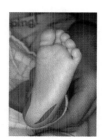

FIGURE **17-3** Sites for heel punctures on an infant.

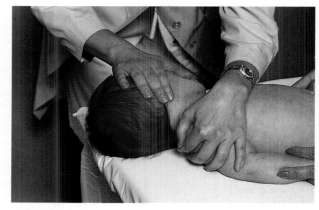

FIGURE **17-4** A child positioned for jugular venipuncture.

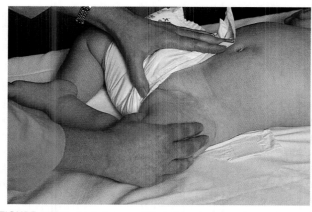

FIGURE **17-5** An infant positioned for femoral venipuncture. This provides exposure of the groin area.

how to position the patient for jugular and femoral venipuncture. Both the jugular and the femoral veins are large; therefore, after venipuncture, the patient is checked frequently to ensure that there is no bleeding. The child is soothed accordingly because crying and thrashing may precipitate oozing. The nurse charts the site used, the name of the blood test, and any untoward developments.

Skill 17-6   Obtaining a Throat Culture

■ Equipment
✓ Throat swab(s)
✓ Tongue depressor
✓ Media culture

■ Safety Issues
• Nurse may need to wear mask/eye goggles for protection.
• Label specimen appropriately.

■ Method
1. Explain procedure to child/parents.
2. Gather equipment.
3. Wash hands; wear gloves.
4. Have child stick out tongue and say "ah."
5. Depress anterior half of tongue with tongue depressor if necessary.
6. Swab area with exudate or redness, one time only per swab (avoid teeth, tongue, cheeks, lips, and palate).
7. Place swab(s) into media culture.
8. Be sure parents or nurse comfort child.
9. Label, obtain requisition.
10. Transport to laboratory.
11. Document procedure, including description of pharyngeal area if you can see it.

■ Skills Checklist
✓ Explain procedure.
✓ Wash hands; glove.
✓ Obtain specimen.
✓ Place in media culture.
✓ Provide comfort.
✓ Label, obtain requisition.
✓ Take to laboratory.
✓ Document procedure.

COLLECTION OF THROAT CULTURES

A throat culture is frequently ordered by the physician when a child has a "sore throat" or a strep infection is suspected (Skill 17-6). The child may need to be temporarily restrained when a throat specimen is obtained. The child needs to stick out the tongue and say "ah" while the nurse swabs the pharyngeal area. If the child is unable to cooperate, a tongue depressor should be used to hold down the tongue while obtaining the swabbed specimen. **If the child has a diagnosis suspicious of epiglottitis, the throat culture should not be done. The airway may become edematous and occlude from the trauma of specimen collection.**

COLLECTION OF NASOPHARYNGEAL CULTURES

A nasopharyngeal culture may be ordered to rule out certain respiratory infections such as pertussis in children. Have the child look up, dip the swab tip into saline, and with the wire bent, insert the swab to the back of the nares and into the nasopharyngeal area. Remove after several seconds, place the swab into the culture media, label, and transport to the lab with specimen requisition form. Comfort the child after the procedure. Record the specimen collection and child's response.

ASSISTING WITH LUMBAR PUNCTURE

The nurse assists the physician with a lumbar puncture, which is also referred to as a *spinal tap*. It is done to obtain cerebrospinal fluid (CSF) for diagnosis and treatment. Disposable lumbar puncture sets are available. EMLA cream should be applied to the site at least 1 hour previous to the spinal tap. Children may require additional analgesia or anesthesia, depending on the physician's orders.

Normal spinal fluid is clear, like water. The pressure ranges from 60 to 180 mm Hg. It is somewhat lower in infants. The procedure for children is essentially the same as for adults. The main difference lies in the patient's ability to cooperate with positioning. The nurse explains that the child must lie quietly and that there will be help in doing this. Sensations during a lumbar puncture include a cool feeling when the skin is cleansed and a feeling of pressure when the needle is inserted.

The patient lies on the side with the back parallel to the side of the treatment table. The knees are flexed, and the head is brought down close to the flexed knees. The nurse can keep the child in this position by placing the child's head in the crook of one arm and the knees in the crook of the other arm. The nurse then clasps hands together at the front of the child and leans forward, gently placing his or her chest against the patient (Figure 17-6). Infants may be supported in the sitting position with their backs curved and head flexed forward. The way in which the child is held can directly affect the success of the procedure. **Always monitor the child's respiratory status during a lumbar puncture. There is a potential for airway obstruction related to neck flexion.**

Once the patient is positioned, the physician cleans the skin and numbs the area for needle insertion. A

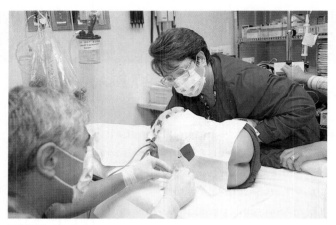

FIGURE **17-6** During a lumbar puncture, the nurse holds the child in a side-lying position with the head flexed and the knees drawn upward toward the chest. This position enlarges the spaces between the vertebral spines, thereby improving access to the spinal fluid spaces.

> **Box 17-1** *Doses for Children Based on Weight in Kilograms*
>
> **STEPS**
> 1. Weigh and record child's weight in kilograms (convert from pounds by dividing by 2.2).
> 2. Determine recommended safe range in milligrams/kilogram (mg/kg) by checking (pediatric) medication reference.
> 3. Multiply child's weight by the lower and upper limits of the dose range.
> 4. Compare child's ordered dose with dose range to determine whether medication dose falls within the "safe range."
> 5. Any dose that does not fall within the "safe range" needs to be verified by the physician.
>
> **EXAMPLE**
> Child weighs 44 lb
> Conversion: 1 kg = 2.2 lb
> 44 lb ÷ 2.2 = 20 kg
> If reference text states that the recommended dose range is 50 to 100 mg/kg of body weight/24 hr in four divided doses:
>   1. 50 mg × 20 kg = 1000 mg/24 hr
>   2. 100 mg × 20 kg = 2000 mg/24 hr
>   3. Safe range = 1000-2000 mg/24 hr
> Child's ordered dose is 400 mg every 6hr
>   4. 400 mg given every 6 hr = 400 × 4 = 1600 mg/24 hr
> Conclusion: Dose falls in safe range

long, hollow spinal tap needle is inserted into the patient's lower back, and the spinal fluid is collected into different test tubes. These are labeled for different studies. Once the procedure is complete, a sterile Band-Aid is applied over the injection site and the child is comforted. The site should be checked for any drainage or redness. Monitor vital signs according to the procedure of the hospital. Specimens are then labeled and taken to the laboratory with the appropriate requisition form.

Children need to be monitored for headaches after a lumbar puncture. Postlumbar puncture headaches may be avoided by having the child lie flat for a period of time after the procedure. Children also need to be monitored for fever or cerebrospinal fluid (CSF) leakage at the puncture site.

The nurse charts the date and time of the lumbar puncture and the name of the attending physician. Also charted are the amount of fluid obtained, its character (cloudy, bloody), whether or not specimens were sent to the laboratory, and the reaction of the patient to the procedure. The nurse then cleans and restocks the treatment room.

ADMINISTERING MEDICATIONS

VARIATIONS IN CHILDREN

The responsibility for giving medications to children is a serious one. Although a full technical description of drug administration is beyond the scope of this book, the following considerations and hazards are applicable to pediatric patients.

Many drugs currently on the market are unsuitable for children because of their toxicity or because of lack of information about their effect on pediatric patients. Children are smaller than adults, and their medications have to be adapted to their size and age. Neonates and preterm infants are in particular jeopardy because of the immaturity of their body systems. In these patients, simply adjusting the dosage is insufficient. Drugs must be individualized and tailored to a multitude of factors (Figure 17-7).

The nurse should always ask whether the calculated dose makes sense. It is also helpful to remember that children usually receive small doses and amounts, and if either of these is large, the nurse should recheck. Most pediatric medications are prescribed in milligrams per kilogram of body weight per 24 hours (Box 17-1). A specific dose per kilogram of body weight may also be prescribed, such as 10 mg/kg. A hospital drug formulary is usually available on the unit to enable the nurse to determine the safety of a particular dose. If there is any question, the nurse should also consult another nurse, the physician who wrote the order, the hospital pharmacist, or the shift supervisor.

The physician may need to calculate a particular dosage of a medication for a certain child. One method, calculation by *body surface area* (BSA), is considered to be a very accurate method. In this method, a **nomogram** is used (Figure 17-8). The child's height is located on the left scale, and weight is located on the right scale. A line is drawn between the two points. The point at which the line transects the surface area (SA) gives the BSA. If the patient is roughly of average size, the SA also can be estimated from the weight alone with the

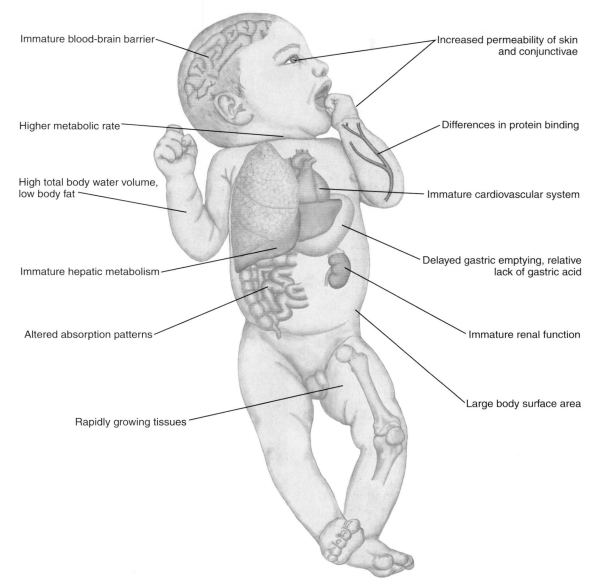

Immature blood-brain barrier

Increased permeability of skin and conjunctivae

Higher metabolic rate

Differences in protein binding

High total body water volume, low body fat

Immature cardiovascular system

Immature hepatic metabolism

Delayed gastric emptying, relative lack of gastric acid

Altered absorption patterns

Immature renal function

Rapidly growing tissues

Large body surface area

FIGURE **17-7** Some of the multiple factors that modify drug interaction in children. Physiological differences in the body systems make the effects of drug interactions more dramatic in the newborn.

enclosed (shaded) area. The results are inserted into a formula. The average adult BSA is approximately 1.7 square meters.

$$BSA\ (child)/BSA\ (adult) \times Average\ adult\ dose = Child's\ dose$$

In addition to knowing the correct amount and route of a drug, the nurse must also be aware of the toxic side effects that might occur. The absorption, distribution, metabolism, and excretion of drugs differ substantially in children, who also react more quickly and violently to medication. Drug reactions are therefore not as predictable as in adult patients. The impact of a drug on normal growth and development must be considered. Drug circulars must be read carefully

to determine suitability of a particular drug for children. **Drugs should be given only by the route indicated**. Double-check with another nurse if using calculated dosages or for any drug or dosage that may give reason for concern. (Some hospitals specify double-checking for digoxin, insulin, heparin, and certain other drugs.)

The child should be correctly identified with the hospital identification band and second identifier, such as the child's birthday. *Never* call out a child's name for identification. The nurse must always know what medications the patient is receiving, whether or not the nurse administers them personally. The nurse should review the medications with the parent prior to administering them. If there is any discrepancy, always

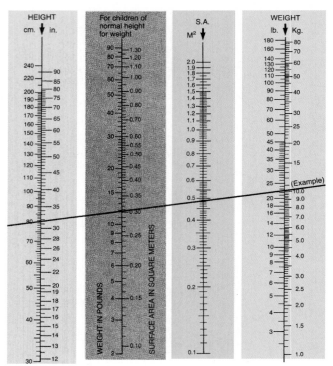

FIGURE **17-8** Nomogram for estimating BSA. The SA is indicated where a straight line that connects the height and weight levels intersects the SA column. If the patient is of average size, the SA can be deduced on the basis of weight alone *(see shaded area)*.

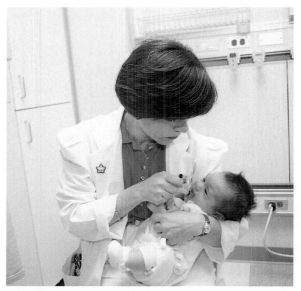

FIGURE **17-9** Administering oral medication to an infant. Note how the nurse can control the infant's movements by holding the infant's left arm (the infant's right arm is tucked under the nurse's left arm) and tucking the infant's head in the crook of her arm.

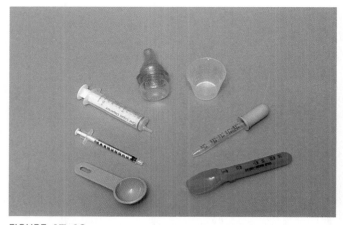

FIGURE **17-10** Medications can be administered to children with a measuring spoon, oral syringe, calibrated nipple, medicine cup, calibrated dropper, or hollowed-handled medicine spoon.

double-check the physician's orders. See Table 17-1 for further considerations about pediatric medications.

ORAL MEDICATIONS

The administration of medication by mouth is preferred in children but is not always possible because of vomiting, malabsorption, or refusal. Children younger than 5 years of age find it difficult to swallow tablets or capsules, so many pediatric medications are available in liquid, suspension, or chewable tablets. Only scored tablets should be divided. Suspensions must be fully shaken before use. Always measure liquid medications with an oral syringe as measuring spoons are inaccurate.

Capsules may have to be emptied and the powder disguised in a pleasant-tasting medium. Be sure to check with the pharmacist to ascertain that capsules can be emptied. This is also necessary when the medication is bitter or otherwise unpalatable. Cherry syrup or jelly may be used. Use of important sources of nutrients such as orange juice, formula, or milk for this purpose is discouraged because the child may develop distaste for them. *Never* refer to the medication as candy. Administer medication slowly, especially if the child is crying. **Elevate the patient's head and shoulders to prevent aspiration**. The child may attempt to push the medicine cup away. In anticipation of this, the child is held in the nurse's lap in a semisitting position with the hands restrained (Figure 17-9). "Chasers" of water,

fruit juice, or carbonated beverage are appreciated. In choosing a chaser, the patient's age, diet, and preference are considered.

If a nasogastric tube is in place, test for proper placement of the tube before pouring medication into the syringe barrel. Administer a small amount of water afterward to cleanse the tube. Record the intake.

For infants, an oral syringe is an excellent device for measuring small quantities. It is easily transported, and medication can be given directly from the syringe. Place the syringe midway back at the side of the mouth. An empty nipple may also be used. Apply a bib to an infant before performing the procedure. Do not place medication in a bottle

Table 17-1	*Selected Considerations in Giving Medications to Children*
AGE	**CONSIDERATIONS**
Infant	Apply bib or use towel under chin
	Support and elevate head and shoulders
	Determine plastic disposable syringe is accurate and safe for oral medications
	Depress chin with thumb to open mouth
	Slowly insert medication along the side of the infant's mouth; this helps prevent gagging
	Allow time for swallowing
	The recommended site for intramuscular (IM) injections is the vastus lateralis muscle
	Avoid use of buttocks because gluteal muscles are undeveloped in infants; danger of injury to sciatic nerve
	As a rule of thumb, give no more than 1 mL of solution in a single site; if in doubt, check hospital policy
	Soothe infant
Toddler	May require help of another person
	May require some type of restraint if no assistance is available
	Let child explore an empty medicine cup
	Explain reasons for medication
	Crush tablets if not chewable variety
	If cooperative, child may hold medicine cup
	Allow child to drink at own pace
	When giving medications IM, carry out injection quickly and gently. IM injections in the dorsogluteal muscle are only given to toddlers who have been walking for one year.
	Be prepared to find that resistive behavior is at its peak, particularly kicking, crying, and thrashing about
	Be prepared to be surprised because some toddlers are very cooperative
Preschool	Chewable tablets and liquids are preferred
	Regression in pill-taking may be seen
	Watch for loose teeth that could be swallowed
	Avoid prolonged reasoning; only give choices when there is one
	Involve parents if appropriate
	Provide puppet play to help child express frustration concerning injections
	Praise child after procedure
School-age	Can take pills and capsules; instruct child to place pill near back of tongue and immediately swallow water or fluid of choice
	Emphasize swallowing of fluid to distract child from swallowing of pill
	Some children continue to have a difficult time swallowing pills and other forms of the medication should be explored (many come in suspensions); never ridicule child
	Children can be unpredictable from day to day in their cooperation; allow more time for the giving of pediatric medications
	Always ascertain that child is fully awake (particularly after nap time and during night shift)
	Always inform child of what you are about to do
	Remain with fearful child after procedure until composure is regained
	When this is not possible or appears prolonged, enlist help of auxiliary personnel
Adolescent	Prepare patient with explanations suitable to understanding
	Always ensure privacy
	Teach adolescent what side effects to report
	Identify adolescents on contraceptives to avoid drug interactions (may have been too embarrassed to provide information during history or may be attempting to keep secret from significant others)
	Remain with patient until medicine is consumed (particularly if the patient has a behavioral disorder)
	Anticipate mood swings in compliance
	Consider possibility of adolescent addiction (drugs, alcohol) even though this may not be presenting problem; many medications are altered by such conditions

of juice, milk, or water; if some of the contents is refused, there is no way to determine how much of the drug was consumed. A plastic medicine dropper is useful and may be provided with the medication by the drug manufacturer (Figure 17-10). Use only for the medication specified because these droppers are not intended for measuring other liquids. A drug ordered in teaspoons should be measured in milliliters to ensure accuracy (5 mL = 1 teaspoon). When administering medications in pediatric units, it is particularly important to keep the medicine cart or tray in sight at all times, so that a child does not take or play with any medications.

NOSEDROPS, EARDROPS, AND EYEDROPS

Except for a few differences, the principles of administering nosedrops, eardrops, and eyedrops to children are essentially the same as for adults. Infants and small children may need to be restrained. If restraint is necessary, a second person can help or a mummy restraint can be used. Warm all medications to room temperature. Explain the procedure to the child in age-appropriate detail.

Nosedrops

To administer nosedrops, first wipe mucus from the nose with a tissue. Position the infant or child lying flat with the

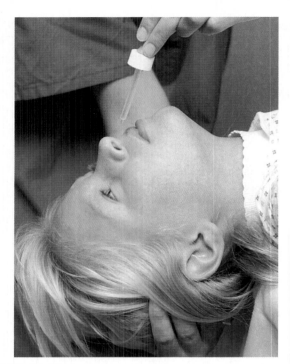

FIGURE **17-11** Technique of instilling nosedrops requires proper positioning for installation.

head over the edge of a pillow. Encircle the child's cheeks and chin with your nondominant arm to hold the head steady. Instill the drops with the dominant hand. Keep the child in this position with head back for 1 minute to allow the drops to reach the proper area (Figure 17-11).

After instilling the drops, chart the time, name of medication, strength, number of drops instilled, how child tolerated the procedure, and untoward reactions.

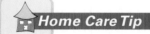

Home Care Tip

Parents and Caregivers Need to Know the Following When Medicating Children:
- Name and purpose of the medication
- The route used to deliver the medication (many medications are given orally but parents may be taught other routes such as IM, subcutaneous (SubQ), or rectal)
- How much is to be given (always measure *accurately*)
- Time(s) of day medication is to be given
- Determine whether it is to be taken with food
- Know possible side effects of the medication
- Know possible drug or food interactions (including herbal medications)
- Follow medication schedule as prescribed (such as completing *all* of an antibiotic)

Parents need to let their doctor know if the medication does not appear to be working or if there are any adverse or side effects.

Eardrops

The doctor may prescribe a drug to be instilled into the ear. Eardrops should be warmed to room temperature

before instilling. The infant and young child may need to be restrained during this procedure. Cooperation may be gained through the use of games and the involvement of parents. In the child under 3 years of age, the infected ear is drawn down and back to straighten the ear canal and the correct number of drops is instilled. In the older child, the earlobe is pulled up and back to obtain a straight canal. The patient remains supine for a few minutes to permit the fluid to be absorbed. The nurse charts the time, name of drug, number of drops administered, the area (right or left ear), untoward reactions, and whether or not the patient obtained relief.

The area in front of the ear may be gently massaged to aid in the entry of the drops into the ear canal. A sterile cotton pledget may be placed in the canal to prevent leakage of medication; however, this should be loose enough to allow for drainage.

Eyedrops

Ophthalmic medication is administered to a child in the same manner as for an adult. Ascertain which eye requires treatment. Gloves are to be worn if drainage or infection is present. Hands are washed well before and after application of eyedrops. The child should be either supine or in the sitting position. The infant and small child may need to be restrained.

With the thumb and index finger, use gentle pressure in opposite directions to open the eye. Instruct the child to "look up." Supporting the hand on the patient's forehead, instill the medication into the center of the lower lid (conjunctival sac). Instruct the child to close the eye but not to squeeze it because this could expel some of the solution. Infants may clench their eyes shut. When this happens, the drops can be placed in the nasal corner where the lids meet. When the child opens the lids, the medication flows onto the conjunctiva.

Ointment is applied into the same conjunctival sac as the eyedrops (Figure 17-12). Excess ointment may be wiped outward with a tissue. If both drops and ointment are ordered, apply drops first, wait 3 minutes, then apply ointment (Hockenberry et al., 2005).

INTRAMUSCULAR INJECTIONS

Intramuscular (IM) injections are rarely administered to children, especially if an intravenous (IV) line is present. However, physicians do order certain medications by the IM route, and most immunizations are still being given by this route.

The recommended injection site for children under 3 years of age is the vastus lateralis. It is well developed at birth, is the largest muscle mass in infants and small children, and has few major nerves and blood vessels. After 18 months, the ventrogluteal site may be used. It is free of major blood vessels and nerves as well. The dorsogluteal site should not be used in any child who has not been walking for at least 1-2 years, and it is generally avoided in children younger than 6 years of age. The deltoid is also avoided in young children because the small muscle mass cannot hold large volumes of medication, nor should it be used if medications need to be injected into deep muscle mass. It should be used only for very small amounts of medication (0.5 mL for the 6-14 year old; 1.0 mL for the older adolescent). Figure 17-13 shows the location of preferred injection sites.

The size of the syringe and needle to be used depends on several factors: the size of the child, the amount of

medication to be given, the amount of muscle tissue available, and the viscosity of the medication. A 23-gauge to 25-gauge needle 0.5 to 1 inch long is usually used. Generally, 1 mL is the maximum volume to be administered at one site in older infants and small children. Figure 17-13 provides guidelines for IM injections.

The nurse should anticipate some protest from children in regard to injections. EMLA cream should be applied 1-2 hours prior to the injection. Whenever possible, a second nurse should be available to distract and restrain the child when necessary. If discomfort is minimized, the patient is less likely to fear a return visit. If a parent chooses to be present, he or she should not be asked to restrain the child but rather should be there for distraction before and comforting after the procedure. The nurse should remain with the child until the child is calm and can focus attention on more pleasant things.

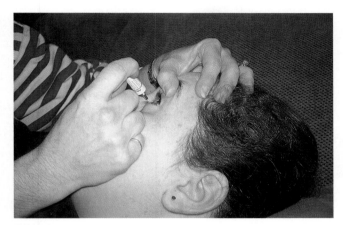

FIGURE **17-12** Administration of eye ointment or eye drops. The eye ointment/eyedrops should fall in the center of the lower conjunctival sac, *never* directly on the eyeball. Wipe excess medication with separate tissues for each eye, from the inner to the outer canthus.

 Communication Alert

When children ask whether a procedure will hurt, the nurse should be truthful. The nurse might say, "Some children say it feels a little like a mosquito bite. I want you to tell me what you think after we are finished." EMLA (eutectic mixture of local anesthetics) cream can be used to reduce pain for procedures such as IV starts or lumbar spinal taps (Figure 17-14).

Ventrogluteal site. Use the hand opposite the side for injection to locate landmarks (e.g., to give in child's left hip, use your right hand to locate landmarks). Locate by placing your palm on the greater trochanter, index finger on the anterior superior iliac spine, and middle finger on the posterior edge of the iliac spine. Inject into center of the V formed by the index and middle fingers.

 Guidelines: Insert needle at 90 degrees but directed slightly upward toward iliac crest. Use in any age. Use $^5/_8$-inch to 1-inch needle. Limit volume injected to 0.5 mL in infant, 1.5 mL in preschooler, 2 mL in older child. Site is free from major nerves and blood vessels.

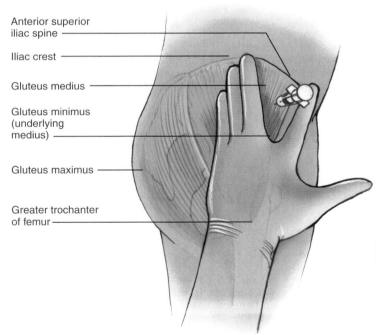

Anterior superior iliac spine

Iliac crest

Gluteus medius

Gluteus minimus (underlying medius)

Gluteus maximus

Greater trochanter of femur

A

FIGURE **17-13** Injection sites. **A,** *Ventrogluteal site.* Use the hand opposite the side for injection to locate landmarks (e.g., to give in child's left hip, use your right hand to locate the landmarks). Locate by placing your palm on the greater trochanter, index finger on the anterior superior iliac spine, and middle finger on the posterior edge of the iliac spine. Inject into center of the V formed by the index and middle fingers. **Guidelines:** Insert needle at 90 degrees but directed slightly upward toward iliac crest. Use in any age. Use $^5/_8$-inch to 1-inch needle. Limit volume injected to 0.5 mL in infant, 1.5 mL in preschooler, 2 mL in older child. Site is free from major nerves and blood vessels.

Continued

Vastus lateralis site. Palpate greater trochanter and knee. Divide into thirds; site is in middle third. Draw two imaginary lines from greater trochanter to knee: one midanteriorly, one midlaterally. Injection site is located between these lines in midlateral, anterior thigh.

 Guidelines: Insert needle at 90 degrees. Largest muscle available in infants and young children. Use $^5/_8$-inch to 1-inch needle. Limit volume injected to 0.5 mL in infant, 1 mL in toddler, 2 mL in school-age child. Site can be used in older children but is more painful than other sites. Site is relatively free from major nerves and blood vessels.

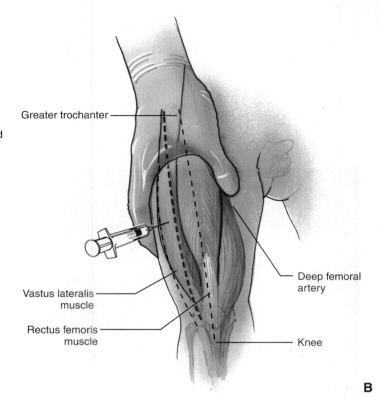

B

Deltoid site. Identify lower edge of acromion process and the point on the arm that is in line with axilla. Site is one to three fingerbreadths (depending on size of child) below the acromion process and just above the axilla. Inject into mid-deltoid region.

 Guidelines: Insert needle into muscle at 90 degrees, pointed slightly toward acromion process. Use $^1/_2$-inch to 1-inch needle. Muscle mass is limited so use small volumes (0.5 to 1 mL) and avoid irritating solutions. Avoid repeated injections. Site provides more rapid medication absorption than gluteal regions. Radial nerve lies under the deltoid muscle.

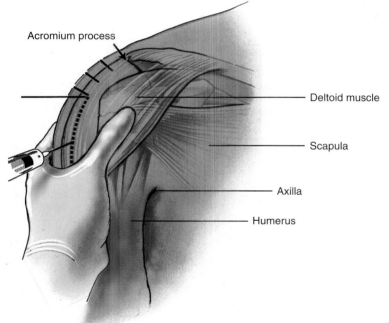

C

FIGURE **17-13, cont'd** Injection sites. **B,** *Vastus lateralis site.* Palpate greater trochanter and knee. Divide into thirds; site is in middle third. Draw two imaginary lines from greater trochanter to knee: one midanteriorly, one midlaterally. Injection site is located between these lines in midlateral, anterior thigh. **Guidelines:** Insert needle at 90 degrees. Largest muscle available in infants and young children. Use $^5/_8$-inch to 1-inch needle. Limit volume injected to 0.5 mL in infant, 1 mL in toddler, 2 mL in school-age child. Site can be used in older children but is more painful than other sites. Site is relatively free from major nerves and blood vessels. **C,** Deltoid site. Identify lower edge of acromion process and the point on the arm that is in line with axilla. Site is one to three fingerbreadths (depending on size of child) below the acromion process and just above the axilla. Inject into mid-deltoid region. **Guidelines:** Insert needle into muscle at 90 degrees, pointed slightly toward acromion process. Use $^1/_2$-inch to 1-inch needle. Muscle mass is limited so use small volumes (0.5 to 1 mL) and avoid irritating solutions. Avoid repeated injections. Site provides more rapid medication absorption than gluteal regions. Radial nerve lies under the deltoid muscle.

Dorsogluteal site. Locate posterior superior iliac spine and the greater trochanter; imagine a line between the two sites. Inject in the upper outer region above the imaginary line into the gluteus medius muscle.

Guidelines: Have the child lie prone and toe-in to relax muscle. Insert needle at 90 degrees perpendicular to surface on which child is lying. Use ¹/₂-inch to 1¹/₂-inch needle depending on the child's size. Site can accommodate larger volumes (1.5 mL in school-age, 2 mL in adolescent). Close to the sciatic nerve and superior gluteal artery.

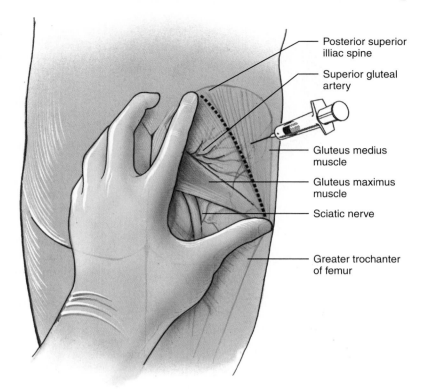

D

FIGURE **17-13, cont'd** Injection sites. **D,** Dorsogluteal site. Locate posterior superior iliac spine and the greater trochanter; imagine a line between the two sites. Inject in the upper outer region above the imaginary line into the gluteus medius muscle. **Guidelines:** Have the child lie prone and toe-in to relax muscle. Insert needle at 90 degrees perpendicular to surface on which child is lying. Should not be used in children younger than 2 years of age (need to have been walking for at least 1 year). The muscle is not well developed, and the margin of error is very small. Use ¹/₂-inch to 1¹/₂-inch needle depending on the child's size. Site can accommodate larger volumes (1.5 mL in school-age child, 2 mL in adolescent). Close to the sciatic nerve and superior gluteal artery.

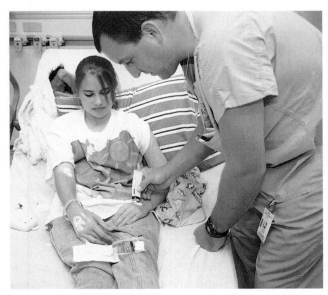

FIGURE **17-14** EMLA cream is placed on the site at least 1 hour before the painful procedure.

SUBCUTANEOUS AND INTRADERMAL MEDICATIONS

Subcutaneous and intradermal medications may also be ordered for children. Subcutaneous injections are given in the dorsum of the upper arm and anterior of the thigh for infants and toddlers. The abdomen and fat pads above the iliac crests and hips may be used. Insulin is one medication ordered subcutaneously. Some vaccines are also ordered by this route. Small needles (25- to 27-gauge) and small amounts (up to 0.5 mL) with short needles (¹/₂- to ⁵/₈-inch) are used. A 90-degree angle is generally used (a 45-degree angle may be preferred if little subcutaneous tissue is present), and aspiration is generally not required. Always check institutional policy.

The intradermal route is ordered for medications such as tuberculin testing. Generally a 25-gauge, ¹/₂-inch needle is used. The amount is small (0.1 mL). Administered at a 10- to 15-degree angle, the needle will barely penetrate the skin on the inner aspect of the forearm. A bleb should be observed if technique is correct. Record the forearm used and patient tolerance.

INTRAVENOUS MEDICATIONS

Medications are routinely administered by the IV route in pediatric patients. IV infusion sites are illustrated in Figure 17-15. Some drugs are effective only if given by this method. The medication is also absorbed more rapidly, which is of value. IV medications usually require a specified dilution and rate of administration. **Always refer to an IV medication book for specific information on pediatric dosages and administration**

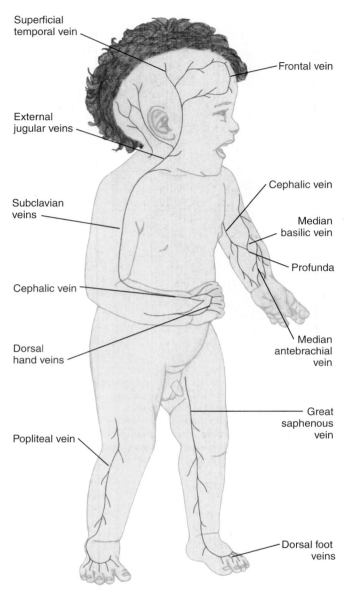

Superficial temporal vein

Frontal vein

External jugular veins

Cephalic vein

Subclavian veins

Median basilic vein

Profunda

Cephalic vein

Dorsal hand veins

Median antebrachial vein

Great saphenous vein

Popliteal vein

Dorsal foot veins

FIGURE **17-15** Sites for IV infusion in children.

information. It is also less traumatic for the child to receive some medications, such as pain medications and antibiotics, IV rather than IM. The nurse assesses the IV site carefully for infiltration, inflammation, and patency, particularly before administration of the medication. **Always check the institution's policy to determine who can administer IV medications.**

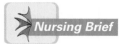

Document the type and rate of infusion, IV line location, and appearance of the site, according to the policy of the institution. Many institutions require hourly notations.

Compatibility is always checked between the fluid that is infusing and the medication to be given. The IV line must be flushed before and after the medication if it is not compatible with the IV solution. If two drugs are ordered to be given at the same time, compatibility must be checked again. Only one antibiotic should be administered at a time. Medication is *never* administered via blood products.

Children should not receive IV fluids without a continuous infusion pump to prevent fluid overload. Medications may be added directly to the IV bag or bottle. More often, medications are added to the Soluset (calibrated burette) or are given with precision-controlled syringe pumps (Figure 17-16). The precision-controlled syringe pump, sometimes called an *autosyringe*, allows a small amount of fluid to be given over a specified period of time. In addition, IV pumps are now being designed specifically for medication administration with children. Although the use of this equipment provides a safety factor, the nurse must remember that it is a machine and is subject to failing. For this reason, children receiving IV fluids must be observed closely. The *piggyback* method is also used in children. In general, antibiotics should infuse within 30 minutes to 1 hour. Always check the IV medication book for time frames.

Long-Term Venous Access

The heparin lock is usually used as an alternative for a keep-open infusion when long-term access is needed for administration of medication. The needle remains in place and is flushed with heparin or saline solution, according to the protocol of the hospital. The child is not continuously connected to IV tubing, which allows the patient more freedom.

PICCs or peripherally inserted central catheters can be used for short- to moderate-term therapy. They are inserted by specially trained nurses or physicians, most commonly above the antecubital area. The catheter is threaded into the superior vena cava and can be used for total parenteral nutrition (TPN), IV fluids, and IV medications.

Indwelling central venous catheters (Broviac or Hickman catheters) and implantable infusion ports (MediPort, Port-A-Cath) are other methods of obtaining long-term venous access. Medications, TPN, chemotherapy, IV fluids, and blood products can be given through the catheter. IV tubing is changed daily on a child with a central line, to reduce the risk for infection. The child and the parents are taught how to care for the catheter at home. They are also taught how the catheters are flushed with saline and heparin, to maintain patency and prevent clotting. The approach to care of these catheters varies, and each institution provides this information. Older children and parents need to be taught signs of infection, regardless of which IV device is used.

RECTAL MEDICATIONS

Some drugs (Tylenol, glycerin) come in the form of suppositories. Children's suppositories are long and

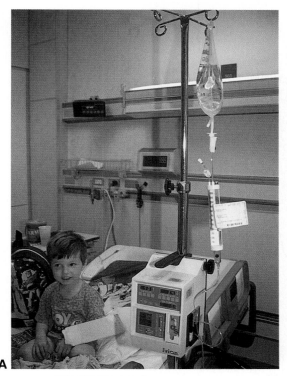
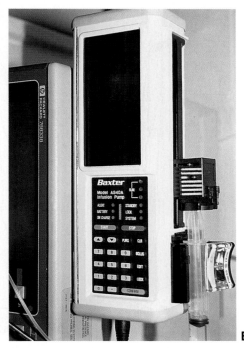

FIGURE **17-16** **A,** Intravenous medication being administered via Buretrol. Note the sticker on the Buretrol to alert all staff that medication is infusing. **B,** Autosyringe.

thin in comparison with the cone-shaped types administered to adults. The nurse, wearing gloves, inserts the lubricated suppository well beyond the anal sphincter; about half as far as the forefinger reaches. The nurse applies pressure to the anus by gently holding the buttocks together until the patient's desire to expel the suppository subsides.

PRINCIPLES OF FLUID BALANCE IN CHILDREN

Infants and small children have different proportions of **body water and body fat** than do adults (Figure 17-17), and the water needs and water losses of the infant, per unit of body weight, are greater. In children under 2 years of age, surface area is particularly important in fluid and electrolyte balance because more water is lost through the skin than through the kidneys. The surface area of the infant is two to three times greater than that of the adult in proportion to body volume or body weight. **Metabolic rate** and **heat production** are also two to three times greater in infants per kilogram of body weight. This produces more **waste products,** which must be diluted to be excreted. It also stimulates respiration, which causes greater evaporation through the lungs. Compared with adults, children less than 2 years old have a greater percentage of body water contained in the **extracellular compartment.**

Fluid turnover is rapid, and dehydration occurs more quickly in infants than in adults. (Signs of dehy-

dration are outlined in Chapter 8.) The infant cannot survive as long as the adult can in the presence of continued water depletion. A sick infant does not adapt as rapidly to **shifts in intake and output** because the **kidneys lack maturity**. Their kidneys are less able to concentrate urine and require more water than an adult's kidneys to excrete a given amount of solute. Disturbances of the gastrointestinal tract frequently lead to vomiting and diarrhea. Electrolyte balance depends on fluid balance and cardiovascular, renal, adrenal, pituitary, parathyroid, and pulmonary regulatory mechanisms. Many of these mechanisms are maturing in the developing child and are unable to react to full capacity under the stress of illness.

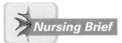
Nursing Brief

One way of determining fluid loss in infants is to weigh the wet diaper (urine or liquid stool), subtract the weight of a comparable dry diaper, and record the difference.

ORAL FLUIDS

Whenever possible, fluids are given by mouth. It is the most natural and satisfactory method. The nurse must use ingenuity to encourage the sick child to take enough fluids because the patient may refuse food and water and cannot understand their relation to recovery. The

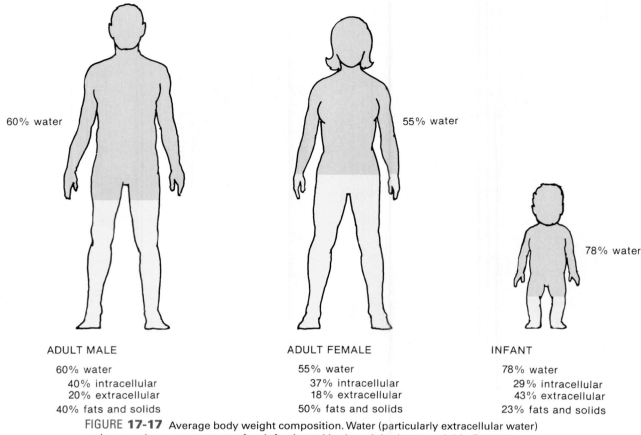

ADULT MALE	ADULT FEMALE	INFANT
60% water	55% water	78% water
40% intracellular	37% intracellular	29% intracellular
20% extracellular	18% extracellular	43% extracellular
40% fats and solids	50% fats and solids	23% fats and solids

FIGURE **17-17** Average body weight composition. Water (particularly extracellular water) makes up a larger percentage of an infant's total body weight than an adult's. Because extracellular water is lost first when water loss occurs in illness, trauma, or environmental stress, the infant is extremely susceptible to fluid and electrolyte imbalances.

infant and small child become dehydrated faster than the adult does. Toddlers and infants are not capable of drinking by themselves. The busy nurse must find time to offer fluids and must be patient and gently persistent. Liquids are offered frequently and in small amounts. Brightly colored containers and drinking straws may be a help. The nurse keeps an accurate record of the patient's intake and output. The doctor cannot determine whether a child needs IV fluids with a partially completed chart. **The importance of this particular responsibility on the pediatric unit cannot be overemphasized.**

Some common clear liquid fluids used to replace fluid lost are Popsicles, lemon-lime drinks, and the oral replacement solutions such as Pedialyte.

PARENTERAL FLUIDS

Parenteral (*para*, beside or apart; *enteron*, intestine) fluids are those given by some route other than the digestive tract. This is necessary when sickness is accompanied by vomiting or loss of consciousness or when the gastrointestinal system requires rest. Use of parenteral fluids is important in severe cases of vomiting and diarrhea in which the excessive loss of water and electrolytes leads to death if untreated. It also provides a means for the safe and effective administration of

selective parenteral medications. Solutions given parenterally must be sterile to prevent a general or local infection. The nurse must be aware of the importance of parenteral therapy and the problems that might arise.

The infant or child receiving parenteral fluids needs the nurse's warmth and affection. Babies still need to be held and derive the pleasures they receive from sucking a pacifier if it is not contraindicated. Older children need suitable diversions and company. Intake and output should be charted on all children receiving parenteral fluids.

Fluids Given via Vein

Intravenous infusion presents certain problems in pediatric patients. The procedure is more complicated and dangerous in infants and small children and is more taxing psychologically. The infant's veins are small and hard to locate. The veins of the scalp may be used, which requires shaving the head. The baby must be effectively restrained to prevent the needle from becoming dislodged. When fluids are given IV, regardless of the site, the infant must be **closely observed.** Fluids given by vein are passing into a closed space that can be distended only to a certain point without serious difficulties. If the circulation becomes overloaded with fluid that is infused too rapidly, cardiac failure can result. IV medications should *always* be administered to a child via an infusion pump. For purposes of calculating fluid volume and IV rate in children, the pediatric patient receives 60 mini- or micro-drops per cubic centimeter rather than the usual 10 or 15 drops from the standard adult set-up.

In-line volume control devices, such as a Buretrol, are an added safety feature in some hospitals. The pump can be set to deliver only what the Buretrol holds (100-150 mL). This also reduces the risk for accidental fluid volume overload. Infusion pumps have an alarm that sounds when difficulties arise. Such safeguards, however, do not replace close observation and charting by the nurse.

The nurse should observe the child for these changes:
- Swelling or redness at the insertion site
- Moisture at the site or on the dressing covering the site
- Complaint of pain or inconsolable crying when fluids or medications are infusing.

A special hourly chart is kept on infants who are being given fluids via vein. The nurse charts such information as time, name and amount of the solution, amount infused, rate of infusion, amount of fluid remaining in the bag, location of infusion site, and condition of the site.

TOTAL PARENTERAL NUTRITION

Intravenous alimentation solutions are complex combinations of crystalline amino acids, glucose, vitamins, trace minerals, and electrolytes. Conditions other than low birth weight that may require their use include severe burns, chronic intestinal obstruction, intractable diarrhea, irradiation, and other life-threatening maladies. Although the beginning student would not be given total responsibility for the child receiving total parenteral nutrition (TPN), all nursing personnel must be alert to the fact that this is not just the usual superficial vein infusion.

A Silastic catheter is passed directly into the superior vena cava by way of the jugular or subclavian vein, with careful surgical technique. It is secured in place. A filter is attached. An infusion pump is essential for hourly monitoring of the flow. The patient receiving TPN must be carefully supervised and evaluated. If an infusion gets behind, it must be reported to the charge nurse; it is *never* adjusted to "catch up." Increasing or decreasing the rate of TPN can cause hyperglycemia or hypoglycemia. Complications of TPN can be serious and are related to both the catheter and the metabolism of the infusate. The bag, IV tubing, and filter (if used) must be changed every 24 hours to prevent infections. Any IV tubing connections to be taken apart must be cleaned with an antiseptic solution before doing so to prevent contamination. All connections should be taped to prevent accidental separation. Contamination via catheter or solution is particularly dangerous because infectious organisms have direct access to body circulation. **Thrombosis** (development of a blood clot), dislodgment of the catheter, or **extravasation** (the escape of fluid into surrounding tissue) can occur. **Metabolic complications** include hyperglycemia because of the high glucose content of the solution, osmotic diuresis, dehydration, and **azotemia** (the presence of nitrogenous bodies in the blood). Home hyperalimentation is being successfully used for selected children. This requires specific instruction and demonstration by specialty teams. Continuous support and supervision are vital to success. The parents' insurance coverage should be reviewed because home hyperalimentation is costly.

Peripheral vein hyperalimentation may be used for short-term therapy or as a supplement to IV alimentation. A more dilute concentration is generally used. Infiltration must be avoided because severe tissue sloughing from dextrose irritation may occur. Because hyperalimentation provides no fatty acids, fat or lipid emulsions may be ordered; these may be administered with a peripheral line or central line. Lipids must be added aseptically below the filter because the fat particles are too large to pass through it.

PROCEDURES TO ASSIST NUTRITION, DIGESTION, AND ELIMINATION

GASTROSTOMY

A gastrostomy (*gastro*, stomach; *stoma*, opening) is made for the purpose of introducing food directly into the stomach through the abdominal wall (Skill 17-7). This is done with a surgically placed tube or button (Figure 17-18). It is used in patients who cannot take food by mouth because of anomalies or corrosive strictures of the esophagus or who are severely debilitated or in coma.

GASTROSTOMY BUTTON FEEDING

The gastrostomy feeding button may be used with children requiring long-term enteral feeding. Buttons are small, flexible silicone devices. The stomach end has a mushroom-like dome. The skin end has a flat surface that allows the child a more normal lifestyle (see Figure 17-18). There is a one-way valve to prevent reflux of stomach contents.

In both the tube and button, skin care is a concern. Special attention should be paid to the area under the wings of the button. The wings are periodically rotated. If breakdown does occur, the button is changed to one that has a longer shaft. The area around the stoma should be cleansed frequently with mild soap and water. If a small gauze dressing is used, it should be kept dry.

ENEMA

Administering an enema to a child is essentially the same as to an adult; however, the amount, type, and

Skill 17-7 Gastrostomy Tube Feeding

■ Equipment

✓ Tray with room-temperature formula
✓ Funnel or syringe barrel
✓ Syringe for aspiration, to flush tube as ordered (may be up to 15 to 30 mL)

NOTE: Equipment should be sterile for premature and newborn infants.

■ Safety Issues

- Cold formula can cause abdominal discomfort—always use formula at room temperature.
- Position child with head elevated unless contraindicated.
- Check for residual volume.
- Do not allow air to get into feeding tube.
- Never force a feeding.
- Stop feeding if signs of respiratory distress, vomiting, cyanosis, or abdominal distention occur.
- Leave patient with head of bed elevated and positioned on right side unless contraindicated.

■ Method

1. Explain procedure.
2. Gather equipment.
3. Wash hands.
4. Position child comfortably, with head slightly elevated if not contraindicated. Provide pacifier to relax a baby. An infant can be held and cuddled during the feeding; an older child can sit in a highchair.
5. Check residual stomach contents by attaching syringe to gastrostomy tube and aspirating. (Authors vary on their approach to checking and replacing residual. Always check the institution's policy on this.) Residual is always checked because overloading the stomach can cause reflux and increase the danger of aspiration. If the residual amount continues or increases, this needs to be reported to the physician.

6. Attach syringe barrel to gastrostomy tube. Fill with formula. Remove clamp. (This prevents air from entering the stomach and causing distention.)
7. Elevate receptacle. Allow formula to flow slowly by gravity—force should *never* be used.
8. Continue to add formula to the syringe before it empties completely. The feeding should take 20 to 25 minutes to complete to prevent regurgitation, vomiting, or aspiration. Always observe for signs of respiratory distress, vomiting, cyanosis, or abdominal distention. Stop feeding if any of these occur and notify the charge nurse.
9. Clamp the tube as the final formula or water is passing through the lower part of the syringe. (Note: In infants, some physicians may prefer that the gastrostomy tube remain open at all times to produce a safety valve in the event that the baby vomits. In such cases, the tube is elevated above the patient's body.)
10. Whenever possible, hold the patient quietly after feeding. Reposition in Fowler's position or on the right side to promote gastric emptying.
11. Record the type (gastrostomy feeding), the amount given, the amount and characteristics of the residual, and how the patient tolerated the procedure. If the patient is on measured fluids, record on intake and output section.

■ Skills Checklist

✓ Explain procedure.
✓ Assemble equipment.
✓ Wash hands.
✓ Check residual.
✓ Attach syringe barrel, add formula.
✓ Elevate receptacle.
✓ Continue to add formula.
✓ Clamp tube at end of procedure.
✓ Position or hold patient.
✓ Document procedure.

insertion depth require modification (Table 17-2). Mineral oil enemas are considered safe, as are saline enemas. Mineral oil enemas can be purchased at the drug store or pharmacy without a prescription. Saline enemas can be made at home by mixing 2 level teaspoons of table salt to a quart of lukewarm distilled water. Do not use soapsuds, hydrogen peroxide, or plain water as an enema (tap water is isotonic and can cause a rapid fluid shift and overload). In addition, Fleet's phosphate enemas (labeled as saline enemas) can cause serious side effects and are not recommended for children.

Always be certain you know what type of solution is intended. This is an invasive procedure for the patient; therefore careful age-appropriate explanations are necessary. Other invasive procedures related to the gastrointestinal tract include barium enema, intestinal biopsy, endoscopy, and colonoscopy. These are performed by the gastroenterologist.

To administer the enema, place a towel under the child, lubricate the enema tube or nozzle with a lubricant such as KY jelly and insert 1½ to 2 inches into the rectum. Instill the solution slowly without pressure

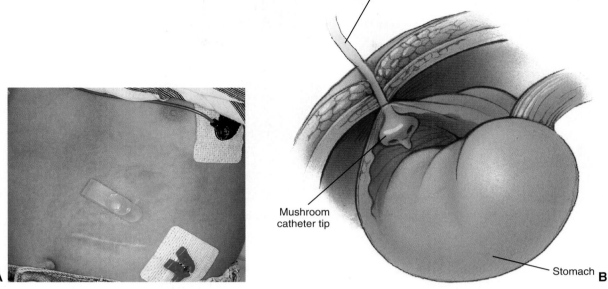

FIGURE **17-18** **A,** A skin-level gastrostomy access device has a low profile and therefore is not as bulky or obvious as gastrostomy tubes. **B,** The gastrostomy mushroom tip prevents the tube from being pulled out.

Table 17-2	*Enema Administration Guidelines*	
AGE	**VOLUME AMOUNT (mL)**	**INSERTION DEPTH (iN)**
Infant	120-240	1
2-4 yr	240-360	2
4-10 yr	360-480	3
11 yr and older	480-720	4

for approximately 10 to 15 minutes; the tubing should be clamped at intervals, especially if the child has cramping. Encourage the older child to "hold" the solution 3 to 5 minutes if possible. The time of procedure; name, amount, and temperature of solution used; amount and character of results; untoward reactions; and child's response should all be recorded.

OSTOMY

An *ostomy* is a general term referring to any operation in which an artificial opening is formed between two hollow organs or between one or more such viscera and the abdominal wall for discharge of intestinal contents or of urine. Conditions requiring a child to have an ostomy (**colostomy,** involving the large intestine, or **ileostomy,** involving the small intestine) include necrotizing enterocolitis, Hirschsprung's disease, imperforate anus, inflammatory bowel syndrome, spina bifida, tumor, or trauma. A **urostomy,** or urinary diversion, is performed if the bladder or urinary tract is involved.

Parents of a child with an ostomy need to understand many things before discharge. They need to know the reason for the surgery, any special nutritional needs, dietary modifications, signs and symptoms of complications, supplies needed for care, and resources in the community. They also need to know how to provide the care. The procedure is similar to the adult procedure with size modification, except that the infant's ostomy is covered with a dressing. Dressings are changed after each bowel movement. Once the stoma has healed and the infant is large enough to wear a pouch, care is similar to that for an adult (Figure 17-19). Skin management can be a challenge with infants and children because of the fragility of the skin. Always provide good skin care to prevent breakdown at the stoma site.

CARE OF THE CHILD WITH A TRACHEOSTOMY

A tracheostomy is a surgical procedure in which an opening is made in the trachea to enable the patient to breathe. This artificial airway may be used in emergency situations, may be an elective procedure, or may be combined with mechanical ventilation. Some of the childhood conditions that may require tracheostomy are acute laryngotracheobronchitis, epiglottitis, head injury, burns, or any condition in which the patient is unconscious or debilitated for an extended period. Nursing care is indispensable to the survival of the patient because blockage of the tube by mucus or other secretions can lead to suffocation. In many hospitals, the patient is placed in the intensive care unit immediately after surgery because this is a critical period requiring frequent suctioning and very close observation. When the condition stabilizes, the child is transferred to a regular unit.

The child with a tracheostomy is placed in an area of high visibility. Infants and small children

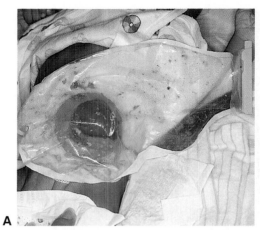
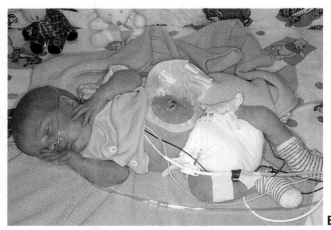

FIGURE **17-19** Note the reduction in the stoma from shortly after surgery (**A**) to several weeks later (**B**).

normally communicate their needs by crying, but the tracheostomy prohibits vocalization. Whenever possible, one person is assigned to the child and to work with the parents. Reinforce preoperative teaching. Explain what has happened in an age-appropriate manner. For example, "You were having a lot of trouble breathing. This operation called a tracheostomy helps you breathe easier. A small opening has been made in your neck. A hollow tube was inserted to keep the area open. It is frightening not to be able to speak. When you are better, the hole will close by itself and your voice will return." An explanation of suction might be, "We have to keep the area in your neck open. This tube goes into the airway and clears it." Demonstrate use of suction in a glass of water. Prepare the child for the unfamiliar sound. "You might feel like gagging, but afterward you will feel better. I know this is difficult for you, and I'm sorry there is no easier way." Another approach is to make up a story involving the child's favorite toy, which goes to the repair shop because the toy is having trouble breathing.

The nursing care of the child with a tracheostomy is a significant responsibility. The anatomical differences between children and adults and the small child's inability to communicate through writing increase the need for close observation. Added moisture and humidity are provided by the use of a special tracheostomy collar, or direct attachment to a mechanical ventilator. This is necessary because the nose and mouth no longer warm and moisten the inspired air. Toddlers and infants often have short, stubby necks that become easily irritated with tracheostomy ties.

Maintaining **patency** of the tracheostomy tube is of utmost importance. Plastic or Silastic tubes are generally used because they are flexible and reduce crust formation. They are lightweight and disposable, and most do not have inner cannulas. Cuffed tubes are not usually necessary in infants and small children because their air passages are smaller and the

tracheostomy tube provides a sufficient seal. The surgeon chooses a tracheostomy tube that is appropriate for the size of the patient's neck and condition.

SUCTIONING

Selection of a suction catheter by the nurse is of importance. Choose one that does not completely block the tube during suctioning. The diameter should be approximately one half that of the tracheostomy tube. Measure the length of the tracheostomy tube (use an extra one) and pass the suction catheter only the measured length to prevent trauma to the mucosa. Instilling a small amount of sterile isotonic saline solution into the tube before suctioning is controversial and currently subject to ongoing research. Findings generally indicate this is not best practice and may contribute to lower respiratory infection.

Suctioning is done when there are signs of secretions in the airway (Skill 17-8). This may include coughing, noisy breathing, or a bubbling sound. When suctioning the tracheostomy tube, do not apply suction as the catheter is introduced. Withdraw the catheter while rotating and applying suction by covering the port on the catheter with the thumb. Hold suction no more than 5 seconds (Hockenberry et al., 2005). The child should be allowed to rest for about a minute (and take two or three breaths) between suctioning. Most institutions advise the use of hyperventilating with 100% oxygen between suctioning to prevent hypoxia. The use of pulse oximetry can provide a measure of the child's oxygenation during and after the procedure. Nurses should be aware of any variations in this procedure that might be unique to the agency in which they are working.

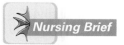

Nursing Brief

Many institutions teach tracheostomy suctioning for home care as a clean rather than sterile technique.

Skill 17-8 Suctioning the Tracheostomy

■ Equipment
✓ Sterile suctioning catheters
✓ Sterile gloves
✓ Bag-valve mask for hyperventilating
✓ Sterile saline solution

■ Safety Issues
• Maintain sterile technique during procedure.
• Monitor the amount of time suction is applied.
• Provide reoxygenation between suctioning attempts.
• Monitor for signs of respiratory distress during procedure.

■ Method
1. Explain procedure.
2. Gather equipment.
3. Wash hands; put on sterile gloves.
4. If necessary, hyperventilate the child with 100% oxygen to prevent hypoxia.
5. Lubricate the tube with sterile saline solution and insert the catheter without applying suction.
6. Withdraw the catheter in a continuous rotating motion while applying suction (5 seconds only).
7. Allow the child to rest. Some children may need a few breaths via a resuscitation bag.

8. Clear the catheter with sterile saline solution between insertions; child may need to be suctioned more than once. Saline solution should also be discarded to prevent growth of *Pseudomonas* in the standing solution.
9. Document: Time and frequency of suctioning, the character of the secretions, the relief afforded the patient, the patient's behavior, the appearance of the stoma, and any other pertinent data.

■ Skills Checklist
✓ Explain procedure.
✓ Gather equipment.
✓ Wash hands; put on sterile gloves.
✓ Instill normal saline solution per institutional policy.
✓ Insert catheter.
✓ Apply suction while withdrawing the catheter.
✓ Allow/provide ventilation.
✓ Rinse catheter tubing.
✓ Repeat as necessary.
✓ Discard equipment and saline solution.
✓ Document procedure.

CARE OF THE TRACHEAL STOMA

The tracheal stoma is treated as a surgical wound. Keep the area free of secretions and exudate to minimize the risk for infection. Nonsterile gloves and eye protection should be used when caring for a tracheostomy. Cotton-tipped applicators dipped in half-strength hydrogen peroxide can be used to remove crusted mucus. Rinse by dipping in sterile water. Change the gauze square or Telfa pad under the tracheostomy site as needed. If this dressing remains wet, it causes skin irritation. Always check the stoma site for signs of infection and breakdown of the skin.

Ties around the child's neck should be snug but loose enough that one finger can be inserted easily. Place the knot to the side of the neck. Assess the condition of the skin beneath the ties. Document the skin condition. Change the ties daily and as necessary. Two people should be used for this procedure, one to hold the cannula and the other to change the ties. It works best if the new ties are looped through the flanges and tied snugly in a triple knot at the side of the neck *before* the soiled ties are cut and removed (Hockenberry et al., 2005).

The nurse observes the patient for such symptoms as restlessness, rising pulse rate, fatigue, apathy, dyspnea,

sternal retractions, pallor, cyanosis, and inflammation or drainage around the incision. Possible complications include tracheoesophageal fistula, stenosis, tracheal ischemia, infection, atelectasis, cannula occlusion, and accidental extubation. Baseline assessment of the patient is done on each shift and before suctioning. The patient's mental status, respirations, pulse rate and rhythm, and chest sounds are of particular importance. Accurate recording of observations is essential to evaluation.

A sterile hemostat is kept at the bedside for emergency use. Accidental **extubation** or expulsion of the tube, although uncommon, can occur from severe coughing if the ties are too loose. Patency of the airway is maintained by spreading the edges of the wound with the sterile clamp until a duplicate tube is inserted. Extra tracheostomy tubes, one the same size and one smaller, and the equipment needed for its replacement are always kept in a visible, easily reached area at the bedside for use in such emergencies. As the child's condition improves, he or she is weaned from the tube. The opening gradually closes with granulation. Children whose tubes must remain in place longer require periodic tube change. This is generally done on a weekly basis once healing has occurred.

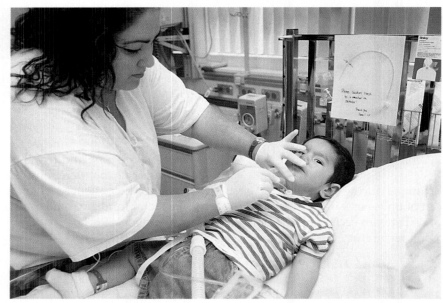

FIGURE **17-20** Caretakers should be given ample opportunity to take care of the child's tracheostomy before the child is discharged.

Additional nursing measures include frequent change of position, the use of arm restraints, oral feedings unless contraindicated, and careful bathing to prevent water from entering the tube. Range-of-motion exercises are a must for long-term patients, and in acute cases, arm restraints are removed one at a time to allow for passive exercises. The diet is ordered by the physician. Although patients initially may have nothing by mouth (NPO), as their condition improves, they progress to a soft or normal diet. Fowler's position is preferred during feedings. Older children can cooperate by holding their head flexed with the chin down. This decreases swallowing difficulties because the esophagus opens and the airway narrows. Monitor feeding of an infant closely so that no food particles are aspirated through the tracheostomy.

Some patients are discharged with a tracheostomy. This should be anticipated, and instruction and demonstration for the parents should begin early (Figure 17-20). Parents who are comfortable with the procedure during hospitalization feel more secure when the child returns home. It is advisable for the parents to be "checked off" on tracheostomy procedures before discharge, and most hospitals now require this. Parents should also learn CPR if their child has a tracheostomy. Information about parent groups and the visiting nurse and other referrals are made before discharge.

OXYGEN THERAPY FOR CHILDREN

GENERAL SAFETY CONSIDERATIONS

It is important that all equipment used for oxygen therapy be inspected periodically to determine that materials are intact and that no pieces are missing. Keep combustible materials and potential sources of fire away from oxygen equipment. These materials are essentially the same as for adults; however, for the child, friction toys are also to be avoided. Know where the nearest fire extinguisher is located.

Infection control is extremely important. It is imperative that cross infection via unclean equipment be prevented. Humidifiers and nebulizers, which are warm and moist, provide excellent niches for the growth of disease-producing organisms. Although most masks, tents, and cannulas that come into direct contact with the child are disposable, other pieces of mechanical equipment cannot be discarded. **They require periodic cleaning if therapy is extended and terminal cleaning according to product direction.**

Prolonged exposure to high oxygen concentrations can be toxic to some body tissues (e.g., the retina in preterm babies and the lungs in the general population) but particularly in children with pulmonary diseases such as asthma or cystic fibrosis. It is therefore necessary to measure oxygen content at regular intervals with an **oxygen analyzer.** This is usually done by the respiratory department; however, the nurse needs to be sure that the procedure is carried out on the assigned patients. Readings should be obtained close to the child's head. The amount of oxygen administered depends on the child's arterial oxygen concentration. Frequent blood gas determinations (PO_2 and PCO_2) ensure safe and accurate therapy. Noninvasive techniques that measure blood oxygen tension via the skin are available. One example is the **pulse oximeter** (Figure 17-21).

Oxygen is a dry gas and requires the addition of moisture to prevent irritation of the respiratory tree. **Oxygen therapy should be terminated gradually.** This allows the patient to adjust to *ambient* (environmental) oxygen. Slowly reduce the liter flow, open the air vents in incubators, or open zippers in the oxygen tent.

Constantly monitor the child's response. An increase in restlessness, a decrease in pulse oximeter readings, and an increase in pulse and respirations indicate that the child is not tolerating withdrawal from the oxygen-enriched environment.

METHODS OF ADMINISTRATION

Oxygen is administered to pediatric patients as age-appropriate via Isolette, nasal cannula, mask, hood, or tent (Table 17-3). The method of delivery is often determined by what method the child tolerates (Figure 17-22). If uncooperative in a tent or with a mask, the child may receive oxygen with the oxygen tubing held near the mouth and nose of the child. Regardless of the method used, the child is observed frequently to determine the effectiveness of the oxygen. **The desired goals include decreased restlessness and improved breathing, vital signs, and color.** The highest concentrations of oxygen are delivered with a plastic hood. Warmed, humidified oxygen is delivered directly over the child's head. It may be used in an incubator or warming unit.

Oxygen tents are available from various manufacturers. Often the respiratory therapy department sets these up. Nurses need to be aware of certain precautions in case they are required to set up the oxygen tent. The directions for the specific apparatus should be closely followed. Before assembling the tent, carefully examine the plastic for tears. Tents consist of a plastic canopy suspended from an overhead rod that is attached to a cabinet containing a machine. When adjusted, the machine regulates the ventilation and temperature of the tent and may also provide increased humidity in connection with the oxygen flow. Following are several general recommendations for the use of tents:

- Prepare bed; place bath blanket and absorbent pad over the mattress.
- Select the tent according to the age and size of the patient. This information should be ascertained before admission for patients in acute respiratory distress.
- Bring the canopy and control unit to the bedside; extend the overhead bar and fold tent out along the bar.
- Plug in control cabinet and turn on unit. If there is a ventilation control on the refrigerator unit, set this halfway between low and high or according to the manufacturer's instructions.
- Connect tubing to oxygen flow meter and flush tent with oxygen for 2 minutes. Reset flow meter to the prescribed number of liters. Another method is to allow oxygen to flow at 15 liters for about 30 minutes. Analyze the concentration.
- Maintain a tight canopy. Provide nursing care through zippered openings; organize nursing care. Oxygen loss is greater at the bottom of the tent because oxygen is heavier than air. The front of the tent may be secured with bath blanket

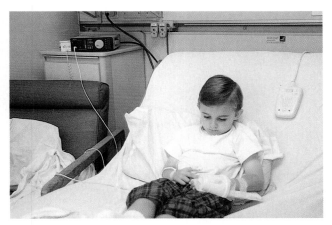

FIGURE **17-21** Child with pulse oximeter. The finger probe has a red sensor light that fascinates some children. Pulse oximetry is a simple, painless, noninvasive means of measuring the oxygen saturation of the blood (SaO_2). The sensor is placed on the toe or the end of the finger, over the nail. The sensor obtains readings either continuously or intermittently. It is available in infant and pediatric sizes.

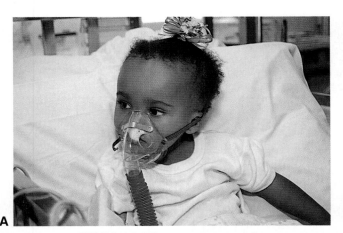

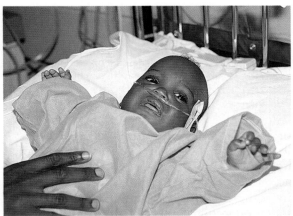

A   B

FIGURE **17-22** Oxygen delivery. **A,** Child receiving oxygen via a face mask. **B,** Infant with a nasal cannula.

Table 17-3 | *Selected Considerations for the Child Receiving Oxygen*

AGE	COMMENTS
General considerations	Signs of respiratory distress include an increase in pulse and respiration, restlessness, flaring nares intercostal and substernal retractions, and cyanosis. In addition, children with dyspnea frequently vomit, which increases the danger of aspiration. Maintain a clear airway with suctioning if needed. Organize nursing care so that interruptions are kept to a minimum. Observe children carefully because your vision may be obstructed by mist and young children are unable to verbalize their needs.
Neonate	Oxygen may be provided via hood, which may be used in incubator or warming unit May be provided via Isolette; keep sleeves closed to decrease oxygen loss Oxygen needs to be warmed to prevent neonatal stress from cold Analyze concentration carefully to avoid pulmonary disease Parents are primary focus of preparations; help develop good parenting skills and self-confidence in their ability to care for the child who is ill
Infant	Nose may need to be suctioned with bulb syringe to remove mucus May benefit from use of infant seat; secure seat to bed frame, watch for slumping in seat Make sure crib sides are up; a canopy often gives the illusion of safety Avoid the use of baby oil, A and D ointment, Vaseline, or other oil-based or alcohol-based substances Anticipate stranger anxiety at around 8 mo; baby clings to parents, turns away from nurse An extremely irritable baby may benefit from comforting in parent's lap, followed by sleeping in tent; clarify at report time Frequently children can be removed from oxygen tent for bathing and eating; determine before proceeding
Toddler	Anticipate that a toddler will be distressed by a tent Anticipate regression A restless and fussy child may pull tent and covers apart Toddler cannot tell nurse if tent is "too hot" or "too cold" Change clothing and bed linen when damp Toddler may be comforted by transitional object such as a blanket Parents may have suggestions as to how to keep child happy in the tent
Preschool	Tent plastic distorts view Because thought processes are immature in preschool children, reality and fantasy are inseparable Prepare child for all procedures to decrease fear Anticipate that child will feel lonely and isolated Child will enjoy stories, puppets, dramatic play An extremely restless and anxious child may benefit from holding parent's hand through small opening in zippers Helpful if child can be out of tent for meals and can eat with peers
School-age	School children usually are less frightened by tent; fears center around body mutilation and loss of control Preparation information continues to focus on what the child will see, hear, feel, and be expected to do Child may benefit from writing a story about the experience; nurse reviews story with child and clarifies misconceptions; posting story on unit affirms child's self-esteem and mastery (always ask permission to post) Allow child to make realistic choices before, during, and after procedures Draw "what it feels like to be in a tent," discuss
Adolescent	Needs more time to process information, needs to know the results of blood studies and other tests Nurse remains available to the patient to answer questions as they arise Trust is extremely important as adolescent attempts to move beyond the nuclear family Anticipate problems of being restricted by apparatus May feel "weird" when visited by peers, wavers between feeling self-confident and feeling ineffective Reiterate no smoking and other safety precautions with patient and peers Include patient in therapy, may be able to manage own oxygen needs Review safe use of oxygen in the home if required for comfort and survival

or sheet. Tent temperature is adjusted to 64° F to 70° F (17.8° C to 21.1° C). The patient should not appear too warm or too cold. Dress the child according to body temperature.

- Inspect connecting tubes periodically for kinks, loose connections, or faulty apparatus. A hissing sound can be heard as oxygen passes through the tubing if the lines are patent. This may also be tested by holding one finger over the end momentarily.
- Empty condensation reservoir as needed.
- Refill distilled water jar as appropriate.
- Select toys that retard absorption and do not produce static electricity.

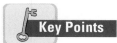

Key Points

- The medical care providers should provide atraumatic care by fostering child-parent relationships, providing information to the patient regarding treatments or procedures, controlling pain, providing privacy, providing play therapy, and giving choices.
- Have someone with the child at all times when bathing.
- Sterile techniques are necessary when obtaining a clean-catch urine specimen or a specimen with catheterization.
- Have an assistant help in the procedure when obtaining specimens from small children who cannot hold still.
- During lumbar puncture, always monitor the child's respiratory status.
- Dosages for children's medications are usually smaller and in lesser amounts. The nurse should determine safe dose ranges of medication before administering.
- Children should be given age-appropriate explanations for impending procedures. If a procedure is painful, the child should be told.
- EMLA cream can be applied to decrease painful insertions of needles.

- When giving medications by the IV route, always check for compatibility of the IV fluid and the medication.
- Dehydration occurs rapidly in infants and children. Intake and output is closely monitored in children with hydration problems.
- Monitoring patency of a tracheostomy tube is a priority. Children should be watched for early signs of respiratory distress. A pulse oximeter can assist in monitoring respiratory distress by providing measurements of blood oxygen.
- Know the hospital policy before performing any procedures.

 Go to your Companion CD-ROM for an Audio Glossary, video clips, and more.

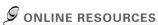 Be sure to visit the companion Evolve site at http://evolve.elsevier.com/Price/pediatric/ for WebLinks and additional online resources.

ONLINE RESOURCES

Mayo Clinic: http://www.mayoclinic.com/health/childrens-health/CC00046

18 End-of-Life Care for Children and Their Families

evolve http://evolve.elsevier.com/Price/pediatric/

Objectives

Upon completion of this chapter, the student will be able to:

1. Define the vocabulary terms listed
2. Discuss legal and ethical issues related to death
3. Discuss measures the nurse can take regarding palliative care
4. Discuss the child's reaction to death
5. Describe the impact death has on the different age groups
6. Discuss fears of the child related to dying
7. Discuss pain management for the dying child
8. Describe how a terminal illness affects the child and family
9. Describe cultural issues related to death
10. Discuss the benefits of hospice
11. Discuss management of symptoms the dying child may have
12. Discuss the nurse's role during the end-of-life care of a child

Key Terms

Be sure to check out the bonus material on the Companion CD-ROM, including selected audio pronunciations.

acceptance (p. 404)
anger (p. 404)
anticipatory grief (ăn-TĬS-ĭ-pă-tō-rē; p. 406)
anxiolytic (ĂNG-zī-ō-LĬ-tĭk; p. 405)
bargaining (p. 404)
bereavement (bĕ-RĒV-mĕnt; p. 406)
denial (p. 404)
depression (p. 404)
ethical (p. 400)
grief (p. 404)
legal (p. 400)
pain (p. 403)
palliative care (PĂL-ē-Ă-tĭv; p. 401)

Facing death with a child and the family is not an easy task. Nurses who become involved with dying patients often express a sense of gratitude to have had the privilege of the experience. This is an area where rules fall short and patience may become stretched. While it can be tiring, discouraging, and sad, it also requires a profound look at acceptance. Nurses who deal with the dying child and his or her family undoubtedly have a special gift. When nurses are able to ease the burden of end-of-life issues for the patient and family, the experience of the child's death and *the nurse* are often remembered for a lifetime (Jacobs, 2005).

SELF-EXPLORATION

One of the most important, if not the most important, preparations for dealing with the dying patient is self-exploration. Our own attitudes about life and death affect our nursing practice. Our attitudes and emotions may be buried deep within us and can form barriers to effective communication unless they are recognized and released. How we have or have not dealt with our own losses affects our present lives and our ability to relate to patients. Nurses must recognize that **coping is an active and ongoing process.** At times we need to lovingly detach ourselves from the patients and their families to be revitalized. We must find constructive outlets such as exercise and music to help maintain our equilibrium. An active support system consisting of nonjudgmental people (professional or personal) who are not threatened by natural expressions of emotions is crucial. Taking time off periodically may be necessary. Even attending the child's funeral may help the nurse in coping and does not detract from professionalism (Hockenberry et al., 2005). Proper channeling of these feelings can be a valuable part of our empathetic response to others.

LEGAL AND ETHICAL ISSUES RELATED TO DEATH

Legal issues related to death revolve around what is made a law by a legally sanctioned group. Legal issues include informed consent, role of a legal guardian, a Do Not Resuscitate (DNR) order, organ donation, and so forth. An ethical issue relates to what is good or moral. Ethical principles include respect for autonomy, benevolence, nonmaleficence, veracity, confidentiality, fidelity, and justice (Table 18-1). For example, life-sustaining medical treatment (such as a ventilator) may have positive and/or negative implications; ethical principles may be used to evaluate the situation. Use of these principles aids the health care team and the family to provide the dying child with a peaceful and dignified death. Through the use of ethical principles, the unique needs of the patient and family can be kept

Table 18-1 | Ethical Principles and Definitions

PRINCIPLE	DEFINITION
Respect for autonomy	The patient's right to self-determination and decision making
Benevolence	Doing what is good, meeting needs, balancing benefits with risk and harm, providing relief of pain and suffering
Nonmaleficence	Doing no harm
Veracity	Being honest, telling the truth
Confidentiality	Respecting privileged information; preserving rights, privacy, and dignity
Fidelity	Keeping promises
Justice	Treating fairly, ensuring distribution of resources

in perspective, as can assisting in resolving dilemmas that can arise during these challenging times.

PALLIATIVE CARE

Palliative care is the care and comfort given to a dying person. Palliative treatment focuses on the "relief of symptoms (e.g., pain, dyspnea) and conditions (e.g., loneliness) that cause distress and detract from the child's enjoyment of life" (American Academy of Pediatrics, 2000). The focus of palliative care is for the individual and the family to experience a comfortable, supported, and dignified end of life. Palliative care is often misunderstood to mean "little or no care." On the contrary, there is a great deal of care involved because palliative care aids the patient who is experiencing death and the family to feel cared for and supported and to have this care performed in the most dignified way. The goal of palliative care is to "add life to the child's years, not simply years to the child's life" (American Academy of Pediatrics, 2000).

When this type of care is needed for a child, it brings with it a great wall of emotional feelings. As parents and primary caregivers to a child, parents expect their children to outlive them. In the world of pediatric nursing, nurses assume that their time will be spent on curing and healing in the pediatric population. Nurses, however, must also recognize the value of caring for the pediatric patient who is dying. The pediatric nurse has much to gain from working with the dying child and assisting the family in confronting issues they must face. In looking back, parents—and indeed, often the child—recall a sense of the time at which living with the disease changed to preparing for death. Health care providers who work with children recognize that open and honest communication is the best approach. Broaching this subject with a child is difficult for all concerned. It is an issue that requires communication skills, empathy, and many discussions. Box 18-1 discusses some issues to consider before the discussion of death with a child.

Box 18-1 | Key Psychosocial Issues in End-of-Life Care

- Death, like birth, is a part of the natural order of things. Some die sooner than others.
- All of us have special feelings for those with whom we share our lives. There are many emotional feelings to express.
- Death is also a separation from family, friends, and siblings. The child who dies is not the only one who loses.
- The loss is never complete. Religion plays an important role in emphasizing that the child still lives on in spirit. The memory of the child is always in our hearts.
- Child is assured he or she will not be alone in death or after death. It is very important for the child to know that the parents are there for support and love.
- At the time of death, everyone needs to know they made a difference and did all they could do with their lives.
- Assure the child that crying is acceptable and feelings of sadness may occur. It is equally all right to feel angry and resentful. Children should not feel pressured to discuss their illness if that is not a choice. However, if a child chooses to express feelings, the support of an adult listener should be present.
- Assure the dying child that silence is acceptable, and no matter how the child chooses to express feelings, or how confused or silly it may sound, it is acceptable.
- Reassure the child that when death comes, it will not hurt. Children are very concerned about pain. They need to be reassured the health care team will reduce their pain to a minimum.
- When someone dies, there is a need to say good-bye and to know the arms and love of the family will surround them.
- Give the child permission to die. Saying it is "okay" to go helps put the child's mind at ease.

Communication Alert

The three main ingredients in communication are words, tone of voice, and body language. The most powerful of these is body language, followed by tone of voice, and then by the words that are actually said. If words are said with an angry tone of voice and with arms crossed, the person receiving this message perceives the sender as angry regardless of the words that are said. Children are keenly adept at reading body language and tone of voice.

For the patient and family to be supported, a multidisciplinary approach is needed. A team approach is most beneficial, particularly one that allows the individual and the family to have input into the decisions that are made. At a minimum, the team includes a physician, nurse, social worker, spiritual advisor, and child life therapist. Needs that should be considered center around physical, psychological, social, and spiritual areas. Table 18-2 lists factors for each of these.

In providing care to the dying child and family, the members of the health care team should see, as a result

Table 18-2 | *Physical, Psychological, Social, and Spiritual Needs*

AREA	NEEDS
Physical	Pain management
	Management of symptoms
	Comfort measures
Psychological	Anxiety/stress
	Guilt/anger
	Depression
	Fear of dying
	Grief/bereavement
Social	Financial concerns
	Insurance concerns
	Role and relationship changes
	Social isolation
Spiritual	Meaning
	Religiosity
	Sense of despair

Table 18-3 | *Children's Concepts of Death*

AGE	CONCEPT
Infant-toddler	Little understanding of death
	Fear and anxiety over separation
Preschooler	Something that happens to others
	Not permanent
	Curious about dead flowers and animals
	Magical thinking
	Believe that "bad thoughts" may come true, harbor guilt
	Believe their thoughts can cause death
	Death is reversible
	Will not happen to them
Early school years	Death is final
	Think they might die, but only in the distant future
	May understand death as a "person"
	Death is universal
	Suspect parents will die "someday"
	Fear of mutilation
Preadolescent-adolescent	Able to understand death in a logical manner
	Understand death is universal
	Understand death is permanent
	Fear of disfigurement and isolation from peers

of their efforts, a reduction of symptoms of pain or discomfort related to the disease; appropriate coping of both the child and the family; satisfaction of the child and family with the care that is being given; a sense of open and honest communication with all involved in the care; the dealing with and resolving of fears, grief, and anger; planning for future events such as the funeral; availability of quality of time for the child and family to enjoy; spiritual problems addressed and reconciled; and the family's grief being resolved after the death has occurred. This care involves a lengthy period of time and may be ongoing. There is so much to consider, and time becomes a friend as well as a foe.

CHILD'S REACTION TO DEATH

Each child, like each adult, approaches death in an individual way, drawing on limited experience (Table 18-3). Nurses must become well-acquainted with patients and view them within the context of their family and social culture. Children's anxiety about death often centers on symptoms. They fear that the treatments necessary to alleviate their problem may be painful, as indeed some of them are. Their sense of trust is precarious. It is important that nurses be honest and inform patients of what is about to be done and why it is necessary. Information should be shared in terms that children can understand. Encourage expression of feelings, such as by saying "You seem angry." Allow sufficient time for a response. It is important that children be allowed to have as much control over what happens to them as possible. This is fostered by including them in decisions that concern their welfare. Do not, however, offer a choice when there is none. Children often communicate symbolically. **Listen** to what they are saying to you, to their toys, and to other children. Provide crayons and paper. Drawing feelings is often therapeutic.

Although age is a factor, the child's cognitive development rather than chronological age per se affects the response to death. Children younger than 5 years are mainly concerned with separation from their parents and abandonment. (Even adults are threatened by thoughts of dying alone.) Preschool children respond to questions concerning death by relying on their experience and by turning to fantasy. They may believe death is reversible or that they are in some way responsible. Children between 6 and 12 years are beginning to be able to make knowledgeable decisions and their wishes should be considered when making health care decisions (Jacobs, 2005). Dying adolescents are faced with conflicts between their treatment regimens and their need to establish independence from their parents and conformity with their peers. Teens may also not want to disappoint their parents by "giving up." This leads to anger and resentment, which are frequently displaced onto hospital staff members. An atmosphere of acceptance and nonjudgmental listening allows patients freedom to express their hostility in a nonthreatening environment. Older children and teenagers also need a voice in decision-making processes, especially in a terminal condition that affords no hope with ongoing treatment.

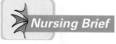
Nursing Brief

Brothers and sisters often feel neglected and lonely. They are frustrated because they are unable to comfort their parents and loved ones.

CHILD'S AWARENESS OF CONDITION

Surprising as it may seem, many investigators have shown that terminally ill children are generally aware of their condition even when careful concealment has been advocated. This is reflected in their drawings and play and can be detected through psychological testing. Failure to be honest with children leaves them to suffer alone, unable to express fears and sadness or even to say goodbye. The prospect of death is frightening to children; it is up to the parents and caregivers to help the child work through their feelings. Evidence has shown that parents who spoke with their child about death before the experience were relieved that they did so (Kreichbergs et al., 2004). Children in turn may try to protect their parents. Many actually try to protect their parents by pretending that they do not know they are dying, and the secrecy everyone tries to maintain keeps all from sharing at a time when closeness is what they all need and most want (Lewis et al., 2002).

Communication Alert

Wishes of the parents are to be respected when it comes to talking to the child or siblings about the prognosis, unless it is decided that this is not in the child's best interest. At that point, legal involvement may be necessary.

FEARS OF THE CHILD

In dealing with death, the child most likely has two major fears: fear of pain and fear of being alone. The child should be comforted and reassured that both of these issues will be managed.

PAIN

In consideration of the child and family, **pain** should be accepted as being "whatever the experiencing person says it is, existing whenever he says it does" (McCaffery & Pasero, 1999). Pain, as discussed previously in Chapter 3, needs to be properly assessed and managed. Dying teenagers often fear symptoms of pain and suffering more than actual death, so they need reassurance that their comfort needs will be met. Narcotic analgesics such as morphine are effective pain relievers in children and adults. Studies have shown that pain is not always well controlled in children, so the nurse needs to be vigilant of the child's needs.

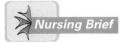

Nursing Brief

In children, the intramuscular or the rectal route may be offensive, so keep this in mind when medications are changed or added.

Box 18-2 | *Complementary Methods*

Relaxation is a method children can be taught to tense and relax different muscle groups. By tensing the muscle first, the child can compare how it feels when the tension is released. The child is then taught to hold the relaxed muscle for a short amount of time.

Distraction is a method used to divert attention from the main portion of an experience. Blowing bubbles is a form of distraction used with children.

Biofeedback is a method of training designed to help an individual control her or his autonomic (involuntary) nervous system.

Guided Imagery is a complementary/alternative therapy that uses pleasant mental images of events, feelings, or sensations. Simple imagery entails using the sounds and sights in the imagination of the child to feel good and be less afraid. An example is having the child visualize a favorite vacation spot.

Barriers to proper management of pain for the terminally ill child can be related to addiction or overdosing. The goal of safe and effective administration of pain medication should revolve around comfort and the ability of the child to function. As the disease worsens or as a tolerance to the medication develops, the amount of pain medication may not be as effective. The dosage may need to be adjusted, other medications added, or a stronger medication begun. Often, *complementary* methods are used along with pharmacologic approaches. Relaxation, distraction, biofeedback, or guided imagery may all be used. The dosage of narcotics can often be reduced, and the adverse effects may be diminished (Box 18-2).

FEAR OF BEING ALONE

Reassure children that they will not be left alone. Allow the child to verbalize concerns, thoughts, and feelings. Encourage the parents and family to take the time to listen. As the child loses the ability to speak, the care and comfort given needs to be verbalized. The parents and family can also speak to the child at the bedside, reflecting on the past and discussing the present as a way of comforting the child. Children love to hear how they made an impact in a loved one's life. They need to know they made a difference (Figure 18-1).

FAMILY ROLES AND NEEDS

The impending death of a child affects every member of the family. Family dynamics and the family's ability to cope and resolve issues are of concern. Parents may be overwhelmed by the decisions they must make. Communication with the family is important, but also family members need ways to express themselves. Parents and family members need to be encouraged and given the opportunity to verbalize. Guilt, anger, and sadness are just some of the emotions that family members are experiencing. They need their feelings

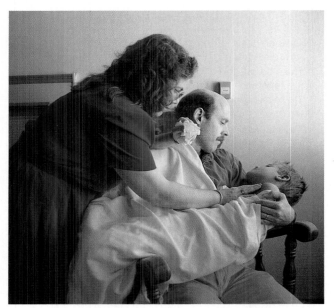

FIGURE **18-1** Parents' wishes to hold their dying child should be respected and facilitated.

validated, and they need to be praised for the care they are giving the child. Help family members see a role they can play in the care and comfort of their loved one. It is also important that they know how to make the final days count and become memorable. Referrals should be made to other disciplines as the need arises. Other health care team members, such as the social worker and chaplain, can help the parents and family in dealing with social, emotional, financial, and spiritual issues.

The stages of dying as detailed by Kübler-Ross (1969)—denial, anger, bargaining, depression, and acceptance—can be applied to parents and siblings as they grieve and to the sick child. It is important to accept and support participants at whatever stage they are in and not try to direct progress. Parents should be encouraged to assist in the care of their child. It is therapeutic for children to be in their own surroundings whenever possible. Siblings involved in the patient's care feel less neglected. They may be able to help with simple things, such as bringing a toy or a food item to the bedside of their dying brother or sister. Parents need to encourage siblings to be open about their own grief as well. It is common for the siblings to feel guilty because they are jealous of the attention paid to the ill child. Parents feel guilty because they cannot give equal time to all of their children. Special time with each of their children is often therapeutic. Discipline and enforcing household rules should not vary because of a dying child. The ill child may not be able to perform the same tasks as before, but they can still be given simple jobs to do (Lewis et al., 2002).

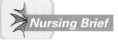

Nursing Brief

A long illness threatens a child's independence. Do not contribute to this with overprotection.

The family's religious associations can be a source of strength and support, as can caring neighbors and friends. Statistics show a high correlation between the death of a child and divorce. Nurses should try to be alert to signs of tension between parents so that suitable interventions may be established. It is important to realize that each parent grieves in his or her own time and way, often making it impossible for spouses to be supportive of each other. The suppression of strong feelings of guilt, helplessness, and outrage can be devastating. The father may be easily overlooked because of his absence during the day or because of a need to conceal his emotions from others.

CULTURAL ISSUES

Depending on the culture, various issues may arise regarding death. Learning about different cultures is an important first step. Customs regarding death are usually unique to a given culture. For example, some cultures believe in an afterlife, and certain customs may need to be followed regarding that belief. Other cultures may have their own funeral and burial customs. Some believe death should occur with only the family present, and others wish an extended group present (Lewis et al., 2002). Many cultures believe religion and faith are important aspects of end-of-life care. Cultural education is thus an important aspect regarding care of the dying child.

Language barriers make it difficult to communicate in any hospital situation, especially when hospice and palliative care are involved. The use of interpreters is not always ideal, and communicating to families in stressful situations may be frustrating for all parties concerned. Patience on the part of the health care provider becomes an important virtue.

HOSPICE CARE

Hospice services are for individuals who no longer can benefit from curative care and treatment. Care is designed to provide sensitivity and support to the individual in the final phase of life. Hospice care refers to a package of palliative care services, such as durable medical equipment, etc. Life is seen as quality time rather than length of time. The entire family unit is considered in hospice care so that the needs of all can be met.

Hospice care began in 1974. In 1977, an 8-year-old boy was denied hospice care because he was a child. In 1983, Children's Hospice International (CHI) was founded, which is a nonprofit organization that provides care and support to children with life-threatening conditions and to their families. This organization's goal is quality of life for the dying child and ongoing strengthened life for the family.

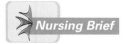

Hospice can offer many positive benefits for the dying child and the family. It is best to investigate it long before it is needed. Hospice services can be life-affirming, and parents may benefit from having this knowledge as early as possible. Children's hospice encourages day-to-day communication so that the family can look back and treasure the time spent together. The support received from hospice enables the family to cope more effectively. Grief is normal, and to cope and recover from grief requires choices. With hospice support, families can be strengthened and can return to positive and productive lives.

PREPARING FOR DEATH

The end of an individual's life is as important as the beginning of that person's life. For a birth, the family plans and educates itself. The experience is visualized and eventually is realized. If the opportunity arises, with an expected death, an individual's preparation for death can likewise be planned. In the case of a child, wishes, dreams, and desires can be planned and accomplished if they are known. If parents and family members have time to identify what is important for them to have during the child's illness and death, then if possible, these can be arranged, leaving the parents and family with positive memories. Parents and family members need to verbalize their fears and beliefs about death. It is important to talk with the child about his or her impending death. By allowing the child to continue to express his or her wishes and emotions, he or she becomes better prepared for the inevitable. Through discussion and education, fears can often be lessened or resolved.

With a sudden and unexpected death, parents and family members do not have the opportunity to plan and so **anticipatory grieving** rarely is able to occur. Unfortunately, some families of children do experience unexpected death. In the case of infants or very young children, they do not have the ability to communicate their wishes, making it difficult for their parents and families. Anytime the life of a child is shortened, parents, family members, health care providers, and all involved struggle to make some sense of it all.

Death is a physiological process, and there are signs and symptoms that cessation of life is occurring. Discomforts associated with the respiratory system can be distressing to the child and family. Dyspnea can be caused by worsening of the disease process, anemia, pneumonia, or heart failure. Coughing can occur because of stimulation of the cough reflex from a build-up of secretions. Nursing interventions can include elevating the head of the bed, using a cool cloth on the forehead, using oxygen, changing positions, and adding morphine. Morphine suppresses the cough reflex and also diminishes the feelings of air hunger, which is the sensation caused by dyspnea. Other medications such as a bronchodilator or an **anxiolytic** may be ordered.

Gastrointestinal system discomforts involve nausea or vomiting, anorexia (lack of desire to eat), dysphagia (difficulty swallowing), dehydration, and constipation. Some of these may be related to the progress of the disease, the slowing down of metabolism, or the result of medication side effects. Consider the discomfort of your patient and seek to remedy the cause. Diet and environment (sights and odors) can be adjusted. Medications may be added to the patient's care to control nausea/vomiting. As the disease progresses, the child may lose his or her appetite. Help parents understand that this is to be expected and that it is okay for the child to have any food or fluid requested. Requests may occur at nonmeal times. Sips of a favorite fluid, ice chips, or a Popsicle can provide comfort. Oral care is needed. Soft-bristled toothbrushes aid in cleansing and soothing the mouth, gums, teeth, and tongue. Lips may also become dry, so a topical preparation may be used. As dehydration occurs and blinking decreases, the eyes may also need moisture and artificial tears are needed.

Weakness and fatigue occur as the disease progresses. The child and family can be assisted to modify events in daily activities. Instead of doing all the care at once, plan on doing segments of it during different parts of the day. Eating is important, so plan a period of rest before and after a meal. Conserve the child's energy by the use of assistance, such as a wheelchair or a wagon for mobility. This conserves energy and yet allows the child to spend time out of the room. It is a natural process that a decrease in activity leads to weakness, so if there is an underlying problem, such as pain, depression, or poor sleeping, these issues need to be addressed for the child to remain active as long as possible.

With a decrease in activity, issues related to the skin arise. Incontinence of urine and feces add to this problem. Special care should center around providing for the child's dignity and keeping the bed linens clean and dry. Because of lack of adequate circulation to the periphery, realize that, if skin breakdown does occur, healing is difficult. Prevention of any type of skin breakdown is important. Turning, positioning, and the use of pillows or other devices to reduce pressure is essential.

Assessment of the mental status of the child is valuable. If depression, fear, anxiety, or confusion occurs, these need to be addressed. Make sure there is adequate pain management.

Box 18-3 summarizes the physical signs of impending death. Parents and caregivers can recognize these. It is essential the nurse provide dignity, comfort, support, guidance, and education to the parents and family members during this time. Comfort and care for the child should continue to be provided while talking to the child, even though the child may not be conscious.

Box 18-3 | *Signs and Symptoms of Impending Death*

LACK OF APPETITE
- May be seen by the family as "giving up"
- Anorexia

WEAKNESS AND FATIGUE
- Caused by disease process
- Lack of energy

DECREASE OF FLUID INTAKE
- Can be useful in keeping lungs less congested
- Care for mucous membranes if they are dry

DECREASE IN CIRCULATORY PERFUSION
- Caused by hypotension and decreased cardiac output
- Causes hands and feet to be cool
- Decrease in urine output

NEUROLOGICAL DYSFUNCTION
- May lead to diminished level of consciousness
- Decreased ability to swallow
- Changes in respirations
- Loss of sphincter control
- Patient may become restless
- Key is to keep patient pain-free

Because the loss of hearing cannot be reliably predicted, the parents and family can gain comfort in the fact that their loved one may still hear them.

Respect and assist the family in their spiritual and cultural needs. This is a time when prayer and the presence of family members can be profoundly meaningful. Be sensitive to the parents' and other family members' needs. Some families need your presence; others may need their privacy. Honor their requests whenever possible. During these last few hours or moments just before death, small things have great meaning for the parents and family. Extend to the parents and family the use of services that they may need, such as calling the spiritual advisor of their choice.

CARE AFTER DEATH

The time of death occurs when there is absence of respiratory, cardiac, and neurological function, pupils are fixed and dilated, body temperature falls, the skin is cool to the touch and pale, sphincter control is lost so there may be passing of urine and stool, and body movement ceases. There is no particular order or time frame in which these events occur. The pronouncement of death is according to the institution's policy.

Once death has occurred, the nurse and the health team members assist the family. Wishes from the parents and family need to be respected and honored. A chaplain or person of the family's choice needs to be with them during this time. Assistance may be needed in notifying other members or making decisions.

In preparing the body for viewing, the nurse should bathe and dress the child in a clean gown. The bed is changed, and the environment is cleaned and made

more peaceful by removing some of the medical equipment. The parents and family are given the opportunity to view and spend time with the child. Holding the newborn, infant, or child may occur; this provides a comfort for the parents, especially if they were unable to do so before death. When the family is ready and has given permission, the body is moved. Parents may want to be present when the mortician comes to remove the body. Honor their requests, if at all possible.

FAMILY COPING

Bereavement is a complex series of reactions that occur during and after the death of a loved one. How an individual grieves is unique. In a situation where death is expected, **anticipatory grief** may occur, which is a sense of loss and grief before death. After the actual death, bereavement can occur for a varied amount of time, and support is needed. Family members need to know that grief has no time frame and that during the first year many changes occur. With the loss of a child, there are likely to be many events that stir the feelings of loss. The first year or two after a child's death are especially difficult for the family. Parents and siblings need support systems in place. Both parents and siblings benefit from reading books about death. Children especially may benefit from activities involving the memory of the child who has died. They may wish to make a memory album or treasure box of mementos about the sibling that died. They may also assist in creating a "memory quilt," each adding a square that depicts how they feel about the person that died (Lewis et al., 2002). In addition, many well-established support groups are available to assist parents and siblings in dealing with loss and grief (Figure 18-2).

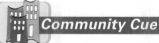
Community Cue

The mission of The Compassionate Friends *(http://compassionatefriends.org)* is to assist families toward the positive resolution of grief following the death of a child of any age and to provide information to help others be supportive.

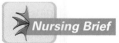
Nursing Brief

Grandparents, teachers, and friends are also grieving. Be alert for all significant others.

REFLECTION

Death is what occurs at the end of life. It is both normal *and* unique. In pediatrics, we as nurses are called on to aid our pediatric patients, parents, and families through

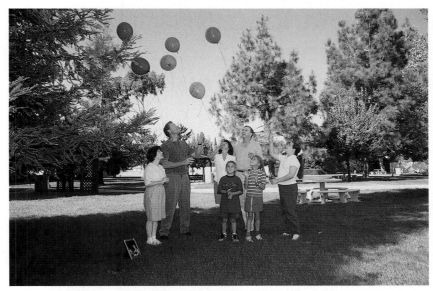

FIGURE **18-2** On the anniversary of a child's death, family members meet to send balloons (non-Mylar) with messages inside up to heaven for the deceased child.

the dying process, with which they may have little or no experience. As nurses, we are responsible for providing dignity, comfort, support, guidance, and education to those in our care. To do this, we must search our own values, beliefs, and judgments. Our experiences have an impact on the choices we make and on how we see the situation. The best time for this searching to happen is before the time it is needed. If we can answer sensitive issues relating to our own concerns, then we are better prepared to care for those patients and families when they most need our care and support. Nurses must also recognize that professional growth comes from our experiences, so with each new event, we learn more about ourselves. Through self-reflection when feelings of conflict arise, identifying whose needs are being met becomes paramount to providing quality patient care.

In dealing with, relating to, coping with, and managing the process of death and dying, a poem by Henry Van Dyke says it very well:

"Time is . . ."
"Too slow for those who wait,"
"Too swift for those who fear,"
"Too long for those who grieve,"
"Too short for those who rejoice,"
"But for those who love,"
"Time is eternity."

Key Points

- Working with a dying child and the family is a difficult task.
- Self-exploration can aid the nurse in identifying values and beliefs.
- There are many legal and ethical decisions to be made during the process of dying and death itself.
- Legal relates to laws, and ethical relates to what is good or moral.

- Palliative care involves comfort and support for physical, psychological, social, and spiritual needs.
- Palliative care is interdisciplinary and involves at least the child, parents, nurse, physician, social worker, spiritual advisor, and child life therapist.
- Communication is an essential aspect of palliative care.
- Cognitive development influences the child's needs in coping with grief and dying.
- Children with a terminal illness often recognize their condition and are aware they are dying.
- Children fear pain and dying alone.
- The stages of grief according to Kübler-Ross are denial, anger, bargaining, depression, and acceptance.
- Grief is subjective and unique for everyone.
- Hospice care provides sensitivity and support for those who are dying and their family.
- Hospice care for children is supported by CHI.
- In an expected death, planning can aid the child and family to complete goals.
- Even though the exact time of death cannot be predicted, there are physiological signs and symptoms that allow us to know death is near.
- The care the family receives after the death of their loved one is one of their lasting memories.
- The family continues to grieve long after the death of a child, and coping mechanisms are vital for the family's welfare.

Go to your Companion CD-ROM for an Audio Glossary, video clips, and more.

evolve   Be sure to visit the companion Evolve site at http://evolve.elsevier.com/Price/pediatric/ for WebLinks and additional online resources.

ONLINE RESOURCES

Children's Hospice International: http://www.chionline.org

National Hospice and Palliative Care Organization: http://www.nhpco

The Compassionate Friends: http://compassionatefriends.org

Recommended Childhood and Adolescent Immunization Schedule—United States, 2007

DEPARTMENT OF HEALTH AND HUMAN SERVICES • CENTERS FOR DISEASE CONTROL AND PREVENTION

Recommended Immunization Schedule for Ages 0–6 Years UNITED STATES • 2007

Vaccine ▼	Age ▶	Birth	1 month	2 months	4 months	6 months	12 months	15 months	18 months	19–23 months	2–3 years	4–6 years
Hepatitis B[1]		HepB	HepB		see footnote 1	HepB				HepB Series		
Rotavirus[2]				Rota	Rota	Rota						
Diphtheria, Tetanus, Pertussis[3]				DTaP	DTaP	DTaP		DTaP				DTaP
Haemophilus influenzae type b[4]				Hib	Hib	Hib[4]	Hib		Hib			
Pneumococcal[5]				PCV	PCV	PCV	PCV				PCV / PPV	
Inactivated Poliovirus				IPV	IPV		IPV					IPV
Influenza[6]						Influenza (Yearly)						
Measles, Mumps, Rubella[7]						MMR						MMR
Varicella[8]						Varicella						Varicella
Hepatitis A[9]						HepA (2 doses)				HepA Series		
Meningococcal[10]										MPSV4		

Range of recommended ages
Catch-up immunization
Certain high-risk groups

This schedule indicates the recommended ages for routine administration of currently licensed childhood vaccines, as of December 1, 2006, for children through age 6 years. For additional information see www.cdc.gov/nip/recs/child-schedule.htm. Any dose not administered at the recommended age should be administered at any subsequent visit when indicated and feasible. Additional vaccines may be licensed and recommended during the year. Licensed combination vaccines may be used whenever any components of the combination are indicated and other components of the vaccine are not contraindicated and if approved by the Food and Drug Administration for that dose of the series. Providers should consult the respective ACIP statement for detailed recommendations. Clinically significant adverse events that follow immunization should be reported to the Vaccine Adverse Event Reporting System (VAERS). Guidance about how to obtain and complete a VAERS form is available at www.vaers.hhs.gov or by telephone, 800-822-7967.

1. Hepatitis B vaccine (HepB). *(Minimum age: birth)*

At birth:
- Administer monovalent HepB to all newborns prior to hospital discharge.
- If mother is HBsAg-positive, administer HepB and 0.5 mL of hepatitis B immune globulin (HBIG) within 12 hours of birth.
- If mother's HBsAg status is unknown, administer HepB within 12 hours of birth. Determine the HBsAg status as soon as possible and if HBsAg-positive, administer HBIG (no later than age 1 week).
- If mother is HBsAg-negative, the birth dose can only be delayed with physician's order and mothers' negative HBsAg laboratory report documented in the infant's medical record.

Following the birth dose:
- The HepB series should be completed with either monovalent HepB or a combination vaccine containing HepB. The second dose should be administered at age 1–2 months. The final dose should be administered at age ≥ 24 weeks. Infants born to HBsAg-positive mothers should be tested for HBsAg and antibody to HBsAg after completion of 3 or more doses in a licensed HepB series, at age 9–18 months (generally at the next well-child visit).

4-month dose of HepB:
- It is permissible to administer 4 doses of HepB when combination vaccines are given after the birth dose. If monovalent HepB is used for doses after the birth dose, a dose at age 4 months is not needed.

2. Rotavirus vaccine (Rota). *(Minimum age: 6 weeks)*
- Administer the first dose between 6 and 12 weeks of age. Do not start the series later than age 12 weeks.
- Administer the final dose in the series by 32 weeks of age. Do not administer a dose later than age 32 weeks.
- There are insufficient data on safety and efficacy outside of these age ranges.

3. Diphtheria and tetanus toxoids and acellular pertussis vaccine (DTaP). *(Minimum age: 6 weeks)*
- The fourth dose of DTaP may be administered as early as age 12 months, provided 6 months have elapsed since the third dose.
- Administer the final dose in the series at age 4–6 years.

4. Haemophilus influenzae type b conjugate vaccine (Hib). *(Minimum age: 6 weeks)*
- If PRP-OMP (PedvaxHIB® or ComVax® [Merck]) is administered at ages 2 and 4 months, a dose at age 6 months is not required.
- TriHiBit® (DTaP/Hib) combination products should not be used for primary immunization but can be used as boosters following any Hib vaccine in ≥ 12 months olds.

5. Pneumococcal vaccine (PCV). *(Minimum age: 6 weeks for Pneumococcal Conjugate Vaccine (PCV); 2 years for Pneumococcal Polysaccharide Vaccine (PPV))*
- Administer PCV at ages 24-59 months in certain high-risk groups. Administer PPV to certain high-risk groups aged ≥ 2 years. See MMWR 2000; 49(RR-9):1-35.

6. Influenza vaccine. *(Minimum age: 6 months for trivalent inactivated influenza vaccine (TIV); 5 years for live, attenuated influenza vaccine (LAIV))*
- All children aged 6–59 months and close contacts of all children aged 0–59 months are recommended to receive influenza vaccine.
- Influenza vaccine is recommended annually for children aged ≥ 59 months with certain risk factors, healthcare workers, and other persons (including household members) in close contact with persons in groups at high risk. See MMWR 2006; 55(RR-10);1-41.
- For healthy persons aged 5–49 years, LAIV may be used as an alternative to TIV.
- Children receiving TIV should receive 0.25 mL if aged 6–35 months or 0.5 mL if aged ≥ 3 years.
- Children aged < 9 years who are receiving influenza vaccine for the first time should receive 2 doses (separated by ≥ 4 weeks for TIV and ≥ 6 weeks for LAIV).

7. Measles, mumps, and rubella vaccine (MMR). *(Minimum age: 12 months)*
- Administer the second dose of MMR at age 4–6 years. MMR may be administered prior to age 4–6 years, provided ≥ 4 weeks have elapsed since the first dose and both doses are administered at age ≥ 12 months.

8. Varicella vaccine. *(Minimum age: 12 months)*
- Administer the second dose of varicella vaccine at age 4–6 years. Varicella vaccine may be administered prior to age 4–6 years, provided that ≥ 3 months have elapsed since the first dose and both doses are administered at age ≥ 12 months. If second dose was administered ≥ 28 days following the first dose, the second dose does not need to be repeated.

9. Hepatitis A vaccine (HepA). *(Minimum age: 12 months)*
- HepA is recommended for all children at 1 year of age (i.e., 12–23 months). The 2 doses in the series should be administered at least 6 months apart.
- Children not fully vaccinated by age 2 years can be vaccinated at subsequent visits.
- HepA is recommended for certain other groups of children including in areas where vaccination programs target older children. See MMWR 2006; 55(RR-7):1-23.

10. Meningococcal polysaccharide vaccine (MPSV4). *(Minimum age: 2 years)*
- Administer MPSV4 to children aged 2–10 years with terminal complement deficiencies or anatomic or functional asplenia and certain other high risk groups. See MMWR 2005;54 (RR-7):1-21.

The Childhood and Adolescent Immunization Schedule is approved by:
Advisory Committee on Immunization Practices www.cdc.gov/nip/acip • American Academy of Pediatrics www.aap.org • American Academy of Family Physicians www.aafp.org

SAFER • HEALTHIER • PEOPLE™

DEPARTMENT OF HEALTH AND HUMAN SERVICES • CENTERS FOR DISEASE CONTROL AND PREVENTION

Recommended Immunization Schedule for Ages 7–18 Years   UNITED STATES • 2007

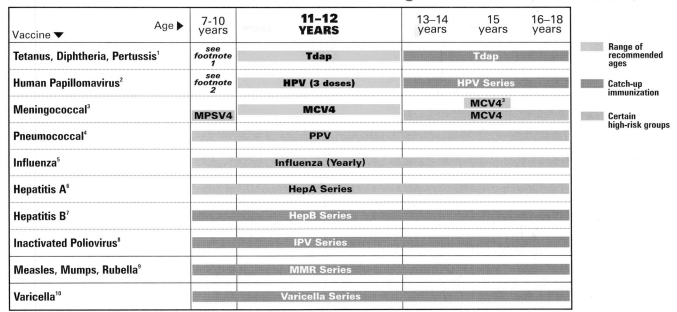

Vaccine ▼ Age ▶	7-10 years	11–12 YEARS	13–14 years	15 years	16–18 years
Tetanus, Diphtheria, Pertussis[1]	see footnote 1	Tdap	Tdap		
Human Papillomavirus[2]	see footnote 2	HPV (3 doses)	HPV Series		
Meningococcal[3]	MPSV4	MCV4	MCV4[3] / MCV4		
Pneumococcal[4]		PPV			
Influenza[5]		Influenza (Yearly)			
Hepatitis A[6]		HepA Series			
Hepatitis B[7]		HepB Series			
Inactivated Poliovirus[8]		IPV Series			
Measles, Mumps, Rubella[9]		MMR Series			
Varicella[10]		Varicella Series			

Legend:
■ Range of recommended ages
■ Catch-up immunization
■ Certain high-risk groups

This schedule indicates the recommended ages for routine administration of currently licensed childhood vaccines, as of December 1, 2006, for children aged 7–18 years. For additional information see www.cdc.gov/nip/recs/child-schedule.htm. Any dose not administered at the recommended earlier age should be administered at any subsequent visit when indicated and feasible. Additional vaccines may be licensed and recommended during the year. Licensed combination vaccines may be used whenever any components of the combination are indicated and other components of the vaccine are not contraindicated and if approved by the Food and Drug Administration for that dose of the series. Providers should consult the respective ACIP statement for detailed recommendations. Clinically significant adverse events that follow immunization should be reported to the Vaccine Adverse Event Reporting System (VAERS). Guidance about how to obtain and complete a VAERS form is available at www.vaers.hhs.gov or by telephone, 800-822-7967.

FOOTNOTES

1. **Tetanus and diphtheria toxoids and acellular pertussis vaccine (Tdap).**
   (Minimum age: 10 years for BOOSTRIX® and 11 years for ADACEL™)
   • Administer at age 11–12 years for those who have completed the recommended childhood DTP/DTaP vaccination series and have not received a Td booster dose.
   • Adolescents 13–18 years who missed the 11–12 year Td/Tdap booster dose should also receive a single dose of Tdap if they have completed the recommended childhood DTP/DTaP vaccination series.

2. **Human papillomavirus vaccine (HPV).** *(Minimum age: 9 years)*
   • Administer the first dose of the HPV vaccine series to females at age 11–12 years.
   • Administer the second dose 2 months after the first dose and the third dose 6 months after the first dose.
   • Administer the HPV vaccine series to females at age 13–18 years if not previously vaccinated.

3. **Meningococcal vaccine.** *(Minimum age: 11 years for meningococcal conjugate vaccine (MCV4); 2 years for meningococcal polysaccharide vaccine (MPSV4))*
   • Administer MCV4 at age 11–12-years and to previously unvaccinated adolescents at high school entry (~15 years of age).
   • Administer MCV4 to previously unvaccinated college freshmen living in dormitories; MPSV4 is an acceptable alternative.
   • Vaccination against invasive meningococcal disease is recommended for children and adolescents aged ≥ 2 years with terminal complement deficiencies or anatomic or functional asplenia and certain other high risk groups. See *MMWR* 2005;54 (RR-7):1-21. Use MPSV4 for children aged 2–10 years and MCV4 or MPSV4 for older children.

4. **Pneumococcal polysaccharide vaccine (PPV).**
   (Minimum age: 2 years)
   • Administer for certain high-risk groups. See *MMWR* 1997; 46(RR-08); 1-24 and *MMWR* 2000; 49(RR-9):1-35.

5. **Influenza vaccine.** *(Minimum age: 6 months for trivalent inactivated influenza vaccine (TIV); 5 years for live, attenuated influenza vaccine (LAIV)*
   • Influenza vaccine is recommended annually for persons with certain risk factors, healthcare workers, and other persons (including household members) in close contact with persons in groups at high risk. See *MMWR* 2006; 55(RR-10);1-41.
   • For healthy persons aged 5–49 years, LAIV may be used as an alternative to TIV.
   • Children aged < 9 years who are receiving influenza vaccine for the first time should receive 2 doses (separated by ≥ 4 weeks for TIV and ≥ 6 weeks for LAIV).

6. **Hepatitis A vaccine (HepA).** *(Minimum age: 12 months)*
   • The 2 doses in the series should be administered at least 6 months apart.
   • HepA is recommended for certain other groups of children including in areas where vaccination programs target older children. See *MMWR* 2006; 55(RR-7):1-23.

7. **Hepatitis B vaccine (HepB).** *(Minimum age: birth)*
   • Administer the 3-dose series to those who were not previously vaccinated.
   • A 2-dose series of Recombivax HB® is licensed for 11–15 year olds.

8. **Inactivated poliovirus vaccine (IPV).** *(Minimum age: 6 weeks)*
   • For children who received an all-IPV or all-oral poliovirus (OPV) series, a fourth dose is not necessary if third dose was administered at age ≥ 4 years.
   • If both OPV and IPV were administered as part of a series, a total of 4 doses should be given, regardless of the child's current age.

9. **Measles, mumps, and rubella vaccine (MMR).**
   (Minimum age: 12 months)
   • If not previously vaccinated, administer 2 doses of MMR during any visit with ≥ 4 weeks between the doses.

10. **Varicella vaccine.** *(Minimum age: 12 months)*
    • Administer 2 doses of varicella vaccine to persons without evidence of immunity.
    • Administer 2 doses of varicella vaccine to persons aged ≤ 13 years at least 3 months apart. Do not repeat the second dose, if administered ≥ 28 days following the first dose.
    • Administer 2 doses of varicella vaccine to persons aged ≥ 13 years at least 4 weeks apart.

The Childhood and Adolescent Immunization Schedule is approved by:
Advisory Committee on Immunization Practices www.cdc.gov/nip/acip • American Academy of Pediatrics www.aap.org • American Academy of Family Physicians www.aafp.org
SAFER • HEALTHIER • PEOPLE™

Activity intolerance
Activity intolerance, Risk for
Airway clearance, Ineffective
Allergy response, Latex
Allergy response, Risk for latex
Anxiety
Anxiety, Death
Aspiration, Risk for
Attachment, Risk for impaired parent/infant/child
Autonomic dysreflexia
Autonomic dysreflexia, Risk for havior, Risk-prone health
Behavior, Risk-prone health
Body image, Disturbed
Body temperature, Risk for imbalanced
Bowel incontinence
Breastfeeding, Effective
Breastfeeding, Ineffective
Breastfeeding, Interrupted
Breathing pattern, Ineffective
Cardiac output, Decreased
Caregiver role strain
Caregiver role strain, Risk for
Comfort, Readiness for enhanced
Communication, Impaired verbal
Communication, Readiness for enhanced
Conflict, Decisional
Conflict, Parental role
Confusion, Acute
Confusion, Chronic
Confusion, Risk for Acute
Constipation
Constipation, Perceived
Constipation, Risk for
Contamination
Contamination, Risk for
Coping, Compromised family
Coping, Defensive
Coping, Disabled family
Coping, Ineffective
Coping, Ineffective community
Coping, Readiness for enhanced
Coping, Readiness for enhanced community
Coping, Readiness for enhanced family
Decision making, Readiness for enhanced
Denial, Ineffective
Dentition, Impaired
Development, Risk for delayed

Diarrhea
Dignity, Risk for Compromised Human
Disuse syndrome, Risk for
Diversional activity, Deficient
Energy field, Disturbed
Environmental interpretation syndrome, Impaired
Failure to thrive, Adult
Falls, Risk for
Family processes: Alcoholism, Dysfunctional
Family processes, Interrupted
Family processes, Readiness for enhanced
Fatigue
Fear
Fluid balance, Readiness for enhanced
Fluid volume, Deficient
Fluid volume, Excess
Fluid volume, Risk for deficient
Fluid volume, Risk for imbalanced
Gas exchange, Impaired
Glucose level, Risk for unstable
Grieving
Grieving, Complicated
Grieving, Risk for Complicated
Growth, Risk for disproportionate
Growth and development, Delayed
Health behavior, Risk Prone
Health maintenance, Ineffective
Health-seeking behaviors
Home maintenance, Impaired
Hope, Readiness for enhanced
Hopelessness
Hyperthermia
Hypothermia
Identity, Disturbed personal
Immunization status, Readiness for enhanced
Incontinence, Functional urinary
Incontinence, Overflow urinary
Incontinence, Reflex urinary
Incontinence, Stress urinary
Incontinence, Total urinary
Incontinence, Urge urinary
Incontinence, Risk for urge urinary
Infant behavior, Disorganized
Infant behavior, Readiness for enhanced organized
Infant behavior, Risk for disorganized
Infant feeding pattern, Ineffective
Infection, Risk for

Injury, Risk for
Injury, Risk for perioperative-positioning
Insomnia
Intracranial adaptive capacity, Decreased
Knowledge, Deficient
Knowledge, Readiness for enhanced
Lifestyle, Sedentary
Liver function, Risk for impaired
Loneliness, Risk for
Memory, Impaired
Mobility, Impaired bed
Mobility, Impaired physical
Mobility, Impaired wheelchair
Moral distress
Nausea
Neglect, Unilateral
Noncompliance
Nutrition, Readiness for enhanced
Nutrition: less than body requirements, Imbalanced
Nutrition: more than body requirements, Imbalanced
Nutrition: more than body requirements, Risk for imbalanced
Oral mucous membrane, Impaired
Pain, Acute
Pain, Chronic
Parenting, Impaired
Parenting, Readiness for enhanced
Parenting, Risk for impaired
Peripheral neurovascular dysfunction, Risk for
Poisoning, Risk for
Poisoning, Risk for perioperative
Post-trauma syndrome
Post-trauma syndrome, Risk for
Power, Readiness for enhanced
Powerlessness
Powerlessness, Risk for
Protection, Ineffective
Rape-trauma syndrome
Rape-trauma syndrome, compound reaction
Rape-trauma syndrome, silent reaction
Religiosity, Impaired
Religiosity, Readiness for enhanced
Religiosity, Risk for impaired
Relocation stress syndrome
Relocation stress syndrome, Risk for
Role performance, Ineffective
Self-care, Readiness for enhanced
Self-care deficit, Bathing/hygiene

Self-care deficit, Dressing/grooming
Self-care deficit, Feeding
Self-care deficit, Toileting
Self-concept, Readiness for enhanced
Self-esteem, Chronic low
Self-esteem, Situational low
Self-esteem, Risk for situational low
Self-mutilation
Self-mutilation, Risk for
Sensory perception, Disturbed
Sexual dysfunction
Sexuality pattern, Ineffective
Skin integrity, Impaired
Skin integrity, Risk for impaired
Sleep, Readiness for enhanced
Sleep deprivation
Social interaction, Impaired
Social isolation
Sorrow, Chronic
Spiritual distress
Spiritual distress, Risk for
Spiritual well-being, Readiness for enhanced
Stress overload
Sudden Infant Death Syndrome, Risk for
Suffocation, Risk for
Suicide, Risk for
Surgical recovery, Delayed
Swallowing, Impaired
Therapeutic regimen management, Effective
Therapeutic regimen management, Ineffective
Therapeutic regimen management, Ineffective community
Therapeutic regimen management, Ineffective family
Therapeutic regimen management, Readiness for enhanced
Thermoregulation, Ineffective
Thought processes, Disturbed
Tissue integrity, Impaired
Tissue perfusion, Ineffective
Transfer ability, Impaired
Trauma, Risk for
Urinary elimination, Impaired
Urinary elimination, Readiness for enhanced
Urinary retention
Ventilation, Impaired spontaneous
Ventilatory weaning response, Dysfunctional
Violence, Risk for other-directed
Violence, Risk for self-directed
Walking, Impaired
Wandering

Recommendations for Preventive Pediatric Health Care

AGE[5]	INFANCY[4]									EARLY CHILDHOOD[4]				
	PRENATAL[1]	NEWBORN[2]	2-4D[3]	BY 1MO	2MO	4MO	6MO	9MO	12MO	15MO	18MO	24MO	3Y	4Y
History														
Initial/Interval	●	●	●	●	●	●	●	●	●	●	●	●	●	●
Measurements														
Height and Weight		●	●	●	●	●	●	●	●	●	●	●	●	●
Head Circumference		●	●	●	●	●	●	●	●	●	●	●	●	●
Blood Pressure														
Sensory Screening														
Vision		S	S	S	S	S	S	S	S	S	S	S	O[6]	O
Hearing		O[7]	S	S	S	S	S	S	S	S	S	S	S	O
Developmental/ Behavioral Assessment[8]		●	●	●	●	●	●	●	●	●	●	●	●	●
Physical Examination[9]		●	●	●	●	●	●	●	●	●	●	●	●	●
Procedures-General[10]														
Hereditary/ Metabolic Screening[11]			← ● →											
Immunization[12]		●	●	●	●	●	●	●	● →	●	●	●		● →
Hematocrit or Hemoglobin[13]								● →		*				→
Urinalysis														
Procedures- Patients at Risk														
Lead Screening[16]								* →				*		
Tuberculin Test[17]									*	*	*	*	*	*
Cholesterol Screening[18]												*	*	*
STD Screening[19]														
Pelvic Exam[20]														
Anticipatory Guidance[21]	●	●	●	●	●	●	●	●	●	●	●	●	●	●
Injury Prevention[22]	●	●	●	●	●	●	●	●	●	●	●	●	●	●
Violence Prevention[23]	●	●	●	●	●	●	●	●	●	●	●	●	●	●
Sleep Positioning Counseling[24]	●	●	●	●	●	●	●							
Nutrition Counseling[25]	●	●	●	●	●	●	●	●	●	●	●	●	●	●
Dental Referral[26]										←		→		

1. A prenatal visit is recommended for parents who are at high risk, for first-time parents, and for those who request a conference. The prenatal visit should include anticipatory guidance, pertinent medical history, and a discussion of benefits of breastfeeding and planned method of feeding per AAP statement "The Prenatal Visit" (1996).
2. Every infant should have a newborn evaluation after birth. Breastfeeding should be encouraged and instruction and support offered. Every breastfeeding infant should have an evaluation 48-72 hours after discharge from the hospital to include weight, formal breastfeeding evaluation, encouragement, and instruction as recommended in the AAP statement "Breastfeeding and the Use of Human Milk" (1997).
3. For newborns discharged in less than 48 hours after delivery per AAP statement "Hospital Stay for Healthy Term Newborns" (1995).
4. Developmental, psychosocial, and chronic disease issues for children and adolescents may require frequent counseling and treatment visits separate from preventive care visits.
5. If a child comes under care for the first time at any point on the schedule, or if any items are not accomplished at the suggested age, the schedule should be brought up to date at the earliest possible time.
6. If the patient is uncooperative, rescreen within 6 months.

	MIDDLE CHILDHOOD[4]			ADOLESCENCE[4]										
5Y	**6Y**	**8Y**	**10Y**	**11Y**	**12Y**	**13Y**	**14Y**	**15Y**	**16Y**	**17Y**	**18Y**	**19Y**	**20Y**	**21Y**
•	•	•	•	•	•	•	•	•	•	•	•	•	•	•
•	•	•	•	•	•	•	•	•	•	•	•	•	•	•
•	•	•	•	•	•	•	•	•	•	•	•	•	•	•
O	O	O	O	S	O	S	S	O	S	S	O	S	S	S
O	O	O	O	S	O	S	S	O	S	S	O	S	S	S
•	•	•	•	•	•	•	•	•	•	•	•	•	•	•
•	•	•	•	•	•	•	•	•	•	•	•	•	•	•
•	•	•	•	•	•	•[14]	•	•	•	•	•	•	•	•
← 14 →														
•						•[15]								
← 15 →														
*	*	*	*	*	*	*	*	*	*	*	*	*	*	*
*	*	*	*	*	*	*	*	*	*	*	*	*	*	*
				*	*	*	*	*	*	*	*	*[20]	*	*
				*	*	*	*	*	*	*	* ← 20 →			*
•	•	•	•	•	•	•	•	•	•	•	•	•	•	•
•	•	•	•	•	•	•	•	•	•	•	•	•	•	•
•	•	•	•	•	•	•	•	•	•	•	•	•	•	•
•	•	•	•	•	•	•	•	•	•	•	•	•	•	•

Continued

7. All newborns should be screened per the AAP Task Force on Newborn and Infant Hearing statement, "Newborn and Infant Hearing Loss: Detection and Intervention" (1999).

8. By history and appropriate physical examination: if suspicious, by specific objective developmental testing. Parenting skills should be fostered at every visit.

9. At each visit, a complete physical examination is essential, with infant totally unclothed, older child undressed and suitably draped.

10. These may be modified, depending upon entry point into schedule and individual need.

11. Metabolic screening (e.g., thyroid, hemoglobinopathies, PKU, Galactosemia) should be done according to state law.

12. Schedule(s) per the Committee on Infectious Diseases, published annually in the January edition of *Pediatrics*. Every visit should be an opportunity to update and complete a child's immunizations.

13. See AAP *Pediatric Nutrition Handbook* (1998) for a discussion of universal and selective screening options. Consider earlier screening for high-risk infants (e.g., premature infants and low—birth weight infants). See also "Recommendations to Prevent and Control Iron Deficiency in the United States. *MMWR*. 1998;47 (RR-3): 1-29.

14. All menstruating adolescents should be screened annually.

15. Conduct dipstick urinalysis for leukocytes annually for sexually active male and female adolescents.

16. For children at risk of lead exposure consult the AAP statement "Screening for Elevated Blood Levels" (1998). Additionally, screening should be done in accordance with state law where applicable.
17. TB testing per recommendations of the Committee on Infectious Diseases, published in the current edition of *Red Book: Report of the Committee on Infectious Diseases*. Testing should be done upon recognition of high-risk factors.
18. Cholesterol screening for high-risk patients per AAP statement "Cholesterol in Childhood" (1998). If family history cannot be ascertained and other risk factors are present, screening should be at the discretion of the physician.
19. All sexually active patients should be screened for sexually transmitted diseases (STDs).
20. All sexually active females should have a pelvic examination. A pelvic examination and routine Pap smear should be offered as part of preventive health maintenance between the ages of 18 and 21 years.
21. Age-appropriate discussion and counseling should be an integral part of each visit for care per the AAP *Guidelines for Health Supervision III* (1998).
22. From birth to age 12, refer to the AAP injury prevention program (TIPP) as described in *A Guide to Safety Counseling in Office Practice* (1994).
23. Violence prevention and management for all patients per AAP statement "The Role of the Pediatrician in Youth Violence Prevention in Clinical Practice and at the Community Level" (1999).
24. Parents and caregivers should be advised to place healthy infants on their backs when putting them to sleep. Side positioning is a reasonable alternative but carries a slightly higher risk of SIDS. Consult the AAP statement "Positioning and Sudden Infant Death Syndrome (SIDS): Update" (1996).
25. Age-appropriate nutrition counseling should be an integral part of each visit per the AAP *Handbook of Nutrition* (1998).
26. Earlier initial dental examinations may be appropriate for some children. Subsequent examinations as prescribed by dentist.

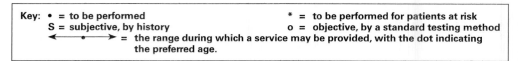

Key: • = to be performed   * = to be performed for patients at risk
S = subjective, by history   o = objective, by a standard testing method
◄——•——► = the range during which a service may be provided, with the dot indicating the preferred age.

NB: Special chemical, immunologic, and endocrine testing is usually carried out upon specific indications. Testing other than newborn (e.g., inborn errors of metabolism, sickle disease, etc.) is discretionary with the physician.

Each child and family is unique; therefore these **Recommendations for Preventive Pediatric Health Care** from the Committee on Practice and Ambulatory Medicine are designed for the care of children who are receiving competent parenting, have no manifestations of any important health problems, and are growing and developing in satisfactory fashion. **Additional visits may become necessary** if circumstances suggest variations from normal.

These guidelines represent a consensus by the Committee on Practice and Ambulatory Medicine in consultation with national committees and sections of the American Academy of Pediatrics. The Committee emphasizes the great importance of **continuity of care** in comprehensive health supervision and the need to avoid **fragmentation of care.**

D Normal Laboratory Values for Children—Reference Ranges

Knowledge of normal laboratory values for children of various ages can greatly assist the pediatric nurse with appropriate data gathering. Laboratory value reference ranges are guides for judging health and disease. The following reference ranges have been determined by examining the distribution of measurements in normal individuals of appropriate age ranges. These ranges have proved to be clinically useful in pediatric settings. For adequate data gathering and analysis, the nurse can use these values to compare clinical presentation to what is expected for the child. Keep in mind that laboratory values are used to augment the assessment of other clinical signs.

ORGANIZATION OF REFERENCE VALUES

I.   Analyses of blood
A.   Formed elements, indices, and coagulation factors
B.   Chemical elements
C.   Analyses of blood for drugs of all classes
II. Analyses of urine
A.   Formed elements
B.   Chemical elements
III. Analyses of feces
A.   Chemical elements
IV. Analyses of cerebrospinal fluid
A.   Formed elements
B.   Chemical elements
V.   Analyses of other body fluids
A.   Chemical analyses

I.   ANALYSES OF BLOOD

A.   Formed Elements, Indices, and Coagulation Factors

ANALYTE OR PROCEDURE	SPECIMEN	REFERENCE VALUES (USA)	CONVERSION FACTOR	REFERENCE VALUES (SI)	COMMENTS
Activated partial thromboplastin time (APTT)	P(C)	25–35 sec Infants < 90 sec	×1	25–35 sec Infants < 90 sec	
Clotting time, Lee-White, 37°C	W	Glass tubes 5–8 min (5–15 min at RT) Silicone tubes ≈30 min prolonged		Glass tubes 5–8 min (5–15 min at RT) Silicone tubes ≈30 min prolonged	
Coagulation factor assays					
Factor I, see *Fibrinogen*					
Factor II	P(C)	0.5–1.5 U/ml or 60–150% of normal	×1	0.5–1.5 kU/L or 60–150 AU	
Factor V		0.5–2.0 U/mL or 60–150% of normal	×1	0.5–2.0 kU/L or 60–150 AU	
Factor VII		65–135% of normal	×1	65–135 AU	
Factor VIII		60–145% of normal	×1	60–145 AU	
Factor VIII antigen		50–200% of normal	×1	50–200 AU	
Factor IX		60–140% of normal	×1	60–140 AU	
Factor X		60–130% of normal	×1	60–130 AU	
Factor XI		65–135% of normal	×1	65–135 AU	
Factor XII		65–150% of normal	×1	65–150 AU	
Factor XII (fibrin-stabilizing factor [FSF])	W(C,0)	Minimal hemostatic level 0.02–0.05 U/mL 1–2% of normal	×1,000 ×1	20–50 U/L or 1–2 AU	
Fibrin degradation products (D-dimer)	P(C)	Adults 68–494 µg/L Mean 207	×1	68–494 µg/L Mean 207	(Pittet et al., 1996)
Fibrinogen	(NaC)	Newborn 125–300 mg/dL Adult 200–400 mg/dL	×0.01	1.25–3.00 g/L 2.00–4.00 g/L	

Erythrocytes

Erythrocyte count (RBC count)	W(E)	Millions of cells/mm³ (µL)		×10¹² cells/L	
		Cord blood	3.9–5.5		3.9–5.5	
		1–3 days (cap)	4.0–6.6		4.0–6.6	
		1 wk	3.9–6.3	×1	3.9–6.3	
		2 wk	3.6–6.2		3.6–6.2	
		1 mo	3.0–5.4		3.0–5.4	
		2 mo	2.7–4.9		2.7–4.9	
		3–6 mo	3.1–4.5		3.1–4.5	
		0.5–2 yr	3.7–5.3		3.7–5.3	
		2–6 yr	3.9–5.3		3.9–5.3	
		6–12 yr	4.0–5.2		4.0–5.2	
		12–18 yr M	4.5–5.3		4.5–5.3	
		F	4.1–5.1		4.1–5.1	

Complete Blood Count

Hematocrit (HCT, Hct) Calculated from mean corpuscular volume (MCV) and RBC count (electronic displacement or laser)	W(E)	% of packed red cells (V red cells/V whole blood cells × 100		Volume fraction (V red cells/V whole blood)	
		1 day (cap)	48–69%	×0.01	0.48–0.69	
		2 days	48–75%		0.48–0.75	
		3 days	44–72%		0.44–0.72	
		2 mo	28–42%		0.28–0.42	
		6–12 yr	35–45%		0.35–0.45	
		12–18 yr M	37–49%		0.37–0.49	
		F	36–46%		0.36–0.46	
		18–49 yr M	41–53%		0.41–0.53	
		F	36–46%		0.36–0.46	
Hemoglobin (Hb)	W(E)	g/dL		mmol/L	
		1–3 days (cap)	14.5–22.5	×0.155	2.25–3.49	MW Hb = 64,500
		2 mo	9.0–14.0		1.40–2.17	
		6–12 yr	11.5–15.5		1.78–2.40	
		12–18 yr M	13.0–16.0		2.02–2.48	
		F	12.0–16.0		1.86–2.48	
		18–49 yr M	13.5–17.5		2.09–2.27	
		F	12.0–16.0		1.86–2.48	
	P(H)	See *Chemical Elements*			

ANALYTE OR PROCEDURE	SPECIMEN	REFERENCE VALUES (USA)		CONVERSION FACTOR	REFERENCE VALUES (SI)	COMMENTS
Erythrocyte indices (RBC indices)						
Mean corpuscular hemoglobin (MCH)	W(E)		pg/cell		fmol/cell	
		Birth	31–37	×0.0155	0.48–0.57	
		1–3 days (cap)	31–37		0.48–0.57	
		1 wk–1 mo	28–40		0.43–0.62	
		2 mo	26–34		0.40–0.53	
		3–6 mo	25–35		0.39–0.54	
		0.5–2 yr	23–31		0.36–0.48	
		2–6 yr	24–30		0.37–0.47	
		6–12 yr	25–33		0.39–0.51	
		12–18 yr	25–35		0.39–0.54	
		18–49 yr	26–34		0.40–0.53	
Mean corpuscular hemoglobin concentration (MCHC)	W(E)		% Hb/cell or g Hb/dL RBC		mmol Hb/L RBC	
		Birth	30–36	×0.155	4.65–5.58	
		1–3 days (cap)	29–37		4.50–5.74	
		1–2 wk	28–38		4.34–5.89	
		1–2 mo	29–37		4.50–5.74	
		3 mo–2 yr	30–36		4.65–5.58	
		2–18 yr	31–37		4.81–5.74	
		>18 yr	31–37		4.81–5.74	
Mean corpuscular volume (MCV)	W(E)		μm³		fL	
		1–3 days (cap)	95–121	×1	95–121	
		0.5–2 yr	70–86		70–86	
		6–12 yr	77–95		77–95	
		12–18 yr M	78–98		78–98	
		F	78–102		78–102	
		18–49 yr M	80–100		80–100	
		F	80–100		80–100	
Erythrocyte sedimentation rate (ESR), Westergren, modified			mm/hr	×1	mm/hr	
		Child	0–10		0–10	
		Adult M < 50	0–15		0–15	
	W(E)	F < 50	0–20		0–20	
Wintrobe		Child	0–13		0–13	
		Adult M	0–9		0–9	
		F	0–20		0–20	
Zeta			41–54%		41–54 AU	
Leukocyte count (WBC count)	W(E)		×1,000 cells/mm³ (μL)		×10⁹ cells/L	
		Birth	9.0–30.0	×1	9.0–30.0	
		24 hr	9.4–34.0		9.4–34.0	
		1 mo	5.0–19.5		5.0–19.5	
		1–3 yr	6.0–17.5		6.0–17.5	
		4–7 yr	5.5–15.5		5.5–15.5	
		8–13 yr	4.5–13.5		4.5–13.5	
		Adult	4.5–11.0		4.5–11.0	
Leukocyte differential	W(E)		%		Number fraction	
Myelocytes			0%	×0.01	0	
Neutrophils ("bands")			3–5%		0.03–0.05	
Neutrophils ("segs")			54–62%		0.54–0.62	
Lymphocytes			25–33%		0.25–0.33	
Monocytes			3–7%		0.03–0.07	
Eosinophils			1–3%		0.01–0.03	
Basophils			0–0.75%		0–0.0075	
			Cells/mm³ (μL)		×10⁶ cells/L	
Myelocytes			0	×1	0	
Neutrophils ("bands")			150–400		150–400	
Neutrophils ("segs")			3,000–5,800		3,000–5,800	
Lymphocytes			1,500–3,000		1,500–3,000	
Monocytes			285–500		285–500	
Eosinophils			50–250		50–250	
Basophils			15–50		15–50	

		Age				
		2–3 mo	4–8 mo	12–23 mo	24–59 mo	
Lymphocyte subsets	W(E)					(Denny et al., 1992)
Median lymphocytes, total		5.68 × 10⁹/L	5.99 × 10⁹/L	5.16 × 10⁹/L	4.06 × 10⁹/L	
5th–95th centiles		2.92–8.84	3.61–8.84	2.18–8.27	2.40–5.89	
Median CD3 lymphocytes		4.03 × 10⁹/L	4.27 × 10⁹/L	3.33 × 10⁹/L	3.04 × 10⁹/L	
5th–95th centiles		2.07–6.54	2.28–6.45	1.46–5.44	1.61–4.23	
Median CD4 lymphocytes		2.83 × 10⁹/L	2.95 × 10⁹/L	2.07 × 10⁹/L	1.80 × 10⁹/L	
5th–95th centiles		1.46–5.11	1.69–4.60	1.02–3.60	0.90–2.86	
Median CD8 lymphocytes		1.41 × 10⁹/L	1.45 × 10⁹/L	1.32 × 10⁹/L	1.18 × 10⁹/L	
5th–95th centiles		0.65–2.45	0.72–2.49	0.57–2.23	0.63–1.91	
Median % lymphocytes		66	64	59	50	
5th–95th centiles		55–78	45–79	44–72	38–64	

ANALYTE OR PROCEDURE	SPECIMEN	REFERENCE VALUES (USA)		CONVERSION FACTOR	REFERENCE VALUES (SI)		COMMENTS
Median % CD3 lymphocytes		72	71	66	72		
5th–95th centiles		60–87	57–84	53–81	62–80		
Median % CD4 lymphocytes		52	49	43	42		
5th–95th centiles		41–64	36–61	31–54	35–51		
Median % CD8 lymphocytes		25	24	25	30		
5th–95th centiles		16–35	16–34	16–38	22–38		
Osmotic fragility test (RBC fragility) pH 7.4, 20°C	W(H)	% NaCl (g/dL)	% hemolysis	×0.01 (hemolyzed fraction)	NaCl (g/L)	Hemolyzed fraction	
		0.30	97–100		3.0	0.97–1.00	
		0.35	90–99		3.5	0.90–0.99	
		0.40	50–95		4.0	0.50–0.95	
		0.45	5–45		4.5	0.05–0.45	
		0.50	0–6		5.0	0.00–0.06	
		0.55	0		5.5	0.00	
Osmotic fragility test (sterile incubation) at 37°C		% NaCl (g/dL)	% hemolysis	×0.01 (hemolyzed fraction)	NaCl (g/L)	Hemolyzed fraction	
		0.20	95–100		2.0	0.95–1.00	
		0.30	85–100		3.0	0.85–1.00	
		0.35	75–100		3.5	0.75–1.00	
		0.40	65–100		4.0	0.65–1.00	
		0.45	55–95		4.5	0.55–0.95	
		0.50	40–85		5.0	0.40–0.85	
		0.55	15–70		5.5	0.15–0.70	
		0.60	0–40		6.0	0.00–0.40	
		0.65	0–10		6.5	0.00–0.10	
		0.70	0–5		7.0	0.00–0.05	
		0.85	0		8.5	0.00	
Partial thromboplastin time (PTT)	W(NaC)						
Nonactivated		60–85 sec (platelin)			60–85 sec		
Activated, see *Activated partial thromboplastin time (APTT)*							
Platelet count (thrombocyte count)	W(E)	×10³/mm³ (μL)		×10⁶	×10⁹/L		(Buck, 1996)
		Newborn 84–478 (after 1 wk, same as adult)			84–478		
		Adult 150–400			150–400		
Prothrombin time (PT)							
One-stage (Quick)	W(NaC)	In general, 11–15 sec (varies with type of thromboplastin)		×1	11–15 sec		
		Newborn prolonged by 2–3 sec			Newborn prolonged by 2–3 sec		
		International normalized ratio (INR) used only for patients receiving coumarin			INR used only for patients receiving coumarin		
		Clinical problem	Target INR		Clinical problem	Target INR	
		Deep venous thrombosis	2.0–3.0		Deep venous thrombosis	2.0–3.0	
		Prosthetic heart valve	2.5–3.0		Prosthetic heart valve	2.5–3.0	
Two-stage modified (Ware and Seegers)	W(NaC)	18–22 sec			18–22 sec		
RBC count, see *Erythrocyte count (RBC count)*							
RBC fragility test, see *Osmotic fragility test (RBC fragility)*							
Red cell volume	W(H)	M 20–36 mL/kg		×0.001	M 0.020–0.036 L/kg		
		F 19–31 mL/kg			F 0.019–0.031 L/kg		
Reticulocyte count	W(E,H,O)	Adults 0.5–1.5% of erythrocytes		×0.01	0.005–0.015 (number fraction)		
		or 25,000–75,000/mm³ (μL)		×10⁶	or 25,000–75,000 × 10⁶/L		
			%		Number fraction		
	W(cap)	1 day	0.4–6.0	×0.01	0.004–0.060		
		7 days	<0.1–1.3		<0.001–0.013		
		1–4 wk	<1.0–1.2		<0.001–0.012		
		5–6 wk	<0.1–2.4		<0.001–0.024		
		7–8 wk	0.1–2.9		0.001–0.029		
		9–10 wk	<0.1–2.6		<0.001–0.026		
		11–12 wk	0.1–1.3		0.001–0.013		
Sedimentation rate, see *Erythrocyte sedimentation rate (ESR), Westergren, modified*							
Sickle cell tests							
Sodium metabisulfite	W(E,H,O)	Negative					
Dithionite test	W(E,H,O)	Negative					
Sucrose hemolysis and sugar-water tests for paroxysmal nocturnal hemoglobinuria (PNH)	W(C,O)	≤5% lysis		×0.01	Lysed fraction ≤ 0.05		
		6–10% lysis questionable			Lysed fraction 0.06–0.10 questionable		
Thrombin time	W(NaC)	Control time ±2 sec when control is 9–13 sec			Control time ±2 sec when control is 9–13 sec		
Thromboplastin time, activated, see *Activated partial thromboplastin time (APTT)*							
Tourniquet test		<5–10 petechiae in 2.5 cm circle on forearm (halfway between systolic and diastolic pressure for 5 min); 0–8 petechiae in 6 cm circle (50 mm Hg for 15 min); 10–20 petechiae in 5 cm circle (80 mm Hg)			<5–10 petechiae in 2.5 cm circle on forearm (halfway between systolic and diastolic pressure for 5 min); 0–8 petechiae in 6 cm circle (50 mm Hg for 15 min); 10–20 petechiae in 5 cm circle (80 mm Hg)		
WBC, see *Leukocyte count*							

ANALYTE OR PROCEDURE	SPECIMEN	REFERENCE VALUES (USA)		CONVERSION FACTOR	REFERENCE VALUES (SI)	COMMENTS
B. Chemical Elements						
Acetone						
Semiquantitative	S,P(O)	Negative (<3 mg/dL)			Negative (<0.5 mmol/L)	
Quantitative		0.3–2.0 mg/dL		×0.1722	0.05–0.34 mmol/L	
Adrenocorticotropic hormone (ACTH)	P(H)		pg/mL		ng/L	
		Cord	130–160	×1	130–160	
		1–7 days postnatal	100–140		100–140	
		Adults 8:00 A.M.	25–100		25–100	
		6:00 A.M.	<50		<50	
Alanine aminotransferase (ALT, SGPT)	S	0–5 days	6–50 U/L	×1	6–50 U/L	37°bw
		1–19 yr	5–45		5–45	(Lockitch, Halstead, and Albersheim, 1988)
Albumin	P	Premature 1 day	1.8–3.0 g/dL	×10	18–30 g/dL	g (Meites, 1989)
		Full term <6 days	2.5–3.4		25–34	
		<5 yr	3.9–5.0		39–50	
		5–19 yr	4.0–5.3		40–53	
Aldolase	S	10–24 mo	3.4–11.8 U/L	×1	3.4–11.8 U/L	j (Visnapu et al., 1989)
		25 mo–16 yr	1.2–8.8		1.2–8.8	
Aldosterone	S,P(H,E)	Supine				(Esoterix Endocrinology)
Ad lib sodium intake						
		Premature infants				
		26–28 wk	5–635 ng/dL	×0.0277	0.14–17.6 nmol/L	
		31–35 wk	19–141		0.53–3.9	
		Full-term infants				
		3 days	7–184 ng/dL		0.19–5.1 nmol/L	
		1 wk	5–175		0.14–4.8	
		1–12 mo	5–90		0.14–2.5	
		Children	Supine			
		1–2 yr	7–54 ng/dL		0.19–1.5 nmol/L	
		2–10 yr	3–35		0.1–0.97	
		10–15 yr	2–22		0.1–0.6	
Alkaline phosphatase, see *Phosphatase, alkaline*						
Amino acids, plasma, quantitative	P(H)			×1		(Shapira et al., 1989)

	Premature 0–6 wk µmol/L	Full-term 0–1 mo µmol/L	1–24 mo µmol/L	2–18 yr µmol/L	Adult µmol/L	Premature 0–6 wk µmol/L	Full-term 0–1 mo µmol/L	1–24 mo µmol/L	2–18 yr µmol/L	Adult µmol/L
1-Methylhistidine	4–28	0–43	0–44	0–42	72–124	4–28	0–43	0–44	0–42	72–124
3-Methylhistidine	5–33	0–5	0–5	0–5	0	5–33	0–5	0–5	0–5	0
Alanine	212–504	131–710	133–439	152–547	177–583	212–504	131–710	133–439	152–547	177–583
Arginine	34–96	6–140	12–133	10–140	15–128	34–96	6–140	12–133	10–140	15–128
Asparagine	90–295	29–132	21–95	23–112	35–74	90–295	29–132	21–95	23–112	35–74
Aspartic acid	24–50	20–129	0–23	1–24	1–25	24–50	20–129	0–23	1–24	1–25
Citrulline	20–87	10–45	3–35	1–46	12–55	20–87	10–45	3–35	1–46	12–55
Cystathionine	5–10	0–3	0–5	0–3	0–3	5–10	0–3	0–5	0–3	0–3
Cystine	15–70	17–98	16–84	5–45	5–82	15–70	17–98	16–84	5–45	5–82
Ethanolamine	ND	0–115	0–4	0–7	0–153	ND	0–115	0–4	0–7	0–153
Glutamic acid	107–276	62–620	10–133	5–150	10–131	107–276	62–620	10–133	5–150	10–131
Glutamine	248–850	376–709	246–1182	254–823	205–756	248–850	376–709	246–1182	254–823	205–756
Glycine	298–602	232–740	81–436	127–341	151–490	298–602	232–740	81–436	127–341	151–490
Histidine	72–134	30–138	41–101	41–125	0–8	72–134	30–138	41–101	41–125	0–8
Hydroxylysine	0	0–7	0–7	0–2	0	0	0–7	0–7	0–2	0
Hydroxyproline	tr–80	0–91	0–63	3–45	0–53	tr–80	0–91	0–63	3–45	0–53
Isoleucine	23–85	26–91	31–86	22–107	30–108	23–85	26–91	31–86	22–107	30–108
Leucine	151–220	48–160	47–155	49–216	72–201	151–220	48–160	47–155	49–216	72–201
Lysine	128–255	92–325	52–196	48–284	0–39	128–255	92–325	52–196	48–284	0–39
Methionine	37–91	10–60	9–42	7–47	10–42	37–91	10–60	9–42	7–47	10–42
Ornithine	77–212	48–211	22–103	10–163	48–195	77–212	48–211	22–103	10–163	48–195
Phenylalanine	98–213	38–137	31–75	26–91	35–85	98–213	38–137	31–75	26–91	35–85
Phosphoethanolamine	5–35	3–27	0–6	0–69	0–40	5–35	3–27	0–6	0–69	0–40
Phosphoserine	10–45	7–47	1–20	1–30	2–14	10–45	7–47	1–20	1–30	2–14
Proline	92–310	110–417	52–298	59–369	97–329	92–310	110–417	52–298	59–369	97–329
Sarcosine	0	0–625	0	0–9	0	0	0–625	0	0–9	0
Serine	127–248	99–395	71–186	69–187	58–181	127–248	99–395	71–186	69–187	58–181
Taurine	151–411	46–492	15–143	10–170	54–210	151–411	46–492	15–143	10–170	54–210
Threonine	150–330	90–329	24–174	35–226	60–225	150–330	90–329	24–174	35–226	60–225
Tryptophan	28–136	0–60	23–71	0–79	10–140	28–136	0–60	23–71	0–79	10–140
Tyrosine	147–420	55–147	22–108	24–115	34–112	147–420	55–147	22–108	24–115	34–112
Valine	99–220	86–190	64–294	74–321	119–336	99–220	86–190	64–294	74–321	119–336
α-Aminoadipic acid	0	0	0	0	0–6	0	0	0	0	0–6
α-Aminobutyric acid	14–52	8–24	3–26	4–31	5–41	14–52	8–24	3–26	4–31	5–41
β-Alanine	0	0–10	0–7	0–7	0–12	0	0–10	0–7	0–7	0–12
β-Aminoisobutyric acid	0	0	0	0	0	0	0	0	0	0
γ-Aminobutyric acid	0	0–2	0	0	0	0	0–2	0	0	0

ANALYTE OR PROCEDURE	SPECIMEN	REFERENCE VALUES (USA)	CONVERSION FACTOR	REFERENCE VALUES (SI)	COMMENTS
Aminolevulinic acid (ALA)	S	15–23 µg/dL (lower in child)	×0.076	1.1–1.8 µmol/L	

ANALYTE OR PROCEDURE	SPECIMEN	REFERENCE VALUES (USA)		CONVERSION FACTOR	REFERENCE VALUES (SI)	COMMENTS
Ammonia	W	<30 days	21–95 µmol/L	×1	21–95 µmol/L	(Diaz et al., 1995)
		1–12 mo	18–74		18–74	
		1–14 yr	17–68		17–68	
		>14 yr	19–71		19–71	
Amylase	S,P	1–19 yr	30–100 U/L	×1	30–100 U/L	(Lockitch, Halstead, and Albersheim et al., 1988; Gillard et al., 1983)
Amylase isoenzymes	S,P(H)		% pancreatic fraction		% pancreatic fraction	
		Cord–8 mo	0–34%	×0.01	0–0.34%	
		9 mo–4 yr	5–56%		0.05–0.56%	
		5–19 yr	23–59%		0.23–0.59%	
Androstenedione	S	Tanner	Age	M		(Esoterix Endocrinology)
		1	<9.8 yr	8–50 ng/dL	×0.03492	0.28–1.75	
		2	9.8–14.5	31–65		1.08–2.27	
		3	10.7–15.4	50–100		1.75–3.49	
		4	11.8–16.2	48–140		1.68–4.89	
		5	12.8–17.3	65–210		2.27–7.33	
		Adult	18–40	75–205		2.62–7.16	
	S	Tanner stage	Age	F		
		1	<9.2 yr	8–50 ng/dL	×0.03492	0.28–1.75	
		2	9.2–13.7	42–100		1.47–3.49	
		3	10.0–14.4	80–190		2.79–6.63	
		4	10.7–15.6	77–225		2.69–7.86	
		5	11.8–18.6	80–240		2.79–8.38	
		Adult	18–40	60–245		2.10–8.56	
		Postmenopausal		30–120		1.05–4.19	
Anion gap (sodium − [chloride + bicarbonate])	P(H)	7–16 mEq/L		×1	7–16 mEq/L	
Anti-deoxyribonuclease B titer (anti-DNase B titer)	S	Age	Upper limit of normal		Upper limit of normal	(Kaplan et al., 1998)
		4–6 yr	240–480 U	×1	240–480 U	
		7–12 yr	480–800 U		480–800 U	
Antidiuretic hormone (hADH, vasopressin)	P(E)	Plasma osmolarity (mOsm/kg)	Plasma ADH (pg/mL)		Plasma ADH ng/L	
		270–280	<1.5	×1	<1.5	
		280–285	<2.5		<2.5	
		285–290	1–5		1–5	
		290–295	2–7		2–7	
		295–300	4–12		4–12	
Antistreptolysin-O titer (ASO titer)	S	Age	Upper limit of normal		Upper limit of normal	(Kaplan et al., 1998)
		2–5 yr	120–160 Todd units	×1	120–160 Todd units	
		6–9 yr	240 Todd units		240 Todd units	
		10–12 yr	320 Todd units		320 Todd units	
α₁-Antitrypsin	S	0–5 days	143–440 mg/dL	×0.01	1.43–4.40 g/L	(Lockitch, Halstead, and Quigley et al., 1988)
		1–9 yr	147–245		1.47–2.45	
		9–19 yr	152–317		1.52–3.17	
Apolipoproteins						(Baroni et al., 1996)
A-1	S	2–12 mo	133 ± 27 mg/dL	×0.01	1.33 ± 0.27 g/L	
		2–10 yr	143 ± 18 mg/dL		1.43 ± 0.18	
B	S	2–12 mo	73 ± 16 mg/dL	×0.01	0.73 ± 0.16 g/L	
		2–10 yr	78 ± 17 mg/dL		0.78 ± 0.17	
CII	S	2–12 mo	47.0 ± 16 mg/L	×1	47.0 ± 16 mg/L	
		2–10 yr	41.0 ± 16 mg/L		41.0 ± 16	
CIII	S	2–12 mo	76.0 ± 29 mg/L	×1	76.0 ± 29 mg/L	
		2–10 yr	69.0 ± 22 mg/L		69.0 ± 22	
E	S	2–12 mo	41.0 ± 9 mg/L	×1	41.0 ± 9 mg/L	
		2–10 yr	39.0 ± 10 mg/L		39.0 ± 10	
Lipoprotein (a)	S	2–12 mo	42.0 ± 36 mg/L	×1	42.0 ± 36 mg/L	
		2–10 yr	64.0 ± 57 mg/L		64.0 ± 57	
		6–16 yr		×10	6–16 yr	
		Median 19 mg/dL			Median 190 mg/L	By immunoturbimetry (Laskowska-Klita et al., 2001)
		Range 11–95 mg/dL			Range 110–950 mg/L	
Ascorbic acid, see *Vitamin C*						
Aspartate aminotransferase (AST, SGOT)	S		U/L		U/L	
		0–5 days	35–140	×1	35–140	37°b(Lockitch, Halstead, and Quigley et al., 1988)
		1–9 yr	15–55		15–55	
		10–19 yr	5–45		5–45	
Base excess	W(H)		mmol/L		mmol/L	
		Newborn	(−10)–(−2)	×1	(−10)–(−2)	
		Infant	(−7)–(−1)		(−7)–(−1)	
		Child	(−4)–(+2)		(−4)–(+2)	
		Thereafter	(−3)–(+3)		(−3)–(−3)	

ANALYTE OR PROCEDURE	SPECIMEN	REFERENCE VALUES (USA)			CONVERSION FACTOR	REFERENCE VALUES (SI)		COMMENTS
Bicarbonate	S,P		mmol/L		×1	mmol/L		
		Arterial	21–28			21–28		
		Venous	22–29			22–29		
Bile acids, total	S, fasting	0.3–2.3 µg/mL			×1	0.3–2.3 µg/L		
	S, 2 hr pc	1.8–3.2 µg/mL				1.8–3.2 µg/L		
	F	120–225 mg/24 hr			×1	120–225 mg/L		
Bilirubin, total	S		Premature (mg/dL)	Full-term (mg/dl)		Premature µmol/L	Full-term (µmol/L)	
	S	Cord blood	<2.0	<2.0	×17.10	<34	<34	
		0–1 day	<8.0	<6.0		<137	<103	
		1–2 days	<12.0	<8.0		<205	<137	
		2–5 days	<16.0	<12.0		<274	<205	
		>5 days	<20.0	<10		<340	<171	
Bilirubin, conjugated	S	0–0.2 mg/dL			×17.10	0–3.4 µmol/L		
Bleeding time (BT)								
Ivy		Normal 2–7 min			×1	2–7 min		
		Borderline 7–11 min				7–11 min		
Simplate		2.75–8 min				2.75–8 min		
Blood volume	W(H)	mL/kg				L/kg		
		M 52–83			×0.001	M: 0.052–0.083		
		F 50–75				F: 0.050–0.075		
B-type natriuretic peptide	P		pg/mL		×1	ng/L		(Koch and Singer, 2003)
		4–6 days	232 (SD 198)			232 (SD 198)		
		<10 yr	48 (SD 49)			48 (SD 49)		
		10–17 yr	25 (95th percentile			25 (95th percentile)		
		M	12 (95th percentile)			12 (95th percentile)		
		F	30 (95th percentile)			30 (95th percentile)		
Brucellosis, agglutinins	S	≤1 : 8			×1	≤1 : 8		
C-peptide of insulin	S	Children 8:00 A.M. fasting	0.4–2.2 ng/mL		×1	0.4–2.2 µg/L		(Esoterix Endocrinology)
C-reactive protein (high sensitivity)	S							(Soldin et al., 2004)
			M (mg/dL)	F (mg/dL)			M (mg/L) F (mg/L)	
		0–90 days	0.08–1.58	0.09–1.58	×10		0.8–15.8 0.9–15.8	
		91 days–12 mo	0.08–1.12	0.05–0.79			0.8–11.2 0.5–7.9	
		13 mo–3 yr	0.08–1.12	0.08–0.79			0.8–11.2 0.8–7.9	
		4–10 yr	0.06–0.79	0.5–1.0			0.6–7.9 0.5–10.0	
		11–14 yr	0.08–0.76	0.06–0.81			0.8–7.6 0.6–8.1	
		15–18 yr	0.04–0.79	0.06–0.79			0.4–7.9 0.6–7.9	
Calcitonin	S,P(H,E)		pg/mL		×0.28	pmol/L		(Basuyau et al., 2004)
		<6 mo	<40			<11.2		
		>6 mo–3 yr	<15			<4.2		
		Adult M	<12			<3.36		
		F	<5			<1.4		
Calcium, ionized (Ca)	S,P(H),W(H)		mg/dL			mmol/L		
		Cord blood	5.0–6.0		×0.25	1.25–1.50		
		Newborn, 3–24 hr	4.3–5.1			1.07–1.27		
		24–48 hr	4.0–4.7			1.00–1.17		
		Thereafter	4.8–4.92			1.12–1.23		
		or	2.24–2.46 Eq/L		×0.5	1.12–1.23		
Calcium, total	S		mg/dL			mmol/L		
		Cord blood	9.0–11.5		×0.25	2.25–2.88		
		Newborn, 3–24 hr	9.0–10.6			2.3–2.65		
		24–48	7.0–12.0			1.75–3.00		
		4–7 days	9.0–10.9			2.25–2.73		
		Child	8.8–10.8			2.20–2.70		
		Thereafter	8.4–10.2			2.10–2.55		
Carbon dioxide, partial pressure (PCO₂)	W(H)		mm Hg			kPa		
		Newborn	27–40		×0.1333	3.6–5.3		
		Infant	27–41			3.6–5.5		
		Thereafter M	35–48			4.7–6.4		
		F	32–45			4.3–6.0		
Carbon dioxide, total (tCo₂)	S,P(H)		mmol/L			mmol/L		
		Cord	14–22		×1	14–22		
		Premature	14–27			14–27		
		Newborn	13–22			13–22		
		Infant	20–28			20–28		
		Child	20–28			20–28		
		Thereafter	23–30			23–30		
Carbon monoxide (carboxyhemoglobin)	W(E)	Nonsmoker	<2% HbCO		×0.01	HbCO fraction < 0.02		
		Smoker	<10%			<0.10		
		Lethal	>50%			>0.5		

ANALYTE OR PROCEDURE	SPECIMEN	REFERENCE VALUES (USA)			CONVERSION FACTOR	REFERENCE VALUES (SI)			COMMENTS
Carnitine	P		μmol/L				μmol/L		(Schmidt-Sommerfeld et al., 1988)
		Age	Total	Free	×1	Age	Total	Free	
		1 day	36.4 ± 10.8	20.1 ± 6.7		1 day	36.4 ± 10.8	20.1 ± 6.7	
		2–7 days	25.2 ± 4.1	14.9 ± 3.0		2–7 days	25.2 ± 4.1	14.9 ± 3.0	
		8–28 days	36.7 ± 10.5	27.6 ± 9.7		8–28 days	36.7 ± 10.5	27.6 ± 9.7	
		29 days–1 yr	47.6 ± 7.7	35.5 ± 6.5		29 days–1 yr	47.6 ± 7.7	35.5 ± 6.5	
		1–6 yr	54.4 ± 9.9	41.7 ± 7.9		1–6 yr	54.4 ± 9.9	41.7 ± 7.9	
		6–10 yr	56.2 ± 11.4	41.4 ± 10.0		6–10 yr	56.2 ± 11.4	41.4 ± 10.0	
		10–17 yr	53.4 ± 9.5	39.4 ± 8.7		10–17 yr	53.4 ± 9.5	39.4 ± 8.7	
		22–60 yr	54.0 ± 12.6	39.1 ± 8.6		22–60 yr	54.0 ± 12.6	39.1 ± 8.6	
Beta-carotene	S		μg/dL				μmol/L		
		Infant	20–70		×0.0186		0.37–1.30		
		Child	40–130				0.74–2.42		
		Thereafter	60–200				1.12–3.72		
Catecholamines, fractionated	P(E)	Norepinephrine	pg/mL						
		Supine	100–400		×5.911	591–2,364 pmol/L			
		Standing	300–900			1,773–5,320			
		Epinephrine	pg/mL						
		Supine	<70		×5.458	<382 pmol/L			
		Standing	<100			<546			
		Dopamine	<30 pg/mL		×6.528	<196 pmol/L			
		(no postural change)				(no postural change)			
Ceruloplasmin	S	0–5 days	5–26 mg/dL		×10	50–260 mg/L			CS (Lockitch, Halstead, and Quigley et al., 1988)
		1–19 yr	20–46 mg/dL			200–460 mg/L			
Chloride	S,P(H)	Cord blood	96–104 mmol/L		×1	96–104 mmol/L			
		Newborn	97–110			97–110			
		Thereafter	98–106			98–106			
Cholesterol, total	S	1–3 yr	45–182 mg/dL		×0.0259	1.15–4.70 mmol/L			j (Lockitch, Halstead, and Albersheim et al., 1988) (Mayo Medical Laboratories)
		4–6 yr	109–189			2.80–4.80			

			M		×0.0259		M		
Age (yr)		5	Percentile 75	95		Age (yr)	5	Percentile 75	95
6–9		126	172	191 mg/dL		6–9	3.26	4.45	4.94 mmol/L
10–14		130	179	204		10–14	3.36	4.63	5.28
15–19		114	167	198		15–19	2.95	4.32	5.12
			F					F	
Age (yr)		5	Percentile 75	95		Age (yr)	5	Percentile 75	95
6–9		122	173	209 mg/dL		6–9	3.16	4.47	5.41 mmol/L
10–14		124	174	217		10–14	3.21	4.50	5.61
15–19		125	175	212		15–19	3.23	4.53	5.48

ANALYTE OR PROCEDURE	SPECIMEN	REFERENCE VALUES (USA)		CONVERSION FACTOR	REFERENCE VALUES (SI)	COMMENTS
Chorionic gonadotropin β-subunit (β-hCG)	S,P(E)	Child and M undetectable				(Abbott Laboratories)
		F, postconception	mIU/mL	×1	IU/L	
		1–2 wk	9–130		9–130	
		2–3 wk	75–2,600		75–2,600	
		3–4 wk	850–20,800		850–20,800	
		4–5 wk	4,000–100,200		4,000–100,200	
		5–10 wk	11,500–289,000		11,500–289,000	
		10–14 wk	18,300–137,000		18,300–137,000	
Complement components						
Total hemolytic complement activity (CH$_{50}$)	P(E)	75–160 U/mL		×1	75–160 IU/L	
Total complement decay rate (functional)	P(E)	<10–20%		×0.01	<0.10–0.20 (fraction of decay rate)	
		Deficiency >50%			> 0.50 (fraction of decay rate)	
Classic pathway components						
C1q	S		mg/dL		mg/L	
		Cord blood	1.0–14.9	×10	10–149	
		1 mo	2.2–6.2		22–62	
		6 mo	1.2–7.6		12–76	
		Adult	5.1–7.9		51–79	
C1r	S	2.5–3.8 mg/dL		×10	25–38	
C1s (C1 esterase)	S	2.5–3.8 mg/dL		×10	25–38	
C2	S		mg/dL		mg/L	
		Cord blood	1.6–2.8	×10	16–28	
		1 mo	1.9–3.9		19–39	
		6 mo	2.4–3.6		24–36	
		Adult	1.6–4.0		16–40	
C3	S		mg/dL	×10	mg/L	s (Meites, 1989)
		Cord blood	57–116		570–1,160	
		1–3 mo	53–131		530–1,310	
		3 mo–1 yr	62–180		620–1,800	
		1 yr–10 yr	77–195		770–1,950	
		Adult	83–177		830–1,770	

ANALYTE OR PROCEDURE	SPECIMEN	REFERENCE VALUES (USA)		CONVERSION FACTOR	REFERENCE VALUES (SI)	COMMENTS
C4	S		mg/dL	×10	mg/L	s (Meites, 1989)
		Cord blood	7–23		70–230	
		1–3 mo	7–27		70–270	
		3 mo–10 yr	7–40		70–400	
		Adult	15–45		150–450	
C5	S		mg/dL		mg/L	
		Cord blood	3.4–6.2	×10	34–62	
		1 mo	2.3–6.3		23–63	
		6 mo	2.4–6.4		24–64	
		Adult	3.8–9.0		38–90	
C6	S		mg/dL		mg/L	
		Cord blood	1.0–4.2	×10	10–42	
		1 mo	2.2–5.2		22–52	
		6 mo	3.7–7.1		37–71	
		Adult	4.0–7.2		40–72	
C7	S	4.9–7.0 mg/dL		×10	49–70 mg/L	
C8	S	4.3–6.3 mg/dL		×10	43–63 mg/L	
C9	S	4.7–6.9 mg/dL		×10	47–69 mg/L	
Alternative pathway components						
C4 binding protein	S	18.0–32.0 mg/dL		×10	180–320 mg/L	
Factor B (C3 proactivator) radial immunodiffusion	P(E)		mg/dL		mg/L	
		Cord blood	7.8–15.8	×10	78–158	
		1 mo	6.2–28.6		62–286	
		6 mo	16.9–29.3		169–293	
		Adult	14.7–33.5		147–335	
Nephelometry	S		mg/dL		mg/L	
		Newborn	14–33	×10	140–330	
		Adult	20–45		200–450	
Properdin	S		mg/dL		mg/L	
		Cord blood	1.3–1.7	×10	13–17	
		1 mo	0.6–2.2		6–22	
		6 mo	1.3–2.5		13–25	
		Adult	2.0–3.6		20–36	
Regulatory protein β_1H-globulin (C3b inactivator accelerator)	S		mg/dL		mg/L	
		Cord blood	26–42	×10	260–420	
		1 mo	24–56		240–560	
		6 mo	33–61		330–610	
		Adult	40–72		400–720	
C1 inhibitor (esterase inhibitor)	P(E)	17.4–24.0 mg/dL		×10	174–240 mg/L	
Complement decay rate (functional)	S	<20% decay		×0.01	<0.20 (fractional decay)	
		Deficiency > 50% decay			>0.50 (fractional decay)	
C3b inactivator (KAF)	S		mg/dL		mg/L	
		Cord blood	1.8–2.6	×10	18–26	
		1 mo	1.5–3.9		15–39	
		6 mo	2.3–4.3		23–43	
		Adult	2.6–5.4		26–54	
Copper	S		µg/dL		µmol/L	cd (Lockitch, Halstead, and Wadsworth et al., 1988)
		0–5 days	9–46	×0.157	1.4–7.2	
		1–9 yr	80–150		12.6–23.6	
		10–14 yr	80–121		12.6–19.0	
		15–19 yr	64–160		11.3–25.2	
Corticosteroid-binding globulin (CBG), see *Transcortin*						
Cortisol	S,P(H)		µg/dL		nmol/L	
		Newborn	1–24	×27.59	28–662	
		Adults, 8:00 A.M.	5–23		138–635	
		4:00 P.M.	3–15		82–413	
		8:00 P.M.	<50% of 8:00 A.M.	×0.01	Fraction of 8:00 A.M. ≤0.50	
Creatine kinase	S	Cord blood	70–380 U/L	×1	70–380 U/L	30° b (Jedeikin et al., 1982)
		5–8 hr	214–1,175		214–1,175	
		24–33 hr	130–1,200		130–1,200	
		72–100 hr	87–725		87–725	
		Adult	5–130		5–130	
Creatine kinase isoenzymes	S		% MB	% BB		
		Cord blood	0.3–3.1	0.3–10.5		
		5–8 hr	1.7–7.9	3.6–13.4		
		24–33 hr	1.8–5.0	2.3–8.6		
		72–100 hr	1.4–5.4	5.1–13.3		
		Adult	0–2	0		

ANALYTE OR PROCEDURE	SPECIMEN	REFERENCE VALUES (USA)			CONVERSION FACTOR	REFERENCE VALUES (SI)		COMMENTS
Creatinine								
Jaffe, kinetic, or enzymatic	S,P			mg/dL			μmol/L	
		Cord blood		0.6–1.2	×88.4		53–106	
		Newborn		0.3–1.0			27–88	
		Infant		0.2–0.4			18–35	
		Child		0.3–0.7			27–62	
		Adolescent		0.5–1.0			44–88	
		Adult M		0.6–1.2			53–106	
		F		0.5–1.1			44–97	
Creatinine clearance (endogenous)	S,P,U	Newborn 40–65 mL/min/1.73 m²						
		<40 YR, M 97–137						
		F 88–128						
		Decreases <6.5 mL/min/decade						
Cyclic adenosine monophosphate	P(E)			ng/mL			nmol/L	
		M		5.6–10.9	×3.04	M	17–33	
		F		3.6–8.9		F	11–27	
Dehydroepiandrosterone	S	M						(Esoterix Endocrinology)
		Tanner stage	Age (yr)	ng/dL			nmol/L	
		1	<9.8	31–345	×0.0347		1.07–11.96	
		2	9.8–14.5	110–495			3.81–17.16	
		3	10.7–15.4	170–585			5.89–20.28	
		4	11.8–16.2	160–640			5.55–22.19	
		5	12.8–17.3	250–900			8.67–31.21	
			Adult	160–800			5.55–27.74	
		F						
		Tanner stage	Age (yr)	ng/dL			nmol/L	
		1	<9.2	31–345			1.07–11.96	
		2	9.2–13.7	150–570			5.20–19.76	
		3	10.0–14.4	200–600			6.93–20.80	
		4	10.7–15.6	200–780			6.93–27.07	
		5	11.8–18.6	215–850			7.46–29.47	
		Adult	Follicular	160–800			5.55–27.74	
			Luteal	160–800			5.55–27.74	
Dehydroepiandrosterone sulfate (DHEA-sulfate, DHEA-S)	S	M						(Esoterix Endocrinology)
		Tanner stage	Age (yr)	μg/dL			μmol/L	
		1	<9.8	13–83	×0.026		0.34–2.16	
		2	9.8–14.5	42–109			1.09–2.83	
		3	10.7–15.4	48–200			1.25–5.20	
		4	11.8–16.2	102–385			2.65–10.01	
		5	12–17.3	120–370			3.12–9.62	
			21–30 yr	100–460			2.60–11.96	
		F						
		Tanner stage	Age (yr)	μg/dL			μmol/L	
		1	<9.2	19–144			0.49–2.96	
		2	9.2–13.7	34–129			0.88–3.35	
		3	10.0–14.4	32–226			0.83–8.48	
		4	10.7–15.6	58–260			1.51–6.76	
		5	11.8–18.6	44–248			1.14–6.45	
			21–30 yr	76–255			1.98–6.63	
Deoxycorticosterone	S				×0.03026			(Esoterix Endocrinology)
		Newborn	Very high			Very high		
		1–12 mo	7–49 ng/dL			0.2–1.5 nmol/L		
		Prepubertal (2–10 yr)	2–34 ng/dL			0.1–1 nmol/L		
		Pubertal and adult	2–19 ng/dL			0.1–0.6 nmol/L		
11-Desoxycortisol Specific compound S	S		ng/dL		×0.02886		nmol/L	(Esoterix Endocrinology)
		Full-term 3 days	13–147				0.38–4.24	
		Full-term 1–12 mo	<10–156				<0.29–4.50	
		Prepubertal child (8:00 A.M.)	20–155				0.58–4.47	
		Pubertal and adult (8:00 A.M.)	12–158				0.35–4.56	
Dihydrotestosterone (DHT)	S	M						(Esoterix Endocrinology)
		Tanner stage	Age (yr)	ng/dL			nmol/L	
		1	<9.8	<3	×0.03443		<0.10	
		2	9.8–14.5	3–17			0.10–0.59	
		3	10.7–15.4	8–33			0.28–1.14	
		4	11.8–16.2	22–52			0.76–1.79	
		5	12.8–17.3	24–65			0.83–2.24	
			Adult	30–85			1.03–2.93	

ANALYTE OR PROCEDURE	SPECIMEN	REFERENCE VALUES (USA)			CONVERSION FACTOR	REFERENCE VALUES (SI)		COMMENTS
	S	F			×0.03443	nmo/L		
		Tanner stage	Age (yr)	ng/dL				
		1	<9.2	<3		<0.10		
		2	9.2–13.7	5–12		0.17–0.41		
		3	10.0–14.4	7–19		0.24–0.65		
		4	10.7–15.6	4–13		0.14–0.45		
		5	11.8–18.6	3–18		0.10–0.62		
		Adult	Follicular	4–22		0.14–0.76		
			Luteal	4–22		0.14–0.76		
Disaccharide absorption test	S	Change in glucose from fasting value				Change in glucose from fasting value		
			mg/dL				mmol/L	
		Normal	>30		×0.055	Normal	>1.67	
		Inconclusive	20–30			Inconclusive	1.11–1.67	
		Abnormal	<20			Abnormal	<1.11	
Electrophoresis, hemoglobin, see *Hemoglobin (Hb) electrophoresis*								
Epinephrine, see *Catecholamines, fractionated*								
Erythropoietin								
Radioimmunoassay	S	<5–20 mU/mL			×1	<5–20 U/L		
Hemagglutination		25–125				25–125		
Bioassay		5–18				5–18		
Estradiol	S	M				pmol/L		(Esoterix Endocrinology)
		Tanner stage	Age (yr)	ng/dL				
		1	<9.8	0.5–1.1	×36.71	18–40		
		2	9.8–14.5	0.5–1.6		18–59		
		3	10.7–15.4	0.5–2.5		18–92		
		4	11.8–16.2	1.0–3.6		37–132		
		5	12.8–17.3	1.0–3.6		37–132		
						29–128		
		Adult		0.8–3.5				
		F						
		Tanner stage	Age (yr)	ng/dL		pmol/L		
		1	<9.2 yr	0.5–2.0		18–73		
		2	9.2–13.7	1.0–2.4		37–88		
		3	10.0–14.4	0.7–6.0		26–220		
		4	10.7–15.6	2.1–8.5		77–312		
		5	11.8–18.6	3.4–17		125–624		
		Adult	Follicular	3–10		110–367		
			Luteal	7–30		257–1,100		
Estriol (E₃), free	S	Gestation (wk)	μg/L			nmol/L		
		25	3.5–10.0		×3.47	12.1–34.7		
		28	4.0–12.5			13.9–43.4		
		30	4.5–14.0			15.6–48.6		
		32	5.0–16.0			17.4–55.5		
		34	5.5–18.5			19.1–64.2		
		36	7.0–25.0			24.3–86.8		
		37	8.0–28.0			27.8–97.2		
		38	9.0–32.0			31.2–111.0		
		39	10.0–34.0			34.7–118.0		
		40–41	10.5–25.0			36.4–86.8		
Estriol (E₃), total	S	Pregnancy (wk)	ng/mL			nmol/L		
		24–28	30–170		×3.467	104–590		
		28–32	40–220			140–760		
		32–36	60–280			208–970		
		36–40	80–350			280–1,210		
		Adult M and nonpregnant F	<2			<7		
Estrogens, total	S		pg/mL			ng/L		
		Child	<30		×1	<30		
		M	40–115			40–115		
		F, cycle-days						
		1–10 days	61–394			61–394		
		11–20 days	122–437			122–437		
		21–30 days	156–350			156–350		
		Prepubertal	≤40			≤40		
Free fatty acids	S	Premature	mmol/L			mmol/L		(Meites, 1989)
		10–55 days	0.15–0.71		×1	0.15–0.71		
			mmol/L			mmol.L		
	W	1–12 mo	0.5–1.6		×1	0.5–1.6		(Bonnefont et al., 1990)
		1–7 yr	0.6–1.5			0.6–1.5		
		7–15 yr	0.2–1.1			0.2–1.1		

ANALYTE OR PROCEDURE	SPECIMEN	REFERENCE VALUES (USA)			CONVERSION FACTOR	REFERENCE VALUES (SI)		COMMENTS
Ferritin	S		ng/mL			μg/L		
		Newborn	25–200		×1	25–200		
		1 mo	200–600			200–600		
		2–5 mo	50–200			50–200		
		6 mo–15 yr	7–140			7–140		
		Adult, M	15–200			15–200		
		F	12–150			12–150		
α-Fetoprotein (AFP)	S	Pregnancy (wk)	Median (ng/mL)			Median (μg/L)		
		15	34		×1	34		
		16	38			38		
		17	44			44		
		18	49			49		
		19	56.5			56.5		
		20	66			66		
Folate	S	Newborn 7.0–32 ng/mL			×2.265	15.9–72.4 nmol/L		
		Thereafter 1.8–9.0				4.1–20.4		
	W(E)	150–450 ng/mL RBCs				340–1,020 nmol/L cells		
Follicle-stimulating hormone (FSH)	S		M					(Esoterix Endocrinology)
		Tanner stage	Age (yr)	mIU/mL		U/L		
		1	<9.8	0.26–3.0	×1	0.26–3.0		
		2	9.8–14.5	1.8–3.2		1.8–3.2		
		3	10.7–15.4	1.2–5.8		1.2–5.8		
		4	11.8–16.2	2.0–9.2		2.0–9.2		
		5	12.8–17.3	2.6–11.0		2.6–11.0		
			Adult	2.0–9.2		2.0–9.2		
			F					
		Tanner stage	Age (yr)	mIU/mL		U/L		
		1	<9.2	1.0–4.2		1.0–4.2		
		2	9.2–13.7	1.0–10.8		1.0–10.8		
		3	10.0–14.4	1.5–12.8		1.5–12.8		
		4	10.7–15.6	1.5–11.7		1.5–11.7		
		5	11.8–18.6	1.0–9.2		1.0–9.2		
		Adult	Follicular	1.8–11.2		1.8–11.2 mIU/mL		
			Midcycle	6–35		6–35		
			Luteal	1.8–11.2		1.8–11.2		
			Postmenopause	30–120		30–120		
Fructosamine	S		mmol/L			mmol/L		w (DeSchepper et al., 1988)
		0–3 yr	1.56–2.27			1.56–2.27		
		3–6 yr	1.73–2.34			1.73–2.34		
		6–9 yr	1.82–2.56			1.82–2.56		
		9–15 yr	2.02–2.63			2.02–2.63		
Galactose	S	Newborn	0–20 mg/dL		×0.0555	0.0–1.11 mmol/L		
	P	5 mo–17 yr	0.0–0.5 mg/dL			0.0–0.03 mmol/L		j (Pesce and Boudorian, 1982)
Galactose-1-PO₄	W(H)	5 mo–17 yr	0–44 μg/g Hb		×0.0038	0.0–0.17 μmol/g Hb		l (Pesce, Boudorian, and Nicholson, 1982)
Galactose-1-PO₄ uridylyltransferase	W (H)	18–26 U/g Hb			×1	18–26 U/g Hb		(Pesce, Boudorian, and Harris, 1977)
Gastrin	S		pg/mL			ng/L		
		Newborn	20–300		×1	20–300		
		Children	<10–125			<10–125		a (Esoterix Endocrinology)
Glucagon	P(E)	Children and adults (fasting)	50–150 pg/mL		×1	50–150 ng/L		(Esoterix Endocrinology)
Glucose	S		mg/dL			mmol/L		
		Cord blood	45–96		×0.0555	2.5–5.3		
		Premature	20–60			1.1–3.3		
		Neonate	30–60			1.7–3.3		
		Newborn						
		1 day	40–60			2.2–3.3		
		>1 day	50–90			2.8–5.0		
		Child	60–100			3.3–5.5		
		Adult	70–105			3.9–5.8		
	W(H)	Adult	65–95			3.6–5.3		
Glucose, 2 hr post	S	<120 mg/dL				<6.7 mmol/L		
Glucose tolerance test (GTT)	S		mg/dL			mmol/L		
Oral dose Adult: 75 g			Normal	Diabetic		Normal	Diabetic	
Child: 1.75 g/kg of ideal weight, up to a		Fasting	70–105	≥126	×0.0555	3.9–5.8	≥7.0	(American Diabetes Association, 1977)
maximum of 75 g		60 min	120–170	≥200		6.7–9.4	≥11	
		90 min	100–140	≥200		5.6–7.8	≥11	
		120 min	70–120	≥200		3.9–6.7	≥11	

ANALYTE OR PROCEDURE	SPECIMEN	REFERENCE VALUES (USA)		CONVERSION FACTOR	REFERENCE VALUES (SI)	COMMENTS
Glucose-6-phosphate dehydrogenase (G6PD) in erythrocytes	W(E,H,C)					
Bishop, modified		**Adult**			**Adult**	
		3.4–8.0 U/g Hb		×0.0645	0.22–0.52 mU/mol Hb	
		98.6–232 U/10¹² RBC		×10⁻³	0.10–0.23 nU/10⁶ RBC	
		1.16–2.72 U/mL RBC		×1	1.16–2.72 kU/L RBC	
		Newborn: 50% higher			Newborn: 50% higher	
γ-glutamyl transpeptidase (GGT, GGTP)	S		U/L		U/L	37°b(Knight and Haymond, 1981)
		Cord blood	37–193	×1	37–193	
		0–1 mo	13–147		13–147	
		1–2 mo	12–123		12–123	
		2–4 mo	8–90		8–90	
		4 mo–10 yr	5–32		5–32	
		10–15 yr	5–24		5–24	
Growth hormone (GH), somatotropin	S,P(E,H)		ng/mL		μg/L	(Esoterix Endocrinology)
		1 day	5–53	×1	5–53	
		1 wk	5–27		5–27	
		1–12 mo	2–10		2–10	
	Fasting, at rest		ng/mL		μg/L	
		Child	<0.7–6.0		<0.7–6.0	
		Adult	<0.7–6.0		<0.7–6.0	
Haptoglobin	S		mg/dL		g/L	(Davis et al., 1996)
		0–1 mo	<5.8–196.0	×0.01	<0.058–1.960	
		1 mo–19 yr	22–164		0.220–1.640	
Hemoglobin total	W	See *Formed Elements, Indices, and Coagulation Factors*				
	P(H)		mg/dL		μmol/L	
			<10	×0.155	<1.55	
		<3 with butterfly setup and 18-gauge needle			<0.47 with butterfly setup and 18-gauge needle	
High-density lipoprotein cholesterol	S		mg/dL		mmol/L	ac (Meites, 1989)
		1–13 yr	35–84	×0.0259	0.9–2.15	
		14–19 yr	35–65		0.90–1.65	
Glycohemoglobin hemoglobin A₁c	W(H)		% of total		Fraction of total Hb	f (Meites, 1989)
			Hb			
		1–5 yr	2.1–7.7	×0.01	0.021–0.077	
		5–16 yr	3.0–6.2		0.030–0.062	
Total glycohemoglobin	W(H)	4–16 yr	6.0–10.0%		0.060–0.100	e (Meites, 1989)
Hemoglobin A (HbA)	W(E,C,H)	>95%		×0.01	Fraction of Hb: >0.95	
Hemoglobin A₂ (HbA₂)	W(E,O)				Mass fraction	
		Adult: 1.5–3.5% (2 SD)			0.015–0.035 (2 SD)	
		Lower in infants <1 yr				
Hemoglobin (Hb) electrophoresis	W(H,E,C)				Mass fraction	
		HbA > 95%		×0.01	HbA > 0.95	
		HbA₂ 1.5–3.5%			HbA₂ 0.015–0.035	
		HbF < 2%			HbF < 0.02	
Hemoglobin F (HbF)	W(E)		%HbF		Mass fraction	
Alkali denaturation		1 day	63–92	×0.01	0.63–0.92	
		5 days	65–88		0.65–0.88	
		3 wk	55–85		0.55–0.85	
		6–9 wk	31–75		0.31–0.75	
		3–4 mo	<2–59		<0.02–0.59	
		6 mo	<2–9		<0.02–0.09	
		Adult	<2		<0.02	
Hemoglobin H (HbH)	W(H,E,C)					
Isopropanol precipitation		No precipitation at 40 min			No precipitation at 40 min	
Homocysteine	P	2 mo–18 yr	3.3–11.3 μmol/L	×1	3.3–11.3 μmol/L	(Vilaseca et al., 1997)
17-Hydroxyprogesterone (17-OHP)	S	Preterm infants	ng/dL		nmol/L	(Esoterix Endocrinology)
		26–28 wk, day 4	124–841	×0.03029	3.76–25.5	
		31–35 wk, day 4	26–568		0.79–17.2	
		Term infants	ng/dL		nmol/L	
		3 days	7–77		0.2–2.33	
		M 1–12 mo	Peak values of 40–200 ng/dL at 30–60 days		Peak values of 1.21–6.1 nmol/L at 30–60 days	
					nmol/L	
		F 1–11 mo	13–106 ng/dL		0.39–3.21	
		Prepubertal children				
		1–10 yr	3–90 ng/dL		0.09–2.73	

	M				
Tanner stage	Age (yr)	ng/dL		nmol/L	
1	<9.8	3–90		0.09–2.73	
2	9.8–14.5	5–115		0.15–3.48	
3	10.7–15.4	10–138		0.30–4.18	
4	11.8–16.2	29–180		0.88–5.45	
5	12.8–17.3	24–175		0.73–5.30	
	Adult	27–199		0.82–6.03	

ANALYTE OR PROCEDURE	SPECIMEN	REFERENCE VALUES (USA)			CONVERSION FACTOR	REFERENCE VALUES (SI)	COMMENTS
		F					
		Tanner stage	Age	ng/dL		nmol/L	
		1	<9.2 yr	3–82		0.09–2.48	
		2	9.2–13.7	11–98		0.33–2.97	
		3	10.0–14.4	11–155		0.33–4.69	
		4	10.7–15.6	18–230		0.55–6.97	
		5	11.8–18.6	20–265		0.61–8.03	
		Adult	Follicular	15–70		0.45–2.12	
			Luteal	35–290		1.06–8.78	
β-Hydroxybutyrate			mmol/L			mmol/L	(Bonnefont et al., 1990)
		1–12 mo	0.1–1.0		×1	0.1–1.0	
		1–7 yr	<0.1–0.9			<0.1–0.9	
		7–15 yr	<0.1–0.3			<0.1–0.3	
Hypoxanthine	W	Age	μmol/L			μmol/L	(Jung et al., 1985)
		12–36 hr	27–11.2		×1	2.7–11.2	
		3 days	1.3–7.9			1.3–7.9	
		5 days	0.6–5.7			0.6–5.7	
Immunoglobulin A (IgA)	S		mg/dL		×10	mg/L	s (Meites, 1989)
		Cord blood	1.4–3.6			14–36	
		1–3 mo	1.3–53			13–530	
		4–6 mo	4.4–84			44–840	
		7 mo–1 yr	11–106			110–1,060	
		2–5 yr	14–159			140–1,590	
		6–10 yr	33–236			330–2,360	
		Adult	70–312			700–3,120	
Immunoglobulin D (IgD)	S	Newborn: none detected				None detected	
		Thereafter: 0–8 mg/dL			×10	0–80 mg/L	
Immunoglobulin E (IgE)	S	M 0–230 IU/mL			×1	0–230 kIU/L	
		F 0–170				0–170	
Immunoglobulin G (IgG)	S		mg/dL			g/L	
		Cord blood	636–1,606		×0.01	6.36–16.06	s (Meites, 1989)
		1 mo	251–906			2.51–9.06	
		2–4 mo	176–601			1.76–6.01	
		5–12 mo	172–1,069			1.72–10.69	
		1–5 yr	345–1,236			3.45–12.36	
		6–10 yr	608–1,572			6.08–15.72	
		Adult	639–1,349			6.39–13.49	

IgG subclasses	S					×10					(Mayo Medical Laboratories, 2001)
			mg/dL				mg/L				
Age		IgG_1	IgG_2	IgG_3	IgG_4		IgG_1	IgG_2	IgG_3	IgG_4	
0–1 mo		240–1,060	87–410	14–55	4.0–55		2,440–10,600	870–4,100	140–550	40–550	
2–3 mo		180–670	38–210	14–70	≤36		1,800–6,700	380–2,100	140–700	≤360	
4–5 mo		180–700	43–210	15–80	≤23		1,800–7,000	340–2,100	150–800	≤230	
6–11 mo		200–770	34–230	15–97	≤43		2,000–7,700	340–2,300	150–970	≤430	
12–17 mo		250–820	38–240	15–107	≤62		2,500–8,200	380–2,400	150–1,070	≤620	
18–23 mo		290–850	45–260	15–113	≤79		2,900–8,500	450–2,600	150–1,130	≤790	
2 yr		320–900	52–280	14–120	≤106		3,200–9,000	520–2,800	140–1,200	≤1,060	
3 yr		350–940	63–300	13–126	≤127		3,500–9,400	630–3,000	130–1,260	≤1,270	
4–5 yr		370–1,000	72–340	13–133	≤158		3,700–10,000	720–3,400	130–1,330	≤1,580	
6–8 yr		400–1,080	85–410	13–142	≤189		4,000–10,800	850–4,100	130–1,420	≤1,890	
9–11 yr		400–1,150	98–480	15–149	3–210		4,000–11,500	980–4,800	150–1,490	30–2,100	
12–17 yr		370–1,280	106–610	18–163	4–230		3,700–12,800	1,060–6,100	180–1,630	40–2,300	
≥18 yr		490–1,140	150–640	20–110	8–140		4,900–11,400	1,500–6,400	200–1,100	80–1,400	

Immunoglobulin M (IgM)	S		mg/dL			mg/L	
		Cord blood	6.3–25	×10	63–250	s (Meites, 1989)
		1–4 mo	17–105		170–1,050	
		5–9 mo	33–126		330–1,260	
		10 mo–1 yr	41–173		410–1,730	
		2–8 yr	43–207		430–2,070	
		9–10 yr	52–242		520–2,420	
		Adult	56–352		560–3,520	
Insulin (12 hr fast)	S		uU/mL	×1.0	mU/L	
		Newborn	3–20		3–20	
		Thereafter	7–24		7–24	
Insulin with oral glucose tolerance test	S	min	uU/mL		mU/L	
		0	7–24	×1	7–24	
		30	25–231		25–231	
		60	18–276		18–276	
		120	16–166		16–166	
		180	4–38		4–38	

ANALYTE OR PROCEDURE	SPECIMEN	REFERENCE VALUES (USA)					CONVERSION FACTOR	REFERENCE VALUES (SI)				COMMENTS
Insulin-like growth factor 1 (IGF-1)	S	*Infants*	*Term (40 wk gestation)*		*Preterm (<40 wk gestation)*		×1	*Term*		*Preterm (birth < 40 wk)*		(Esoterix Endocrinology)
			Range (ng/mL)	Mean (ng/mL)	Range (ng/mL)	Mean (ng/mL)		Range (µg/L)	Mean (µg/L)	Range (µg/L)	Mean (µg/L)	
		Birth	15–109	59	21–93	51		15–109	59	21–93	51	
		2 mo	15–109	55	23–163	81		15–109	55	23–163	81	
		4 mo	7–124	50	23–171	74		7–124	50	23–171	74	
		6 mo	7–93	41	15–132	61		7–93	41	15–132	61	
		12 mo	15–101	56	15–179	77		15–101	56	15–179	77	
		Children and young adults	Range M	Mean	Range F	Mean		Range M	Mean	Range F	Mean	
		Age (yr)	ng/mL	ng/mL	ng/mL	ng/mL		(µg/L)	(µg/L)	(µg/L)	(µg/L)	
		1–2 yr	30–122	76	56–144	100		30–122	76	56–144	100	
		3–4 yr	54–178	116	74–202	138		54–178	116	74–202	138	
		5–6 yr	60–228	144	82–262	172		60–228	144	82–262	172	
		7–8 yr	113–261	187	112–276	194		113–261	187	112–276	194	
		9–10 yr	123–275	199	140–308	224		123–275	199	140–308	224	
		11–12 yr	139–395	267	132–376	254		139–395	267	132–376	254	
		13–14 yr	152–540	346	192–640	416		152–540	346	192–640	416	
		15–16 yr	257–601	429	217–589	403		257–601	429	217–589	403	
		17–18 yr	236–524	380	176–452	314		236–524	380	176–452	314	
		19–20 yr	281–510	371	217–475	323		281–510	371	217–475	323	
		21–30 yr	155–432	289	87–368	237		155–432	289	87–368	237	
Interleukin 6	S	Age (mo)	pg/mL					ng/L				(Berdat et al., 2003)
		0–3 mo	9.00 ± 7.48					9.00 ± 7.48				
		4–12 mo	3.41 ± 1.11					3.41 ± 1.11				
		13–24 mo	1.75 ± 0.36				×1	1.75 ± 0.36				
		25–36 mo	5.78 ± 2.06					5.78 ± 2.06				
		37–48 mo	5.41 ± 2.49					5.41 ± 2.49				
		49–60 mo	9.19 ± 5.18					9.19 ± 5.18				
		Adult	0–149					0–149				
Interleukin 10	S	0–60 mo	3.3–5.9 pg/mL					3.3–5.9				
		Adult	0–14.1 pg/mL				×1	0–14.1 ng/L				(Berdat et al., 2003)
Iron	S	All ages	22–184 µg/dL				×0.1791	4–33 µmol/L				(Lockitch, Halstead, and Wadsworth et al., 1988)
Iron-binding capacity, total (TIBC)	S	Infant 100–400 µg/dL					×0.179	17.90–71.60 µmol/L				
		Thereafter 250–400						44.75–71.60				
Ketone bodies, qualitative	S	Negative					×1	Negative				(Bonnefont et al., 1990)
Ketone bodies, quantitative	W		mmol/l					mmol/l				Sum of acetone, β-hydroxybutyrate and acetoacetate
		1–12 mo	0.1–1.5					0.1–1.5				
		1–7 yr	0.15–2.0					0.15–2.0				
		7–15 yr	<0.1–0.5					<0.1–0.5				
Low-density lipoprotein cholesterol (LDLC)	S,P(E)		mg/dL					mmol/L				
			M	F				M	F			
		Cord blood	10–50	10–50			×0.0259	0.26–1.30	0.26–1.30			
		1–9 yr	60–140	60–150				1.55–3.63	1.55–3.89			
		10–19 yr	50–170	50–170				1.30–4.40	1.30–4.40			
		20–29 yr	60–175	60–160				1.55–4.53	1.55–4.14			
		30–39 yr	80–190	70–170				2.07–4.92	1.81–4.40			
		40–49 yr	90–205	80–190				2.33–5.31	2.07–4.92			
		Recommended (desirable) range for adults: <100 mg/dL						1.68–4.53				
L+lactate	W		mmol/L					mmol/L				(Bonnefont et al., 1990)
		1–12 mo	1.1–2.3				×1	1.1–2.3				
		1–7 yr	0.8–1.5					0.8–1.5				
		7–15 yr	0.6–0.9					0.6–0.9				
D-lactate	P(H)											j (Rosenthal and Pesce, 1985)
		6 mo–3 yr	0.0–0.3				×1	0.0–0.3				
Lactate dehydrogenase	S		U/L					U/L				
		<1 yr	170–580				×1	170–580				37° a (Meites, 1989)
		1–9 yr	150–500					150–500				
		10–19 yr	120–330					120–330				
Isoenzymes	S		% of total activity									
			1–6 yr	7–19 yr								
		LD1	20–38	20–35								
		LD2	27–38	31–38								
		LD3	16–26	19–28								
		LD4	5–16	7–13								
		LD5	3–13	5–12								
Lead	W(H)		µg/dL					mmol/L				
		Child	<10				×0.0483	<0.48				
		Toxic	≥70					≥3.38				
Lipase	P,S	1–18 yr	145–216 U/L				×1	145–216 U/L				(Ghoshal and Soldin, 2003)

ANALYTE OR PROCEDURE	SPECIMEN	REFERENCE VALUES (USA)			CONVERSION FACTOR	REFERENCE VALUES (SI)		COMMENTS
Lipoprotein electrophoresis	S	Distinct β band; negligible chylomicron and pre-β bands						
Long-acting thyroid-stimulating hormone (LATS)	S	Undetectable				Undetectable		
Luteinizing hormone (LH)	S	**M**				U/L		(Esoterix Endocrinology)
		Tanner stage	Age (yr)	mIU/mL				
		1	<9.8	0.02–0.3	×1	0.02–0.3		
		2	9.8–14.5	0.2–4.9		0.2–4.9		
		3	10.7–15.4	0.2–5.0		0.2–5.0		Referred to WHO 2nd
		4–5	11.8–17.3	0.4–7.0		0.4–7.0		International
		Adult		1.5–9		1.5–9		Standard
		F				U/L		
		Tanner stage	Age (yr)	mIU/mL				
		1	<9.2	0.02–0.18		0.02–0.18		
		2	9.2–13.7	0.02–4.7		0.02–4.7		
		3	10.0–14.4	0.10–12.0		0.10–12.0		
		4–5	10.7–15.6	0.4–11.7		0.4–11.7		
		Adult	Follicular	2–9		2–9		
			Midcycle	18–49		18–49		
			Luteal	2–11		2–11		
Magnesium	P(H)	mg/dL				mmol/L		w (Meites, 1989)
		0–6 days	1.2–2.6		×0.411	0.48–1.05		
		7 days–2 yr	1.6–2.6			0.65–1.05		
		2–14 yr	1.5–2.3			0.60–0.95		
Methemoglobin (MetHb)	W(E,H,C)	0.06–0.24 g/dL or			×155	9.3–37.2 µmol/L		
		0.78 ± 0.37% of total Hb			×0.01	0.0078 ± 0.0037 (mass fraction)		
Methylmalonic acid	S	4–14 yr	0.03–0.26 µmol/L		×1	0.03–0.26 µmol/L		(Straczek et al., 1993)
Microsomal antibodies, thyroid, see *Thyroid microsomal antibodies*								
Myoglobin	S	6–85 ng/mL			×1	6–85 µg/L		
N-TERMINAL PRO-B-type natriuretic peptide	P	pg/mL				ng/L		(Bar-Oz et al., 2005)
		Maternal blood	89 (SD 45)			89 (SD 45)		(Nir et al., 2004)
		Cord blood	579 (SD 351)			579 (SD 351)		
		1–4 days	3042 (SD 1783)		×1	3042 (SD 1783)		
		4 mo–15 yr	349 (95th percentile)			349 (95th percentile)		
Osmolality	S	Child, adult						
		275–295 mOsmol/kg H₂O						
Oxygen, partial pressure (Po₂)	W(H), arterial	mmHg				kPa		
		Birth	8–24		×0.133	1.1–3.2		
		5–10 min	33–75			4.4–10.0		
		30 min	31–85			4.1–11.3		
		>1 hr	55–80			7.3–10.6		
		1 day	54–95			7.2–12.6		
		Thereafter decreases with age	83–108			11–14.4		
Oxygen saturation	W(H), arterial	% saturation				Fraction saturated		
		Newborn	85–90		×0.01	0.85–0.90		
		Thereafter	95–99			0.95–0.99		
Po₂, see *Oxygen, partial pressure (Po₂)*								
Po₂ at half saturation (Po₂[0.5] or P₅₀)	W(H), arterial	25–29 mm Hg			×0.133	3.3–3.9 kPa		
Parathyroid hormone (PTH)	S	pg/mL				pmol/L		(Nichols Institute Diagnostics)
		Cord blood	≤3.0		×0.1053	≤0.32		
Intact (IRMA)		2 yr–adult	9–65			0.95–6.8		
pH	W(H), arterial	pH				H⁺ concentration (nmol/L)		
		Premature (48 hr)	7.35–7.50			31–44		
		Birth, full term	7.11–7.36			43–77		
		5–10 min	7.09–7.30			50–81		
		30 min	7.21–7.38			41–61		
		>1 hr	7.26–7.49			32–54		
		1 day	7.29–7.45			35–51		
		Thereafter	7.35–7.45			35–44		
		Must be corrected for body temperature						
Phenylalanine	S	mg/dL				µmol/L		
		Premature	2.0–7.5		×60.54	120–450		
		Newborn	1.2–3.4			70–210		
		Thereafter	0.8–1.8			50–110		
Phosphatase, tartrate-resistant acid	S	Children	3.4–9.0 u/L		×1	3.4–9.0 u/L		
Phosphatase, alkaline	S	U/L				U/L		37°C aw
		1–9 yr	145–420		×1	145–420		(Lockitch, Halstead, and
		10–11 yr	130–560			130–560		Albersheim et al.,
			M	**F**		**M**	**F**	1988)
		12–13 yr	200–495	105–420		200–495	105–420	
		14–15 yr	130–525	70–230		130–525	70–230	
		16–19 yr	65–260	50–130		65–260	50–130	

ANALYTE OR PROCEDURE	SPECIMEN	REFERENCE VALUES (USA)			CONVERSION FACTOR	REFERENCE VALUES (SI)		COMMENTS
Phospholipids, total	S,P(E)		mg/dL			g/L		
		Newborn	75–170		×0.01	0.75–1.70		
		Infant	100–275			1.00–2.75		
		Child	180–295			1.80–2.95		
		Adult	125–275			1.25–2.75		
Phosphorus, inorganic	S,P(H)		mg/dL			mmol/L		w (Meites, 1989)
		0–5 days	4.8–8.2		×0.3229	1.55–2.65		
		1–3 yr	3.8–6.5			1.25–2.10		
		4–11 yr	3.7–5.6			1.20–1.80		
		12–15 yr	2.9–5.4			0.95–1.75		
		16–19 yr	2.7–4.7			0.90–1.50		
Plasma volume	P(H)	M 25–43 mL/kg			×0.001	M 0.025–0.043 L/kg		
		F 28–45				F 0.028–0.045		
Potassium	S		mmol/L			mmol/L		r (Meites, 1989)
		<2 mo	3.0–7.0		×1	3.0–7.0		Increased by hemolysis;
		2–12 mo	3.5–6.0			3.5–6.0		serum values
		>12 mo	3.5–5.0			3.5–5.0		systematically higher
								than plasma values
	P(H)	3.5–4.5 mmol/L				3.5–4.5 mmol/L		
Prealbumin (transthyretin)	P		mg/L			mg/L		s (Sherry et al., 1988)
		2–6 mo	142–330		×1	142–330		
		6–12 mo	120–274			120–274		
		1–3 yr	108–259			108–259		
Progesterone	S	M						(Esoterix Endocrinology)

M

Tanner stage	Age (yr)	ng/dL		nmol/L
1	<9.8	<10–33	×0.03180	<0.32–1.05
2	9.8–14.5	<10–33		<0.32–1.05
3	10.7–15.4	<10–48		<0.32–1.53
4	11.8–16.2	10–108		0.32–3.43
5	12.8–17.3	21–82		0.67–2.61
	Adult	13–97		0.41–3.08

F

Tanner stage	Age	ng/dL		nmol/L
1	<9.2 yr	<10–33		<0.32–1.05
2	9.2–13.7	10–55		<0.32–1.75
3	10.0–14.4	10–450		0.32–14.31
4	10.7–15.6	10–1,300		0.32–41.34
5	11.8–18.6	10–950		0.32–30.21
Adult	Follicular	15–70		0.48–2.23
	Luteal	200–2,500		6.36–79.50

ANALYTE OR PROCEDURE	SPECIMEN	REFERENCE VALUES (USA)			CONVERSION FACTOR	REFERENCE VALUES (SI)		COMMENTS
Prolactin	S	M	F			M	F	(Esoterix Endocrinology)
		3–18	3–24 ng/mL		×0.0426	0.13–0.77	0.13–1.02 nmol/L	
		Higher in newborn infants				Higher in newborn infants		
Protein, total	S		g/dL			g/L		(Meites, 1989)
		Premature	4.3–7.6		×10	43–76		
		Newborn	4.6–7.4			46–74		
		1–7 yr	6.1–7.9			61–79		
		8–12 yr	6.4–8.1			64–81		
		13–19 yr	6.6–8.2			66–82		
Protein electrophoresis	S	Albumin	g/dL			g/L		
		Premature	3.0–4.2		×10	30–42		
		Newborn	3.6–5.4			36–54		
		Infant	4.0–5.0			40–50		
		Thereafter	3.5–5.0			35–50		
		α_1-globulin						
		Premature	0.1–0.5			1–5		
		Newborn	0.1–0.3			1–3		
		Infant	0.2–0.4			2–4		
		Thereafter	0.2–0.3			2–3		
		α_2-globulin						
		Premature	0.3–0.7			3–7		
		Newborn	0.3–0.5			3–5		
		Infant	0.5–0.8			5–8		
		Thereafter	0.4–1.0			4–10		
		β-globulin						
		Premature	0.3–1.2			3–12		
		Newborn	0.2–0.6			2–6		
		Infant	0.5–0.8			5–8		
		Thereafter	0.5–1.1			5–11		
		γ-globulin						
		Premature	0.3–1.4			3–14		
		Newborn	0.2–1.0			2–10		
		Infant	0.3–1.2			3–12		
		Thereafter	0.7–1.2			7–12		
		Higher in blacks				Higher in blacks		

ANALYTE OR PROCEDURE	SPECIMEN	REFERENCE VALUES (USA)		CONVERSION FACTOR	REFERENCE VALUES (SI)		COMMENTS
Pyruvate	W	7–17 yr	0.076 ± 0.026 mmol/L	×1	0.076 ± 0.026 mmol/L		(Pianosi et al., 1995)
Renin (renin activity, plasma [PRA])	P(E)		ng/mL/hr		µg/L/hr		
		0–3 yr	<16.6	×1	<16.6		
		3–6 yr	<6.7		<6.7		
		6–9 yr	<4.4		<4.4		
		9–12 yr	<5.9		<5.9		
		12–15 yr	<4.2		<4.2		
		15–18 yr	<4.3		<4.3		
		Normal sodium diet					
		Supine	0.2–2.5		0.2–2.5		
		Upright	0.3–4.3		0.3–4.3		
		Low-sodium diet					
		Upright	2.9–24.0		2.9–24.0		
Retinol-binding protein (RBP)	S		mg/dL		mg/L		s(Lockitch, Halstead, and Quigley et al., 1988)
		0–5 day	0.8–4.5	×10	8–45		
		1–9 yr	1.0–7.8		10–78		
		10–13 yr	1.3–9.9		13–99		
		14–19 yr	3.0–9.2		30–92		
Reverse triiodothyronine (rT$_3$)	S		ng/dL		nmol/L		
		1–5 yr	15–71	×0.0154	0.23–1.10		
		5–10 yr	17–79		0.26–1.20		
		10–15 yr	19–88		0.29–1.36		
		Adults	30–80		0.46–1.23		
S100B protein	P		µg/L (25th–75th percentiles)		µg/l (25th–75th percentiles)		(Gazzolo et al., 2003)
		0–1 yr	0.44–2.55	×1	0.44–2.55		
		2–7 yr	0.44–1.06		0.44–1.06		
		9–11 yr	0.91–1.74		0.91–1.74		
		11–12 yr	0.39–0.45		0.39–0.45		
		13–14 yr	1.12–2.01		1.12–2.01		
		14–15 yr	0.5–0.87		0.50–0.87		
Selenium	S		µg/dL		µmol/L		(Muntau, et al., 2002)
		<1 mo	1.5–10.6	×0.127	0.19–1.35		
		1–12 mo	1.0–11.6		0.13–1.47		
		1–5 yr	3.4–12.8		0.43–1.63		
		5–18 yr	4.2–12.4		0.53–1.57		
Sodium	S,P (LiH,NH$_4$H)		mmol/L		mmol/L		
		Newborn	134–146	×1	134–146		
		Infant	139–146		139–146		
		Child	138–145		138–146		
		Thereafter	136–146		136–146		

Somatomedin C, see *Insulin-like growth factor 1 (IGF-1)*

T$_3$, see *Triiodothyronine total*

T$_4$, see *Thyroxine*

ANALYTE OR PROCEDURE	SPECIMEN				CONVERSION FACTOR			COMMENTS
Testosterone	S	M				nmol/L		(Esoterix Endocrinology)
		Tanner stage	Age (yr)	ng/dL				
		1	<9.8	<3–10	×0.03467	<0.1–0.35		
		2	9.8–14.5	18–150		0.62–5.20		
		3	10.7–15.4	100–320		3.47–11.10		
		4	11.8–16.2	220–620		7.63–21.50		
		5	12.8–17.3	350–970		12.14–3,363.0		
			Adult	350–1,030		12.14–35.71		
		F						
		Tanner stage	Age (yr)	ng/dL		nmol/L		
		1	<9.2	<3–10		<0.1–0.35		
		2	9.2–13.7	7–28		0.24–0.97		
		3	10.0–14.4	15–35		0.52–1.21		
		4	10.7–15.6	13–32		0.45–1.11		
		5	11.8–18.6	20–38		0.69–1.32		
			Adult	10–55		0.35–1.91		
Testosterone, free	S	M				M		(Esoterix Endocrinology)
			pg/mL	% free		pmol/L	Fraction free	
		1–15 days	1.5–31.0	0.9–1.7	×3.4673	5.2–107	0.009–0.017	
		1–2 mo	3.3–18.0	0.4–0.8		11.4–62	0.004–0.008	
		3–4 mo	0.7–14.0	0.4–1.1		2.4–49	0.004–0.011	
		5–6 mo	0.4–4.8	0.4–1.0		1.4–16.6	0.004–0.011	
		1–10 yr	0.15–0.60	0.4–0.9		0.5–2.1	0.004–0.009	
		Pubertal	Not defined			Not defined		
		Adult	52–280	1.5–3.2		180–971	0.015–0.032	

ANALYTE OR PROCEDURE	SPECIMEN	REFERENCE VALUES (USA)			CONVERSION FACTOR	REFERENCE VALUES (SI)		COMMENTS
		F				**F**		
			pg/mL	% Free		pmol/L	Fraction free	
		1–15 days	0.5–2.5	0.8–1.5		1.7–8.7	0.008–0.015	
		1–2 mo	0.1–1.3	0.4–1.1		0.3–4.5	0.004–0.011	
		3–4 mo	0.3–1.1	0.5–1.0		1.1–3.8	0.005–0.01	
		5–6 mo	0.2–0.6	0.5–0.8		0.7–2.1	0.005–0.008	
		1–10 yr	0.15–0.60	0.4–0.9		0.5–2.1	0.004–0.009	
		Pubertal	Not defined			Not defined		
		Adult	1.1–6.3	0.8–1.4		3.8–21.8	0.008–0.014	
Thiamine (vitamin B$_1$)	S	0.0–2.0 µg/dL			×37.68	0.0–75.4 nmol/L		
Thyrolobulin	S	2–16 yr	2.3–39.6 ng/mL		×1	2.3–39.6 µg/L		(Nichols Institute Diagnostics)
		Adult	3.5–56.0			3.5–56.0		
Thyroid microsomal antibodies	S	Nondetectable(hemagglutination)				Nondetectable (hemagglutination) or		
Thyroid thyroglobulin	S	or < 1:10				< 1:10		
Tanned RBC agglutination test		Children ≤ 1:4 dilution				≤ 1:4 dilution		
		Thereafter ≤ 1:10				≤ 1:10		
Thyroid-stimulating hormone	S	Premature (28–36 wk)	mIU/L			mIU/L		
		1st wk of life	0.7–27.0		×1	0.7–27.0		(Nichols Institute Diagnostics)
		Term infants						
		Cord blood	2.3–13.2			2.3–13.2		
		1–2 days	3.2–34.6			3.2–34.6		
		3–4 days	0.7–15.4			0.7–15.4		
		2–20 wk	1.7–9.1			1.7–9.1		
		21 wk–20 yr	0.7–6.4			0.7–6.4		
Thyroid uptake of radioactive iodine	Activity over thyroid gland	2 hr	<6%		×0.01	2 hr <0.06		
		6 hr	3–20%			6 hr 0.03–0.20		
		24 hr	8–30%			24 hr 0.08–0.30		
Thyroid uptake of technetium 99 m	Activity over thyroid gland	After 24 hr	0.4–3.0%		×0.01	Fractional uptake 0.004–0.030		
Thyrotropin-releasing hormone (hTRH)	P	5–60 pg/mL			×2.759	14–165 pmol/L		
Thyroxine-binding globulin (TBG)	S		mg/dL			mg/L		
		Cord blood	1.4–9.4		×10	14–94		
		1–4 wk	1.0–9.0			10–90		
		1–12 mo	2.0–7.6			20–76		
		1–5 yr	2.9–5.4			29–54		
		5–10 yr	2.5–5.0			25–50		
		10–15 yr	2.1–4.6			21–46		
		Adult	1.5–3.4			15–34		
Thyroxine, total	S	Full-term infants			×12.9	Full-term infants		(Esoterix Endocrinology)
			µg/dL				nmol/L	
		1–3 days	8.2–19.9			1–3 days	106–256	
		1 wk	6.0–15.9			1 wk	77–205	
		1–12 mo	6.1–14.9			1–12 mo	79–192	
		Prepubertal children				Prepubertal children		
		1–3 yr	6.8–13.5			1–3 yr	88–174	
		3–10 yr	5.5–12.8			3–10 yr	71–165	
		Pubertal children and adults				Pubertal children and adults		
			4.2–13.0				54–167	
Thyroxine, free	S	Newborn infants	ng/dL		×12.9	Full-term infants	pmol/L	(Esoterix Endocrinology)
		3 days	2.0–4.9			3 days	26–63	
		Infants	0.9–2.6			Infants	12–33	
		Prepubertal children	0.8–2.2			Prepubertal children	10–28	
		Pubertal children and adults	0.8–2.3			Pubertal children and adults	10–30	
Thyroxine, total	W	Newborn screen (filter paper) 6.2–22.0 µg/dL			×12.9	80–283 nmol/L		
Tumor necrosis factor-α	S		pg/mL			ng/L		(Berdat et al., 2003)
		0–60 mo	2.2–3.5		×1	2.2–3.5		
		Adults	0–1.3			0.0–1.3		
Transcortin	S		mg/dL			mg/L		
		M	1.5–2.0		×10	15–20		
		F, follicular	1.7–2.0			17–20		
		Luteal	1.6–2.1			16–21		
		Postmenopausal	1.7–2.5			17–25		
		Pregnancy						
		21–28 wk	4.7–5.4			47–54		
		33–40 wk	5.5–7.0			55–70		
Transferrin isoforms (test for congenital disorders of glycosylation)	S	Mono-oligosaccharide/≤0.074 Dioligosaccharide 0.075–0.109 Indeterminate A-oligosaccharide/≤0.022 Dioligosaccharide			×1	Mono-oligosaccharide/≤0.074 Dioligosaccharide 0.075–0.109 Indeterminate A-oligosaccharide/≤0.022 Dioligosaccharide		(Mayo Medical Laboratories)
Transferrin (siderophilin)	S	95–385 mg/dL			×0.01	0.95–3.85 g/L		(Davis et al., 1996)

ANALYTE OR PROCEDURE	SPECIMEN	REFERENCE VALUES (USA)		CONVERSION FACTOR	REFERENCE VALUES (SI)		COMMENTS
Triglycerides	S, after ≥ 12 hr fast	mg/dL			g/L		
		M	F		M	F	
		Cord blood 10–98	10–98	×0.01	0.10–0.98	0.10–0.98	
		0–5 yr 30–86	32–99		0.30–0.86	0.32–0.99	
		6–11 yr 31–108	35–114		0.31–1.08	0.35–1.14	
		12–15 yr 36–138	41–138		0.36–1.38	0.41–1.38	
		16–19 yr 40–163	40–128		0.40–1.63	0.40–1.28	
		20–29 yr 44–185	40–128		0.44–1.85	0.40–1.28	
		Recommended (desirable) levels					
Recommended (desirable)		Adults			Adults		
		mg/dL			g/L		
		M 40–160			M 0.40–1.60		
		F 35–135			F 0.35–1.35		
Triidothyronine, free	S	pg/dL			pmol/L		
		Cord blood 20–240		×0.01536	0.3–3.7		
		1–3 dys 200–610			3.1–9.4		
		6 wk 240–560			3.7–8.6		
		Adult (20–50 yr) 230–660			3.5–10.0		
Triiodothyronine resin uptake test (T₃RU)	S				Fractional uptake		
		Newborn 26–36%		×0.01	0.26–0.36		
		Thereafter 26–35%			0.26–0.35		
Triiodothyronine, total	S	ng/dL			nmol/L		
		Cord blood 30–70		×0.0154	0.46–1.08		
		Newborn 75–260			1.16–4.00		
		1–5 yr 100–260			1.54–4.00		
		5–10 yr 90–240			1.39–3.70		
		10–15 yr 80–210			1.23–3.23		
		Thereafter 115–190			1.77–2.93		
Troponin I	S	ng/mL			μg/L		
		0–30 days <8.4		×1	<8.4		(Ghoshal and Soldin, 2003)
		31–90 days <0.7			<0.7		
		3–6 mo <0.5			<0.5		
		7–12 mo <0.3			<0.3		
		1–18 yr <0.1			<0.1		
Troponin T	S	Full-term newborn		×1	Full-term newborn		k
		Median: 0 ng/mL			Median: 0 μg/L		(Mäkikallio et al., 2000)
		Range: 0–0.14 ng/mL			Range: 0–0.14 μg/L		
Tyrosine	S	mg/dL			mmol/L		
		Premature 7.0–24.0		×0.0552	0.39–1.32		
		Newborn 1.6–3.7			0.088–0.20		
		Adult 0.8–1.3			0.044–0.07		
Urea nitrogen	S,P	mg/dL			mmol urea/L		
		Cord blood 21–40		×0.357	7.5–14.3		
		Premature (1 wk) 3–25			1.1–9.0		
		Newborn 3–12			1.1–4.3		
		Infant or child 5–18			1.8–6.4		
		Thereafter 7–18			2.5–6.4		
Uric acid	S	mg/dL			μmol/L		j (Meites, 1989)
		1–5 yr 1.7–5.8		×59.48	100–350		
		6–11 yr 2.2–6.6			130–390		
		M 12–19 yr 3.0–7.7			180–460		
		F 12–19 yr 2.7–5.7			160–340		
Vitamin A (retinol)	S	μg/dL			μmol/L		p (Lockitch, Halstead, and Wadsworth et al., 1988)
		1–6 yr 20–43		×0.0349	0.70–1.5		
		7–12 yr 25–48			0.9–1.7		
		13–19 yr 26–72			0.9–2.5		
Vitamin B₁, see Thiamine (Vitamin B₁)							
Vitamin B₂, see Riboflavin							
Vitamin B₆	P(E)	3.6–18.0 ng/mL		×4.046	14.6–72.8 nmol/L		
					pmol/L		
Vitamin B₁₂	S	Newborn 175–800 pg/mL		×0.738	129–590		
		Thereafter 140–700			103–157		
Vitamin C	P(O,H,E)	0.6–2.0 mg/dL		×56.78	34–113 μmol/L		
					μg/L		
Vitamin D, 25-hydroxy vitamin D	S	1–30 days 1.9–33.4 ng/mL		×1	1.9–33.4		(Soldin et al., 1997)
		31 days–1 yr 7.4–53.3			7.4–53.3		
Vitamin D₃, 1,25-dihydroxy vitamin D (calcitriol)	S	25–45 pg/mL		×2.4	60–108 nmol/L		
					μmol/L		
Vitamin E (tocopherol)	S	1–6 yr 3.0–9.0 mg/L		×2.32	7–21		p (Lockitch, Halstead, and Wadsworth et al., 1988)
		7–19 yr 4.4–10.4			10–24		

ANALYTE OR PROCEDURE	SPECIMEN	REFERENCE VALUES (USA)		CONVERSION FACTOR	REFERENCE VALUES (SI)	COMMENTS
Xylose absorption test (0.5 g/kg in H_2O, 25 g maximum)	S		mg/dL		mmol/L	
		Child:1 hr	>20	×0.0667	>1.33	
		Adult:2 hr	>25		>1.67	
Zinc	S	1–19 hr	64–118 µg/dL	×0.1530	9.8–18.1 µmol/L	d (Lockitch, Halstead, and Wadsworth et al., 1988)

C. Analyses of Blood for Drugs of All Classes

ANTIBIOTICS		Peak		Trough		Conversion	SI Peak		SI Trough		
	Specimen	Therapeutic	Toxic	Therapeutic	Toxic	Factor	Therapeutic	Toxic	Therapeutic	Toxic	Comment
Amikacin	S	20–25 µg/mL	>30 µg/mL	1–4 µg/mL	>8 µg/mL	×1.708	34–43 µmol/L	>51 µmol/L	1.7–6.8 µmol/L	>14 µmol/L	kn (Taylor and Caviness, 1986)
Chloramphenicol	S	10–20 µg/mL	>25 µg/mL			×3.095	31–62 µmol/L	>77 µmol/L			k (Taylor and Caviness, 1986)
Gentamicin	S	6–10 µg/mL	>12 µg/mL	0.5–2.0 µg/mL	>2.0 µg/mL	×2.064	12–21 µmol/L	>25 µmol/L	1.0–4.1 µmol/L	>4.1 µmol/L	kn (Taylor and Caviness, 1986)
Netilmicin	S	6–10 µg/mL	>12 µg/mL	0.5–2.0 µg/mL	>2 µg/mL	×2.103	13–21 µmol/L	>25 µmol/L	1.1–4.2 µmol/L	>4.2 µmol/L	kn (Taylor and Caviness, 1986)
Tobramycin	S	6–10 µg/mL	>12 µg/mL	0.5–2.0 µg/mL	>2 µg/mL	×2.139	13–21 µmol/L	>26 µmol/L	1.1–4.3 µmol/L	>4.3 µmol/L	kn (Taylor and Caviness, 1986)
Vancomycin	S	30–40 µg/mL	>60 µg/mL	5–10 µg/mL	>20 µg/mL	×0.303	9.1–12.1 µmol/L	>18.2 µmol/L	1.5–3.0 µmol/L	>6.1 µmol/L	kn (Syva, Company, 1986)

OTHER DRUGS						
Acetaminophen	S,P(H,E)	Therapeutic	10–30 µg/mL	×6.62	66–200 µmol/L	n
		Toxic	>200 µg/mL		>1,300 µmol/L	
Amphetamine	S,P(H,E)	Therapeutic	20–30 ng/mL	×7.396	150–220 nmol/L	
		Toxic	>200 ng/mL		>1,500 nmol/L	
Amitriptyline (includes nortriptyline)	S	Therapeutic	100–250 ng/mL	×1	100–250 µg/L	(Syva, Company, 1986)
Nortriptyline (only)		Therapeutic	50–150 ng/mL	×1	50–150 µg/L	
Caffeine	S,P	Therapeutic for neonatal apnea	5–20 µg/mL	×5.150	26–103 µmol/L	k (Syva, Company, 1986)
Carbamazepine	S,P(H,E) at trough	Therapeutic	4–10 µg/mL	×4.233	17–42 µmol/L	kn
		Toxic	>12 µg/mL		>51 µmol/L	
Chloral hydrate	S	As trichloroethanol				
		Therapeutic	2–12 µg/mL	×6.694	13–80 µmol/L	
		Toxic	>20 µg/mL		>134	
Diazepam	S,P(H,E) at trough	Therapeutic	100–1,000 ng/mL	×3.512	350–3,500 nmol/L	
		Toxic	>5,000 ng/mL		>17,500 nmol/L	
Digitoxin	S,P(H,E) 6 hr post dose	Therapeutic	20–35 ng/mL	×1.307	26–46 nmol/L	n
		Toxic	>45 ng/mL		>59 nmol/L	
Digoxin	S,P(H,E) 12 hr post dose					kn
			ng/mL		nmol/L	
		Therapeutic	0.5–2.0	×1.281	1–1.9	
					0.6–2.6	
		Toxic				
		Child	>2.5		>3.2	
		Adult	>3.0		>3.8	
Diphenylhydantoin, see *Phenytoin*						
Doxepin (includes desmethyldoxepine)	S,P	Therapeutic	110–250 ng/mL	×1	110–250 µg/L	(Syva, Company, 1986)
Ethanol	W(O),S	Toxic	50–100 mg/dL	×0.2171	11–22 nmol/L	
		Depression of central nervous system	>100		>22 nmol/L	
Ethosuximide	S,P(H,E) at trough	Therapeutic	40–100 µg/mL	×7.084	280–700 µmol/L	kn
		Toxic	>150 µg/mL		>1,060 µmol/L	
Imipramine (includes desipramine)	S	Therapeutic	150–250 ng/mL	×1	150–250 µg/L	k (Syva, Company, 1986)
Lithium	S,P (not LiH) 12 hr after dose					
		Therapeutic	0.6–1.2 mmol/L	×1	0.6–1.2 mmol/L	
		Toxic	>2 mmol/L		>2 mmol/L	
Lysergic acid diethylamide	P(E)		After hallucinogenic dose		After hallucinogenic dose	
	U		0.005–0.009 µg/mL	×3,089	15.5–27.8 nmol/L	
			0.001–0.050 µg/mL		3.1–155.0 nmol/L	
Methotrexate	S,P		After high-dose therapy		After high-dose therapy	kn
		Toxic	>5 µmol/L at 24 hr	×1	>5 µmol/L at 24 hr	
		Toxic	>1 µmol/L at 48 hr		>1 µmol/L at 48 hr	
Paraldehyde	S,P(H,E)		µg/mL		µmol/L	
		Sedative	10–100	×7.567	75–750	(Koren et al., 1986)
		Anticonvulsant	100–200		>750–1,500	
		Toxic	>200		>1,500	
		Lethal	>500		>3,750	
Phenacetin	P(E)		µg/mL		µmol/L	
		Therapeutic	1–20	×5.580	5.6–110	
		Toxic	50–250		280–1,400	

ANALYTE OR PROCEDURE	SPECIMEN	REFERENCE VALUES (USA)		CONVERSION FACTOR	REFERENCE VALUES (SI)	COMMENTS
Phenobarbital	S,P(H,E) at trough	Therapeutic	µg/mL 15–40	×4.306	µmol/L 65–170	kn
		Toxic				
		Slowness, ataxia, nystagmus	35–80		150–345	
		Coma with reflexes	65–117		280–504	
		Coma without reflexes	>100		>430	
Phensuximide (both parent and N-desmethyl metabolite)	S,P(H,E)	Therapeutic	40–60	×5.71	228–343 µmol/L	
Phenytoin	S,P(H,E)	Therapeutic	10–20	×3.964	40–80 µmol/L	
Primidone	S,P(H,E) at trough		µg/mL		µmol/L	(Taylor and Caviness, 1986)
		Therapeutic	5–12	×4.582	23–55	
		Toxic	>15		>69	
		Toxic (neonatal)	>20		>92	
Procainamide	S,P(H,E)	Therapeutic	4–10	×4.25	17–42	
		Toxic	>10–12		>42–51	
		(Also consider concentration of metabolite N-acetylprocainamide [NAPA])				
Propranolol	S,P(H,E) at trough	Therapeutic 50–100 ng/mL		×3.856	190–380 nmol/L	
Quinidine	S,P(H,E)	Therapeutic	2–5 µg/mL	×3.083	6.2–15.5 µmol/L	
		Toxic	>6 µg/mL		>18.5 µmol/L	
Salicylate	S,P(H,E) at trough	Therapeutic	15–30 mg/dL	×0.0724	1.1–2.2 mmol/L	
		Toxic	>30 mg/dL		>2.2 mmol/L	
Theophylline	S,P(H,E)					
		Therapeutic	µg/mL		µmol/L	kn
		Bronchodilator	10–20	×5.550	56–110	
		Neonatal apnea	5–10		28–56	
		Toxic	>20		>110	
Valproic acid	S,P(H,E) at trough	Therapeutic	50–100	×6.934	350–700 µmol/L	
		Toxic	>100		>700 µmol/L	

II. ANALYSES OF URINE
A Formed Elements

Sediment casts	U	Hyaline occasional (0–1) casts/hpf		Hyaline occasional (0–1) casts/hpf
		RBCs not seen		RBCs not seen
		WBCs not seen		WBCs not seen
		Tubular epithelial not seen		Tubular epithelial not seen
		Transitional and squamous epithelial not seen		Transitional and squamous epithelial not seen
Cells		RBC 0–2/hpf		RBC 0–2/hpf
		WBC		WBC
		M 0–3/hpf		M 0–3/hpf
		F and children 0–5/hpf		F and children 0–5/hpf
		Epithelial: few; more frequent in newborn		Epithelial: few; more frequent in newborn
		Bacterial: unspun; no organisms per oil immersion field		Bacterial: unspun; no organisms per oil immersion field
		Spun: <20 organisms/hpf		Spun: <20 organisms/hpf
Specific gravity	U	Adult 1.002–1.030		Adult 1.002–1.030
		After 12 hr fluid restriction >1.025		After 12 hr fluid restriction >1.025
	U, 24 hr	1.015–1.025		

Urine volume	U, 24 hr		mL/24 hr		L/24 hr
		Newborn	50–300	×0.001	0.050–0.300
		Infant	350–550		0.350–0.550
		Child	500–1,000		0.500–1.000
		Adolescent	700–1,400		0.700–1.400
		Adult, M	800–1,800		0.800–1.800
		F	600–1,600		0.600–1.600
		(varies with intake and other factors)			

B. Chemical Elements

Acetone, semiquantitative	U		Negative		Negative	
Albumin	U	4–16 yr	3.35–18.3 mg/24 hr/1.73 m²			(Meites, 1989)
Aldosterone	U	Newborn (1–3 days)	20–140 µg/g Cr	×0.3139	6.28–43.94 nmol/mmol Cr	
			0.5–5 µg/24 hr	×2.775	1.39–13.88 nmol/day	
		Prepubertal (4–10 yr)	4–22 µg/g Cr	×0.3139	1.26–6.91 nmol/mmol Cr	
			1–8 µg/24 hr	×2.775	2.78–22.20 nmol/day	
		Adults	1.5–20 µg/g Cr	×0.3139	0.47–6.28 nmol/mmol Cr	
			3–19 µg/24 hr	×2.775	8.32–52.72 nmol/day	

ANALYTE OR PROCEDURE	SPECIMEN	REFERENCE VALUES (USA)					CONVERSION FACTOR		REFERENCE VALUES (SI)				COMMENTS
Amino acids, urine, quantitative	U												
		Premature	Full-term										
		0–6 wk (μmol/g Cr)	0–1 mo (μmol/g Cr)	1–24 mo (μmol/g Cr)	2–18 yr (μmol/g Cr)	Adult (μmol/g Cr)	0–6 wk (mmol/mol Cr)	0–1 mo (mmol/mol Cr)	1–24 mo (mmol/mol Cr)	2–18 yr (mmol/mol Cr)	Adult (mmol/mol Cr)		(Shapira, et al., 1989)
1-Methylhistidine		170–880	96–499	106–1,275	170–1,688	170–1,680	19–100	11–56	12–144	19–191	19–190		
3-Methylhistidine		420–1,340	189–680	147–391	182–365	160–520	48–152	21–77	17–44	21–41	18–59		
Alanine		1,320–4,040	982–3,055	767–6,090	231–915	240–670	149–457	11–346	87–689	26–103	27–76		
Anserine			0–3	0–5	0	0	0	0	0–1	0	0		
Arginine		190–820	35–214	38–165	31–109	10–90	21–93	4–24	4–19	4–12	1–10		
Asparagine		1,350–5,250	185–1,550	252–1,280	72–332	99–470	153–594	21–175	29–145	8–38	11–53		
Aspartic acid		580–1,520	336–810	230–685	0–120	60–240	66–172	38–92	26–77	0–14	7–27		
Carnosine		260–370	97–665	203–635	72–402	10–90	29–42	11–75	23–72	8–45	1–10		
Citrulline		240–1,320	27–181	22–180	10–99	8–50	27–149	3–20	2–20	1–11	1–6		
Cystathionine		260–1,160	16–147	33–470	0–26	20–50	29–131	2–17	4–53	0–3	2–6		
Cystine		480–1,690	212–668	68–710	25–125	43–210	54–191	24–76	8–80	3–14	5–24		
Ethanolamine			840–3,400	0–2,230	0–530	0–520	0	95–385	0–252	0–60	0–59		
Glutamic acid		380–3,760	70–1,058	54–590	0–176	39–330	43–425	8–120	6–67	0–20	4–37		
Glutamine		520–1,700	393–1,042	670–1,562	369–1,014	190–510	59–192	44–118	76–177	42–115	21–58		
Glycine		7,840–23,600	5,749–16,423	3,023–11,148	897–4,500	730–4,160	887–2,669	650–1,858	342–1,261	101–509	83–470		
Histidine		1,240–7,240	908–2,528	815–7,090	644–2,430	460–1,430	140–819	103–286	92–802	73–275	52–162		
Hydroxylysine			10–125	10–97	40–102	40–90	0	1–14	1–11	5–12	5–10		
Hydroxyproline		560–5,640	40–440	0–4,010	0–3,300	0–26	63–638	5–50	0–454	0–373	0–3		
Isoleucine		250–640	125–390	38–642	10–126	16–180	28–72	14–44	4–73	1–14	2–20		
Leucine		190–790	78–195	70–570	30–500	30–150	21–89	9–22	8–64	3–57	3–17		
Lysine		1,860–16,460	270–1,850	189–850	153–634	145–634	210–1,862	31–209	21–96	17–72	16–72		
Methionine		500–1,230	342–880	174–1,090	16–114	38–210	57–139	39–100	20–123	2–13	4–24		
Ornithine		260–3,350	118–554	55–364	31–91	20–80	29–379	13–63	6–41	4–10	2–9		
Phenylalanine		920–2,280	91–457	175–1,340	61–314	51–250	104–258	10–52	20–152	7–36	6–28		
Phosphoethanolamine		80–340	0–155	108–533	18–150	20–100	9–38	0–18	12–60	2–17	2–11		
Phosphoserin		500–1,690	150–339	112–304	70–138	40–510	57–191	17–38	13–34	8–16	5–58		
Proline		1,350–10,460	370–2,323	254–2,195	0	0	153–1,183	42–263	29–248	0	0		
Sarcosine		0	0–56	30–358	0–26	0–80	0	0–6	3–40	0–3	0–9		
Serine		1,680–6,000	1,444–3,661	845–3,190	362–1,100	240–670	190–679	163–414	96–361	41–124	27–76		
Taurine		5,190–23,620	1,650–6,220	545–3,790	639–1,866	380–1,850	587–2,671	187–703	62–429	72–211	43–209		
Threonine		840–5,700	445–1,122	252–1,528	121–389	130–370	95–645	50–127	29–173	14–44	15–42		
Tryptophan		0	0	0–93	0–108	0–70	0	0	0–11	0–12	0–8		
Tyrosine		1,090–6,780	220–1,650	333–1,550	122–517	90–290	123–767	25–187	38–175	14–58	10–33		
Valine		180–890	113–369	99–316	58–143	27–260	20–101	13–42	11–36	7–16	3–29		
α-Aminobutyric acid		50–710	8–65	30–136	0–77	0–90	6–80	1–7	3–15	0–9	0–10		
α-Aminoadipic acid		70–460	0–180	45–268	2–88	40–110	8–52	0–20	5–30	0–10	5–12		
β-Alanine		1,020–3,500	25–288	0–297	0–65	0–130	115–396	3–33	0–34	0–7	0–15		
β-Aminoisobutyric acid		50–470	421–3,133	802–4,160	291–1,482	10–510	6–53	48–354	91–470	33–168	1–58		
γ-Aminoisobutyric acid		20–260	0–15	0–105	15–30	0–32	2–29	0–2	0–12	2–3	0–4		

ANALYTE OR PROCEDURE	SPECIMEN	REFERENCE VALUES (USA)		CONVERSION FACTOR	REFERENCE VALUES (SI)	COMMENTS
Aminolevulinic acid (ALA)	U	1.3–7.0 mg/24 hr		×7.626	9.9–53.4 μmol/24 hr	
Ammonia	U	500–1,200 mg N/24 hr		×0.0714	36–86 mmol N/24 hr	
Bilirubin	U	Negative			Negative	
Calcium, total	U	Ca in diet	mg/24 hr		mmol/24 hr	
		Ca free	5–40	×0.025	0.13–1.0	
		Low–average	50–150		1.25–3.8	
		Average (20 mmol/24 hr)	100–300		2.5–7.5	
Catecholamines, fractionated	U	Norepinephrine	μg/24 hr	×5.911	nmol/24 hr	
		0–1 hr	0–10		0–59	
		1–2 hr	0–17		0–100	
		2–4 hr	4–29		24–171	
		4–7 hr	8–45		47–266	
		7–10 hr	13–65		77–384	
		Thereafter	15–80		87–473	
	U	Epinephrine	μg/24 hr		nmol/24 hr	
		0–1 hr	0–2.5	×5.458	0–13.6	
		1–2 hr	0–3.5		0–19.1	
		2–4 hr	0–6.0		0–32.7	
		4–7 hr	0.2–10		1.1–55.0	
		7–10 hr	0.5–14		2.7–76.0	
		Thereafter	0.5–20		2.7–109	
		Dopamine	μg/24 hr		nmol/24 hr	
		0–1 hr	0–85	×6.528	0–555	
		1–2 hr	10–140		65–914	
		2–4 hr	40–260		261–1,697	
		Thereafter	65–400		424–2,611	
Catecholamines, total, free	U		μg/24 hr		μg/24 hr	
		0–1 yr	10–15	×1	10–15	
		1–5 yr	15–40		15–40	
		6–15 yr	20–80		20–80	
		Thereafter	30–100		30–100	

ANALYTE OR PROCEDURE	SPECIMEN	REFERENCE VALUES (USA)		CONVERSION FACTOR	REFERENCE VALUES (SI)	COMMENTS
Chloride	U	Infant	2–10 mmol/24 hr	×1	2–10 mmol/24 hr	
		Child	15–40		15–40	
		Thereafter	110–250		110–250	
		(varies greatly with chloride intake)				
Copper	U	5–18 yr : 0.36–7.56 mg/mol creatinine		×15.7	6–119 μmol/mol creatinine	cd (Lockitch, Halstead, and Wadsworth et al., 1988)
Coproporphyrin	U	34–234 μg/24 hr		×1.5	51–351 nmol/24 hr	
Cortisol, free	U		μg/24 hr		nmol/day	
		Child	2–27	×2.759	5.5–74	
		Adolescent	5–55		14–152	
		Adult	10–100		27–276	
Creatinine	U		mg/kg/24 hr		μmol/kg/24 hr	aw (Meites, 1989)
		Premature	8.1–15.0	×8.84	72–133	
		Full term	10.4–19.7		92–174	
		1.5–7 yr	10–15		88–133	
		7–15 yr	5.2–41.0		46–362	
Cyclic AMP adenosine monophosphate	U	<3.3 mg/24 hr or		×3.040	<10 μmol/24 hr	
		<1.64 mg/g creatinine			<600 μmol	
					cyclic adenosine monophosphate/mol creatinine	
Estradiol, urinary	U		μg/24 hr		nmol/day	
		Adult M	0–6	×3.671	0–22	
		Adult F				
		Follicular	0–3		0–11	
		Ovulatory peak	4–14		15–51	
		Luteal	4–10		15–37	
Estriol (E₃), total	U	Pregnancy (wk)	mg/24 hr		μmol/24 hr	
		30	6–18	×3.467	21–62	
		35	9–28		31–97	
		40	13–42		45–146	
		Decrease of > 40% of previous value			Fraction of previous value of < 0.60	
		suggests fetus at risk			suggests fetus at risk	
Estrogen, total	U, 24 hr		μg/24 hr		μg/24 hr	
		Child	<10	×1	<10	
		Adult M	5–25		5–25	
		Adult F				
		Preovulation	5–25		5–25	
		Ovulation	28–100		28–100	
		Luteal peak	22–80		22–80	
		Pregnancy	<45,000		<45,000	
		Postmenopausal	<10		<10	
Ferric chloride test	U	Negative			Negative	
Galactose	U	Newborn	≤60 mg/dL	×0.0555	≤33 mmol/L	
		Thereafter	<14 mg/24 hr	×0.00555	<0.08 mmol/24 hr	
Glucose						
Quantitative, enzymatic	U	<0.5 g/24 hr		×5.55	<2.8 mmol/24 hr	
Qualitative	U	Negative			Negative	
Hemoglobin (Hb)	U	Negative			Negative	
Homovanillic acid	U, 24 hr		mg/g Cr		mmol/mol Cr	p (Meites, 1989)
		0–1 yr	<32.2	×0.62	<20	
		2–4 yr	<22		<14	
		5–19 yr	<14		<8	
5-Hydroxyindole acetic acid (5-HIAA)	U		mg/24 hr		μmol/24 hr	(Nichols Institute Diagnostics)
		2–10 yr	≤8.0		≤70.4	
		>10 yr	≤6.0	×8.8	≤52.8	
Hydroxyproline, free and bound	U		μmol/24 hr	×1	μmol/24 hr	w (Meites, 1989)
		3 days	33–112		33–112	
		10 days	148–225		148–225	
		20 days	229–310		229–310	
17-Hydroxycorticosteroids (17-OHCS)	U		mg/24 hr		μmol/24 hr	(Conversion based on hydrocortisone, MW = 362)
		0–1 yr	0.5–1.0	×2.76	1.4–2.8	
		Child	1.0–5.6		2.8–15.5	
		Adult, M	3.0–10.0		8.2–27.6	
		F	2.0–8.0		5.5–22.0	
		or 3–7 mg/g Cr		×0.312	or 0.9–2.5 mmol/mol Cr	
17-Ketogenic steroids (17-KGS)	U		mg/24 yr		μmol/24 hr	(Conversion based on dehydroepiandrosterone, MW = 288)
		0–1 yr	<1.0	×3.467	<3.5	
		1–10 yr	<5		<17	
		11–14 yr	<12		<42	
		Thereafter, M	5–23		17–80	
		F	3–15		10–52	
Ketone bodies, qualitative	U	Negative			Negative	

ANALYTE OR PROCEDURE	SPECIMEN	REFERENCE VALUES (USA)		CONVERSION FACTOR	REFERENCE VALUES (SI)	COMMENTS
17-Ketosteroid (17-KS), total	U		mg/24 hr		μmol/24 hr	Zimmerman reaction (conversion based on dehydroepiandrosterone, MW = 288)
		14 days–2 yr	<1	×3.467	<3.5	
		2–6 yr	<2		<7	
		6–10 yr	1–4		3.5–14	
		10–12 yr	1–6		3.5–21.0	
		12–14 yr	3–10		10–35	
		14–16 yr	5–12		17–42	
		Thereafter,				
		M 18–30 yr	9–22		31–76	
		M > 30 yr	8–20		28–70	
		F	6–15		21–52	
Lead	U, 24 hr	<80 μg/L		×0.00483	<0.39 μmol/L	
Magnesium	U, 24 hr	1–6 mo				
			mmol/L		mmol/L	
		breast milk	0.04–1.55	×1	0.04–1.55	
		formula	0.04–1.40		0.04–1.40	
Metanephrine, total	U, 24 hr		μmol/g Cr		mmol/mol Cr	(Meites, 1989)
		<1 yr	<15.9	×0.1131	<1.80	
		1–2 yr	<14.8		<1.67	
		3–4 yr	<12.8		<1.45	
		5–8 yr	<11.7		<1.32	
		9–13 yr	<10.5		<1.19	
Methylmalonic acid	U	6–12 wk	0–57 mg/g Cr	×0.9579	0–55 mmol/mol Cr	o (Meites, 1989)
Mucopolysaccharides	U		μg/g Cr		mg/mmol Cr	
		<2 yr	<50	×0.1131	<5.7	(Meites, 1989)
		2–4 yr	<25		<2.8	
		4–15 yr	<20		<2.3	
Myoglobin	U	Negative			Negative	
Niacin (nicotinic acid)	U	0.3–1.5 mg/24 hr		×8.113	2.43–12.17 μmol/24 hr	
Occult blood	U	Negative			Negative	
Organic acids	U	Adult μmol/g Cr			mmol/mol Cr	(Hoffman et al., 1989)
Lactic		115–407		×0.1132	13–46	
2-Hydroxyisobutyric		Not detected			Not detected	
Glycolic		159–486			18–55	
3-Hydroxybutyric		Not detected–18			Not detected–2.0	
3-Hydroxyisobutyric		36–168			4.1–19.0	
2-Hydroxyisovaleric		Not detected			Not detected	
3-Hydroxyisovaleric		61–221			6.9–25.0	
Methylmalonic		Not detected			Not detected	
4-Hydroxybutyric		2.7–51.0			0.3–5.8	
Ethylmalonic		3.57–37.0			0.4–4.2	
Succinic		4.4–141.0			0.5–16.0	
Fumaric		1.8–7.0			0.2–0.8	
Glutaric		5.3–23.0			0.6–2.6	
3-Methylglutaric		Not detected			Not detected	
Adipic		7–309			0.8–35.0	
Pyruvic		23–70			2.6–7.9	
Pyroglutamic		8–557			0.9–63.0	
2-Oxoisovaleric		Not detected			Not detected	
Acetoacetic		Not detected			Not detected	
Mevalonic		0.5–1.9			0.06–0.22	
2-Hydroxyglutaric		7–460			0.8–52.0	
3-Hydroxy-3-methyl-glutaric		Not detected–88			Not detected–10	
p-Hydroxyphenylacetic		31–195			3.5–22.0	
2-Oxoisocaproic		Not detected			Not detected	
Suberic		Not detected–26			Not detected–2.9	
Orotic		Not detected			Not detected	
cis-Aconitic		24–389			2.7–44.0	
Homovanillic		8–49			0.9–5.5	
Azeleic		11–137			1.3–5.5	
Isocitric		318–743			36–84	
Citric		619–1998			70–226	
Sebacic		Not detected			Not detected	
4-Hydroxyphenyllactic		1.8–23.0			0.2–2.6	
2-Oxoglutaric		35–654			4–74	
5-Hydroxyindoleacetic		Not detected–64			Not detected–72	
Succinylacetone		Not detected			Not detected	
Orotic acid	U	0–20.1 mg/g Cr		×0.7247	0–14.6 mmol/mol Cr	aw (Meites, 1989)
Osmolality	U	50–1400 mOsmol/kg H₂O, depending on fluid intake After 12 hr fluid restriction, >850 mOsmol/kg H₂O			50–1400 mOsmol/kg H₂O, depending on fluid intake After 12 hr fluid restriction, >850 mOsmol/kg H₂O	
	U, 24 hr	300–900 mOsmol/kg H₂O			300–900 mOsmol/kg H₂O	

ANALYTE OR PROCEDURE	SPECIMEN	REFERENCE VALUES (USA)		CONVERSION FACTOR	REFERENCE VALUES (SI)	COMMENTS
pH and acidity	U		pH		H+ concentration	
		Newborn or neonate	5–7		0.1–10.0 µmol/L	
		Thereafter	4.5–8.0		0.01–32.0 µmol/L	
			(average 6)		(average 1.0 µmol/L	
Phenylalanine	U	10 days–2 wk	1–2 mg/24 hr	×6.054	6–12 µmol/24 hr	
		3–12 yr	4–18 yr		24–110	
		Thereafter	trace–17		trace–103	
Phenylpyruvic acid, qualitative	U	Negative by FeCl₃ test			Negative by FeCl₃ test	
Porphobilinogen (PBG)						
Quantitative	U	0–2.0 mg/24 hr		×4.42	0–8.8 µmol/24 hr	
Qualitative	U	Negative			Negative	
Potassium	U, 24 hr	2.5–125.0 mmol/L		×1	2.5–125 mmol/L	
		Varies with diet			Varies with diet	
Pregnanetriol	U		mg/24 hr		µmol/24 hr	
		2 wk–2 hr	0.02–0.20	×2.972	0.06–0.6	
		2–5 yr	<0.5		<1.5	
		5–15 yr	<1.5		<4.5	
		>15 yr	<2.0		<5.9	
Protein, total	U, 24 hr	1–14 mg/dL		×10	10–140 mg/L	
		50–80 mg/24 hr (at rest)		×1	50–80 mg/24 hr	
		<250 mg/24 hr after intense exercise			<250 mg/24 hr after intense exercise	
Electrophoresis			Average % total protein		Fraction of total	
		Albumin	37.9	×0.01	0.379	
		α₁-globulin	27.3		0.273	
		α₂-globulin	19.5		0.195	
		β-globulin	8.8		0.088	
		γ-globulin	3.3		0.033	
Riboflavin (vitamin B₂)	U		µg/g Cr		µmol/mol Cr	
		1–3 yr	500–900		150–270	
		4–6 yr	300–600	×0.3	90–180	
		7–9 yr	270–500		81–150	
		10–15 yr	200–400		60–1200	
		Adult	80–269		24–81	
Sodium	U, 24 hr	40–220 (diet-dependent) mmol/24 hr		×1	40–220 mmol/24 hr	
Thiamine (vitamin B₁)	U, acidified with HCl		µg/g Cr		µmol/mol Cr	
		1–3 yr	176–200	×0.426	75–85	
		4–6 yr	121–400		52–170	
		7–9 yr	181–350		77–149	
		10–12 yr	181–300		77–128	
		13–15 yr	151–250		64–107	
		Thereafter	66–129		28–55	
Vanillylmandelic acid (VMA)	U		mg/g Cr		mmol/mol Cr	
		0–1 yr	<18.8	×0.5709	<11	p (Meites, 1989)
		2–4 yr	<11		<6	
		5–19 yr	<8		<5	
Xylose absorption test	U, 5 hr	Child	16–33% of ingested dose	×0.01	Fraction ingested dose 0.16–0.33	
		(0.5 g/kg, 25 g maximum)				
		Adult	g/5 hr		mmol/5 hr	
		5 g dose	>1.2	×6.66	>8.00	
		25 g dose	>4.0		>26.64	
Zinc	U	5–18 yr:10.1–95.9 mg/mol Cr		×0.0153	0.15–1.47 mmol/mol Cr	d (Lockitch, Halstead, and Wadsworth et al., 1988)

III. ANALYSIS OF FECES
A. Chemical Elements

α₁-antitrypsin	F	<1 yr	mg/g solid			u (Meites, 1989)
		Breast milk	<4.4			
		Formula	<2.9			
		6 mo–44 yr (cow's milk, regular diet)	<1.7			
Bile acids, total	F	120–225 mg/24 hr		×1	120–225 mg/24 hr	
Calcium, total	F	Average 0.64 g/24 hr		×25	16 mmol/24 hr	
Elastase I	F	7–12 days	>180 µg/g stool	×1	>180 µg/g stool	(Kori et al., 2003)
Coproporphyrin	F 24 hr	<30 µg/g dry weight		×1.5	<45 nmol/g dry weight	
		400–1,200 µg/24 hr			600–1,800 nmol/day	

ANALYTE OR PROCEDURE	SPECIMEN	REFERENCE VALUES (USA)		CONVERSION FACTOR	REFERENCE VALUES (SI)	COMMENTS
Fat, fecal	F 72 hr collection		g/24 hr		g/24 hr	
		Infant, breast-fed	<1	×1	<1	
		0–6 yr	<2		<2	
		Adult	<7		<7	
		Adult (fat-free diet)	<4		<4	
		Coefficient of fat absorption	%	×0.01	Absorbed fraction	
		Infant, breast-fed	>93		>0.93	
		Infant, formula-fed	>83		>0.83	
		>1 yr	≥95		≥0.95	
Occult blood	F	Negative			Negative	
		<2 mL blood/24 hr in < 100–200 g stool				
pH and acidity	F	pH 7.0–7.5			H+ concentration 31–100 nmol/L	

IV. ANALYSES OF CEREBROSPINAL FLUID
A. Formed Elements

Cell count	CSF		cells/mm³ (µL)	×10⁶	×10⁶ cells/L	
		Premature	0–25 mononuclear		0–25	
			0–10 polymorphonuclear		0–10	
			0–1,000 RBCs		0–1,000	
		Newborn	0–20 mononuclear		0–20	
			0–10 polymorphonuclear		0–10	
			0–800 RBCs		0–800	
		Neonate	0–5 mononuclear		0–5	
			0–10 polymorphonuclear		0–10	
			0–50 RBCs		0–50	
		Thereafter	0–5 mononuclear		0–5	

(Numbers of cells in very young infants are greater than those in older individuals' CSF, without substantial implication for growth and development in most instances)

Leukocyte differential count	CSF		%		Fraction	
		Lymphocytes	62 ± 34	×0.01	0.62 ± 0.34	
		Monocytes	36 ± 20		0.36 ± 0.20	
		Neutrophils	2 ± 5		0.02 ± 0.05	
		Histiocytes	0–rare		0–rare	
		Ependymal cells (includes pia-arachnoid mesothelial cells)	0–rare		0–rare	
		Eosinophils	0–rare		0–rare	
Cerebrospinal fluid pressure	CSF	70–180 mm water			70–180 mm water	
Cerebrospinal fluid volume	CSF	Child	60–100 mL	×0.001	0.06–0.10 L	
		Adult	100–160		0.10–0.16	

B. Chemical Elements

Amino acids in CSF	CSF		µmol/L		µmol/L	f (Dickinson and Hamilton, 1966)
		Taurine	6.3 ± 1.8	×1	6.3 ± 1.8	
		Aspartic acid	0.9 ± 0.5		0.9 ± 0.5	
		Threonine	25 ± 10		25 ± 10	
		Serine and asparagine	38 ± 23		38 ± 23	
		Glutamine	509 ± 144		509 ± 144	
		Proline	0.6		0.6	
		Glutamic acid	7.0 ± 4.9		7.0 ± 4.9	
		Glycine	6.6 ± 1.8		6.6 ± 1.8	
		Alanine	23 ± 9.4		23.0 ± 9.4	
		Valine	14 ± 5.5		14.0 ± 5.5	
		Half cystine	0.2		0.2	
		Methionine	2.6 ± 1.6		2.6 ± 1.6	
		Isoleucine	4.4 ± 1.3		4.4 ± 1.3	
		Leucine	11 ± 3.6		11.0 ± 3.6	
		Tyrosine	9.1 ± 5.0		9.1 ± 5.0	
		Phenylalanine	9.2 ± 5.8		9.2 ± 5.8	
		Ornithine	5.7 ± 1.8		5.7 ± 1.8	
		Lysine	19 ± 6.6		19.0 ± 6.6	
		Histidine	13 ± 4.4		13.0 ± 4.4	
		Arginine	20 ± 5.8		20.0 ± 5.8	
Calcium, total	CSF	2.1–2.7 mEq/L or		×0.50	1.05–1.35 mmol/L	
		4.2–5.4 mg/dL		×0.25	1.05–1.35 mmol/L	
Chloride	CSF	118–132 mmol/L		×1	118–132 mmol/L	
Glucose	CSF	Adult	40–70 mg/dL	×0.0555	2.2–3.9 mmol/L	
Hypoxanthine	CSF	0–1 mo	1.8–5.5 µmol/L	×1	1.8–5.5 µmol/L	(Jung et al., 1985)
Lactate	CSF	Infant–2 yr	Up to 1.8 mmol/L	×1	Up to 1.8 mmol/L	(Benoist et al., 2003)
Pyruvate	CSF	Infant–2 yr	Up to 0.147 mmol/L	×1	Up to 0.147 mmol/L	(Benoist et al., 2003)
S100B protein	CSF	Infant	0.11–0.33 µg/L	×1	0.11–0.33 µg/L	(Gazzolo et al., 2004)

ANALYTE OR PROCEDURE	SPECIMEN	REFERENCE VALUES (USA)		CONVERSION FACTOR	REFERENCE VALUES (SI)	COMMENTS
Total protein		(25–75th percentile)			(25–75th percentile)	
Turbidimetry	CSF, lumbar	mg/dL			mg/L	
		Premature	40–300	×10	400–3,000	
		Newborn	45–120		450–1,200	
		Child	10–20		100–200	
		Adolescent	15–20		150–200	
		Thereafter	15–45		150–450	
Electrophoresis	CSF	% of total			Fraction of total	
		Prealbumin	2–7	×0.01	0.02–0.07	
		Albumin	56–76		0.56–0.76	
		α_1-globulin	2–7		0.02–0.07	
		α_2-globulin	4–12		0.04–0.12	
		β-globulin	8–18		0.08–0.18	
		γ-globulin	3–12		0.03–0.12	

V. ANALYSES OF OTHER BODY FLUIDS
A. Chemical Analyses
1. Amniotic fluid analysis

ANALYTE OR PROCEDURE	SPECIMEN	REFERENCE VALUES (USA)		CONVERSION FACTOR	REFERENCE VALUES (SI)	COMMENTS
Amnionic fluid Ab450 nm	AF	28 wk 0–0.048 Absorbance		×1	0–0.048 Absorbance	t
		40 wk 0–0.002 Absorbance			0–0.002 Absorbance	
Bilirubin	AF	28 wk <0.075 mg/dL		×17.10	<1.3 µmol/L	
		(or Ab450 <0.048)			(or Ab450 <0.048)	
		40 wk <0.025 mg/dL			<0.43 µmol/L	
		(or Ab450 <0.02)			(or Ab450 <0.02)	
Creatinine	AF	After 37 wk gestation >2.0 mg/dL		×88.4	After 37 wk gestation >180 µmol/L	
Estriol (E₃), free	AF	Gestation	ng/mL		nmol/L	
		(wk)	(95% range)		(95% range)	
		16–20	1.0–3.2	×3.47	3.5–11.1	
		20–24	2.1–7.8		7.3–27.1	
		24–28	2.1–7.8		7.3–27.1	
		28–32	4.0–13.6		13.9–47.2	
		32–36	3.6–15.5		12.5–53.8	
		36–38	4.6–18.0		16.0–62.5	
		38–40	5.4–19.8		18.7–68.7	
α-fetoprotein (AFP)	AF	wk	Amniotic fluid Median, µg/mL			
		15	20.1			
		16	16.2			
		17	13.1			
		18	10.6			
		19	8.6			
		20	6.9			
Lecithin : sphingomyelin (L : S) ratio	AF	2.0–5.0 indicates probable fetal lung maturity (>3.0 in infants or diabetic mothers)			2.0–5.0 indicates probable fetal lung maturity (>3.0 in infants of diabetic mothers)	
Lecithin phosphorus	AF	>0.10 mg/dL indicates probable adequate fetal lung maturity		×0.3229	>0.032 mmol/L indicates probable adequate fetal lung maturity	

2. Sweat

ANALYTE OR PROCEDURE	SPECIMEN	REFERENCE VALUES (USA)		CONVERSION FACTOR	REFERENCE VALUES (SI)	COMMENTS
Chloride	Sweat	mmol/L			mmol/L	
		Normal	<40	×1	<40	(Gibson et al., 1985)
		Indeterminate	40–60		40–60	
		Cystic fibrosis	>60		>60	
Sodium	Sweat	mmol/L			mmol/L	
		Normal	<40	×1	<40	(Gibson et al., 1985)
		Indeterminate	40–60		40–60	
		Cystic fibrosis	>60		>60	

[†]In preparing the reference range listings, a number of abbreviations, symbols, and codes were used (see Table 715.2)

Abbott Laboratories, Diagnostic Division, Abbott Park, IL, 1996.

American Diabetes Association: Report of the Expert Committee on the Diagnosis and Classification of Diabetes Mellitus. *Diabetes Care* 1997;20:1183–1197.

Bar-Oz B, Sagie-Lev A, Arad I, et al: N terminal pro B-type natriuretic peptide concentrations in mothers just before delivery, in cord blood, and in newborns. *Clin Chem* 2005;51:926–927.

Baroni S, Scribano D, Valentini P, et al: Serum apolipoproteins A1, B CII, CIII, E, and lipoprotein (a) in children. *Clin Biochem* 1996;29:603–605.

Basuyau JP, Mallet E, Leroy M, et al: Reference intervals for serum calcitonin in men, women, and children. *Clin Chem* 2004;50:1828–1830.

Benoist JF, Alberti C, Leclercq S, et al: Cerebrospinal fluid lactate and pyruvate concentrations and their ratio in children: Age-related reference intervals. *Clin Chem* 2003;49:487–494.

Berdat P, Wehrle T, Kung A, et al: Age-specific analysis of normal cytokine levels in healthy infants. *Clin Chem Lab Med* 2003;41:1335–1339.

Bonnefont JP, Specola NB, Vassault A, et al: The fasting test in children: Application to the diagnosis of pathological hypo- and hyperketotic states. *Eur J Pediatr* 1990;150:80–85.

Buck ML: Anticoagulation with warfarin in infants and children. *Ann Pharmacother* 1996;30:1316–1322.

Davis ML, Austin C, Messner BL, et al: IFCC-standardized pediatric reference intervals for 10 serum proteins using the Beckman Array 360 System. *Clin Biochem* 1996;29:489–492.

Denny T, Yogev R, Gelman R, et al: Lymphocyte subsets in healthy children during the first five years of life. *JAMA* 1992;267:1484–1488.

De Schepper J, Derde MP, Goubert P, et al: Reference values for fructosamine concentrations in children's sera: Influence of protein concentration, age and sex. *Clin Chem* 1988;34:2444–2447.

Diaz J, Tornel PL, Martinez P: Reference intervals for blood ammonia in healthy subjects, determined by microdiffusion. *Clin Chem* 1995;41:1048.

Dickinson JC, Hamilton PB: The free amino acids of human spinal fluid determined by ion exchange chromatography. *J Neurochem* 1966;13:1179–1185.

Esoterix Endocrinology, Calabasas Hills, CA 91301.

Gazzolo D, Grutzfeld D, Michetti F, et al: Increased s100b in cerebrospinal fluid of infants with bacterial meningitis: Relationship to brain damage and routine cerebrospinal fluid findings. *Clin Chem* 2004;50:941–944.

Gazzolo D, Michetti F, Bruschettini M, et al: Pediatric concentrations of s100b protein in blood: Age- and sex related changes. *Clin Chem* 2003;49:967–970.

Ghoshal A, Soldin S: Evaluation of the Dade Behring Dimension RxL: Integrated chemistry system-pediatric reference ranges. *Clin Chim Acta* 2003;331:135–146.

Gibson LE, di Sant'Agnese PA, Schwachman H: Procedure for the Quantitative Iontophoretic Sweat Test for Cystic Fibrosis. Rockville, MD, Cystic Fibrosis Foundation, 1985, pp 1–4.

Gillard BK, Simbala JA, Goodglick L: Reference intervals for amylase isoenzymes in serum and plasma of infants and children. *Clin Chem* 1983;29:1119–1123.

Hoffman G, Aramaki S, Blum-Hoffman E, et al: Quantitative analysis for organic acids in biological samples: Batch isolation followed by gas chromatographic-mass spectrometric analysis. *Clin Chem* 1989;35:587–595.

Jedeikin R, Makela SK, Shennan AT, et al: Creatine kinase isoenzymes in serum from cord blood and the blood of healthy full-term infants during the first three postnatal days. *Clin Chem* 1982;28:317–322.

Jung D, Lun L, Zinsmeyer J, et al: The concentration of hypoxanthine and lactate in the blood of healthy and hypoxic newborns. *J Perinat Med* 1985;13:43–50.

Kaplan EL, Rothermel CD, Johnson DR: Antistreptolysin O and anti-deoxyribonuclease B titers: Normal values for children ages 2 to 12 in the United States. *Pediatrics* 1998;101:86–88.

Knight JA, Haymond RE: γ-Glutamyltransferase and alkaline phosphatase activities compared in serum of normal children and children with liver disease. *Clin Chem* 1981;27:48–51.

Koch A, Singer H: Normal values of B type natriuretic peptide in infants, children and adolescents. *Heart* 2003;89:875–878.

Koren G, Butt W, Rajchgot P, et al: Intravenous paraldehyde for seizure control in neonates. *Neurology* 1986;36:108–111.

Kori M, Metzger AM, Shamir R, et al: Fecal elastase 1 levels in premature and full term infants. *Arch Dis Child Fetal Neonatal Ed* 2003;88:F106–F108.

Laskowska-Klita T, Szymczak E, Radomyska B: Serum homocysteine and lipoprotein (a) concentrations in hypercholesterolemic and normocholesterolemic children. *Clin Pediatr* 2001;40:149–154.

Lockitch G, Halstead AC, Albersheim S, et al: Age and sex specific pediatric reference intervals for biochemistry analytes as measured on the Ektachem-700 analyzer. *Clin Chem* 1988;34:1622–1625.

Lockitch G, Halstead AC, Quigley G, et al: Age- and sex-specific pediatric reference intervals: Study design and methods illustrated by measurement of serum proteins with the Behring LN Nephelometer. *Clin Chem* 1988;34:1618–1621.

Lockitch G, Halstead AC, Wadsworth L, et al: Age- and sex-specific pediatric reference intervals and correlations for zinc, copper, selenium, iron, vitamins A and E, and related proteins. *Clin Chem* 1988;34:1625–1628.

Mäkikallio K, Vuolteenaho O, Jouppila P, et al: Association of severe placental insufficiency and systemic venous pressure rise in the fetus with increased neonatal cardiac troponin T levels. *Am J Obstet Gynecol* 2000;183:726–731.

Mayo Medical Laboratories, Rochester, MN 55905.

Meites S (editor): *Pediatric Clinical Chemistry, Reference (Normal) Values*, 3rd ed. Washington, DC, American Association for Clinical Chemistry, 1989.

Muntau A, Streiter M, Kappler M, et al: Age-related reference values for serum selenium concentrations in infants and children. *Clin Chem* 2002;48:555–560.

Nichols Institute Diagnostics, San Juan Capistrano, CA 92675.

Nir A, Bar-Oz B, Perles Z, et al: N-terminal pro-B-type natriuretic peptide: Reference plasma levels from birth to adolescence. Elevated levels at birth and in infants and children with heart diseases. *Acta Paediatr* 2004;93:603–607.

Pesce MA, Boudourian S: Clinical significance of plasma galactose and erythrocyte galactose-1-phosphate measurements in transferase-deficient galactosemia and in individuals with below-normal transferase activity. *Clin Chem* 1982;28:301–305.

Pesce MA, Bodourian S, Nicholson JF: A new microfluorometric method for the measurement of galactose-1-phosphate in erythrocytes. *Clin Chim Acta* 1982;118:177–189.

Pesce MA, Bodourian S, Harris RC, et al: Enzymatic micromethod for measuring galactose-1-phosphate uridylyltransferase in erythrocytes. *Clin Chem* 1977;23:1711–1717.

Pianosi P, Seargeant L, Haworth JC: Blood lactate and pyruvate concentrations, and their ratio during exercise in healthy children: Developmental perspective. *Eur J Appl Physiol Occup Physiol* 1995;71:518–522.

Pittet JL, de Moerloose P, Reber G, et al: VIDAS D-dimer: Fast quantitative ELISA for measuring D-dimer in plasma. *Clin Chem* 1996;42:410–415.

Rosenthal P, Pesce MA: Long-term monitoring of D-lactic acidosis in a child. *J Pediatr Gastroenterol Nutr* 1985;4:674–676.

Schmidt-Sommerfeld E, Werner D, Penn D: Carnitine plasma concentrations in 353 metabolically healthy children. *Eur J Pediatr* 1988;147:356–360.

Shapira E, Blitzer MG, Miller JB, et al: *Biochemical Genetics: A Laboratory Manual*. New York, Oxford University Press, 1989.

Sherry B, Jack RM, Weber A, et al: Reference interval for prealbumin for children two to 36 months old. *Clin Chem* 1988;34:1878–1880.

Soldin O, Bierbower L, Choi J, et al: Serum iron, ferritin, transferrin, total iron binding capacity, hs-CRP, LDL cholesterol and magnesium in children: New reference intervals using the Dade Dimension Clinical Chemistry System. *Clin Chim Acta* 2004;342:211–217.

Soldin SJ, Hicks JM, Bailey J, et al: Pediatric reference ranges for 25 hydroxy vitamin D during the summer and winter. *Clin Chem* 1997;43:S200.

Straczcek J, Felden F, Dousset B, et al: Quantification of methylmalonic acid in serum measured by capillary gas chromatography-mass chromatography astert-butyldimethylsilyl derivatives. *J Chromatogr* 1993;620:1–7.

Syva Company: *TDM Serum Sample Guide*. Palo Alto, CA, 1986.

Taylor WJ, Caviness MHD (editors): *A Textbook for the Clinical Application of Therapeutic Drug Monitoring*. Irving, TX, Abbott Laboratories, Diagnostic Division, 1986.

Vilaseca MA, Moyano D, Ferrer I, et al: Total homocysteine in pediatric patients. *Clin Chem* 1997;43:690–692.

Visnapu LA, Karlson LK, Dubinsky EJ, et al: Pediatric reference ranges for serum aldolase. *Am J Clin Pathol* 1989;91:476–477.

From Behrman, R., Kliegman, R., & Arvin, A. (2007). Nelson's textbook of pediatrics. (18th ed.). Philadelphia: WB Saunders.

Standard Precautions

HISTORICAL PERSPECTIVES

For many years, hospitals and health care providers have been struggling with infection control, trying to incorporate control procedures that prevent infection transmission not only from patient to patient but also from patient to personnel and personnel to patient. The movement of patients with infectious diseases from specialty hospitals to general hospitals during the middle of the twentieth century prompted the U.S. Department of Health and Human Services, Centers for Disease Control and Prevention (CDC), to issue detailed guidelines addressing isolation techniques to be used in the general hospital. This manual was updated twice to reflect changes in microorganisms, appearance of new organisms, new epidemiologic information, and the increase in nosocomial infection.

The identification and increasing prevalence of HIV in the early 1980s radically changed infectious disease control approaches. Because of the HIV risk to health care personnel and because of research that indicated that the asymptomatic incubation period for AIDS could be years, in 1985 the CDC published a new strategy for infection control called *Universal Precautions (UP)*. The underlying premise for UP applied blood and body fluid precautions to all persons regardless of whether their infection status was known. In 1991 the Occupational Safety and Health Administration (OSHA) issued guidelines for all health care employers to prevent employee occupational exposure to blood-borne pathogens.

Confusion about definitions of contaminated fluids and substances, as well as the fact that UP and other approaches did not adequately address transmission of illnesses such as tuberculosis and newly identified diseases, prompted the CDC to work with the Hospital Infection Control Practices Advisory Committee (HIC-PAC) to revise the *CDC Guidelines for Isolation Precautions in Hospitals*. The new guidelines, issued in 1996, are divided into three sections: standard precautions (to be applied to all), transmission-based precautions (to reduce airborne, droplet, and contact infection), and temporary precautions (to be used for patients suspected to have certain infections).

SUMMARY OF THE RECOMMENDATIONS FOR ISOLATION PRECAUTIONS IN HOSPITALS— STANDARD PRECAUTIONS

Standard precautions are used for all patients, regardless of infection status. "Standard precautions apply to (1) blood, (2) all body fluids, secretions, and excretions *except sweat*, regardless of whether they contain visible blood, (3) nonintact skin, and (4) mucous membranes" (Hospital Infection Control Practices Advisory Committee & Centers for Disease Control and Prevention, 1996). *Contaminated equipment* or *surfaces* refers to contamination by the previous substances.

FUNDAMENTALS

1. Wash hands with a nonantimicrobial soap after touching blood, body fluids, secretions, excretions, and contaminated articles, *regardless* of whether gloves are worn. Wash hands between patients and between performing different procedures on the same patient (if appropriate). Wash hands immediately after removing gloves. Use an antimicrobial soap for special circumstances to control certain disease outbreaks.
2. Wear clean, nonsterile gloves when touching blood, body fluids, secretions, excretions, and contaminated articles, and before contacting mucous membranes or nonintact skin. Change gloves between patients and between procedures on the same patient if gloves have been in contact with an area likely to contain a high concentration of microorganisms. Remove gloves promptly after use and before touching noncontaminated articles.
3. Wear a clean gown, shoe covers, and mask, goggles, or face shield during procedures and activities likely to generate splashes or sprays of blood, body fluids, secretions, or excretions likely to cause soiling of clothing or exposure to skin and mucous membranes. Remove equipment promptly and wash hands immediately.
4. Handle used, contaminated patient care equipment in a manner that prevents exposure to skin, mucous membranes, and clothing, and that prevents transmission of organisms to others. Properly clean and reprocess all contaminated equipment or properly discard all single-use articles.

5. Ensure that all hospital procedures for the cleaning and disinfection of environmental surfaces are followed.
6. Handle and process contaminated linens in a way that prevents skin and mucous membrane exposure, prevents contamination of clothing, and avoids transmission of microorganisms to others.
7. No special precautions are needed for dishes and eating utensils.
8. Follow OSHA blood-borne pathogen standards for occupational exposure and injury prevention.
   a. Use care in the handling, cleaning, and disposal of sharp instruments and devices.
   b. *Never* recap needles with two hands or point a needle in the direction of the body—may use a one-handed "scoop" procedure or syringes mechanically designed to cover an exposed needle after use.
   c. Do not try to break the needle after use. Dispose of all sharps in an appropriately marked puncture-resistant container placed close to the area of use.
   d. Appropriately mark and handle blood and contaminated fluids for transport (leak-proof containers).
   e. Use mouthpieces, resuscitation bags, or other ventilation devices instead of mouth-to-mouth resuscitation. Keep equipment available in each patient room.
   f. Arrange to have cleaned all contaminated environmental surfaces as soon as possible after the contamination occurs.
   g. Dispose of contaminated articles in properly marked containers designed to handle regulated waste.

OSHA regulations provide for the annual review of all procedures related to the implementation of the blood-borne pathogen standard and mandates employers to provide all equipment necessary to ensure employee safety. OSHA also delineates procedures after an accidental exposure in the workplace.

SUMMARY OF THE RECOMMENDATIONS FOR TRANSMISSION-BASED PRECAUTIONS

See Box E-1 for types of precautions and patient categories.
1. Airborne precautions (5 μm or smaller)
   a. Adhere to standard precautions.
   b. Patient should be in a private room with (1) monitored negative air pressure in relation to the surrounding areas, (2) 6 to 12 air changes per hour, and (3) appropriate discharge of air outdoors or monitored high-efficiency filtration of room air before the air is circulated to other areas of the hospital. May be in room with patient who has active infection with same microorganism but no other infections. Door should stay closed and patient should leave room only if transport is necessary. Have patient wear a mask during transport.
   c. Wear respiratory protection (N95 respirator) when entering the room of a person with known or suspected infectious pulmonary tuberculosis. Susceptible persons should not enter the room of patients known or suspected to have measles (rubeola) or varicella (chickenpox) if other immune caregivers are available. If susceptible persons must enter the room of a patient known or suspected to have measles (rubeola) or varicella, they should wear respiratory protection (N95 respirator). Persons immune to measles (rubeola) or varicella need not wear respiratory protection.
2. Droplet precautions (larger than 5 μm)
   a. Adhere to standard precautions.
   b. Patient should be in private room or in a room with a patient who has active infection with same microorganism but no other infection. Door can remain open.
   c. Wear a mask if working within 3 feet of the patient.
   d. Have patient wear a mask during transport.
3. Contact precautions
   a. Adhere to standard precautions.
   b. Patient should be in private room or with patient who has active infection with same microorganism but no other infections.
   c. In addition to wearing gloves as outlined under standard precautions, wear gloves (clean) when entering the room. During the course of providing care for the patient, change gloves after having contact with infectious material that may contain high concentrations of microorganisms (fecal material and wound drainage). Remove gloves before leaving patient's room. Wash hands immediately with an antimicrobial agent or waterless antiseptic agent. Do not touch any potentially contaminated surfaces after hand-washing.
   d. Wear a gown if you anticipate patient contact, contact with environmental surfaces, or contact with items in the patient's room or if patient is incontinent or has diarrhea, an ileostomy, a colostomy, a urostomy, or wound drainage not contained by a dressing. Remove gown before leaving patient's room but do not allow clothing to become contaminated.
   e. Avoid risk for transmission of microorganisms to other patients and equipment if transported.
   f. Adequately clean and disinfect any equipment before use by another patient.

Box E-1 | *Synopsis of Types of Precautions and Patients Requiring the Precautions*

STANDARD PRECAUTIONS
Use standard precautions for the care of all patients.

AIRBORNE PRECAUTIONS
In addition to standard precautions, use airborne precautions for patients known or suspected to have serious illnesses transmitted by airborne droplet nuclei. Examples of such illnesses include:

- Measles
- Varicella (including disseminated zoster)*
- Tuberculosis†
- Smallpox

DROPLET PRECAUTIONS
In addition to standard precautions, use droplet precautions for patients known or suspected to have serious illnesses transmitted by large particle droplets. Examples of such illnesses include:

- Invasive *Haemophilus influenzae* type b disease, including meningitis, pneumonia, epiglottitis, and sepsis
- Invasive *Neisseria meningitidis* disease, including meningitis, pneumonia, and sepsis
- Other serious bacterial respiratory infections spread by droplet transmission, including:
  Diphtheria (pharyngeal)
  Mycoplasma pneumonia
  Pertussis
  Pneumonic plague
  Streptococcal pharyngitis, pneumonia, or scarlet fever in infants and young children
- Serious viral infections spread by droplet transmission, including:
  Adenovirus*
  Influenza
  Mumps
  Parvovirus B19
  Rubella

CONTACT PRECAUTIONS
In addition to standard precautions, use contact precautions for patients known or suspected to have serious illnesses easily transmitted by direct patient contact or by contact with items in the patient's environment. Examples of such illnesses include:

- Gastrointestinal, respiratory, skin, or wound infections or colonization with multidrug-resistant bacteria judged by the infection control program, based on current state, regional, or national recommendation, to be of special clinical and epidemiologic significance
- Enteric infections with a low infectious dose or prolonged environmental survival, including:
  Clostridium difficile
  For diapered or incontinent patients:
     enterohemorrhagic *Escherichia coli* O157:H7,
     Shigella, hepatitis A, or rotavirus
- Respiratory syncytial virus, parainfluenza virus, or enteroviral infections in infants and young children
- Skin infections that are highly contagious or that may occur on dry skin, including:
  Diphtheria (cutaneous)
  Herpes simplex virus (neonatal or mucocutaneous)
  Impetigo
  Major (noncontained) abscesses, cellulitis, or decubiti
  Pediculosis
  Scabies
  Smallpox
  Staphylococcal furunculosis in infants and young children
  Zoster (disseminated or in the immunocompromised host)*
- Viral/hemorrhagic conjunctivitis
- Viral hemorrhagic infections (Ebola, Lassa, or Marburg)

*Certain infections require more than one type of precaution.
†See CDC *Guidelines for Preventing the Transmission of Tuberculosis in Health-Care Facilities.*

REFERENCES
Hospital Infection Control Practices Advisory Committee and the Centers for Disease Control and Prevention. (1996). Guideline for isolation precautions in hospitals. *Am J Infect Cont, 24,* 24-52.

Occupational Safety and Health Act. (1991). Blood-borne pathogen standard, *Fed Register, 56*(2), 40-46.

F Growth Charts

Appendix F includes several groupings of charts related to the growth of a child. The first chart, used at birth, is the Maturational Assessment of Gestational Age, also sometimes referred to as the Ballard Scoring System. This growth chart is used to determine the gestational age of a newborn by neuromuscular and physical characteristics. Using this chart aids the health care practitioner in determining the gestational development of the newborn. Those newborns who are less than 37 weeks' gestation will need further assessment and possible interventions. The second part of the Ballard Scoring System allows for the newborn's gestational age to be compared with weight, head circumference, and length. These measurements will show the newborn to be one of the following: large for gestational age, appropriate for gestational age, or small for gestational age. The newborn whose measurements are large for gestational age or small for gestational age will need further assistance and interventions.

In 2000 the Centers for Disease Control and Prevention (CDC) released new growth charts for children. These growth charts allow the health care practitioner to plot the child's measurements according to the child's age to determine how the child measures up against the national mean. The child's growth should progress, and the growth charts allow the health care practitioner and the family to quickly see how the child is growing.

The CDC growth charts begin with those for boys, birth to 36 months. The criteria that are measured in percentiles are Weight for Age, Length for Age, Head Circumference for Age, and Weight for Length.

After age 2 years, growth slows and the child is measured less frequently. The charts are still identified for boys and girls and can be used until the age of 20 years. The CDC charts for boys 2 to 20 years are Weight for Age, Stature for Age, Weight for Stature, and Body Mass Index for Age. The CDC charts for girls 2 to 20 years follow the same format as for boys. New to the growth charts is the body mass index (BMI). After age 2 years, BMI is useful in determining whether a child is progressing toward obesity.

In summary, growth charts are a quick and accurate way to measure and monitor the growth of a child as well as to compare the child's growth with the national mean. In using the growth charts, anticipatory guidance, nutrition, and health care issues can be addressed.

MATURATIONAL ASSESSMENT OF GESTATIONAL AGE (New Ballard Score)

NAME _____   SEX _____

HOSPITAL NO. _____   BIRTH WEIGHT _____

RACE _____   LENGTH _____

DATE/TIME OF BIRTH _____   HEAD CIRC. _____

DATE/TIME OF EXAM _____   EXAMINER _____

AGE WHEN EXAMINED _____

APGAR SCORE: 1 MINUTE _____   5 MINUTES _____   10 MINUTES _____

NEUROMUSCULAR MATURITY

NEUROMUSCULAR MATURITY SIGN	SCORE							RECORD SCORE HERE
	-1	0	1	2	3	4	5	
POSTURE								
SQUARE WINDOW (Wrist)	>90°	90°	60°	45°	30°	0°		
ARM RECOIL		180°	140°-180°	110°-140°	90°-110°	<90°		
POPLITEAL ANGLE	180°	160°	140°	120°	100°	90°	<90°	
SCARF SIGN								
HEEL TO EAR								

TOTAL NEUROMUSCULAR MATURITY SCORE

PHYSICAL MATURITY

PHYSICAL MATURITY SIGN	SCORE							RECORD SCORE HERE
	-1	0	1	2	3	4	5	
SKIN	sticky friable transparent	gelatinous red translucent	smooth pink visible veins	superficial peeling &/or rash, few veins	cracking pale areas rare veins	parchment deep cracking no vessels	leathery cracked wrinkled	
LANUGO	none	sparse	abundant	thinning	bald areas	mostly bald		
PLANTAR SURFACE	heel-toe 40-50 mm:-1 <40 mm:-2	>50 mm no crease	faint red marks	anterior transverse crease only	creases ant. 2/3	creases over entire sole		
BREAST	imperceptible	barely perceptible	flat areola no bud	stippled areola 1-2 mm bud	raised areola 3-4 mm bud	full areola 5-10 mm bud		
EYE/EAR	lids fused loosely: -1 tightly: -2	lids open pinna flat stays folded	sl. curved pinna; soft; slow recoil	well-curved pinna; soft but ready recoil	formed & firm instant recoil	thick cartilage ear stiff		
GENITALS (Male)	scrotum flat, smooth	scrotum empty faint rugae	testes in upper canal rare rugae	testes descending few rugae	testes down good rugae	testes pendulous deep rugae		
GENITALS (Female)	clitoris prominent & labia flat	prominent clitoris & small labia minora	prominent clitoris & enlarging minora	majora & minora equally prominent	majora large minora small	majora cover clitoris & minora		

Ballard JL, Khoury JC, Wedig K, et al: New Ballard Score, expanded to include extremely premature infants, *J Pediatr* 119:417-423, 1991. Reprinted by permission of Dr Ballard and Mosby.

TOTAL PHYSICAL MATURITY SCORE

SCORE

Neuromuscular _____

Physical _____

Total _____

MATURITY RATING

score	weeks
-10	20
-5	22
0	24
5	26
10	28
15	30
20	32
25	34
30	36
35	38
40	40
45	42
50	44

GESTATIONAL AGE (weeks)

By dates _____

By ultrasound _____

By exam _____

CLASSIFICATION OF NEWBORNS (BOTH SEXES)
BY INTRAUTERINE GROWTH AND GESTATIONAL AGE [1,2]

NAME _____ DATE OF EXAM _____ LENGTH _____

HOSPITAL NO. _____ SEX _____ HEAD CIRC. _____

RACE _____ BIRTH WEIGHT _____ GESTATIONAL AGE _____

DATE OF BIRTH _____

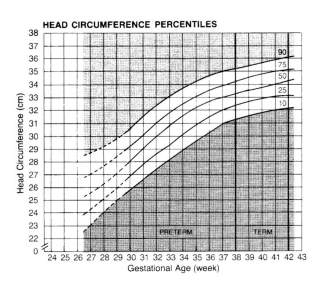

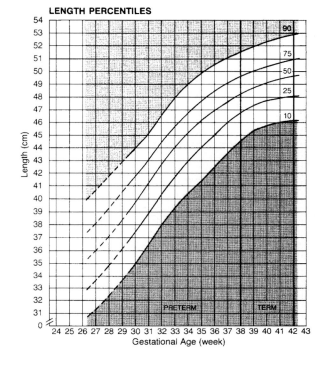

CLASSIFICATION OF INFANT*	Weight	Length	Head Circ.
Large for Gestational Age (LGA) (>90th percentile)			
Appropriate for Gestational Age (AGA) (10th to 90th percentile)			
Small for Gestational Age (SGA) (<10th percentile)			

*Place an "X" in the appropriate box (LGA, AGA or SGA) for weight, for length, and for head circumference.

1. Battaglia FC, Lubchenco LO: A practical classification of newborn infants by weight and gestational age, *J Pediatr* 71:159-163, 1967.
2. Lubchenco LO, Hansman C, Boyd E: Intrauterine growth in length and head circumference as estimated from live births at gestational ages from 26 to 42 weeks, *Pediatrics*; 37:403-408, 1966.

Reprinted by permission from Dr Battaglia, Dr Lubchenco, *Journal of Pediatrics* and *Pediatrics*.

Birth to 36 months: Boys
Length-for-age and Weight-for-age percentiles

NAME _____

RECORD # _____

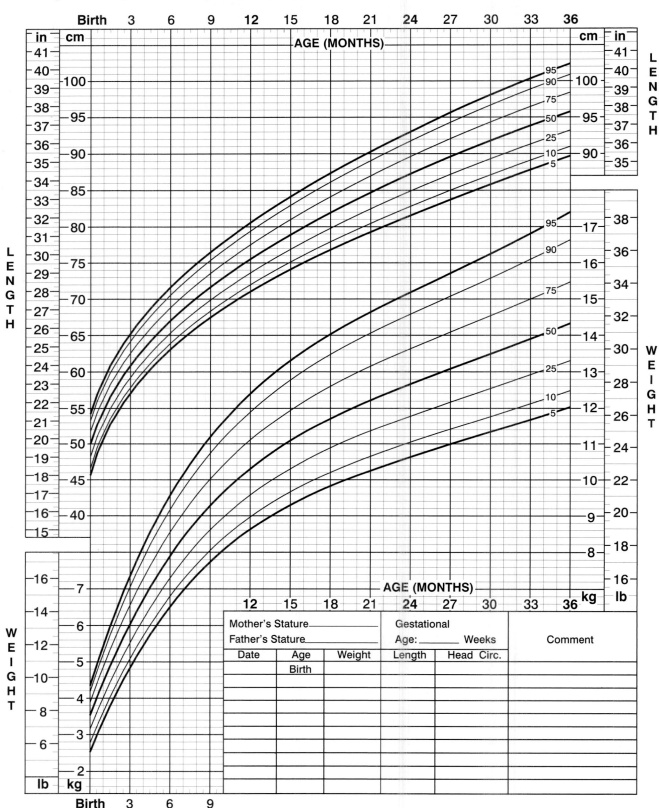

Pubished May 30, 2000 (modified 4/20/01).
SOURCE: Developed by the National Center for Health Statistics in collaboration with
the National Center for Chronic Disease Prevention and Health Promotion (2000).
http://www.cdc.gov/growthcharts

CDC

SAFER · HEALTHIER · PEOPLE™

Birth to 36 months: Girls
Length-for-age and Weight-for-age percentiles

NAME _____

RECORD # _____

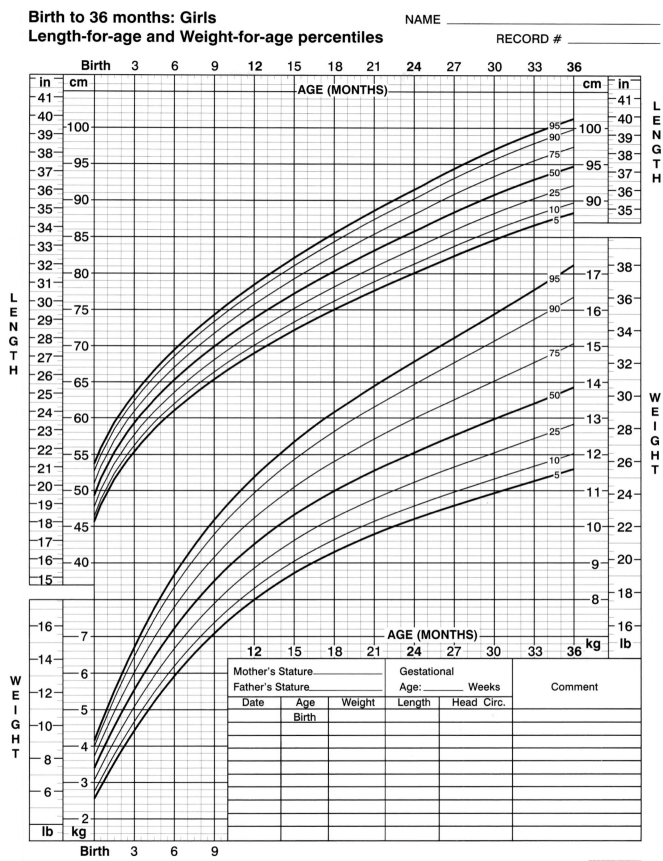

Mother's Stature_____
Father's Stature_____

Gestational
Age: _____ Weeks

Date	Age	Weight	Length	Head Circ.	Comment
	Birth				

Published May 30, 2000 (modified 4/20/01).
SOURCE: Developed by the National Center for Health Statistics in collaboration with
the National Center for Chronic Disease Prevention and Health Promotion (2000).
http://www.cdc.gov/growthcharts

SAFER · HEALTHIER · PEOPLE™

Birth to 36 months: Boys
Head circumference-for-age and
Weight-for-length percentiles

NAME _____

RECORD # _____

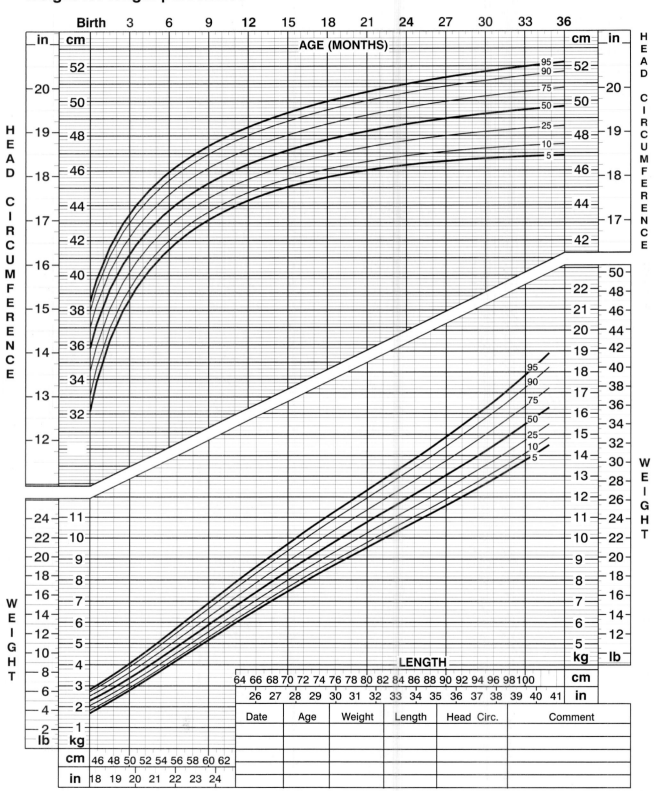

Published May 30, 2000 (modified 10/16/00).
SOURCE: Developed by the National Center for Health Statistics in collaboration with
       the National Center for Chronic Disease Prevention and Health Promotion (2000).
       http://www.cdc.gov/growthcharts

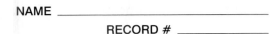

SAFER · HEALTHIER · PEOPLE™

Birth to 36 months: Girls
Head circumference-for-age and
Weight-for-length percentiles

NAME _____

RECORD # _____

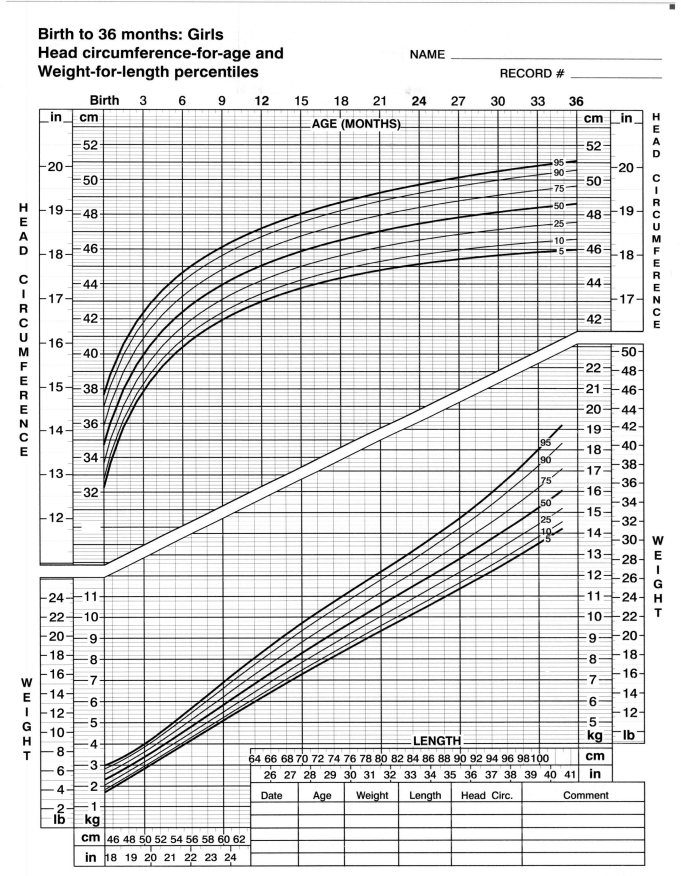

Published May 30, 2000 (modified 10/16/00).

SOURCE: Developed by the National Center for Health Statistics in collaboration with
the National Center for Chronic Disease Prevention and Health Promotion (2000).
http://www.cdc.gov/growthcharts

SAFER · HEALTHIER · PEOPLE™

2 to 20 years: Boys
Stature-for-age and Weight-for-age percentiles

NAME _____

RECORD # _____

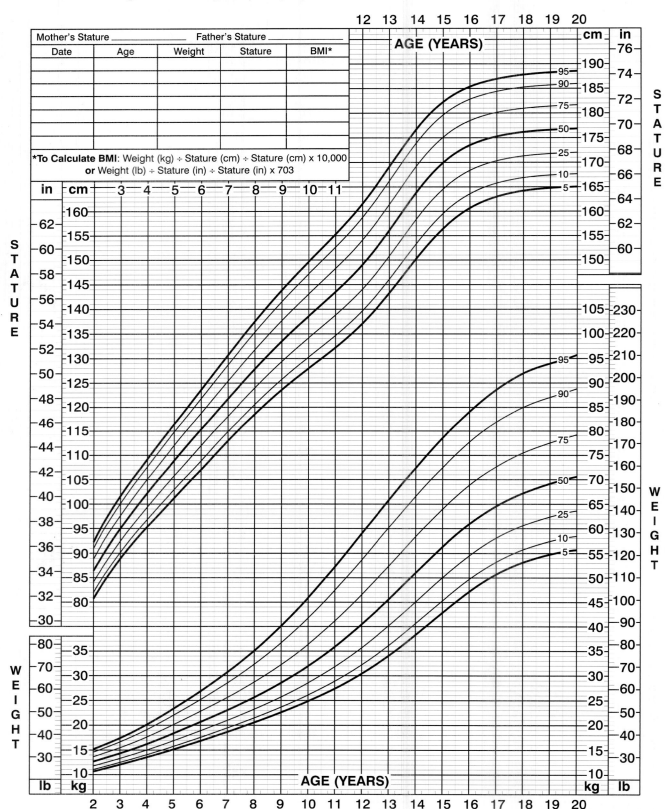

Mother's Stature _____	Father's Stature _____

Date	Age	Weight	Stature	BMI*

*To Calculate BMI: Weight (kg) ÷ Stature (cm) ÷ Stature (cm) x 10,000
  or Weight (lb) ÷ Stature (in) ÷ Stature (in) x 703

AGE (YEARS)

Published May 30, 2000 (modified 11/21/00).
SOURCE: Developed by the National Center for Health Statistics in collaboration with
   the National Center for Chronic Disease Prevention and Health Promotion (2000).
   http://www.cdc.gov/growthcharts

SAFER • HEALTHIER • PEOPLE™

2 to 20 years: Girls
Stature-for-age and Weight-for-age percentiles

NAME _____

RECORD # _____

Mother's Stature _____		Father's Stature _____		
Date	Age	Weight	Stature	BMI*

*To Calculate BMI: Weight (kg) ÷ Stature (cm) ÷ Stature (cm) x 10,000
or Weight (lb) ÷ Stature (in) ÷ Stature (in) x 703

AGE (YEARS)

12 13 14 15 16 17 18 19 20

STATURE

95
90
75
50
25
10
5

STATURE

WEIGHT

95
90
75
50
25
10
5

AGE (YEARS)

2 3 4 5 6 7 8 9 10 11 12 13 14 15 16 17 18 19 20

Published May 30, 2000 (modified 11/21/00).
SOURCE: Developed by the National Center for Health Statistics in collaboration with
the National Center for Chronic Disease Prevention and Health Promotion (2000).
http://www.cdc.gov/growthcharts

SAFER·HEALTHIER·PEOPLE™

2 to 20 years: Boys
Body mass index-for-age percentiles

NAME _____

RECORD # _____

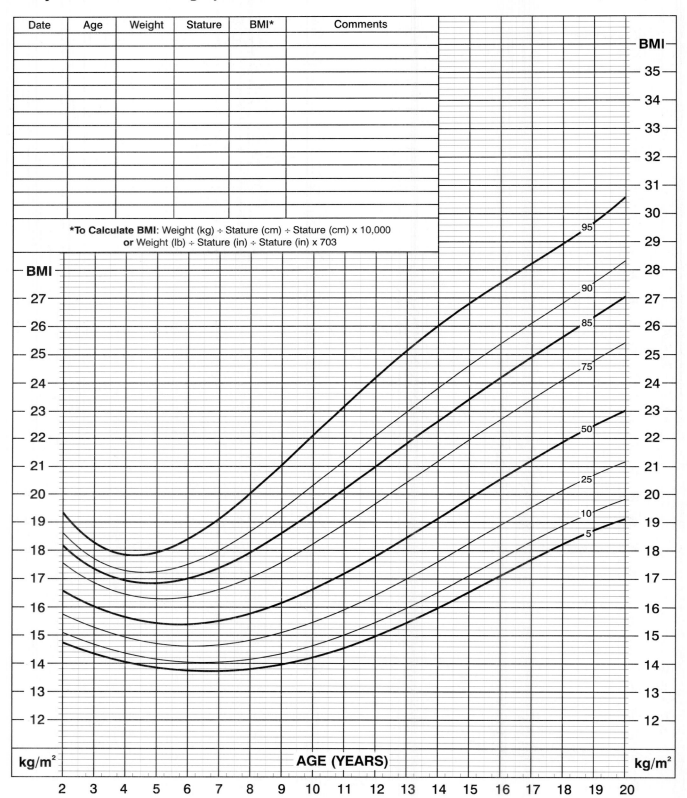

Date	Age	Weight	Stature	BMI*	Comments

*To Calculate BMI: Weight (kg) ÷ Stature (cm) ÷ Stature (cm) x 10,000
or Weight (lb) ÷ Stature (in) ÷ Stature (in) x 703

BMI

AGE (YEARS)

kg/m²

Published May 30, 2000 (modified 10/16/00).
SOURCE: Developed by the National Center for Health Statistics in collaboration with
the National Center for Chronic Disease Prevention and Health Promotion (2000).
http://www.cdc.gov/growthcharts

CDC

SAFER · HEALTHIER · PEOPLE™

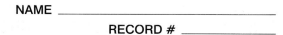

2 to 20 years: Girls
Body mass index-for-age percentiles

NAME _____

RECORD # _____

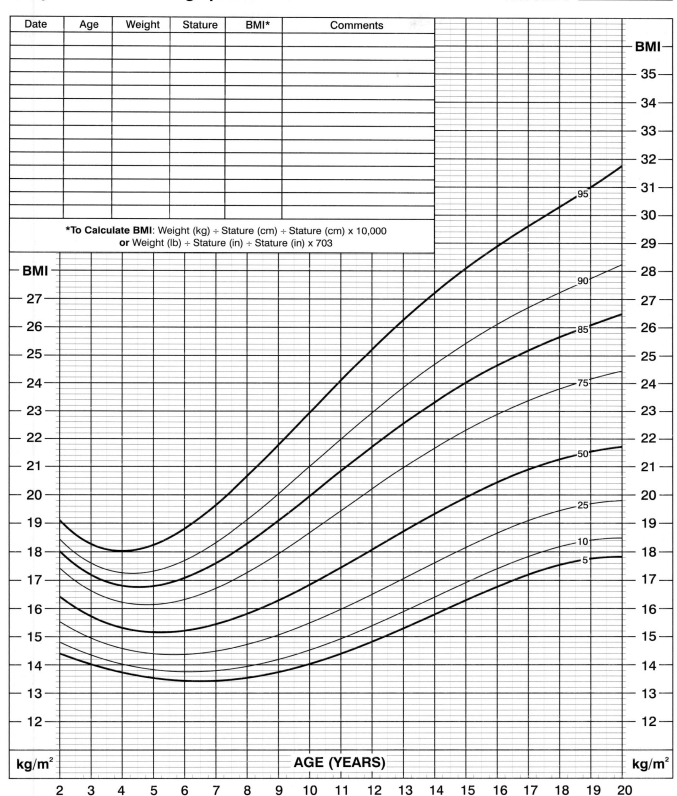

Date	Age	Weight	Stature	BMI*	Comments

*To Calculate BMI: Weight (kg) ÷ Stature (cm) ÷ Stature (cm) x 10,000
or Weight (lb) ÷ Stature (in) ÷ Stature (in) x 703

BMI

kg/m²   AGE (YEARS)   kg/m²

2 3 4 5 6 7 8 9 10 11 12 13 14 15 16 17 18 19 20

Published May 30, 2000 (modified 10/16/00).
SOURCE: Developed by the National Center for Health Statistics in collaboration with
the National Center for Chronic Disease Prevention and Health Promotion (2000).
http://www.cdc.gov/growthcharts

SAFER · HEALTHIER · PEOPLE™

NAME _____

Weight-for-stature percentiles: Boys

RECORD # _____

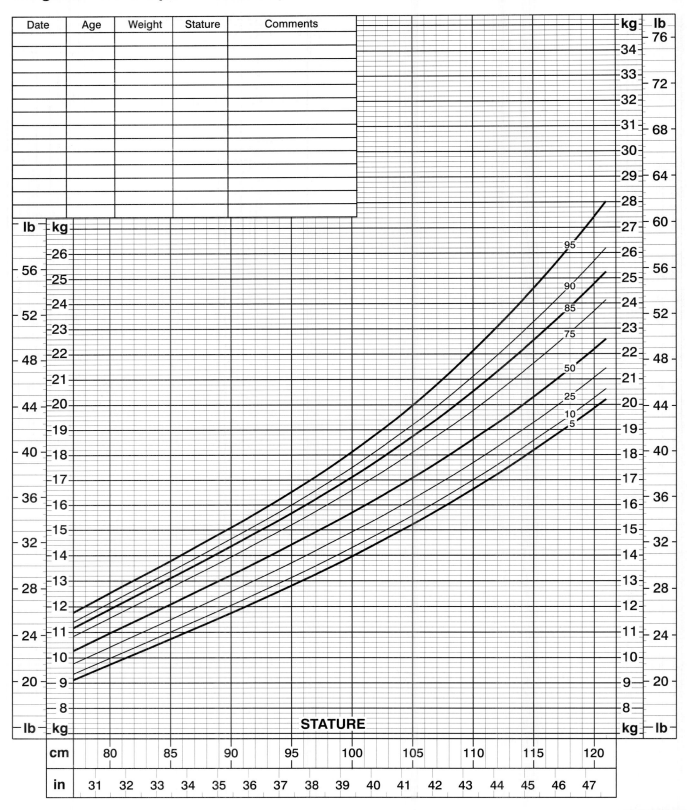

Date	Age	Weight	Stature	Comments

STATURE

Published May 30, 2000 (modified 10/16/00).
SOURCE: Developed by the National Center for Health Statistics in collaboration with
the National Center for Chronic Disease Prevention and Health Promotion (2000).
http://www.cdc.gov/growthcharts

CDC
SAFER · HEALTHIER · PEOPLE™

Weight-for-stature percentiles: Girls

NAME _____

RECORD # _____

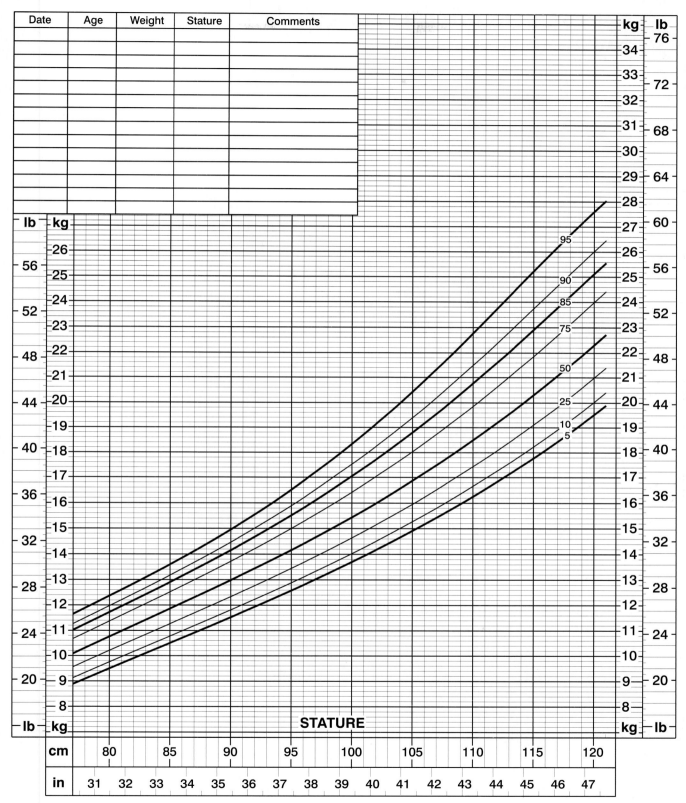

Date	Age	Weight	Stature	Comments

STATURE

Published May 30, 2000 (modified 10/16/00).
SOURCE: Developed by the National Center for Health Statistics in collaboration with
the National Center for Chronic Disease Prevention and Health Promotion (2000).
http://www.cdc.gov/growthcharts

SAFER·HEALTHIER·PEOPLE™

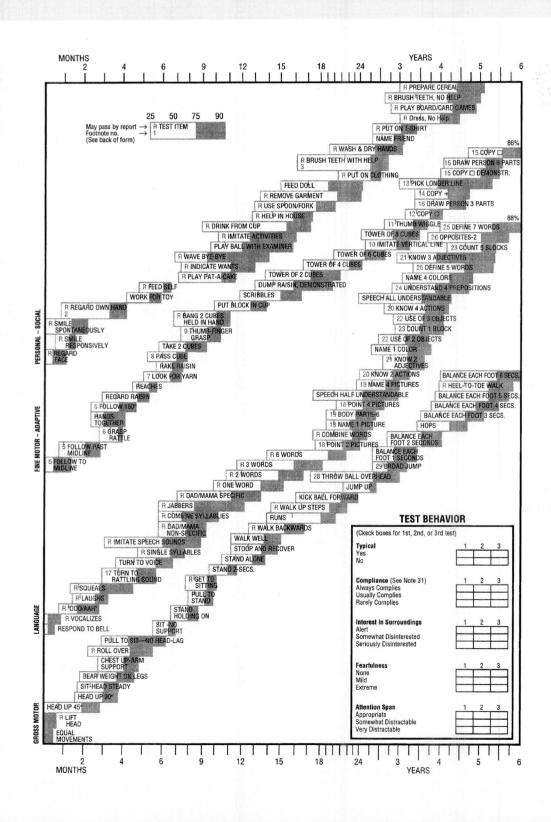

DIRECTIONS FOR ADMINISTRATION

1. Try to get child to smile by smiling, talking or waving. Do not touch him/her.
2. Child must stare at hand several seconds.
3. Parent may help guide toothbrush and put toothpaste on brush.
4. Child does not have to be able to tie shoes or button/zip in the back.
5. Move yarn slowly in an arc from one side to the other, about 8" above child's face.
6. Pass if child grasps rattle when it is touched to the backs or tips of fingers.
7. Pass if child tries to see where yarn went. Yarn should be dropped quickly from sight from tester's hand without arm movement.
8. Child must transfer cube from hand to hand without help of body, mouth, or table.
9. Pass if child picks up raisin with any part of thumb and finger.
10. Line can vary only 30 degrees or less from tester's line.
11. Make a fist with thumb pointing upward and wiggle only the thumb. Pass if child imitates and does not move any fingers other than the thumb.

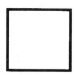

12. Pass any enclosed form. Fail continuous round motions.

13. Which line is longer? (Not bigger.) Turn paper upside down and repeat. (pass 3 of 3 or 5 of 6)

14. Pass any lines crossing near midpoint.

15. Have child copy first. If failed, demonstrate.

When giving items 12, 14, and 15, do not name the forms. Do not demonstrate 12 and 14.

16. When scoring, each pair (2 arms, 2 legs, etc.) counts as one part.
17. Place one cube in cup and shake gently near child's ear, but out of sight. Repeat for other ear.
18. Point to picture and have child name it. (No credit is given for sounds only.)
    If less than 4 pictures are named correctly, have child point to picture as each is named by tester.

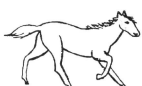

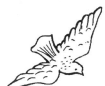

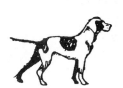

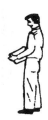

19. Using doll, tell child: Show me the nose, eyes, ears, mouth, hands, feet, tummy, hair. Pass 6 of 8.
20. Using pictures, ask child: Which one flies?... says meow?... talks?... barks?... gallops? Pass 2 of 5, 4 of 5.
21. Ask child: What do you do when you are cold?... tired?... hungry? Pass 2 of 3, 3 of 3.
22. Ask child: What do you do with a cup? What is a chair used for? What is a pencil used for?
    Action words must be included in answers.
23. Pass if child correctly places <u>and</u> says how many blocks are on paper. (1, 5).
24. Tell child: Put block **on** table; **under** table; **in front of** me, **behind** me. Pass 4 of 4.
    (Do not help child by pointing, moving head or eyes.)
25. Ask child: What is a ball?... lake?... desk?... house?... banana?... curtain?... fence?... ceiling? Pass if defined in terms
    of use, shape, what it is made of, or general category (such as banana is fruit, not just yellow). Pass 5 of 8, 7 of 8.
26. Ask child: If a horse is big, a mouse is __? If fire is hot, ice is __? If the sun shines during the day, the moon shines
    during the __? Pass 2 of 3.
27. Child may use wall or rail only, not person. May not crawl.
28. Child must throw ball overhand 3 feet to within arm's reach of tester.
29. Child must perform standing broad jump over width of test sheet (8 1/2 inches).
30. Tell child to walk forward, ⚭⚭⚭⚭➔ heel within 1 inch of toe. Tester may demonstrate.
    Child must walk 4 consecutive steps.
31. In the second year, half of normal children are non-compliant.

OBSERVATIONS:

Reprinted with permission from *AAP News,* July 1991. Copyright © 1991, American Academy of Pediatrics.

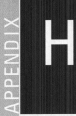

Conversion Charts

Weight and Length Conversion

WEIGHT				LENGTH			
LB	**KG**	**KG**	**LB**	**IN**	**CM**	**CM**	**IN**
1	0.5	1	2.2	1	2.5	1	.4
2	0.9	2	4.4	2	5.1	2	.8
4	1.8	3	6.6	4	10.2	3	1.2
6	2.7	4	8.8	6	15.2	4	1.6
8	3.6	5	11.0	8	20.3	5	2.0
10	4.5	6	13.2	12	30.5	6	2.4
20	9.1	8	17.6	18	46	8	3.1
30	13.6	10	22	24	61	10	3.9
40	18.2	20	44	30	76	20	7.9
50	22.7	30	66	36	91	30	11.8
60	27.3	40	88	42	107	40	15.7
70	31.8	50	110	48	122	50	19.7
80	36.4	60	132	54	137	60	23.6
90	40.9	70	154	60	152	70	27.6
100	45.4	80	176	66	168	80	31.5
150	68.2	90	198	72	183	90	35.4
200	90.8	100	220	78	198	100	39.4

1 lb = 0.454 kg
1 kg = 2.204 lb

1 in = 2.54 cm
1 cm = 0.3937 in

Temperature Equivalents (Celsius and Fahrenheit)*

C	F	C	F
0	32.0	39.0	102.2
20	68.0	39.2	102.6
30	86.0	39.4	102.9
31	87.8	39.6	103.3
32	89.6	39.8	103.7
33	91.4	40.0	104.0
34	93.2	40.2	104.4
35	95.0	40.4	104.7
36	96.8	40.6	105.1
37	98.6	40.8	105.4
37.2	99.0	41.0	105.8
37.4	99.3	41.2	106.2
37.6	99.7	41.4	106.5
37.8	100.1	41.6	106.9
38.0	100.4	41.8	107.2
38.2	100.8	42	107.6
38.4	101.2	43	109.4
38.6	101.5	44	111.2
38.8	101.8	100	212.0

*To convert Celsius (centigrade) readings to Fahrenheit, multiply by 1.8 and add 32. To convert Fahrenheit readings to Celsius, subtract 32 and divide by 1.8.

The Joint Commission List of Dangerous Abbreviations, Acronyms, and Symbols

Table I-1 | The Joint Commission Minimum Do Not Use List of Abbreviations

SET	ITEM	ABBREVIATION	POTENTIAL PROBLEM	PREFERRED TERM
1.	1.	U (for unit)	Mistaken as *zero, four* or *cc.*	Write *unit.*
2.	2.	IU (for international unit)	Mistaken as *IV* (intravenous) or *10* (ten).	Write *international unit.*
3.	3.	Q.D.	Mistaken for each other. The period after the "Q" can be mistaken for an "I," and the "O" can be mistaken for "I."	Write *daily* and *every other* day.
	4.	Q.O.D. (Latin abbreviation for once daily and every other day)		
4.	5.	Trailing zero (X.0 mg)	Decimal point is missed.	Never write a zero by itself after a decimal point (X mg), and always use a zero before a decimal point (0.X mg).
	6.	[NOTE: Prohibited only for medication-related notations]; Lack of leading zero (.X mg)		
5.	7.	MS	Confused for one another. Can mean morphine sulfate or magnesium sulfate.	Write *morphine sulfate* or *magnesium sulfate.*
	8.	MSO$_4$		
	9.	MgSO$_4$		

Table I-2 | The Joint Commission Additional Abbreviations to Avoid

ABBREVIATION	POTENTIAL PROBLEM	PREFERRED TERM
µg (for microgram)	Mistaken for *mg* (milligrams) resulting in 1000-fold dosing overdose.	Write *mcg.*
H.S. (for half-strength or Latin abbreviation for bedtime)	Mistaken for either half-strength or hour of sleep (at bedtime). *q.H.S.* mistaken for every hour. All can result in a dosing error.	Write out *half-strength* or *at bedtime.*
T.I.W. (for three times a week)	Mistaken for three times a day or twice weekly, resulting in an overdose.	Write *3 times weekly* or *three times weekly.*
S.C. or S.Q. (for subcutaneous)	Mistaken as *SL* for sublingual, or "5 every."	Write *Sub-Q, subQ,* or *subcutaneously.*
D/C (for discharge)	Interpreted as discontinue whatever medications follow (typically discharge meds).	*Write discharge.*
c.c. (for cubic centimeter)	Mistaken for *U* (units) when poorly written.	Write *ml* for milliliters.
A.S., A.D., A.U. (Latin abbreviations for left, right, or both ears)	Mistaken for *OS, OD,* and *OU,* etc.).	Write: *left ear, right ear,* or *both ears.*

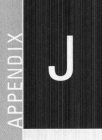
The Fourth Report on the Diagnosis, Evaluation, and Treatment of High Blood Pressure in Children and Adolescents

Blood Pressure Levels for Boys by Age and Height Percentile*

AGE (YEAR)	BP PERCENTILE	SYSTOLIC BP (mm HG) ← PERCENTILE OF HEIGHT →							DIASTOLIC BP (mm HG) ← PERCENTILE OF HEIGHT →						
		5th	10th	25th	50th	75th	90th	95th	5th	10th	25th	50th	75th	90th	95th
1	50th	80	81	83	85	87	88	89	34	35	36	37	38	39	39
	90th	94	95	97	99	100	102	103	49	50	51	52	53	53	54
	95th	98	99	101	103	104	106	106	54	54	55	56	57	58	58
	99th	105	106	108	110	112	113	114	61	62	63	64	65	66	66
2	50th	84	85	87	88	90	92	92	39	40	41	42	43	44	44
	90th	97	99	100	102	104	105	106	54	55	56	57	58	58	59
	95th	101	102	104	106	108	109	110	59	59	60	61	62	63	63
	99th	109	110	111	113	115	117	117	66	67	68	69	70	71	71
3	50th	86	87	89	91	93	94	95	44	44	45	46	47	48	48
	90th	100	101	103	105	107	108	109	59	59	60	61	62	63	63
	95th	104	105	107	109	110	112	113	63	63	64	65	66	67	67
	99th	111	112	114	116	118	119	120	71	71	72	73	74	75	75
4	50th	88	89	91	93	95	96	97	47	48	49	50	51	51	52
	90th	102	103	105	107	109	110	111	62	63	64	65	66	66	67
	95th	106	107	109	111	112	114	115	66	67	68	69	70	71	71
	99th	113	114	116	118	120	121	122	74	75	76	77	78	78	79
5	50th	90	91	93	95	96	98	98	50	51	52	53	54	55	55
	90th	104	105	106	108	110	111	112	65	66	67	68	69	69	70
	95th	108	109	110	112	114	115	116	69	70	71	72	73	74	74
	99th	115	116	118	120	121	123	123	77	78	79	80	81	81	82
6	50th	91	92	94	96	98	99	100	53	53	54	55	56	57	57
	90th	105	106	108	110	111	113	113	68	68	69	70	71	72	72
	95th	109	110	112	114	115	117	117	72	72	73	74	75	76	76
	99th	116	117	119	121	123	124	125	80	80	81	82	83	84	84
7	50th	92	94	95	97	99	100	101	55	55	56	57	58	59	59
	90th	106	107	109	111	113	114	115	70	70	71	72	73	74	74
	95th	110	111	113	115	117	118	119	74	74	75	76	77	78	78
	99th	117	118	120	122	124	125	126	82	82	83	84	85	86	86
8	50th	94	95	97	99	100	102	102	56	57	58	59	60	60	61
	90th	107	109	110	112	114	115	116	71	72	72	73	74	75	76
	95th	111	112	114	116	118	119	120	75	76	77	78	79	79	80
	99th	119	120	122	123	125	127	127	83	84	85	86	87	87	88
9	50th	95	96	98	100	102	103	104	57	58	59	60	61	61	62
	90th	109	110	112	114	115	117	118	72	73	74	75	76	76	77
	95th	113	114	116	118	119	121	121	76	77	78	79	80	81	81
	99th	120	121	123	125	127	128	129	84	85	86	87	88	88	89
10	50th	97	98	100	102	103	105	106	58	59	60	61	61	62	63
	90th	111	112	114	115	117	119	119	73	73	74	75	76	77	78
	95th	115	116	117	119	121	122	123	77	78	79	80	81	81	82
	99th	122	123	125	127	128	130	130	85	86	86	88	88	89	90

BP, Blood pressure

* The 90th percentile is 1.28 SD, 95th percentile is 1.645 SD, and the 99th percentile is 2.326 SD over the mean. For research purposes, the standard deviations in Appendix Table B-1 allow one to compute BP Z-scores and percentiles for boys with height percentiles given in Table 3 (i.e., the 5th, 10th, 25th, 50th, 75th, 90th, and 95th percentiles). These height percentiles must be converted to height Z-scores given by (5% = −1.645; 10% = −1.28; 25% = −0.68; 50% = 0; 75% = 0.68; 90% = 1.28; 95% = 1.645) and then computed according to the methodology in steps 2-4 described in Appendix B. For children with height percentiles other than these, follow steps 1-4 as described in Appendix B.

Continued

Blood Pressure Levels for Boys by Age and Height Percentile—cont'd

AGE (YEAR)	BP PERCENTILE	SYSTOLIC BP (mm HG) ← PERCENTILE OF HEIGHT →							DIASTOLIC BP (mm HG) ← PERCENTILE OF HEIGHT →						
		5th	10th	25th	50th	75th	90th	95th	5th	10th	25th	50th	75th	90th	95th
11	50th	99	100	102	104	105	107	107	59	59	60	61	62	63	63
	90th	113	114	115	117	119	120	121	74	74	75	76	77	78	78
	95th	117	118	119	121	123	124	125	78	78	79	80	81	82	82
	99th	124	125	127	129	130	132	132	86	86	87	88	89	90	90
12	50th	101	102	104	106	108	109	110	59	60	61	62	63	63	64
	90th	115	116	118	120	121	123	123	74	75	75	76	77	78	79
	95th	119	120	122	123	125	127	127	78	79	80	81	82	82	83
	99th	126	127	129	131	133	134	135	86	87	88	89	90	90	91
13	50th	104	105	106	108	110	111	112	60	60	61	62	63	64	64
	90th	117	118	120	122	124	125	126	75	75	76	77	78	79	79
	95th	121	122	124	126	128	129	130	79	79	80	81	82	83	83
	99th	128	130	131	133	135	136	137	87	87	88	89	90	91	91
14	50th	106	107	109	111	113	114	115	60	61	62	63	64	65	65
	90th	120	121	123	125	126	128	128	75	76	77	78	79	79	80
	95th	124	125	127	128	130	132	132	80	80	81	82	83	84	84
	99th	131	132	134	136	138	139	140	87	88	89	90	91	92	92
15	50th	109	110	112	113	115	117	117	61	62	63	64	65	66	66
	90th	122	124	125	127	129	130	131	76	77	78	79	80	80	81
	95th	126	127	129	131	133	134	135	81	81	82	83	84	85	85
	99th	134	135	136	138	140	142	142	88	89	90	91	92	93	93
16	50th	111	112	114	116	118	119	120	63	63	64	65	66	67	67
	90th	125	126	128	130	131	133	134	78	78	79	80	81	82	82
	95th	129	130	132	134	135	137	137	82	83	83	84	85	86	87
	99th	136	137	139	141	143	144	145	90	90	91	92	93	94	94
17	50th	114	115	116	118	120	121	122	65	66	66	67	68	69	70
	90th	127	128	130	132	134	135	136	80	80	81	82	83	84	84
	95th	131	132	134	136	138	139	140	84	85	86	87	87	88	89
	99th	139	140	141	143	145	146	147	92	93	93	94	95	96	97

Blood Pressure Levels for Girls by Age and Height Percentile*

AGE (YEAR)	BP PERCENTILE	SYSTOLIC BP (mm HG) ← PERCENTILE OF HEIGHT →							DIASTOLIC BP (mm HG) ← PERCENTILE OF HEIGHT →						
		5th	10th	25th	50th	75th	90th	95th	5th	10th	25th	50th	75th	90th	95th
1	50th	83	84	85	86	88	89	90	38	39	39	40	41	41	42
	90th	97	97	98	100	101	102	103	52	53	53	54	55	55	56
	95th	100	101	102	104	105	106	107	56	57	57	58	59	59	60
	99th	108	108	109	111	112	113	114	64	64	65	65	66	67	67
2	50th	85	85	87	88	89	91	91	43	44	44	45	46	46	47
	90th	98	99	100	101	103	104	105	57	58	58	59	60	61	61
	95th	102	103	104	105	107	108	109	61	62	62	63	64	65	65
	99th	109	110	111	112	114	115	116	69	69	70	70	71	72	72
3	50th	86	87	88	89	91	92	93	47	48	48	49	50	50	51
	90th	100	100	102	103	104	106	106	61	62	62	63	64	64	65
	95th	104	104	105	107	108	109	110	65	66	66	67	68	68	69
	99th	111	111	113	114	115	116	117	73	73	74	74	75	76	76
4	50th	88	88	90	91	92	94	94	50	50	51	52	52	53	54
	90th	101	102	103	104	106	107	108	64	64	65	66	67	67	68
	95th	105	106	107	108	110	111	112	68	68	69	70	71	71	72
	99th	112	113	114	115	117	118	119	76	76	76	77	78	79	79
5	50th	89	90	91	93	94	95	96	52	53	53	54	55	55	56
	90th	103	103	105	106	107	109	109	66	67	67	68	69	69	70
	95th	107	107	108	110	111	112	113	70	71	71	72	73	73	74
	99th	114	114	116	117	118	120	120	78	78	79	79	80	81	81
6	50th	91	92	93	94	96	97	98	54	54	55	56	56	57	58
	90th	104	105	106	108	109	110	111	68	68	69	70	70	71	72
	95th	108	109	110	111	113	114	115	72	72	73	74	74	75	76
	99th	115	116	117	119	120	121	122	80	80	80	81	82	83	83
7	50th	93	93	95	96	97	99	99	55	56	56	57	58	58	59
	90th	106	107	108	109	111	112	113	69	70	70	71	72	72	73
	95th	110	111	112	113	115	116	116	73	74	74	75	76	76	77
	99th	117	118	119	120	122	123	124	81	81	82	82	83	84	84
8	50th	95	95	96	98	99	100	101	57	57	57	58	59	60	60
	90th	108	109	110	111	113	114	114	71	71	71	72	73	74	74
	95th	112	112	114	115	116	118	118	75	75	75	76	77	78	78
	99th	119	120	121	122	123	125	125	82	82	83	83	84	85	86
9	50th	96	97	98	100	101	102	103	58	58	58	59	60	61	61
	90th	110	110	112	113	114	116	116	72	72	72	73	74	75	75
	95th	114	114	115	117	118	119	120	76	76	76	77	78	79	79
	99th	121	121	123	124	125	127	127	83	83	84	84	85	86	87
10	50th	98	99	100	102	103	104	105	59	59	59	60	61	62	62
	90th	112	112	114	115	116	118	118	73	73	73	74	75	76	76
	95th	116	116	117	119	120	121	122	77	77	77	78	79	80	80
	99th	123	123	125	126	127	129	129	84	84	85	86	86	87	88

BP, Blood pressure

* The 90th percentile is 1.28 SD, 95th percentile is 1.645 SD, and the 99th percentile is 2.326 SD over the mean. For research purposes, the standard deviations in Appendix Table B-1 allow one to compute BP Z-scores and percentiles for girls with height percentiles given in Table 4 (i.e., the 5th, 10th, 25th, 50th, 75th, 90th, and 95th percentiles). These height percentiles must be converted to height Z-scores given by (5% = −1.645; 10% = −1.28; 25% = −0.68; 50% = 0; 75% = 0.68; 90% = 1.28; 95% = 1.645) and then computed according to the methodology in steps 2-4 described in Appendix B. For children with height percentiles other than these, follow steps 1-4 as described in Appendix B.

Continued

Blood Pressure Levels for Girls by Age and Height Percentile—cont'd

AGE (YEAR)	BP PERCENTILE	SYSTOLIC BP (mm HG) ← PERCENTILE OF HEIGHT →							DIASTOLIC BP (mm HG) ← PERCENTILE OF HEIGHT →						
		5th	10th	25th	50th	75th	90th	95th	5th	10th	25th	50th	75th	90th	95th
11	50th	100	101	102	103	105	106	107	60	60	60	61	62	63	63
	90th	114	114	116	117	118	119	120	74	74	74	75	76	77	77
	95th	118	118	119	121	122	123	124	78	78	78	79	80	81	81
	99th	125	125	126	128	129	130	131	85	85	86	87	87	88	89
12	50th	102	103	104	105	107	108	109	61	61	61	62	63	64	64
	90th	116	116	117	119	120	121	122	75	75	75	76	77	78	78
	95th	119	120	121	123	124	125	126	79	79	79	80	81	82	82
	99th	127	127	128	130	131	132	133	86	86	87	88	88	89	90
13	50th	104	105	106	107	109	110	110	62	62	62	63	64	65	65
	90th	117	118	119	121	122	123	124	76	76	76	77	78	79	79
	95th	121	122	123	124	126	127	128	80	80	80	81	82	83	83
	99th	128	129	130	132	133	134	135	87	87	88	89	89	90	91
14	50th	106	106	107	109	110	111	112	63	63	63	64	65	66	66
	90th	119	120	121	122	124	125	125	77	77	77	78	79	80	80
	95th	123	123	125	126	127	129	129	81	81	81	82	83	84	84
	99th	130	131	132	133	135	136	136	88	88	89	90	90	91	92
15	50th	107	108	109	110	111	113	113	64	64	64	65	66	67	67
	90th	120	121	122	123	125	126	127	78	78	78	79	80	81	81
	95th	124	125	126	127	129	130	131	82	82	82	83	84	85	85
	99th	131	132	133	134	136	137	138	89	89	90	91	91	92	93
16	50th	108	108	110	111	112	114	114	64	64	65	66	66	67	68
	90th	121	122	123	124	126	127	128	78	78	79	80	81	81	82
	95th	125	126	127	128	130	131	132	82	82	83	84	85	85	86
	99th	132	133	134	135	137	138	139	90	90	90	91	92	93	93
17	50th	108	109	110	111	113	114	115	64	65	65	66	67	67	68
	90th	122	122	123	125	126	127	128	78	79	79	80	81	81	82
	95th	125	126	127	129	130	131	132	82	83	83	84	85	85	86
	99th	133	133	134	136	137	138	139	90	90	91	91	92	93	93

Bibliography and Reader References

Chapter 1

American Academy of Pediatrics. (2005). Reaffirmation of policy statement: Recommendations for pediatricians who discuss alternative, complementary, and unproven therapies with families. Original policy statement, 2001. *Pediatrics, 107*(3), 598-601.

Bowden, V., Dickey, S., & Greenberg, C. (1998). *Children and their families: The continuum of care.* Philadelphia: Saunders.

Centers for Disease Control and Prevention. (2003). LCWK2. Deaths, percent of total deaths, and death rates for the 15 leading causes of death in 10-year age groups: United States.

Fosarelli, P. (2003). Children and the development of faith: Implications for pediatric practice. *Contemp Pediatr, 20*(1), 85-98.

Giger, J., & Davidhizar, R. (2004). *Transcultural nursing* (4th ed.). St. Louis: Mosby.

Going Without: America's Uninsured Children. (2005). Prepared for the Robert Wood Johnson Foundation by the State Health Access Data Assistance Center (SHADAC) and the Urban Institute using data from the U.S. Centers for Disease Control and Prevention National Center for Health Statistics and the U.S. Census Bureau's Current Population Survey (CPS). Washington, DC: Robert Wood Johnson Foundation.

Gustafson, E. (2005). History and overview of school-based health centers in the U.S. *Nurs Clin N Am, 40*(4), 595-606.

Hockenberry, M., & Wilson, D. (2005). *Wong's essentials of pediatric nursing* (7th ed.). St. Louis: Mosby.

Hockenberry, M., & Wilson, D. (2007). *Wong's nursing care of infants and children* (8th ed.). St. Louis: Mosby.

Markenson, D. (2005). The treatment of children exposed to pathogens linked to bioterrorism. *Infect Dis Clin North Am, 19*(3), 731-745.

Markenson, D., & Reynolds, S. (2006). The pediatrician and disaster preparedness. (AAP Policy) *Pediatrics, 117*(2), 340-362.

McEvoy, M. (2005). Are there universal parenting concepts among culturally diverse families in an inner-city pediatric clinic? *J Pediatr Health Care, 19*(3), 142-150.

McIntyre, A. (2005). *Herbal treatment of children.* Philadelphia: Elsevier, Butterworth, Heinemann.

National Center for Complementary and Alternative Medicine (NCCAM) Fact Sheets. National Institutes of Health (Black Cohosh NCCAM Publication No. D268, July 2005; Echinacea NCCAM Publication No. D271, July 2005; Ginkgo NCCAM Publication No. 290, September 2005; Kava NCCAM Publication No. D314, May 2006; St. John's Wort NCCAM Publication No. D269, July 2005). Bethesda, MD: National Institutes of Health.

Nemours Foundation. (2003). *Alternative medicine and your child.* Article reviewed by Steven Dowshen, MD, and Sandra Hassink, MD. Retrieved from http://kidshealth.org/parent/general/sick/alternative_medicine.html.

Sandler, A. (2003). Chairperson of Committee on Children with Disabilities, 2000-2001. Counselling families who choose complementary and alternative medicine for their child with chronic illness or disability. *Pediatrics, 107*(3), 598-601.

U.S. Department of Health and Human Services (2003). *Preventing infant mortality.* Last revised June 19, 2003. Retrieved from http://www.hhs.gov/news/press/2002pres/infant.html

Windle, P. (2003). Understanding evidence-based practice. *J Perianesth Nurs, 18*(5); 360-362.

ONLINE RESOURCES

Centers for Disease Control and Prevention: http://www.cdc.gov/

Federal Emergency Management Agency: http://www.fema.gov/kids

National Center for Complementary and Alternative Medicine: http://altmed.od.nih.gov/

National Center for Health Statistics: http://www.cdc.gov/nchs/fastats/infmort.htm

The Society of Pediatric Nursing: http://www.pedsnurses.org

U.S. Department of Health and Human Services: http://www.hhs.gov/news

Chapter 2

Behrman, R., Kliegman, R., & Jenson, H. (2004). *Nelson's textbook of pediatrics* (17th ed.). Philadelphia: Saunders.

Centers for Disease Control and Prevention. (2006). *Prevalence of overweight among children and adolescents: United States, 2003-2004.* National Center for Health Statistics. Retrieved June 2, 2006, from www.cdc.gov/nccdphp/dnpa/obesity/trend/index.htm.

Cortes, R.A. (2004). Recent advances in fetal surgery. *Semin Perinatol, 28*(3), 199-211.

Freeman, D.S., Dietz, W.H., Srinivasan, S.R., & Berenson, G.S. (2001). The relation of overweight to cardiovascular risk factors among children and adolescents: The Bogalusa Heart Study. *Pediatrics, 108*, 712-718.

Hockenberry, M.J., & Wilson, D. (2007). *Wong's nursing care of infants and children* (8th ed.). St. Louis: Mosby.

James, S.R., Ashwill, J.W., & Droske, S.C. (2002). *Nursing care of children: Principles and practice.* Philadelphia: Saunders.

March of Dimes. (2006). *Quick reference: fact sheets Chorionic villus sampling.* Retrieved June 2, 2006, from http://www.marchofdimes.com.

ONLINE RESOURCES

Abraham Maslow: http://www.ship.edu/~cgboeree/maslow.html

Erik Erikson: http://www.ship.edu/~cgboeree/erikson.html

Genetic disease information: http://www.cdc.gov/genomics/

Growth charts: http://www.cdc.gov/nchs/about/major/nhanes/growthcharts/clinical_charts.htm

Major personality theories: http://www.ship.edu/~cgboeree/perscontents.html

March of Dimes: http://www.marchofdimes.org

National Center for Health Statistics: http://www.cdc.gov/nchs/

New York Online Access to Health (NOAH): http://www.noah-health.org

Chapter 3

Alford, D. (2003). The Clinical Record. *Geriatr Nurs, 24*(4), 228-230.

American Academy of Pediatrics (AAP) Policy Statement, September. (2001). The assessment and management of acute pain in infants, children, and adolescents (0793). *Pediatrics, 108*(3), 793-797.

Behrman, R., Kliegman, R. (2004). *Nelson's textbook of pediatrics* (17th ed.). Philadelphia: Saunders.

Dochterman, J., & Bulechek, G.M. (2004). *Nursing interventions classification (NIC)* (4th ed.). St. Louis: Mosby.

Hockenberry, M., Wilson, D., & Winkelstein, M. (2005). *Wong's essentials of pediatric nursing* (7th ed.). St. Louis: Mosby.

Kemper, K., Sarah, R., Silver-Highfield, E., Xiarhos, E., Barnes, L., & Berde, C. (2000). On pins and needles? Pediatric patients' experience with acupuncture. *Pediatrics, 105*(4), 941-947.

McKinney, E., James, S., Murray, S., & Ashwill, J. (2005). *Maternal child nursing* (2nd ed.). St. Louis: Saunders.

Merkel, S., Voepel-Lewis, T., & Malviya, S. (2002). Pain control. *Am J Nurs, 102*(10), 55-57.

National High Blood Pressure Education Program (NHBPEP) Working Group on High Blood Pressure in Children and Adolescents. (2004). The fourth report on the diagnosis, evaluation, and treatment of high blood pressure in children and adolescents. *Pediatrics, 114*(2), 555-576.

The National Pain Foundation. *Using complementary therapy to relieve pain.* Retrieved June 12, 2006, from http://www. nationalpainfoundation.org/MyTreatment/News_Complementary.asp.

U.S. Dept of Health and Human Services, National Institutes of Health, National Heart, Lung, and Blood Institute, & National High Blood Pressure Education Program. (2005). The fourth report on the diagnosis, evaluation, and treatment of high blood pressure in children and adolescents. NIH Publication No. 05-5267. Originally printed September 1996. Revised May 2005. Washington, DC: U.S. Government Printing Office.

Wollin, S., Plummer, S., Owen, H., Hawkins, R., Materazzo, F., & Morrison, V. (2004). Anxiety in children having elective surgery. *J Pediatr Nurs, 19*(2), 128-132.

Zempsky, W., Cravero, J., & Committee on Pediatric Emergency Medicine and Section on Anesthesiology and Pain Medicine (2004). Relief of pain and anxiety in pediatric patients in emergency medical systems. *Pediatrics, 114*(5), 1348-1356.

ONLINE RESOURCES

AAP (American Academy of Pediatrics), APS (American Pain Society) policy statement on pain: http://www.aap.org/policy/9933.html

Centers for Disease Control and Prevention: http://www.cdc.gov

Children's Health: http://www.kidshealth.org

Chapter 4

American Academy of Pediatrics. (2005). The Changing concept of sudden infant death syndrome: Diagnostic coding shifts, controversies regarding the sleeping environment, and new variables to consider in reducing risk. *Pediatrics, 116*(5), 1245-1255. Retrieved from http://aappolicy.aappublications.org/cgi/content/full/pediatrics;116/5/1245.

American Academy of Pediatrics Policy Statement. (2005). Breastfeeding and the use of human milk. *Pediatrics, 115*(2), 496-506.

Behrman, R., Kliegman, R., & Jenson, H. (2004). *Nelson's textbook of pediatrics* (17th ed.). Philadelphia: Saunders.

Burke, M. (2006). A pacifier reduces the risk of SIDS. *Contemporary Pediatrics,* January 1, 2006. Retrieved from http://www.contemporarypediatrics.com/contpeds/content/.

Gartner, L., & Greer, F. (2003). American Academy of Pediatrics, Section on Breastfeeding and Committee on Nutrition. Prevention of rickets and vitamin D deficiency: New guidelines for vitamin D intake. *Pediatrics, 111,* 908-910.

Hirji, H., Charlton, R., & Sarmah, S. (2005). Male circumcision: A review of the evidence. *The J Men's Health & Gender, 2*(1), 21-30.

Joint Committee on Infant Hearing. (2000). Year 2000 position statement: Principles and guidelines for early hearing detection and intervention programs. *Pediatrics, 106*(4), 798-817.

Kenner, C., & Moran, M. (2005). Newborn screening and genetic testing. *J Midwifery Womens Health, 50*(3), 219-226.

McKinney, E., James, S., Murray, S., & Ashwill, J. (2005). *Maternal-child nursing* (2nd ed.). St. Louis: WB Saunders.

National Institutes of Health: National Institute of Child Health and Human Development (2005). SIDS Back to Sleep Campaign. Retrieved from http://www.nichd.nih.gov/sids/sids.cfm.

Rhead, W., & Irons, M. (2004). The call from the newborn screening laboratory: Frustration in the afternoon. *Pediatr Clin North Am, 51*(3), 803-818.

Schmitt, B. (2005). Breast-feeding essentials. Pediatric Advisor. McKesson Provider Technologies. Retrieved December 8,

2006, from http://www.uofmchildrenshospital.org/library/content/pa_svbreast_hhg.htm.

Zitelli, B., & Davis, H. (2002). *Atlas of pediatric physical diagnosis* (4th ed.). Philadelphia: Mosby.

ONLINE RESOURCES

Joint Committee on Infant Hearing (JCIH): http://www.jcih.org

La Leche League for breastfeeding mothers: http://www.lalecheleague.org

Newborn Screenings: http://www.pediatrix.com

Chapter 5

Behrman, R., Kliegman, R., & Jenson, H. (2004). *Nelson's textbook of pediatrics* (17th ed.). Philadelphia: Saunders.

Chiang, M.F., & Flynn, J.T. (2006). Retinopathy of prematurity. In F.D. Burg, J.R. Ingelfinger, R.A. Polin, & A.A. Gershon (Eds.), *Current pediatric therapy* (18th ed.). Philadelphia: Saunders.

Committee on Fetus and Newborn. (2003). Apnea, sudden infant death syndrome, and home monitoring. *Pediatrics, 111,* 914-917.

Furman, L., Minich, N., & Hack, M. (2002). Correlates of lactation in mothers of very low birth weight infants. *Pediatrics, 109*(4), e57.

Hockenberry, M., & Wilson, D. (2007). *Wong's nursing care of infants and children* (8th ed.). St. Louis: Mosby.

Juppner, H.W., & Carpenter, T.O. (2006). Disorders of the parathyroids, hypocalcemia, and hypercalcemia. In F.D. Burg, J.R. Ingelfinger, R.A. Polin, & A.A. Gershon (Eds.), *Current pediatric therapy* (18th ed.). Philadelphia: Saunders.

Kliegman, R.M., Jenson, H.B., Marcdante, K.J., & Behrman, R.E. (2006). *Nelson essentials of pediatrics* (5th ed.). Philadelphia: WB Saunders.

Maisels, M.J., Baltz, R.D., Bhutani, V.K., Newman, T. B., Palmer, H., Rosenfeld, W., Stevenson, D.K., & Weinblatt, H.B. (2004). Management of hyperbilirubinemia in the newborn infant 35 or more weeks of gestation. *Pediatrics, 114*(1), 297-316.

Moloney-Harmon, P.A. (2005). Pediatric sepsis: The infection unto death. *Crit Care Nurse Clin North Am, 17*(4), 417-429.

Noerr, B. (2003). Current controversies in the understanding of necrotizing enterocolitis. *Adv Neonatal Care, 3*(3), 107-120.

Poland, R.L. (2006). Treatment of neonatal hyperbilirubinemia. In F.D. Burg, J.R. Ingelfinger, R.A. Polin, & A.A. Gershon (Eds.), *Current pediatric therapy* (18th ed.). Philadelphia: Saunders.

Reber, K.M. (2004). Necrotizing enterocolitis: Preventative strategies. *Clin Perinatal, 31*(1), 157-167.

Schmitt, B. (2006). Caffeine therapy for apnea of prematurity. *N Engl J Med, 354*(20), 2112-2121.

Short, M. (2004). Guide to a systematic physical assessment in the infant with suspected infection and/or sepsis. *Adv Neonatal Care, 4*(3), 141-153.

Smith, M., Durkin, M., Hinton, V., & Bellinger, D. (2003). Initiation of breastfeeding among mothers of very low birth weight infants. *Pediatrics, 111*(6), 1337-1342.

Stokowski, L.A. (2005a). A parents' guide to understanding apnea. *Adv Neonatal Care, 5*(3), 175-176.

Stokowski, L.A. (2005b). A primer on apnea of prematurity. *Adv Neonatal Care, 5*(3), 155-170.

Stout, A.U. (2003). Retinopathy of prematurity. *Pediatr Clin North Am, 50*(1), 77-87.

ONLINE RESOURCES

Premature Infant: http://www.premature-infant.com/

Chapter 6

American Academy of Pediatrics. (1999). Folic acid for prevention of neural tube defects. *Pediatrics, 104*(2), 325-327.

American Academy of Pediatrics. (2000). Policy statement: Infection control in the physician's office. *Pediatrics, 10*(6), 1361-1369.

Amieva, M.R. (2005). Important bacterial gastrointestinal pathogens in children: A pathogenesis perspective. *Pediatr Clin North Am, 52*(3), 749-777.

Behrman, R., Kliegman, V., & Jenson, H.B. (2004). *Nelson's textbook of pediatrics* (17th ed.). Philadelphia: Saunders.

Boyer, S.G. (2004). Update in TORCH infections in the newborn infant. *NAINR, 4*(1), 70-80.

Brady, M.T. (2005). Infectious disease in pediatric out of home child care. *Am J Infect Control, 33*(5), 276-285.

Centers for Disease Control (CDC). (2005). Quick facts: Perinatal. April 2003-March 2005. Retrieved June 5, 2006, from http://www.cdc.gov.

Cleft Palate Foundation. (2001). *Cleft lip and palate: The first four years.* Chapel Hill, NC: Author.

Cleft Palate Foundation. (2002). *Feeding an infant with a cleft.* Chapel Hill, NC: Author.

Cowles, R.A., & Stolar, C.J. (2006). Abdominal wall defects and disorders of the umbilicus. In F.D. Burg, J.R. Ingelfinger, R.A. Polin, & A.A. Gershon (Eds.), *Current pediatric therapy* (18th ed.). Philadelphia: Saunders.

Curley, M.A., & Moloney-Harmon, P.A. (2001). *Critical care nursing of infants and children* (2nd ed.). Philadelphia: Saunders.

Dennehy, P.H. (2005). Acute diarrheal disease in children: Epidemiology, prevention, and treatment. *Infect Dis Clin North Am, 19*(3), 585-602.

Feja, K. (2005). Tuberculosis in children. *Clin Chest Med, 26*(2), 295-312.

Feldstein, N.A., & Anderson, R.C. (2006). Diagnosis and management of hydrocephalus. In F.D. Burg, J.R. Ingelfinger, R.A. Polin, & A.A. Gershon (Eds.), *Current pediatric therapy* (18th ed.). Philadelphia: Saunders.

Gore, A.I., & Spencer, J.P. (2004). Newborn foot. *Am Fam Physician, 69*(4), 865-872.

Guntheroth, W.G. (2006). Congenital heart disease. In F.D. Burg, J.R. Ingelfinger, R.A. Polin, & A.A. Gershon (Eds.), *Current pediatric therapy* (18th ed.). Philadelphia: Saunders.

Hockenberry, M.J., Wilson, D., Winkelstein, M.L., & Kline, N.E. (2003). *Wong's nursing care of infants and children* (6th ed.). St. Louis: Mosby.

Johnson, M.P., Gerdes, M., Rintoul, N., Pasquariello, P., Melchionni, J., Sutton, L.N., & Adzick, N.S. (2006). Maternal-fetal surgery for myelomeningocele: Neurodevelopmental outcomes at 2 years of age. *Am J Obstet & Gynecol, 194*(4), 1145-1152.

Johnson, M.P., Sutton, L.N., Rintonl, N., Crombleholme, T.M., Flake, A.W., Howell, L.J., Hendrick, H.L., Wilson, R.D., & Adzick, N.S. (2003). Fetal myelomeningocele repair: Short term clinical outcomes. *Am J Obstet & Gynecol, 189*(2), 482-487.

Kaufman, B.A. (2004). Neural tube defects. *Pediatr Clin North Am, 51*(2), 389-419.

Kestle, J.R. (2003). Pediatric hydrocephalus: Current management. *Neurol Clin, 21*(4), 88-895.

Kliegman, R.M., Jenson, H.B., Marcdante, K.J., & Behrman R.E. (2006). *Nelson essentials of pediatrics* (5th ed.). Philadelphia: Elsevier.

Maisels, M.J., Baltz, R.D., Bhutani, V.K., Newman, T. B., Palmer, H., Rosenfeld, W., Stevenson, D.K., & Weinblatt, H.B. (2004). Management of hyperbilirubinemia in the newborn infant 35 or more weeks of gestation. *Pediatrics, 114*(1), 297-316.

March of Dimes. (2006). *News Desk: U.S. infant mortality rate fails to improve.* Retrieved June 2006 from www.marchofdimes.com

March of Dimes. (2006). *Professional quick reference and fact sheet: Birth defects.* Retrieved June 2006 from www.marchofdimes.com.

Mathews, T.J., Mencacker, F., & MacDorman, M.F. (2002). Infant mortality statistics from the 2000 period linked birth/infant death data set. *Natl Vital Stat Rep, 50*(12), 1-28.

Merritt, L. (2005). Part 2. Physical assessment of the infant with cleft lip and/or palate. *Adv Neonatal Care, 5*(3), 125-134.

Mitchell, J.C., & Wood, R.J. (2000). Management of cleft lip and palate in primary care. *J Pediatr Health Care, 14*(1), 13-19.

Muir, T.L. (1999). Successful feeding interventions for infants with cleft lip and palate and craniofacial anomalies. Presented at the 56th Annual Meeting of the American Cleft Palate-Craniofacial Association, Scottsdale, AZ.

Murthy, K., & Evans, J.R. (2006). Patent ductus arteriosus. In F.D. Burg, J.R. Ingelfinger, R.A. Polin, & A.A. Gershon (Eds.), *Current pediatric therapy* (18th ed.). Philadelphia: Saunders.

Pham, J.T., & Carlos, M.A. (2002). Current treatment strategies of symptomatic patent ductus arteriosus. *J Pediatr Health Care, 16*(6), 307-312.

Pye, S. (2003). Caring for your baby after heart surgery. *Adv Neonatal Care, 3*(3), 157-158.

Reiser, D.J. (2004). Neonatal jaundice: Physiologic variation or pathologic process. *Crit Care Nurs Clin North Am, 16*(2), 257-269.

Ringer, S.A. (2006). Hemolytic disease of the newborn. In F.D. Burg, J.R. Ingelfinger, R.A. Polin, & A.A. Gershon (Eds.), *Current pediatric therapy* (18th ed.). Philadelphia: Saunders.

Robinson, L., & El-Sadr, W.M. (2006). Tuberculosis. In F.D. Burg, J.R. Ingelfinger, R.A. Polin, & A.A. Gershon (Eds.), *Current pediatric therapy* (18th ed.). Philadelphia: Saunders.

Rome, J.J., & Kreutzer, J. (2004). Pediatric interventional catheterization; reasonable expectations and outcomes. *Pediatr Clin North Am, 51*(6), 1589-1610.

Schaaf, H.S., Gie, R.P., Kennedy, M., Beyers, N., Hesseling, P.B., & Donald, P.R. (2002). Evaluation of young children in contact with adult multidrug-resistant pulmonary tuberculosis: A 30-month follow-up. *Pediatrics, 109*(5), 765-771.

Stokowski, L.A. (2005). A primer on apnea of prematurity. *Adv Neonatal Care, 5*(3), 155-170.

Thurber F., & Berry, B. (1990). Children with AIDS: Issues and future direction. *J Pediatr Nur 5,* 168-177.

Tweddell, J.S., & Spray, T.L. (2004). Newborn heart surgery: Reasonable expectations and outcomes. *Pediatr Clin North Am, 51*(6), 1611-1623.

Tworetzkey, W., & Marshall, A.C. (2004). Fetal interventions for cardiac defects. *Pediatr Clin North Am, 51*(6), 1503-1513.

Tyler, C., & Edman, J.C. (2004). Down syndrome, Turner syndrome, Klinefelter syndrome: Primary care throughout the lifespan. *Prim Care, 31*(3), 627-648.

VanCleve, S.N. (2006). Part 1: clinical guidelines for the children with Down syndrome from birth to 12 years. *J Pediatr Health Care, 20*(1), 47-54.

Zeigler, V.L. (2003). Ethical principles and parental choice: Treatment options for neonates with hypoplastic left heart syndrome. *Pediatr Nurs, 29*(1), 65-69.

ONLINE RESOURCES

American Academy of Pediatrics: http://www.aap.org

American Cleft Palate—Craniofacial Association: http://www.cleftline.org

Centers for Disease Control and Prevention: http://www.cdc.gov

Cleft Palate Foundation: http://www.cleftline.org

Congenital Heart Defects: www.americanheart.org

March of Dimes: http://www.marchofdimes.com

Spina Bifida Association of America: http://www.sbaa.org

Chapter 7

Atkinson, W., Pickering, L., Schwartz, B., Weniger, B., Iskander, J., & Watson, J. (2002). General Recommendations on Immunization. Centers for Disease Control MMWR Recommendations and Reports. February 8, 2002, 1-36.

Behrman, R., Kliegman, R., & Jenson, H. (2004). *Nelson's textbook of pediatrics* (17th ed.). Philadelphia: Saunders.

Centers for Disease Control and Prevention. (2003). National Immunization Program. *Vaccines and autism theory.* Retrieved from www.cdc.gov/nip/vacsafe/concerns/autism/default.htm

Centers for Disease Control and Prevention. (2007). Recommended immunization schedules for persons aged 0 to 18 years—United States. *MMWR, 55*(51-52), Q1-Q4.

Hockenberry, M., & Wilson, D. (2007). *Wong's nursing care of infants and children* (8th ed.). St. Louis: Mosby.

Levine, M., Carey, W., & Crocker, A. (1999). *Developmental-behavioral pediatrics* (3rd ed.). Philadelphia: Saunders.

Mahan, L.K., & Escott-Stump, S. (2003). *Krause's food, nutrition, and diet therapy* (11th ed.). Philadelphia: Saunders.

Peckenpaugh, N. (2003). *Nutrition essentials and diet therapy* (9th ed.). St. Louis: Saunders.

ONLINE RESOURCES

American Academy of Pediatrics: http://aap.org

Centers for Disease Control and Prevention: http://www.cdc.gov

Immunization Action Coalition: http://www.immunize.org

Vaccine Adverse Events Reporting System (VAERS): http://www.vaers.org

Chapter 8

Allen, J.L. (2006). Bronchitis and bronchiolitis. In F.D. Burg, J.R. Ingelfinger, R.A. Polin, & A.A. Gershon (Eds.), *Current pediatric therapy* (18th ed.). Philadelphia: Saunders.

American Academy of Pediatrics. (2003). In L.K. Pickering, C.J. Baker, S.S. Long, & J.A. McMillan (Eds.), *Red Book: 2006 Report of the Committee on Infectious Diseases* (27th ed.). Elk Grove Village, IL: American Academy of Pediatrics.

American Academy of Pediatrics & American Academy of Family Physicians. (2004). Clinical practice guidelines: Subcommittee on management of acute otitis media. Diagnosis and management of acute otitis media. *Pediatrics, 113*(5), 1451-1465.

American Academy of Pediatrics, Task Force on Sudden Infant Death Syndrome. (2005). The changing concept of sudden infant death syndrome: diagnostic coding shifts, controversies regarding the sleeping environment, and new variables to consider in reducing risk. *Pediatrics, 116*(5), 1245-1255.

Balkrishnan, R., Manuel, J., Clark, J., Caroll, C.L., Houseman, T.S., & Fleischer, A.B. (2003). Effects of an episode of specialist care on the impact of childhood atopic dermatitis on the child's family. *J Pediatr Health Care, 17*(2), 184-189.

Barkin, R.M., & Gausche-Hill, M. (2001). Sudden infant death syndrome. In *Rosen's emergency medicine: Concepts of clinical practice* (5th ed.). St. Louis: Mosby.

Behrman, R., Kliegman, V., & Jenson, H. (2004). *Nelson's textbook of pediatrics* (17th ed.). Philadelphia: Saunders.

Belcastro, M.R. (2004). Bronchopulmonary dysplasia: A new look at an old problem. *NAINA, 4*(2), 121-125.

Bell, L.M. (2005). The new clinical practice guidelines for acute otitis media: An editorial. *Ann Emerg Med, 45*(5), 514-516.

Bhumbra, N.A., & McCullough, S.G. (2003). Skin and subcutaneous infections. *Prim Care, 30*(1), 1-24.

Bissenger, R.L., & Carlson, C.A. (2006). Surfactant. *NAINR, 6*(2) 106-107.

Black, S., Shienfield, H., Baxter, R., Austrian, R., Brocken, L., Hansen, J., Lewis, E., & Freeman, B. (2004). Post licensure surveillance for pneumococcal invasive disease after use of heptavalent pneumococcal conjugate vaccine in northern California Kaiser Permanente. *Pediatr Infect Dis J, 23*(6), 485-595.

Bradin, S.A. (2006). Croup and bronchiolitis: Classic childhood maladies still pack a punch. *Consultant for Pediatricians, 5*(1), 22-30.

Brady, M.T. (2005). Health care-associated infections in the neonatal intensive care unit. *Am J Infect Control, 33*(5), 268-276.

Briggs, W.S., & Dery, W.H. (2006). Evaluation and treatment of constipation in infants and children. *Am Fam Physician, 73*(3), 469-477.

Cardona, I., Boguniewics, M., & Leung, D.Y. (2006). Atopic dermatitis. In F.D. Burg, J.R. Ingelfinger, R.A. Polin, & A.A. Gershon (Eds.), *Current pediatric therapy* (18th ed.). Philadelphia: Saunders.

Centers for Disease Control and Prevention (2002). Guidelines for hand hygiene in the healthcare setting. Retrieved from www.cdc.gov/od/media/pressrel/fs021025.htm.

Chavez-Bueno, S., & McCracken, G.H. (2005). Bacterial meningitis in children. *Pediatr Clin North Am, 52*(3), 795-810.

Cheigh, N.H. (2003). Managing a common disorder in children: Atopic dermatitis. *J Pediatr Health Care, 17*(2), 84-88.

Dovey, M.E. (2006). Cystic fibrosis. In F.D. Burg, J.R. Ingelfinger, R.A. Polin, & A.A. Gershon (Eds.), *Current pediatric therapy* (18th ed.). Philadelphia: Saunders.

Fixler, J., & Styles, L. (2002). Sickle cell disease. *Pediatr Clin North Am, 49*(6), 1193-1210.

Flatte, T.R., & Laube, B.L. (2001). Gene therapy in cystic fibrosis. *Chest, 120*(3), 1248-1315.

Friedman, N.R. (2006). Development of a practical tool for assessing the severity of acute otitis media. *Pediatr Infect Dis J, 25*(2), 101-107.

Halter, J.M., Baese, T., Nicolette, L., & Ratner, M. (2004). Common gastrointestinal problems and emergencies in neonates and children. *Clin Fam Pract, 6*(3), 731.

Hornor, G. (2005). Physical abuse: Recognition and reporting. *J of Pediatr Health Care, 19*(1), 4-11.

Hunt, C.E., & Hauck, F.R. (2006). Sudden infant death syndrome. *CMAJ, 174*(13), 1861-1869.

Jurgrau, A. (1990). How to spot child abuse. *RN, 53*(10), 26-32.

Kemp, C. (1962). The battered-child syndrome. *JAMA, 181,* 17-24.

Keating, J.P. (2006). Intussusception. In F.D. Burg, J.R. Ingelfinger, R.A. Polin, & A.A. Gershon (Eds.), *Current pediatric therapy* (18th ed.). Philadelphia: Saunders.

Kellog, N. (2005). The evaluation of sexual abuse in children. *Pediatrics, 116*(2), 506-512.

Kliegman, R.M., Jenson, H.B., Marcdante, K.J., & Behrman, R.E. (2006). *Nelson essentials of pediatrics* (5th ed.). Philadelphia: Saunders.

Lane, P.A., Buchanan, G.R., Deposito, F., Pegelow, C.H., Vichinsky, E.P., Wethers, D.L., & Woods, G.M. (2002). Health supervision for children with sickle cell disease. *Pediatrics, 109*(3), 526-535.

Long, L.E. (2003). Stress in families of children with sepsis. *Crit Care Nurs North Am, 15*(1), 47-53.

Mack, E. (2006). Oxygen administration in the neonate. *NAINR, 6*(2), 63-67.

McPherson, M., & Tender, J. (2006). Iron-deficiency anemia. In F.D. Burg, J.R. Ingelfinger, R.A. Polin, & A.A. Gershon (Eds.), *Current pediatric therapy* (18th ed.). Philadelphia: Saunders.

Middlesworth W., & Kadenhe-Chiweshe, A. (2006). Neonatal intestinal obstruction. In F.D. Burg, J.R. Ingelfinger, R.A. Polin, & A.A. Gershon (Eds.), *Current pediatric therapy* (18th ed.). Philadelphia: Saunders.

Miniati, D.N., & Albanese, C.T. (2004). Pyloric stenosis. *OTGS, 6*(4), 296-306.

Nelms, B.C. (2003). Keeping children safe. *J Pediatr Health Care, 17*(6),

Office on Child Abuse and Neglect. (2003). User Manual Series. *A coordinated response to child abuse and neglect: The foundation for practice.* Retrieved from www.childwelfare.gov.

Rosenfeid, R.M. (2006). Otitis media. In F.D. Burg, J.R. Ingelfinger, R.A. Polin, & A.A. Gershon (Eds.), *Current pediatric therapy* (18th ed.). Philadelphia: Saunders.

Sandoval, C. (2004). Trends in diagnosis and management of iron deficiency during infants and early childhood. *Hematol Oncol Clin North Am, 18*(6), 1423-1438.

Saririan, S. (2006). New recommendations to reduce the risks of SIDS: What should we advise parents. *Am Fam Physician, 74*(11), 1839-1840.

Schnitzer, J.J. (2006). Hernias and hydroceles. In F.D. Burg, J.R. Ingelfinger, R.A. Polin, & A.A. Gershon (Eds.), *Current pediatric therapy* (18th ed.). Philadelphia: Saunders.

Shah, B.R., & Laude, T.A. (2000). *Atlas of pediatric clinical diagnosis.* Philadelphia: Saunders.

Smith, M.A. (2005). Antibiotic resistance. *Nurs Clin North Am, 40*(1), 63-75.

Stokowski, L.A. (2006a). Latest guidelines for prevention of sudden infant death syndrome. *Adv Neonatal Care, 6*(2), 64-65.

Stokowski, L.A. (2006b). Pacifiers may offer some protection against sudden infant death syndrome. *Adv Neonatal Care, 6*(2), 63.

Stulberg, D.L., Penrod, M.A., & Blatney, R.A. (2002). Caring for common skin conditions: Common bacterial skin infections. *Am Fam Physician, 66*(1), 119-124.

Swenson, O. (2002). Hirschsprung's disease: A review. *Pediatrics, 109*(5), 914-918.

Talbot, D., Lankford, D., & Dodge, D. (2003). Nasal cannula home oxygen. *Adv Neonatal Care, 3*(2), 98-101.

Thoman, E. (2006). Co-sleeping, an ancient practice: Issues of the past and present, and possibilities for the future. *Sleep Med Rev, 10*(6), 407-417.

Thomas, K.A. (2005). Research guiding neonatal care. *NAINR, 5*(3), 105-106.

Toff, B. (2006). Beyond MRSA: VISA and VRSA. *Am J Nurs, 106*(4), 28-29.

U.S. Department of Health and Human Services. Administration on Child, Youth, and Families. (2006). *Child maltreatment 2004.* Washington, DC: U.S. Government Printing Office.

Walterspiel, J.N., & Baltimore, R.S. (2006). Cellulitis. In F.D. Burg, J.R. Ingelfinger, R.A. Polin, & A.A. Gershon (Eds.), *Current pediatric therapy* (18th ed.). Philadelphia: Saunders.

Watterberg, K.L., & Perkett, E.A. (2006). Bronchopulmonary dysplasia in the neonate. In F.D. Burg, J.R. Ingelfinger, R.A. Polin, & A.A. Gershon (Eds.), *Current pediatric therapy* (18th ed.). Philadelphia: Saunders.

Zitelli, B.J., & Davis, H.W. (2002). *Atlas of pediatric physical diagnosis* (4th ed.). St. Louis: Saunders.

Zlotkin, S. (2003). Clinical nutrition: 8. The role of nutrition in the prevention of iron deficiency anemia in infants, children, and adolescents. *CMAJ, 16*(1), 59-63.

ONLINE RESOURCES

American SIDS Institute: http://www.sids.org

Child Abuse Prevention Network: http://child-abuse.com

Directory of Health, Medicine, and Human Life Sciences: http://www.medlina.com

Eczema: http://www.vh.org

National Clearinghouse on Child Abuse and Neglect Information: http://www.calllib.com/nccanch/

National SIDS Resource Center: http://www.sidscenter.org

SIDS Alliance: http://www.sidsalliance.org

SIDS Network: http://sids-network.org

Chapter 9

American Academy of Pediatrics, Policy Statement. (2001). The use and misuse of fruit juice in pediatrics (RE0047). *Pediatrics, 107*(5), 1210-1213. Current as of July 5, 2006.

American Academy of Pediatrics Summer Safety Tips—Part 1. (2006). Retrieved July 2006 from http://www.aap.org/advocacy/releases/summertips.htm.

American Dental Association. *Facts on fluoride* (1995-2006). Retrieved July 2006 from http://www.ada.org.

Behrman, R., Kliegman, R., & Jenson, H. (2004). *Nelson's textbook of pediatrics* (17th ed.). Philadelphia: Saunders.

Briefel, R., Reidy, K., Karwe, V., Jankowski, L., & Hendricks, K. (2004). Toddler's transition to table foods impact on nutrient intakes and food patterns. *J Am Dietetic Assoc, 104*(S1), 38-44.

Food and Nutrition Board, Institute of Medicine. (2002). *Dietary reference intakes for energy, carbohydrate, fiber, fat, fatty acids, cholesterol, protein, and amino acids,* Washington, DC: National Academies Press.

Hockenberry, M., & Wilson, D. (2007). *Wong's nursing care of infants and children* (8th ed.). St. Louis: Mosby.

Peckenpaugh, N. (2003). *Nutrition essentials and diet therapy* (9th ed.). Philadelphia: Saunders.

Schmitt, B. (2005a). Shoes. Pediatric Advisor. McKesson Corporation. Retrieved from http://www.med.umich.edu/1libr/pa/pa_shoes_hhg.htm.

Schmitt, B. (2005b). Temper tantrums, biting, bedtime resistance or refusal, hitting and spitting, nightmares, and sibling quarrels. Pediatric Advisor. McKesson Corporation. Retrieved from http://www.med.umich.edu/1libr/pa/pa_index.htm#T.

U.S. Department of Agriculture. Center for Nutrition Policy and Promotion, April 2005. Retrieved July 2006 from http://www.MyPyramid.gov.

ONLINE RESOURCES

American Academy of Pediatrics: http://www.aap.org

National Safe Kids Campaign: http://www.safekids.org

U.S. Department of Agriculture: http://www.usda.gov/cnpp

Chapter 10

American Academy of Pediatrics Practice Guidelines, & Ressel, G.W. (2004). AAP releases policy statement on poison treatment in the home. *Am Fam Physician, 69*(3). Retrieved from http://home.mdconsult.com/das/article/body/66414754-2/jorg=journal&source=MI&sp=143.

Behrman, R., Kliegman, R., & Jenson, H. (2004). *Nelson's textbook of pediatrics* (17th ed.). Philadelphia: Saunders.

Burg, F.D., Ingelfinger, J.R., Polin, R.A., & Gershon, A.A (Eds). (2006). *Current pediatric therapy* (18th ed.). Philadelphia: Saunders.

Centers for Disease Control and Prevention. (2001). National Immunization Program: Facts about autism. Retrieved from www.cdc.gov/nip/vacsafe/concerns/autism/autism-facts.htm.

Hockenberry, M., & Wilson, D. (2007). *Wong's nursing care of infants and children* (8th ed.). St. Louis: Mosby.

James, H.E., Anas, N., & Perkin, R.M. (1985). *Brain insults in infants and children.* Orlando, FL: Grune & Stratton.

National Institute of Neurological Disorders and Stroke. (2006). Cerebral palsy: Hope through research. Bethesda, MD: NIH. Retrieved from www.ninds.nih.gov/disorders/cerebral_palsy/detail_cerebral_palsy.htm.

National Institute of Neurological Disorders and Stroke. (2006). NINDS cerebral palsy information page. Retrieved from www.ninds.nih.gov/disorders/cerebral_palsy/cerebral_palsy.htm.

ONLINE RESOURCES

Alexander Graham Bell Association for the Deaf and Hard of Hearing: http://www.agbell.org/information/brochures_faq.cfm

Cerebral palsy website: http://www.ninds.nih.gov/health_and_medical/disorders/cerebral_palsy.htm

Head injury website (Virtual Children's Hospital): http://www.vh.org/pediatric/patient/pediatrics/cqqa/headinjuries.html

Poison prevention website: http://www.aapcc.org

Chapter 11

American Academy of Pediatrics, Policy Statement. (1998). Guidance for effective discipline (RE9740). *Pediatrics, 101*(4), 723-728. Statement of reaffirmation published October 1, 2004.

American Academy of Pediatrics, Policy Statement. (1999). Trampolines at home, school, and recreational centers. *Pediatrics, 103*(5), 1053-1056. Statement of reaffirmation published May 1, 2006.

Anderson, J. (2006). Sibling rivalry: When a family circle becomes a boxing ring. *Contemporary Pediatrics,* February 1, 2006. Retrieved from http://www.contemporarypediatrics.com/contpeds/article/articleDetail.jsp?id=306594&pageID=1&sk=&date.

Behrman, R.E., Kliegman, R.M., & Jenson, H.B. (2004). *Nelson's textbook of pediatrics* (17th ed.). Philadelphia: Saunders.

Driessnack, M. (2006). Children's drawings as facilitators of communication: A meta-analysis. *J Pediatr Nurs, 20*(6), 415-423.

Helms, D., & Turner, J. (1978). *Exploring child behavior: Basic principles* (p. 447). Philadelphia: Saunders.

Hockenberry, M.J., & Wilson, D. (2007). *Wong's nursing care of infants and children* (8th ed.). St. Louis: Mosby.

Kelly, D., & Janine, S. (1999). In Levine, M., Carey, W., & Crocker, A (Eds). *Developmental-behavioral pediatrics* (3rd ed.). Philadelphia: Saunders.

Larsen, M., & Tentis, E. (2003). The art and science of disciplining children. *Pediatr Clin North Am, 50*(4), 817-840.

Levine, M., Carey, W., & Crocker, A (Eds). (1999). *Developmental-behavioral pediatrics* (3rd ed.). Philadelphia: Saunders.

Schmitt, B. (2005). Discipline basics. Pediatric Advisor. McKesson Corporation. Retrieved from http://www.med.umich.edu/1libr/pa/pa_bdisbasc_hhg.htm.

U.S. Department of Agriculture. MyPyramid. Retrieved July 10, 2006, from www.mypyramid.com

ONLINE RESOURCES

Bright Futures: http://www.brightfutures.org

Chapter 12

American Academy of Pediatrics. (2006). *Red Book Online.* Retrieved from www.aapredbook.org.

American Association on Mental Retardation (AAMR). (2002, 2005). *Definition of mental retardation.* Available on the AAMR website: www.aamr.org.

Behrman, R., Kliegman, R., & Jenson, H. (2004). *Nelson's textbook of pediatrics* (17th ed.). Philadelphia: Saunders.

Blume, W. (2003). Diagnosis and management of epilepsy. *Can Med Assoc J, 168*(4), 441-448.

Burg, F.D., Ingelfinger, J.R., Polin, R.A., & Gershon, A.A (Eds). (2006), *Current pediatric therapy* (18th ed.). Philadelphia: Saunders.

Centers for Disease Control and Prevention. (2005). *Department of Health and Human Services.* Retrieved online at http://www.cdc.gov/ncbddd/dd/mr2.htm.

Committee on Trauma, American College of Surgeons. (1999). Guidelines for the operations of burn units. In *Resources for optimal care of the injured patient 1999* (pp. 55-62). Chicago: Authors.

Deitch, E., & Rutan, R. (2001). *The challenges of children: the first 40 hours.* Chicago: American Burn Association.

Duffy, B., McLaughlin, P., & Eichelberger, M. (2006). Assessment, triage, and early management of burns in children. *Clin Pediatr Emer Med, 7*(2), 82-93.

Greenbaum, L., & Mesrobian, H. (2006). Vesicoureteral reflux. *Pediatr Clin North Am, 53*(3), 413-427.

Hockenberry, M., & Wilson, D. (2007). *Wong's nursing care of infants and children* (8th ed.). St. Louis: Mosby.

McKinney, E., James, S., Murray, S., & Ashwill, J. (2005). *Maternal child nursing* (2nd ed.). St. Louis: Saunders.

Messner, A. (2003). Treating pediatric patients with obstructive sleep disorders: An update. *Otolaryngol Clin North Am, 36*(3), 519-530.

National Institute of Neurological Disorders and Stroke Fact Sheet. (2006). U.S. Department of Health and Human Services: National Institutes of Health. Retrieved from www.ninds.nih.gov.

Patient Information Collection. (2002). Information from your family doctor. Celiac disease. *Am Fam Physician, 66*(12), 2269-2270.

Ticho, B.H. (2003). Strabismus. *Pediatr Clin North Am, 50*(1), 173-188.

Warden, C., Zibulewsky, J., Mace, S., Gold, C., & Gausche-Hill, M. (2003). Evaluation and management of febrile seizures in the out-of-hospital and emergency department settings. *Ann Emerg, 41*(2), 215-222.

Wells, J. (2003). Blood relations. *South Central Nurse Week, July 14,* 10-12.

ONLINE RESOURCES

American Association on Mental Retardation: http://www.aamr.org

American Burn Association: http://www.ameriburn.org/

Centers for Disease Control and Prevention: http://www.cdc.gov/

Hemophilia One (a patient resource website): http://www.hemophiliaone.com/

National Association for Retarded Citizens (ARC of the United States): http://www.thearc.org/

Chapter 13

American Academy of Pediatrics. (2006). Statement of reaffirmation for policy statement on in-line skating injuries in children and adolescents. *Pediatrics, 117*(5), 1846-1847.

American Academy of Pediatrics: Committee on Injury and Poison Prevention. (2000). All-terrain vehicle injury prevention in two, three, four wheeled unlicensed motor vehicles. *Pediatrics, 105*(6), 1352-1354.

American Academy of Pediatrics: Committee on Injury and Poison Prevention. (2004). Statement of reaffirmation for policy statement for firearm related injuries affecting the pediatric population. *Pediatrics, 114*(4), 1126.

American Academy of Pediatrics: Committee on Psychosocial Aspects of Child and Family Health. (2001). The new morbidity revisited: A renewed commitment to the psychosocial aspect of pediatric care. *Pediatrics, 108*(5), 1227-1230.

American Academy of Pediatrics: Committee on Public Education. (2001). Media violence. *Pediatrics, 108*(5), 1222-1226.

Behrman, R., Kliegman, R., & Jenson, H. (2004). *Nelson textbook of pediatrics* (17th ed.). Philadelphia: Saunders.

Chen, T.L., Brenner, R.A., Wright, J.L., Sachs, H.C., Moyer, P., & Roa, M.R. (2004). Children's violent television viewing: Are parents monitoring? *Pediatrics, 114*(1), 94-99.

Cohen, G.J. (2002). Helping children and families deal with divorce and separation. *Pediatrics, 110*(5), 1019-1023.

Hockenberry, M.J., & Wilson, D. (2007). *Wong's nursing care of infants and children* (8th ed.). St. Louis: Mosby.

Howard, B.J., Broughton, D.D., & Committee on Psychosocial Aspect of Child and Family Health. (2004). The pediatrician's role in prevention of missing children. *Pediatrics, 114*(4), 1100-1105.

Schmitt, B. (2005). Divorce: Helping children cope. Pediatric Advisor. McKesson Corporation. Retrieved from http://home.mdconsult.com.

Schmitt, B. (2005). Television: Reducing the negative impact. Pediatric Advisor. McKesson Corporation. Retrieved from http://home.mdconsult.com.

Schmitt, B. (2005). Video games. Pediatric Advisor. McKesson Corporation. Retrieved from http://home.mdconsult.com.

Schor, E.L. (1999). *Caring for your school-age children.* New York: Bantam Books.

Scott, J.U., Hague-Armstrong, K., & Downes, K.L. (2003). Teaching and bullying: What can pediatricians do? *Contemp Pediatr, 20*(4), 105-120.

U.S. Department of Agriculture. MyPyramid. Retrieved July 10, 2006, from www.mypyramid.com

Vossekuil, B., Fein, R.A., Reddy, M., Borum, R., & Modzeleski, W. (May 2002). *The final report and findings of the Safe School Initiative: Implications for the prevention of school attacks in the United States.* Washington, DC: U.S. Department of Education and U.S. Secret Service. Retrieved from www.secretservice.gov/ntac_ssi.shtml.

ONLINE RESOURCES

American Academy of Pediatrics: www.aap.org

Bright Futures: www.brightfutures.org

Entertainment Software Rating Board: www.esrb.org

Missing Children: www.pollyklaas.org

National Resource for Safe Schools: www.safetyzone.org

U.S. Department of Agriculture: www.usda.gov

U.S. Department of Agriculture: Food Pyramid: www.mypryamid.com

Chapter 14

American Academy of Pediatrics: Council on Sport Medicine and Fitness and Council on School Health. (2006). Policy Statement: Active healthy living: Prevention of childhood obesity through increased physical activity. *Pediatrics, 117*(5), 1834-1842.

American Academy of Pediatrics: Diabetes in Children and Adolescents Work Group of the National Diabetes Education Program. (2004). An update on type 2 diabetes in youth from the National Diabetes Education. *Pediatrics, 114*(1), 259-263.

American Psychiatric Association. (2000). *Diagnostic and statistical manual of mental disorders (DSM-IV-TR)* (4th ed.). Text revision. Washington, DC: The Association.

Anthony, K.K., & Schabberg, L.E. (2005). Pediatric pain syndromes and management of pain in children and adolescents with rheumatic disease. *Pediatr Clin North Am, 52*(2), 611-639.

Behrman, R., Kliegman, R., & Jenson, H. (2004). *Nelson's textbook of pediatrics* (17th ed.). Philadelphia: Saunders.

Berkhof, J., Melnyk, B.M., & Parker, K. (2003). The effectiveness of anti-leukotriene agents in childhood asthma: Evidence to guide clinical practice. *Pediatr Nurs, 29*(1), 60-62.

Bolte, R.G. (2004). Emergency department management of pediatric asthma. *CPEM, 5*(4), 256-269.

Brown, L.W. (2006). Reye's syndrome. In F.D. Burg, J.R. Ingelfinger, R.A. Polin, & A.A. Gershon (Eds.), *Current pediatric therapy* (18th ed.). Philadelphia: Saunders.

Frankowski, B.L., & Weiner, L.B. (2002). Head lice. *Pediatrics, 110*(3), 638-643.

Gahagan, S., Agarival, I., Brenneman, G., Fargot-Campagne, A., Moore, K., Raymer, T., & Silverstein, J. (2003). Prevention and treatment of type 2 diabetes mellitus in children, with special emphasis on American Indian and Alaskan native children [Electronic version]. *Pediatrics, 112*(4), 328.

Gibbs, I.C., Tuamokumo, N., & Yock, T.I. (2006). Role of radiation therapy in pediatric cancer. *Hematol Oncol Clinc North Am, 20*(2), 455-470.

Greydanus, D.E., Pratt, H.D., Sloane, M.A., & Rappley, M.D. (2003). Attention-deficit/hyperactivity disorder in children and adolescents: Intervention for a complex costly clinical conundrum. *Pediatr Clin North Am, 50*(5), 1049-1092.

Dale, D.E. (2004). Type 2 diabetes and diabetic risk factors in children and adolescents. *Clin Cornerstone, 6*(2), 17-30.

Hockenberry, M.J., & Wilson, D. (2007). *Wong's nursing care of infants and children* (8th ed.). St. Louis: Mosby.

Hockenberry, M.J., & Wong, D.L. (2004). *Wong's clinical manual of pediatric nursing* (6th ed.). St. Louis: Mosby.

Ilowite, N.T. (2002). Current treatment of juvenile rheumatoid arthritis. *Pediatrics, 109*(1), 109-115.

Kahn, P.J., & Immundo, L. (2006). Juvenile rheumatoid arthritis and spondyloarthropathy syndromes. In F.D. Burg, J.R. Ingelfinger, R.A. Polin, & A.A. Gershon (Eds.), *Current pediatric therapy* (18th ed.). Philadelphia: Saunders.

Kinane, T.B., & Scirica, C.V. (2006). Asthma. In F.D. Burg, J.R. Ingelfinger, R.A. Polin, & A.A. Gershon (Eds.), *Current pediatric therapy* (18th ed.). Philadelphia: Saunders.

Kliegman, R.M., Marcdante, K.J., Jenson, H.B, & Behrman, R.E. (2006). *Nelson essentials of pediatrics* (5th ed.). Philadelphia: Saunders.

McKesson Provider Technologies. (2005). Peak flow meter. Pediatric Advisor. Retrieved from http://home.mdconsult.com

Miller, J. (2004). Childhood obesity. *J Clin Endocrinol Metab, 89*(9), 4211-4218.

National Diabetes Education Program. (2006). Overview of diabetes in children and adolescents. Retrieved July 12, 2006, from http://www.ndep.nih.gov/diabetes/youth/youth.htm

Ostrom, N.K. (2006). Outpatient pharmacotherapy for pediatric asthma. *Pediatrics, 148*(1), 108-114.

Pearlman, D.L. (2004). A simple treatment for head lice: Dry-on, suffocation-based pedicalicide. [Electronic version]. *Pediatrics, 114*(3), 275-279.

Shah, S.A., & Stankovits, L.M. (2006). The hip. In F.D. Burg, J.R. Ingelfinger, R.A. Polin, & A.A. Gershon (Eds.), *Current pediatric therapy* (18th ed.). Philadelphia: Saunders.

Simon, H. (2003). Asthma in children and adolescents. Pediatric Advisor. Retrieved from http://home.mdconsult.com.

Stein, M.T., & Perrin, J.M. (2003). Diagnosis and treatment of ADHD in school-age children in primary care settings: A synopsis of the AAP practice guidelines. *Pediatr Rev, 24*(3), 92-98.

Svoren, B.M., & Laffel, L.M.B. (2006). Diabetes mellitus in children and adolescents. In F.D. Burg, J.R. Ingelfinger, R.A. Polin, & A.A. Gershon (Eds.), *Current pediatric therapy* (18th ed.). Philadelphia: Saunders.

Weiss, J.E., & Ilowite, N.T. (2005). Juvenile idiopathic arthritis. *Pediatr Clin North Am, 52*(2), 413-442.

Yock, T.I., & Tarbell, N.J. (2006). Pediatric brain tumors. In F.D. Burg, J.R. Ingelfinger, R.A. Polin, & A.A. Gershon (Eds.), *Current pediatric therapy* (17th ed.). Philadelphia: Saunders.

Young, T.W., & Strong, W.B. (2006). Acute rheumatic fever. In F.D. Burg, J.R. Ingelfinger, R.A. Polin, & A.A. Gershon (Eds.), *Current pediatric therapy* (18th ed.). Philadelphia: Saunders.

ONLINE RESOURCES

American Diabetes Association: http://www.diabetes.org/home.jsp

Arthritis Foundation: http://www.arthritis.org/conditions/DiseaseCenter/jra.asp

Children and Adults with Attention Deficit Disorder: http://www.chadd.org//AM/Template.cfm?Section=Home

National Asthma Education and Prevention Program: www.nhlbi.nih.gov/about/naepp

National Attention Deficit Disorder Association: http://www.add.org/

National Diabetes Education Program: www.ndep.nih.gov

National Institute of Mental Health: www.nimh.nih.gov/

Chapter 15

American Academy of Pediatrics. (2006). Academy lends expertise on web safety service for children. *AAP News 27*(5), 17.

American Academy of Pediatrics: Committee on Adolescence. (1999). Adolescent pregnancy—current trends and issues: 1998. *Pediatrics, 103*(2), 516-520.

Anderson, J., & Martel, S. (2002). Decorating the "human canvas": Body art and your patients. *Contemp Pediatr, 8*, 86. Retrieved from http://www.contemporarypediatrics.com/contpeds/

Broughton, D.D. (2005). Keeping children safe in cyberspace. *AAP News, 26*(8), 11.

Carakushansky, M., O'Brien, K., & Levine, M. (2003). Vitamin D and calcium: Strong bones for life through better nutrition. *Contemp Pediatr, 3*, 37. Retrieved from http://www.contemporarypediatrics.com/contpeds/.

Centers for Disease Control and Prevention. (2006). Youth risk behavior surveillance USA—2005. *MMWR, 55*(SS-5), 1-108.

Hockenberry, M.J., & Wilson, D. (2007). *Wong's nursing care of infants and children* (87th ed.). St. Louis: Mosby.

James, S.R., Ashwill, J.W., & Droske, S.C (Eds). (2002). *Nursing care of children*. Philadelphia: Saunders.

Orr, D.P. (1998). Helping adolescents towards adulthood. *Contemp Pediatr, 15*(5), 55-76.

Schmitt, B. (2006). Instructions for pediatric patients. Pediatric Advisor. McKesson Corporation. Retrieved from http://home.mdconsult.com.

Scott, J.U., Hague-Armstrong, K., & Downes, K.L. (2003). Teasing and bullying: What can pediatricians do? *Contemp Pediatr, 20*(4), 105-120.

Selekman, J. (2003). A new era of body decoration: What are kids doing to their bodies? *Pediatr Nurs, 29*(1) 77-79.

Verkler, E. (2005). Upping the ante: Poker craze puts glamorous spin on gambling, but betting is not risk-free for youths. *AAP News, 26*(5), 1.

ONLINE RESOURCES

American Academy of Pediatrics: www.aap.org

Bright Futures: www.brightfutures.org

Safe Sitter: http://www.safesitter.org

Teen Gambling: www.nati.org

Chapter 16

American Academy of Child and Adolescent Psychiatry. (2001). Practice parameter for the assessment and treatment of children and adolescents with suicide behavior. *J Am Acad Child Adolesc Psychiatry, 40*(7 Suppl), 24S-51S.

American Academy of Pediatrics. (2005) Revised Policy Statement on tobacco, alcohol, and others drugs: The role of the pediatrician in prevention and management of substance abuse (RE9801). *Pediatrics, 115*(3), 816-821.

American Academy of Pediatrics: Committee on Infectious Disease. (2006). *Red Book: 2006 Report of the Committee on Infectious Diseases* (27th ed.). Elk Grove Village, IL: American Academy of Pediatrics.

American Academy of Pediatrics: Committee on Nutrition Policy Statement. (2003). Prevention of pediatric overweight and obesity. *Pediatrics, 112*(2), 424-430.

American Academy of Pediatrics: Committee on Sports Medicine and Fitness. (2001). Medical conditions affecting sports participation. *Pediatrics, 107*(5), 1205.

American Academy of Pediatrics: Committee on Sports Medicine and Fitness, Committee on School Health. (2000). Physical fitness and activity in schools. *Pediatrics, 105*(5), 1156.

American Psychiatric Association. (2000). *Diagnostic and statistics manual of mental disorders ±DSM-IV-TR)* (4th ed.) text revised. Washington, DC: The Association.

Auwaerter, P.G. (2004). Infectious mononucleosis: Return to plan. *Clin Sports Med, 23*(3), 485-497.

Behrman, R.E., Kliegman, R., & Jensen, H. (2004). *Nelson's textbook of pediatrics* (17th ed.). Philadelphia: Saunders.

Braveman, P.K. (2003). Sexually transmitted diseases in adolescents. *CPEM, 4*(1), 21-36.

Burstein, G.R., & Murray, P.J. (2003). Diagnosis and management of sexually transmitted disease pathogens among adolescents. *Pediatr Rev, 24*(3), 75-81.

Diehl, V., Thomas, R.K., & Re, D. (2004) Part II: Hodgkin's lymphoma—diagnosis and treatment. *Lancet Oncol, 5*(1), 19-26.

Ebell, M.H. (2004). Epstein-Barr virus infectious mononucleosis. *Am Fam Physician, 70*(7), 1279-1287.

Feldman, S., Careccia, R.E., Barham, K.L., & Hancox, J. (2004). Diagnosis and treatment of acne. *Am Fam Physician, 69*(9), 2123-2130.

Gibbs, I.C., Tuamokumo, N., & Yock, T.I. (2006). Role of radiation therapy in pediatric cancer. *Hematol Oncol Clinc North Am, 20*(2), 455-470.

Harper, J.C. (2004). An update on pathogenesis and management of acne vulgaris. *J Am Acad Dermatol, 51*(suppl 1), S36-38.

Hillard, P.A. (2005). Overview of contraception. *Adol Med Clin, 16*(3), 485-493.

Hull, P.R., & D'Arcy, C. (2005). Acne, depression and suicide. *Dermatol Clin, 23*(4), 665-674.

Katz, B.Z. (2006) Infectious mononucleosis. In F.D. Burg, J.R. Ingelfinger, R.A. Polin, & A.A. Gershon (Eds.), *Current pediatric therapy* (18th ed.). Philadelphia: Saunders.

Kliegman, R.M., Marcdante, K.J., Jenson, H.B. & Behrman, R.E. (2006). *Nelson essentials of pediatrics* (5th ed.). Philadelphia: Saunders.

Kulig, J.W., Jaffe, A., Behnke, M., Knight, J.R., Kokotailo, P.K., & Williams, J.F. (2005). Tobacco, alcohol, and other drugs: The role of the pediatrician in prevention, identification, and management of substance abuse. *Pediatrics, 115*(4), 816-821.

Lamontagne, L.L. (2004). Adolescent scoliosis: Effects of corrective surgery, cognitive-behavioral interventions, and age on activity outcomes. *Appl Nurs Res, 17*(3), 168-177.

Macsween, K.E. (2003). Epstein-Barr virus: Recent advances. *Lancet Infect Dis, 3*(3), 131-140.

McClain, N. (2003). Adolescent suicide attempt: Undisclosed secrets. *Pediatr Nurs, 29*(1), 52-53.

Miller, J. (2004). Childhood obesity. *J Clin Endocrinol Metab, 89*(9), 4211-4218.

National Institute on Drug Abuse. (2006). *NIDA Infofax.* Retrieved July 10, 2006, from www.drugabuse.gov.

National Campaign to Prevent Teen Pregnancy. (2005). Teen pregnancy: General facts and stats. Retrieved July 10, 2005, from www.teenpregnancy.org.

Polizzotto, M.J. (2005). Prevention of sexually transmitted diseases. *Clin Fam Pract, 7*(1), 127-137.

Sidbury, R. (2006). Acne vulgaris. In F.D. Burg, J.R. Ingelfinger, R.A. Polin, & A.A. Gershon (Eds). *Current pediatric therapy* (18th ed.). Philadelphia: Saunders.

Speiser, P.W., Rudolf, M.C., Anholt, H., Camocho-Hubner, C., Chiarelli, F., Eliakin, A., Freemark, M., Gruters, A., Hershkovitz, E., Iughetti, L., Krude, H., Latzer, Y., Lustig, R.H., Pescovitz, O.H., Pinhas-Hamil, O., Rogol, A.D., Shalitin, S., Sultan, C., Stein, D., Vardi. P., Werther, G.A., Zadik. Z., & Zuckerman-Levin, N. (2005). Childhood obesity. *J Clin Endocrinol Metab, 90*(3), 1871-1887.

Sturdevant, M.S., & Spear, B.A. (2006). Eating disorders and obesity. In F.D. Burg, J.R. Ingelfinger, R.A. Polin, & A.A. Gershon (Eds.), *Current pediatric therapy* (18th ed.). Philadelphia: Saunders.

Taft, E. (2003). Evaluation and management of scoliosis. *J Pediatr Health Care, 17*(1), 42-44.

Toombs, E.L. (2005). Cosmetics in treatment of acne vulgaris. *Dermatol Clin, 23*(3), 575-581.

Wolfe, B.E. (2003). Caring for the hospitalized patient with an eating disorder. *Nurs Clin North Am, 38*(1), 75-99.

ONLINE RESOURCES

American Academy of Child and Adolescent Psychiatry: www.aacap.org

American Association of Suicidology: www.suicidology.org

American Foundation for Suicide Prevention: www.afsp.org

National Institute on Drug Abuse: www.drugabuse.gov

Chapter 17

American Academy of Pediatrics. (2002). Fever—Making your child comfortable. Retrieved June 12, 2006 from http://www.aap.org/pubed/ZZZX3N5Q25D.htm?&sub_cat=1.

American Urological Association. (2002). Retrieved June 12, 2006, from UrologyHealth.org.

Behrman, R., Kliegman, R., & Jenson, H. (2004). *Nelson's textbook of pediatrics* (17th ed.). Philadelphia: Saunders.

Hockenberry, M., Wilson, D., & Winkelstein, M. (2005). *Wong's essentials of pediatric nursing* (7th ed.). St. Louis: Mosby.

ONLINE RESOURCES

Mayo Clinic: http://www.mayoclinic.com/health/childrens-health/CC00046

Chapter 18

American Academy of Pediatrics. (2000). Policy statement. Palliative care for children. *Pediatrics, 106*(2), 351-357.

Hockenberry, M., Wilson, D., & Winkelstein, M. (2005). *Wong's essentials of pediatric nursing* (7th ed.). St. Louis: Mosby.

Jacobs, H. (2005). Ethics in pediatric end of life care: A nursing perspective. *J Pediatr Nurs, 20*(5), 360-369.

Kemp, C. (2005). Cultural issues in palliative care. *Seminars in Oncology Nurs, 21*(1), 44-52.

Kreichbergs, U., Valdimarsdottir, U., Onelov, E., Henter, J., & Steineck, G. (2004). Talking about death with children who have severe malignant disease. *N Engl J Med, 351*, 1175-1186.

Kübler-Ross, E. (1969). *On death and dying.* New York: Macmillan.

Lewis, L. Brecher, M., Reaman, G., & Sahler, L.J., consultants. (2002). How you can help meet the needs of dying children. *Contemp Pediatr, 19*(4), 147-159.

McCaffery, M., & Pasero, C. (1999). *Pain: Clinical manual.* St. Louis: Mosby.

ONLINE RESOURCES

Children's Hospice International: http://www.chionline.org

National Hospice and Palliative Care Organization: http://www.nhpco

The Compassionate Friends: http://www.compassionatefriends.org

Illustration Credits

Chapter 1
Figures 1-1, 1-2: From Bowden, V., Dickey, S., & Greenberg, C. (1998). *Children and their families: The continuum of care.* Philadelphia: Saunders.

Chapter 2
Figures 2-1, 2-3, 2-4, 2-5: From Bowden, V., Dickey, S., & Greenberg, C. (1998). *Children and their families: The continuum of care.* Philadelphia: Saunders.

Figure 2-2: From Mattson, S., & Smith, J.E. (2000): *Core curriculum for maternal-newborn nursing.* Philadelphia: Saunders, p. 139.

Chapter 3
Figures 3-1, 3-2, 3-3, 3-4, 3-5, 3-6, 3-7, 3-12, 3-14, 3-15, 3-17: From Bowden, V., Dickey, S., & Greenberg, C. (1998). *Children and their families: The continuum of care.* Philadelphia: Saunders.

Figure 3-9: From Wong, D.L., Hockenberry-Eaton, M., Wilson, D., Winkelstein, M.L., Ahmann, E., & DiVito-Thomas, P.A. (1999). *Whaley and Wong's nursing care of infants and children.* (6th ed.). St. Louis: Mosby.

Figure 3-10: From National Institutes of Health, National Heart, Lung, Blood Institute. (Sept. 1996). *Update on the Task Force Report [1987] on High Blood Pressure in Children and Adolescents: A Working Group Report from the National High Blood Pressure Education Program.* NIH Pub. No. 96-3790.

Figure 3-16: In Hockenberry, J. (2005). *Wong's essentials of pediatric nursing* (7th ed.). St. Louis: Mosby.

Chapter 4
Figures 4-2, 4-19: From James, S., Ashwill J., & Droske S. (2002). *Nursing care of children: Principles and practice.* (2nd ed.). Philadelphia: Saunders.

Figure 4-3: From Thompson, E. (1995). *Introduction to maternity and pediatric nursing* (2nd ed.). Philadelphia: Saunders.

Figures 4-4, 4-7, 4-8, 4-9: From Zitelli, B., & Davis, H. (2002). *Atlas of pediatric physical diagnosis* (4th ed.). Philadelphia: Mosby.

Figures 4-5, 4-11, 4-13: From Bowden, V., Dickey, S., & Greenberg, C. (1998). *Children and their families: The continuum of care.* Philadelphia: Saunders.

Figures 4-6, 4-14, 4-18: From Hockenberry, M., Wilson, D., Winkelstein, M., & Kline, N. (2003). *Wong's nursing care of infants and children* (7th ed.). St. Louis: Mosby.

Figures 4-10, 4-12, 4-15, 4-17: From Murray S., McKinney E., & Gorrie T. (2002). *Foundations of maternal-newborn nursing* (3rd ed.). Philadelphia: Saunders.

Figure 4-16: From Peckenpaugh, N. (2003). *Nutrition essentials and diet therapy.* (9th ed.). St. Louis: Saunders.

Chapter 5
Figure 5-1, *A:* From Korones, S.B. (1986). *High-risk newborn infants: The basis for intensive care* (4th ed.). St. Louis: Mosby.

Figure 5-1, *B:* Modified from Battaglia, F.C., & Lubchenko, L.C. (1967). A practical classification of newborn infants by weight and gestational ages. *J Pediatr, 71,* 159.

Figure 5-2: Modified from the American Academy of Pediatrics; and Silverman, W., & Andersen, D. (1956). A cold clinical trial of effects of water mist on obstructive respiratory signs, death rate, and necropsy findings among premature infants. *Pediatrics, 17,* 4.

Figures 5-3, 5-4, 5-5: From Murray S., McKinney E., & Gorrie T. (2002). *Foundations of maternal-newborn nursing* (3rd ed.) Philadelphia: Saunders.

Figure 5-6: From Hockenberry, M., Wilson, D., Winkelstein, M., & Kline, N. (2003). *Wong's nursing care of infants and children* (7th ed.). St. Louis: Mosby.

Chapter 6
Figures 6-1, 6-2, 6-3, 6-4, 6-5, 6-6, 6-7, 6-8, 6-9, 6-10, 6-13, 6-14, 6-15, 6-20, 6-25, 6-26: From Bowden, V., Dickey, S., & Greenberg, C. (1998). *Children and their families: The continuum of care.* Philadelphia: Saunders.

Figure 6-11: Courtesy Paul Vincent Kuntz, Texas Children's Hospital. From Hockenberry, M., & Wilson, D. (2007). *Wong's nursing care of infants and children* (8th ed.). St. Louis: Mosby.

Figures 6-12, 6-18, in Skill 6-2: From McKinney, E.S., Ashwill, J., Murray, S.S., James, S.R., Gorrie, T.M., & Droske, S.C. (2000). *Maternal-child nursing.* Philadelphia: Saunders.

Figure 6-16: From Tachdjean, M. (1999). *Pediatric orthopedics.* Philadelphia: Saunders.

Figure 6-17: Courtesy Wheaton Brace Co. From Bowden, V., Dickey, S., & Greenberg, C. (1998). *Children and their families: The continuum of care.* Philadelphia: Saunders.

Figure 6-19: From Zitelli, B., & Davis, H. (2002). *Atlas of pediatric physical diagnosis* (4th ed.). Philadelphia: Mosby.

Figure 6-21: Courtesy Albert Biglan, MD, Children's Hospital of Pittsburgh. From Zitelli, B., & Davis, H. (2002). *Atlas of pediatric physical diagnosis* (4th ed.). Philadelphia: Mosby.

Figure 6-23: From Ashwill, J.W., & Droske, S.C. (2002). *Nursing care of children: Principles and practice.* Philadelphia: Saunders.

Figure 6-24: From Hockenberry, M., & Wilson, D. (2007). *Wong's nursing care of infants and children* (8th ed.). St. Louis: Mosby.

Chapter 7
Figure 7-1, Unnumbered figures 7-1, 7-2, 7-3, 7-4, 7-8, 7-9, 7-10, 7-12 in Box 7-1: From Bowden, V., Dickey, S., & Greenberg, C. (1998). *Children and their families: The continuum of care.* Philadelphia: Saunders.

Figure 7-2, Unnumbered figures 7-5, 7-6, 7-7, 7-11, 7-13, 7-16, 7-17 in Box 7-1: From James, S., Ashwill, J., & Droske, S. (2002). *Nursing care of children: Principles and practice* (2nd ed.). Philadelphia: Saunders.

Unnumbered figures 7-14, 7-15 in Box 7-1: From Hockenberry, M., Wilson, D., Winkelstein, M., & Kline, N. (2003). *Wong's nursing care of infants and children* (7th ed.). St. Louis: Mosby.

Chapter 8
Figures 8-1, *A,* 8-3, 8-4, *B,* 8-5, 8-7, 8-12, 8-18, 8-20, 8-22, 8-23: From Zitelli, B., & Davis, H. (2002). *Atlas of pediatric physical diagnosis.* (4th ed.). Philadelphia: Mosby.

Figure 8-1, *B:* From Fireman, P., & Slavin, R.G. (1991). *Atlas of allergies.* New York: Gower.

Figures 8-2, 8-4, *A and C:* From Shah, B.R., & Laude, T.A. (2000). *Atlas of pediatric clinical diagnosis.* Philadelphia: Saunders.

Figures 8-6, 8-8, 8-9, 8-13, 8-15, 8-17: From Bowden, V., Dickey, S., & Greenberg, C. (1998). *Children and their families: The continuum of care.* Philadelphia: Saunders.

Figures 8-10, 8-19: From James, S., Ashwill, J., & Droske, S. (2002). *Nursing care of children: Principles and practice.* (2nd ed.). Philadelphia: Saunders.

Figures 8-11, 8-14, 8-16: From Liebert, P.S. (1996). *Color atlas of pediatric surgery* (2nd ed.). Philadelphia: Saunders.

Figure 8-21: Adapted from Betz, C.L., Hunsberger, M.M., & Wright, S. (Eds.). (1994). *Family-centered nursing care of children* (2nd ed.). Philadelphia: Saunders. In Bowden, V., Dickey,

S., & Greenberg, C. (1998). *Children and their families: The continuum of care.* Philadelphia: Saunders.

Unnumbered snapshot 8-1 in Nursing Care Plan 8-1: Weston, W.L., Lane, A.T., & Morelli, J.G. (2002). *Color textbook of pediatric dermatology* (3rd ed.). St. Louis, Mosby.

Chapter 9

Figures 9-1, 9-2, 9-3, 9-4, 9-6, 9-7, 9-8, 9-9, 9-10: From Bowden, V., Dickey, S., & Greenberg, C. (1998). *Children and their families: The continuum of care.* Philadelphia: Saunders.

Figure 9-5: From U.S. Department of Agriculture, Center for Nutrition Policy and Promotion, March, 1999.

Figure 9-12: From James, S., Ashwill, J., & Droske, S. (2002). *Nursing care of children: Principles and practice* (2nd ed.). Philadelphia: Saunders.

Figure 9-15, *A*: From Chandra, N.C., & Hazinski, M.F. (Eds.). (2005). *Textbook of basic life support for healthcare providers.* Dallas: American Heart Association.

Figure 9-15, *B*: Courtesy Safe Sitter®, Inc., Indianapolis, IN.

Chapter 10

Figures 10-1, 10-2, 10-4, 10-7: From James, S., Ashwill, J., & Droske, S. (2002). *Nursing care of children: Principles and practice* (2nd ed.). Philadelphia: Saunders.

Figure 10-3, Unnumbered figures in Table 10-1: From Bowden, V., Dickey, S., & Greenberg, C. (1998). *Children and their families: The continuum of care.* Philadelphia: Saunders.

Figures 10-5, 10-8: From Hockenberry, M., Wilson, D., Winkelstein, M., & Kline, N. (2003). *Wong's nursing care of infants and children* (7th ed.). St. Louis: Mosby.

Figure 10-6: From Zitelli B., & Davis, H. (2002). *Atlas of pediatric physical diagnosis* (4th ed.). Philadelphia: Mosby.

Unnumbered snapshot 10-1 in Nursing Care Plan 10-1: McKinney, E.S. (2004). *Maternal child nursing* (2nd ed.). Philadelphia: Saunders.

Chapter 11

Figures 11-1, 11-2, 11-3, 11-4, 11-5: From Bowden, V., Dickey, S., & Greenberg, C. (1998). *Children and their families: The continuum of care.* Philadelphia: Saunders.

Chapter 12

Figure 12-1: From Deitch, E., & Rutan R. (2001). *The challenges of children: The first 48 hours.* Chicago: American Burn Association.

Figures 12-2, 12-4, 12-5, 12-6: From Hockenberry, M., Wilson, D., Winkelstein, M., & Kline, N. (2003). *Wong's nursing care of infants and children* (7th ed.). St. Louis: Mosby.

Figures 12-3, 12-7, 12-8: From Zitelli, B., & Davis, H. (2002). *Atlas of pediatric physical diagnosis* (4th ed.). Philadelphia: Mosby.

Figures 12-9, 12-10, Unnumbered figures in Table 12-1: From James, S., Ashwill J., & Droske, S. (2002). *Nursing care of children: Principles and practice* (2nd ed.). Philadelphia: Saunders.

Figure 12-11, *A*: From Lookingbill, D.P., & Marks, J.G. (2000). *Principles of dermatology* (3rd ed.). Philadelphia: Saunders.

Figure 12-11, *B*: From Fenner, F., Henderson, D.A., Arita, I., Jezek, Z., & Ladnyi, I. (1988). *Smallpox and its eradication.* Geneva: World Health Organization.

Chapter 13

Figures 13-1, 13-2, 13-3, 13-4, 13-5, 13-6, 13-8, 13-11: From Bowden, V., Dickey, S., & Greenberg, C. (1998). *Children and their families: The continuum of care.* Philadelphia: Saunders.

Figures 13-7: From Hockenberry, M., Wilson, D., Winkelstein, M., & Kline, N. (2003). *Wong's nursing care of infants and children* (7th ed.). St. Louis: Mosby.

Figures 13-19, 13-10: From Hockenberry, M., & Wilson, D. (2007). *Wong's nursing care of infants and children* (8th ed.). St. Louis: Mosby.

Figure 13-13: From U.S. Department of Agriculture/U.S. Department of Health and Human Services (August 1992).

Chapter 14

Figure 14-1: Courtesy Michael Sherlock, MD. In Zitelli, B., & Davis, H. (2002). *Atlas of pediatric physical diagnosis.* (4th ed.). St. Louis: Mosby.

Figure 14-2: From Travis, L.B., Brouhard, B., & Schreiner, B. (1987). *Diabetes in children and adolescents.* Philadelphia: Saunders.

Figure 14-3 and "Metered-dose inhaler with spacer" figure in Skill 14-2: From Hockenberry, M., Wilson, D. (2007). *Wong's nursing care of infants and children* (8th ed.). St. Louis: Mosby.

Figures 14-4, 14-5, 14-6, and "Metered-dose inhaler" figure in Skill 14-2: From Bowden, V., Dickey, S., & Greenberg, C. (1998). *Children and their families: The continuum of care.* Philadelphia: Saunders.

Figure 14-7: From James, S., Ashwill, J., & Droske, S. (2002). *Nursing care of children: Principles and practice* (2nd ed.). Philadelphia: Saunders. Data from Behrman, R., Kliegman, R., & Arvin, A. (1996). *Nelson's textbook of pediatrics* (15th ed.). Philadelphia: Saunders.

Figure 14-9: From Zitelli, B., & Davis, H. (2002). *Atlas of pediatric physical diagnosis* (4th ed.). St. Louis: Mosby.

Figure 14-8: From Shah, B.R., & Laude, T.A. (2000). *Atlas of pediatric clinical diagnosis.* Philadelphia: Saunders.

"Mixing insulin" figures in Skill 14-1: From Price, M.J. (1983). Insulin and oral hypoglycemic agents. *Nurs Clin North Am, 18*(4), 687-706.

Chapter 15

Figures 15-1, 15-2, 15-3, 15-5, 15-6, 15-7, 15-8, 15-9, 15-11: From Bowden, V., Dickey, S., & Greenberg, C. (1998). *Children and their families: The continuum of care.* Philadelphia: Saunders.

Figure 15-4: From Hockenberry, M., Wilson, D., Winkelstein, M., & Kline, N. (2003). *Wong's nursing care of infants and children* (7th ed.). St. Louis: Mosby.

Figure 15-10: Courtesy Jared Isaacs. In Bowden, V., Dickey, S., & Greenberg, C. (1998). *Children and their families: The continuum of care.* Philadelphia: Saunders.

Chapter 16

Figures 16-1, 16-2, and "Gonorrhea" and "Herpes genitalis" figures in Table 16-2: From Zitelli, B., & Davis, H. (2002). *Atlas of pediatric physical diagnosis.* (4th ed.). Philadelphia: Mosby.

Figures 16-3, 16-4, 16-5, 16-6, 16-7, 16-8: From Bowden, V., Dickey, S., & Greenberg, C. (1998). *Children and their families: The continuum of care.* Philadelphia: Saunders.

"Genital warts" and "Syphilis" figures in Table 16-2: From Shah, B.R., & Laude, T.A. (2000). *Atlas of pediatric clinical diagnosis.* Philadelphia: Saunders.

Chapter 17

Figures 17-1, 17-16, *B*, 17-22, *B*: Courtesy Parkland Health and Hospital System, Dallas, Texas.

Figures 17-2, 17-4, 17-5, 17-10, 17-11, "Nurse bathing infant" figure in Skill 17-1: From Hockenberry, M., Wilson, D., Winkelstein, M., & Kline, N. (2003). *Wong's nursing care of infants and children* (7th ed.). St. Louis: Mosby.

Figures 17-3, 17-6, 17-9, 17-12, 17-13, 17-14, 17-16, *A*, 17-18, 17-19, 17-20, 17-21, 17-22, *A*, "Urine bags" figures in Skill 17-1: From Bowden, V., Dickey, S., & Greenberg, C. (1998). *Children and their families: The continuum of care.* Philadelphia: Saunders.

Figures 17-7, 17-15: From James, S., Ashwill, J., & Droske, S. (2002). *Nursing care of children: Principles and practice* (2nd ed.). Philadelphia: Saunders.

Figure 17-8: Nomogram modified from data of E. Boyd by C.D. West. From Behrman, R., Kliegman, R., & Jenson, H. (2004). *Nelson's textbook of pediatrics,* (17th ed.). Philadelphia: Saunders.

Chapter 18

Figures 18-1, 18-2: From Bowden, V., Dickey, S., & Greenberg, C. (1998). *Children and their families: The continuum of care.* Philadelphia: Saunders.

Glossary

Pronunciation of Terms* The markings ¯ and ˘ above the vowels (a, e, i, o, and u) indicate the proper sounds of the vowels. When ¯ is above a vowel, its sound is long, that is, exactly like its name. For example:

a as in ape
e as in even
i as in ice
o as in open
u as in unit

The ˘ marking indicates a short vowel sound, as in the following examples:

a as in apple
e as in every
i as in interest
o as in pot
u as in under

A

acceptance The act or process of taking something offered. The condition of being accepted or acceptable. The final stage in Elizabeth Kübler-Ross's stages of grief and dying.

acrocyanosis Peripheral blueness of the hands and feet, which is normal in newborn infants.

acromion The lateral, triangular projection of the spine of scapula, forming the point of the shoulder and articulating with the clavicle.

acute rheumatic fever A systemic disease that involves the joints, heart, central nervous system, skin, and subcutaneous tissues. It follows an infection by certain strains of group A, B-hemolytic streptococci.

adolescence The period from the beginning of puberty until maturity.

adventitious Accidental or acquired; not natural or hereditary.

AIDS (acquired immune deficiency syndrome) Characterized by depression of the immune system and opportunistic infection. Seen in neonates and infants who live in high-risk populations and in children with hemophilia and other conditions who have received contaminated blood products.

alimentation The process of nourishing the body, which includes mastication, swallowing, digestion, absorption, and assimilation.

alkalosis Excessive alkalinity of body fluids from accumulation of alkalis or reduction of acids.

amblyopia (lazy eye) A decrease in or loss of vision, usually in one eye.

amniocentesis A needle is placed into the uterus of an expectant mother to obtain a specimen of amniotic fluid for analysis. This is done to determine possible damage to the fetus by Rh incompatibility, to determine Down syndrome, and for other tests.

anastomosis A natural communication between two vessels or surgical or pathological connection of two tubular structures.

androgen Any steroid hormone that promotes male characteristics. The two main androgens are androsterone and testosterone.

anger A feeling of extreme hostility, indignation, or exasperation; rage; wrath. The second stage in Elizabeth Kübler-Ross's stages of grief and dying.

angioma A tumor, usually benign, that is made up chiefly of blood and lymph vessels.

animism A period of cognitive development in which the child attributes life to inanimate objects.

anorexia nervosa A syndrome most often seen in adolescent girls, characterized by an extreme form of poor appetite or self-starvation. Although its onset may be acute, the underlying emotional problem develops over a relatively long period of time.

anticipatory grief Grief that occurs before a loss or a perceived loss.

anticipatory guidance Providing families with information on normal growth and development and nurturing child-rearing practices before the child enters that stage of development. Injury prevention is an area of anticipatory guidance typically addressed in the care of children.

anuria The cessation of urine production or a urinary output of less than 100 mL/day.

anxiolytics A classification of drugs used to decrease anxiety. The action of these drugs decreases anxiety and does not cause excessive sedation.

Apgar scoring chart A standardized chart used to evaluate the condition of the neonate immediately after delivery. The following five objective signs are evaluated: heart rate, respiration, muscle tone, reflexes, and color.

aplastic anemia Anemia caused by deficient red blood cell production because of bone marrow dysfunction.

arthroscopy A surgical procedure designed to assess joint damage. A small scope is inserted into the joint for visualization of joint structures.

artificialism A period of cognitive development in which the child believes the world and everything in it are created by human beings.

ascariasis Roundworm infestation.

asplenia Absence of the spleen.

asymmetry One side of the body looking different from the other.

asynchrony Lack of concurrence in time. The appearance of a growing child may be gangling because of asynchrony of growth (i.e., different body parts maturing at different rates).

ataxia Failure of muscular coordination.

atelectasis Incomplete expansion of the lungs at birth or a collapse after expansion because of a mucous plug, tumor, pressure from organs, or other causes.

atresia A congenital anomaly in which a normal opening is absent (e.g., atresia of the esophagus).

attention-deficit hyperactivity disorder (ADHD) Refers to specific patterns of behavior that include inattention and impulsivity, which may or may not involve hyperactivity.

audiometry Measurement of hearing.

auditory brainstem response (ABR) An electrophysiologic test used to measure hearing sensitivity and evaluate the integrity of ear structures from the auditory nerve through the brainstem.

aura A subjective sensation or motor phenomenon that precedes and marks the onset of an episode of a neurological condition, particularly an epileptic seizure or a migraine.

*From Chabner, D-E. (2001). *The language of medicine* (6th ed.). Philadelphia: Saunders.

autism A mental state in which the child becomes absorbed in the self, excluding reality.

autoimmunity A condition in which antibodies are produced against the body's own tissues.

autonomy The state of functioning independently, without extraneous influence.

autosome Any of the chromosomes other than sex (X and Y) chromosomes.

B

baby bottle tooth decay Damage to teeth as a result of exposure to sugary acids (from constant access to a bottle of milk or juice).

bacterial agent Pertaining to bacteria (in former systems of classification, a division of the kingdom *Procaryotae*, including all prokaryotic organisms except the blue-green algae).

bargaining To negotiate the terms or conditions of a transaction. The third stage in Elizabeth Kübler-Ross's stages of grief and dying.

barrier technique A method of medical asepsis with use of various types of isolation.

bereavement An acute state of intense psychological sadness experienced after the loss of a loved one or some prized possession.

blast Immature stage in cellular development before appearance of the definitive characteristics of the cell.

bleb An irregular shaped elevation of the epidermis; a blister or bulla.

body mass index (BMI) An index for estimating obesity.

bonding Attachment; the process whereby a unique relationship is established between two people. Used in conjunction with parent-newborn infant ties.

bone marrow transplant Transplantation of bone marrow from one person to another. Currently used to treat aplastic anemia and leukemia.

booster injection Administration of a substance to renew or increase the effectiveness of a prior immunization injection (e.g., a tetanus booster).

Bradford frame A special oblong frame made of 1-inch pipe, covered with canvas strips, and supported by blocks to raise it from the mattress. The canvas strips are movable; thus the patient can urinate and defecate without moving the spine.

Broviac catheter A central venous line used in small children who need total parenteral or continuous intravenous infusion.

Bryant traction A type of traction apparatus commonly used for toddlers with a fractured femur. Vertical suspension is used. Child may not weigh more than 32 pounds.

bulimia A neurotic disorder seen in female adolescents and young women who wish to remain thin. Characterized by overeating and induced vomiting, fasting, and use of purgatives. Also called *bulimorexia*.

C

cafe-au-lait spots Light brown patch spots on the skin characteristic of neurofibromatosis (condition of tumors of various sizes on peripheral nerves).

caput succedaneum A localizing, pitting edema in the scalp of a fetus that may overlie sutures of the skull.

cardiac decompression Heart failure.

cariogenic Conducive to caries or decay.

case manager One (generally a nurse) who provides appropriate services to individuals and families through a problem-solving process.

catecholamines A group of compounds, including epinephrine and dopamine, that have a marked effect on nervous, cardiovascular, and other systems.

celiac syndrome An inability to absorb fats, which results in malnutrition, vitamin deficiency, foul bulky stools, and a distended abdomen.

cellulitis A bacterial infection of the skin, which can spread.

centering The tendency to concentrate on a single outstanding characteristic of an object while excluding its other features.

cephalhematoma Swelling caused by subcutaneous bleeding and accumulation of blood.

cephalocaudal The orderly development of muscular control, which proceeds from head to foot and from the center of the body to the periphery.

cerebral palsy A term used to describe a group of nonprogressive disorders that affect the motor centers of the brain.

cerumen Ear wax.

chickenpox A communicable disease of childhood, also known as *varicella*. It is caused by a virus and is characterized by successive crops of macules, papules, vesicles, and crusts.

Children's Bureau Government agency for child welfare.

chordee A congenital anomaly in which a fibrous strand of tissue extends from the scrotum of the penis, preventing urination with the penis in the normal elevated position. Commonly associated with hypospadias.

chorionic villi sampling (CVS) A procedure by which a sample of chorionic villa is obtained, which can provide information used in evaluation of the chromosomal, enzymatic, and DNA status of the fetus.

choroid plexus A highly vascularized area that protrudes into the lateral ventricle of the brain. Similar areas are present in the third ventricle.

chromosome A DNA-containing structure found in the nuclei of plant and animal cells and responsible for the transmission of hereditary characteristics.

chronic ulcerative colitis A serious chronic inflammatory disease of the large intestine.

circumcision The surgical removal of the foreskin of the penis.

cleft lip and palate Congenital anomalies caused by failure of the embryonic structures of the face to unite. Characterized by an opening in the upper lip or palate.

clubfoot A congenital orthopedic anomaly, characterized by a foot that has been twisted inward or outward.

cluster suicide A situation in which one suicide precipitates several others. Becoming more prevalent in the adolescent population.

coarctation of the aorta A constriction of the aortic arch or of the descending aorta.

cognition The mental process by which knowledge is acquired; awareness with perception, reasoning, judgment, intuition, and memory.

cold stress A condition that can occur in a newborn due to the inability to produce or conserve heat; can result in metabolic and physiologic problems.

comedo A skin lesion caused by a plug of keratin, sebum, and bacteria. The two types are blackheads and whiteheads.

compartment syndrome Pressure on tissues from edema or swelling, resulting in compromised circulation.

compulsive overeating An eating disorder in which people eat not because they are hungry but because they use food to satisfy emotional, rather than physical, needs.

congenital anomaly A malformation present at birth.

congenital syphilis Syphilis passed from an infected mother to the fetus. Causes multiple organ system problems including growth retardation and mucocutaneous, skeletal, hematologic, central nervous system, and ocular involvement.

contaminated Soiled, stained, or polluted; rendered unfit for use through introduction of a substance that is harmful or injurious.

cooperative play Children play with each other, often to achieve a goal, as in team sports.

corrosive A caustic agent.

cover test One eye is covered, and movement of the uncovered eye is observed while the child looks at a distant object. If the uncovered eye does not move, it is aligned. Both eyes are checked. This test is used to detect strabismus.

cradle cap A common seborrheic dermatitis of infants that consists of thick, yellow, greasy scales on the scalp.

craniosynostosis Premature closure of the cranial sutures that produces a head deformity and damage to the brain and eyes; also called *craniostenosis.*

cretinism A congenital defect in the secretion of the thyroid hormones, characterized by physical and mental retardation.

critical or clinical pathway Multidisciplinary plan that schedules clinical interventions over an anticipated time frame for high-risk, high-volume, high-cost types of cases.

critical thinking Advanced way of thinking that emphasizes process, inquiry, reasoning, creativity, and ingenuity. It is a form of analyzing and problem solving.

Crohn's disease (regional enteritis) Inflammation most often found in the anus and ileum.

croup A nonspecific term applied to a number of conditions, the chief symptom of which is a brassy (croupy) cough and varying degrees of inspiratory stridor.

cryptogenic Idiopathic (of unknown cause or spontaneous origin).

cryptorchidism Failure of the testicles to descend into the scrotum.

cystic fibrosis A generalized disorder of the exocrine glands, especially the mucous and sweat glands. The lungs and pancreas in particular are involved.

cystic hygroma A lymphangioma most frequently seen in the neck and the axillae.

D

DDST (Denver Developmental Screening Test) Used to assess the developmental status of a child during the first 6 years of life in five areas: personal, social, fine motor adaptive, language, and gross motor activities.

deciduous teeth Baby teeth.

defecate Eliminate wastes and undigested food as feces from the rectum.

denial An unconscious defense mechanism used to allay anxiety and to deny the existence of important conflicts or troublesome impulses. The first stage in Elizabeth Kübler-Ross's stages of grief and dying.

Denis Browne splint Two separate footplates attached to a crossbar and fitted to a child's shoes, used in the correction of clubfeet.

Denver II Test used to assess the developmental status of children during their first 6 years of life.

depression A temporary mental state characterized by feelings of sadness, loneliness, despair, low self-esteem, and self-reproach; accompanying signs include psychomotor retardation, withdrawal from social contact, and loss of appetite and insomnia. The fourth stage in Elizabeth Kübler-Ross's stages of grief and dying.

development Growth to full size or maturity.

diagnosis-related groups (DRGs) A group of patients classified for measuring a medical facility's delivery of care. These classifications determine Medicare insurance payments for inpatient care.

diaphoresis Profuse sweating.

disinfected Free of pathogenic organisms.

disseminated intravascular coagulation (DIC) A secondary disease characterized by abnormal overstimulation of the coagulation process.

DNA (deoxyribonucleic acid) A complex protein believed to be the storehouse of hereditary information. It is present in the chromosomes of cell nuclei.

domestic mimicry Imitation of activities parents perform such as doing the dishes.

Down syndrome A form of mental retardation caused by chromosomal defects; formerly known as *mongolism.*

dramatic play Play in which children act out roles and experiences that may have happened to them, that they fear will happen to them, or that they have observed happening to someone else.

DSM-IV Classification system for mental disorders that is clinically focused. Allows for the clinicians to diagnosis, study, and treat mental disorders. It is also used for reimbursement.

Duchenne muscular dystrophy A genetically determined progressive muscular disorder.

ductus arteriosus, patent A congenital anomaly in which the opening between the aorta and the pulmonary artery fails to close after birth.

dysarthria A speech disorder consisting of imperfect articulation due to loss of muscular control after damage to the central or peripheral nervous system.

dyscrasia A disease that is usually undefined and associated with blood disorders.

dysfunctional Inadequate, abnormal.

dysmenorrhea Pain in association with menstruation.

E

eczema An inflammation of the skin, frequently associated with an allergy to food protein or environment.

egocentrism A kind of thinking in which a child has difficulty seeing anyone else's point of view; this self-centering is normal in young children.

emancipated minor A term that generally refers to an adolescent less than 18 years of age who is no longer under parental authority.

empyema Pus, especially in the chest cavity.

encephalitis An inflammation of the brain.

encephalopathy Any degenerative disease of the brain.

encopresis The passage of stools in a child's underwear or other inappropriate places after the age of 4 years. Some children display concurrent behavioral problems.

enuresis Abnormal inability to control urine; may be the result of organic, allergic, or psychological problems.

epidemiology Study of factors that determine and influence the frequency and distribution of disease, injury, and other health-related events and their causes in a defined human population for the purpose of establishing programs to prevent and control their development and spread.

epiglottitis Inflammation and swelling of the tissues above the vocal cords. Can be life-threatening to children.

epilepsy A convulsive disease, characterized by seizures and loss of consciousness.

epispadias A congenital anomaly in which the urethral meatus is located on the upper (dorsal) surface of the penis.

erythroblastosis fetalis Physiological hemolytic anemia as the result of blood incompatibility. Associated with babies born of Rh-positive fathers and Rh-negative mothers.

esotropia An inward deviation of one or both eyes.

estrogen A generic term for estrus-producing compounds; the female sex hormones, including estradiol, estriol, and estrone.

ethical Pertaining to what is good or moral. In accordance with accepted principles governing the conduct of a group.

Ewing sarcoma Endothelioma that occurs in long bones and in flat bones such as pelvis, ribs, and scapulae.

exotropia Outward deviation of one or both eyes.

extrusion reflex Reflex that occurs in infancy when food is pushed out of the mouth by the tongue; generally disappears by about 4 months.

F

family Apgar Screening test that reveals how a member of the family perceives its function.

fetoscopy A procedure that utilizes an optical scope to visualize the fetus in the uterus.

fluorosis Condition due to exposure to excessive amounts of fluorine or its compounds.

fontanels Opening at the point of union of skull bones, often referred to as "soft spots."

foreskin The fold of loose skin covering the end of the penis; also called *prepuce*.

fulminating Occurring rapidly, usually said of a disease.

G

gavage Feeding the patient with a stomach tube or with a tube passed through the nose, pharynx, and esophagus into the stomach.

"gel" phenomenon Joint stiffness that occurs mainly in the morning or after a period of inactivity.

gender Sex; the category to which an individual is assigned on the basis of sex.

genetics The study of heredity.

geographic tongue Unusual patterns of papilla formation and denuded areas on the tongue.

glioma Sarcoma involving the support tissue or glial cells of the brain.

glomerulus A tuft or cluster; used in anatomic nomenclature as a general term to designate such a structure, as one composed of blood vessels or nerve fibers.

glucometer A meter used to measure blood glucose.

gluten The protein of wheat and other grains; it gives the dough its tough, elastic character.

grasp reflex Reflex that occurs in infancy when the palms of the infant's hands are touched and flexion occurs; generally disappears by about 3 months of age.

greenstick fracture An incomplete fracture in which one side of the bone is broken and the other is bent. A common type of fracture in children.

grief Deep sadness, as over a loss. An emotional response to an external loss.

growth The progressive development or increase in size of a living thing.

grunting Abnormal short, deep, hoarse sounds in exhalation; grunting occurs because the glottis briefly stops the flow of air.

H

habilitation A term used to describe a treatment on a patient who is handicapped from birth and therefore is learning, not relearning, a task.

Healthy People 2010 Government document listing health-related objectives for Americans.

hemangioma A benign tumor of the skin that consists of blood vessels.

hemarthrosis Extravasation of blood into a joint or its synovial cavity.

hemodynamics A study of the forces involved in circulating blood through the body.

hemophilia A hereditary disease, characterized by an abnormal tendency to bleed.

Henoch-Schönlein purpura An allergic purpura seen in children generally between the ages of 2 and 8 years. Can be caused by medication, insect bites, or other factors.

heparin lock A type of intermittent intravenous device for the administration of heparin. It does not require a continuous flow of fluids; the intravenous flow can be disconnected and the heparin lock filled with a heparin solution that maintains patency of the needle.

hernia Protrusion of an organ through an abnormal opening in the muscle wall of the cavity that surrounds it.

Hickman catheter A tiny rubber catheter that is inserted into a chest vein to establish a long-term or short-term central venous line. Used mainly in adults and teenagers. See Broviac catheter.

high risk (infant) Any neonate, regardless of birth weight, size, or gestational age, who has a greater than average chance of morbidity or mortality, especially within the first 28 days of life.

HIPAA—Health Insurance Portability and Accountability Act (1996) Designed to ensure health insurance portability for workers and families when they change or lose jobs; main focus is protection of privacy.

Hirschsprung's disease Megacolon; enlargement of the colon without evidence of mechanical obstruction. There is a congenital absence of ganglionic cells in the distal segment of the colon.

holistic An approach to caring for a child that recognizes and adapts to the physical, intellectual, emotional, and spiritual natures; a way of relating to the patient as a whole or biopsychosocial individual rather than just a person with an ailment.

homeostasis State of equilibrium of the internal environment of the body that is maintained by dynamic processes of feedback and regulation.

hospice A facility that provides palliative and supportive care for terminally ill patients and their families, either directly or on a consulting basis.

hyaline membrane disease Respiratory distress often seen in premature babies in which a membranous substance lines the alveoli of the lungs, preventing the exchange of gases.

hydrocarbon An organic compound that contains carbon and hydrogen only.

hydrocele An abnormal collection of fluid that surrounds the testicles, causing the scrotum to swell.

hydrocephalus A congenital anomaly, characterized by an increase of cerebrospinal fluid in the ventricles of the brain, which results in an increase in the size of the head and in pressure changes in the brain.

hyperbilirubinemia Excessive amount of bilirubin in the blood.

hypercapnia Increased amount of carbon dioxide in the blood.

hypernatremia Excess sodium in the blood.

hypnosis A state of altered consciousness, usually artificially induced, characterized by focusing of attention; heightened responsiveness to suggestions and commands; suspension of disbelief with lowering of critical judgment; the potential of alteration in perceptions, motor control, or memory in response to suggestions; and the subjective experience of responding involuntarily.

hypokalemia Potassium deficit in the blood.

hypospadias A developmental anomaly in which the urethra opens on the lower surface of the penis.

hypotonic Pertinent to defective muscular tone or tension. A solution of lower osmotic pressure than that of a reference solution or of an isotonic solution.

I

identification A defense mechanism by which an individual unconsciously takes as his or her own the characteristics, postures, achievements, or other identifying traits of other persons or groups.

identity The aggregate of characteristics by which an individual is recognized by herself or himself and others.

idiopathic Of unknown cause or spontaneous origin.

imaginary friends Made-up friends to which preschoolers talk and behave as though they are really present in the room.

immunization Induction of immunity, which is the protection against infectious disease.

imperforate anus A congenital anomaly in which there is no anal opening.

impetigo An infectious disease of the skin, caused by staphylococci or streptococci.

in vitro fertilization Test tube fertilization in which the ripe ovum is collected and fertilized in vitro (glass) with sperm. The embryo is then transferred to the woman's uterus.

incarcerated Confined, constricted.

incest Sexual activities among family members. Often seen in father-daughter relationships, less frequently in mother-son or sibling relationships.

infant mortality The ratio between the number of deaths of infants less than 1 year of age during any given year and the number of live births occurring in the same year.

infanticide The killing of an infant.

infarct An area of tissue in an organ or part that undergoes necrosis after cessation of blood supply.

infectious mononucleosis A generalized disease that causes enlargement of the lymph tissues throughout the body. The number of mononuclear leukocytes in the blood is increased. It occurs mainly in older children and adolescents.

intention tremor When beginning a voluntary movement, there is a resultant trembling that affects the body part being used and worsens as the individual gets nearer to the desired object; often seen in patients with cerebral palsy.

interatrial septal defect An abnormal opening between the right and left atria of the heart. Blood that contains oxygen is forced from the left to the right atrium.

intertrigo A superficial dermatitis in the folds of the skin.

interventricular septal defect An opening between the right and left ventricles of the heart. Blood passes directly from the left to the right ventricle.

intimacy Of a very personal, private nature.

intussusception The slipping of one part of the intestine into another part just below it, often noted in the ileocecal region.

iridocyclitis An inflammation of the iris and ciliary body of the eye.

J

Jones criteria Cluster of major and minor manifestations that help in the diagnosis of acute rheumatic fever.

juvenile rheumatoid arthritis (JRA) A collection of inflammatory diseases that involve the joints, connective tissues, and viscera.

K

karyotype The chromosomal makeup of a normal body cell.

kernicterus A grave form of jaundice of the neonate, accompanied by brain damage.

ketogenic (diet) Diet used in seizure patients in which ketone bodies are formed.

Kohlberg Theorist who described moral development in children

kwashiorkor Extreme protein malnutrition seen in infants and children living in poverty.

L

lanugo Soft downy hair covering a normal fetus beginning in the fifth month of gestation and almost entirely shed by the ninth month.

laryngotracheobronchitis Inflammation of the larynx, trachea, and bronchi.

latchkey child A child who comes home to an empty house (after school) because the parent(s) are at work.

latent Dormant or concealed; not manifest.

lecithin/sphingomyelin or L/S (ratio) The ratio of two components of amniotic fluid; used for predicting fetal lung maturity.

legal Of or relating to the law. Authorized or based on law. Established by law. In conformity with or permitted by law.

Legg-Calvé-Perthes disease Inadequate blood supply to the head of the femur, characterized by pain in the hip joint; also called *flat hip.*

lichenification Cutaneous thickening and hardening of the skin as a result of continual irritation.

Lonalac Low-salt formula.

lumbar puncture Insertion of a hollow needle into the subarachnoid space between the third and fourth vertebrae; also called *spinal puncture* and *spinal tap.*

lupus erythematosus A chronic inflammatory disease of collagen or connective tissue that may be life-threatening.

M

macrosomia Abnormally large size.

Maslow's hierarchy of needs Maslow was a humanistic theorist who theorized that basic human needs are organized into a hierarchy of relative priority from lower-order requirements to higher-order needs.

maturation The full development of adult characteristics (e.g., the development of adult organs or tissue); the development of emotional maturity.

mature minor doctrine Recognizes that individuals mature at different rates.

Meckel's diverticulum A congenital blind pouch, sometimes seen in the lower part of the ileum. A cord may continue to the umbilicus, or a fistula may open at the umbilicus. An intestinal obstruction may occur if the cord becomes strangulated. Corrected with surgery.

meconium The first stool of the newborn; a mixture of amniotic fluid and secretions of the intestinal glands.

meconium ileus A deficiency of pancreatic enzymes in the intestinal tract of the fetus in which the meconium becomes excessively sticky and adheres to the intestinal wall, causing obstruction. Occasionally seen in babies born with cystic fibrosis.

mediastinum The mass of tissues and organs separating the two pleural sacs, between the sternum anteriorly and the vertebral column posteriorly and from the thoracic inlet superiorly to the diaphragm inferiorly. It contains the heart and pericardium, the bases of the great vessels, the trachea and bronchi, esophagus, thymus, lymph nodes, thoracic duct, phrenic and vagus nerves, and other structures and tissues.

megacolon *See* Hirschsprung's disease.

menarche Establishment or beginning of the menstrual function.

meningocele A congenital anomaly, characterized by a protrusion of the meninges or membranes through an opening in the spinal column.

meningomyelocele A congenital anomaly, characterized by a protrusion of the membranes and spinal cord through an opening in the spinal column.

metabolic rate The rate of utilization of energy.

microcephaly A congenital anomaly in which the head of the newborn infant is abnormally small.

miliaria Prickly heat; an inflammation of the skin caused by sweating.

mittelschmerz Abdominal pain midway between menstrual periods, occurring at time of ovulation and from the ovulation site.

modeling A behavior modification technique in which the patient is taught to imitate the desired behavior of another.

mongolism *See* Down syndrome.

morbidity Illness, chronic disease, disability.

Moro reflex When newborn infants are jarred, they draw the legs up and fold the arms across the chest in an embrace position.

mucoviscidosis *See* Cystic fibrosis.

multifactorial The result of many factors, such as a disease resulting from the combined action of several conditions.

murmur A sound heard when listening to the heart, caused by blood leaking through openings that have not closed before birth as they normally do.

muscular dystrophy Wasting away and atrophy of muscles. There are several forms, all with some common characteristics.

mutation A change in genetic material.

myelinization Production of myelin around an axon (of certain nerve fibers).

N

negativism Opposition to suggestions or advice; an attitude or behavior opposite to that appropriate to a specific situation.

nephroblastoma Kidney tumor.

neural tube defects (NTDs) Defective closures of the neural tube during early embryogenesis. Included are fetal anencephaly, spina bifida, lumbar meningomyelocele, and meningocele.

neutropenic Having a decrease in the number of neutrophils (mature granular leukocytes) in the blood.

nevus (pl. nevi) A congenital discoloration of an area of the skin, such as a strawberry mark or mole.

Niemann-Pick disease A hereditary disease in which there is a disturbance in the metabolism of lipids (substances resembling fats), causing physical and mental retardation.

nomogram Representation by graphs, diagrams, or charts of the relationship between numerical variables.

nuchal Pertaining to the neck.

nurse practitioner A registered nurse who has well-developed competencies in utilization of a broad range of cues. These cues are used for prescribing and implementing both direct and indirect nursing care and for articulating nursing therapies with other planned therapies. They demonstrate expertise in nursing practice and ensure ongoing development of expertise through clinical experience and continuing education.

Nursing Interventions Classifications (NIC) A comprehensive, standardized grouping of interventions or actions that nurses perform.

Nursing Outcomes Classifications (NOC) Outcomes that serve as criteria against which to judge the success of nursing interventions.

nystagmus Constant, involuntary, cyclical movement of the eyeball.

O

occlusion Obstruction.

olecranon A large process of the ulna projecting behind the elbow joint and forming the bony prominence of the elbow.

omphalocele A herniation of the abdominal contents through the umbilicus.

ophthalmia neonatorum Acute conjunctivitis of the newborn infant, often caused by *Neisseria gonorrhoeae* and *Chlamydia trachomatis.*

opisthotonos A form of spasm in which head and heels are bent backwards and body is bowed forward. Caused by titanic spasm.

orthopnea A disorder in which the patient has to sit up to breathe.

Osgood-Schlatter disease Tendinitis of the knee, seen in adolescents and adults who participate in sports.

ossification Formation of bone substance.

osteochondroma Benign tumor composed of cartilage and bone.

osteogenesis imperfecta A congenital bone disease in which the bones fracture easily.

osteosarcoma The malignant bone tumor most frequently encountered in children.

otitis media Inflammation of the middle ear.

ototoxic Causing damage to the vestibulocochlear nerve or the organs of hearing and balance.

P

pain An unpleasant sensation arising from injury, disease, or emotional disorder. Pain is whatever the person experiencing it says it is and existing whenever he/she says it does.

palliative care Care and comfort at the end of life. Reducing the severity of the symptoms. Alleviation of symptoms without curing the underlying disease.

palpation The act of feeling with the hand; the application of the fingers with tight pressure to the surface of the body for the purpose of determining the consistency of the parts beneath in physical diagnosis.

papilledema Edema and inflammation of the optic nerve at its point of entrance into the eyeball.

parachute reflex Protective arm extension that occurs when an infant is suddenly thrust downward when prone.

parallel play A type of play that emerges in toddlerhood when children play side by side with similar or different toys, demonstrating little or no social interaction.

paraphimosis Impaired circulation of the uncircumcised penis caused by improper retraction of the foreskin.

patent ductus arteriosus One of the most common cardiac anomalies, in which the ductus arteriosus fails to close. Blood continues to flow from the aorta into the pulmonary artery.

peak expiratory flow rate (PEFR) The force of expiration from maximum lung inflation.

pectus excavatum A variation in the normal configuration of the chest in which the lower portion of the sternum is depressed.

pediatric nurse practitioner Master's-prepared nurse that cares for children generally in an outpatient setting; often collaborates with the physician.

pediatrics Branch of medicine that deals with children.

percutaneous umbilical blood sample (PUBS) A procedure that involves the aspiration of a sample of fetal blood from the umbilical vein of the fetus.

petechiae Small, purplish, hemorrhagic spots on the skin that appear in certain severe fevers and are indicative of great prostration. May be caused by abnormality of blood-clotting mechanisms.

phagocytosis The engulfing of microorganisms or other cells and foreign particles by phagocytes (any cell capable of ingesting particulate matter).

phenylketonuria (PKU) An inborn error of metabolism causing retardation; the body is unable to use phenylalanine, an amino acid.

phimosis A tightening of the prepuce of the uncircumcised penis.

physiologic anorexia A decrease in appetite manifested when the extremely high metabolic demands of infancy slow to keep pace with the more moderate growth of toddlerhood.

Piaget Swiss philosopher and psychologist (1896-1980) whose work provided understanding of how children's thinking differs from adults' and of how children learn.

pica Abnormal appetite, or compulsive ingestion of nonfood substances such as paint, clay, or crayons.

pincer grasp The thumb and index finger are coordinated, and grasping is achievable.

play therapy A technique used in child psychotherapy in which play is used to reveal unconscious material.

plumbism Lead poisoning.

poliomyelitis An acute infectious disease of the brain stem and spinal cord.

polydactyly A developmental anomaly characterized by the presence of extra fingers or toes.

postictal Occurring after a seizure.

prehension Use of hands to pick up small objects; grasping.

premenstrual syndrome (PMS) A syndrome that occurs several days before the onset of menstruation and ends a short time after the onset of menstruation.

previability Fetus incapable of extrauterine existence.

primary dysmenorrhea Painful menstruation associated with the menstrual cycle in the absence of organic pelvic disease.

prodromal (symptoms) Indicating the onset of disease.

prognosis A forecast of the probably outcome of an attack of disease.

proximodistal development Directional pattern of growth where development proceeds from the center of the body to the periphery.

puberty Period in life at which members of both genders become functionally capable of reproduction.

pulse oximeter Photoelectric apparatus for determining the amount of oxygen in the blood with measurement of the amount of light transmitted through a translucent part of the skin.

pulse oximetry A pulse oximeter is a photoelectric device that uses an infrared light to measure the amount of saturated arterial hemoglobin (oxyhemoglobin) during a pulse. Accuracy is influenced by adequate blood flow.

pyloric stenosis A congenital narrowing of the pylorus of the stomach as the result of an enlarged muscle.

R

rapport Harmonious relationship.

rectal prolapse A dropping or protrusion of the mucosa of the rectum through the anus.

respiratory distress syndrome An acute lung disease of the newborn, caused by a deficiency of pulmonary surfactant.

respiratory syncytial virus (RSV) A virus that induces formation of syncytial masses in infected cell cultures. A major cause of acute respiratory disease in children.

respite care Health care providers who assist parents in the home setting care for children with chronic or developmental illness.

retrolental fibroplasia Blindness usually found in preterm infants that is associated with high oxygen concentrations and in which the blood vessels of the retina become damaged.

Reye syndrome Acute encephalopathy with fatty degeneration of the liver, characterized by fever and impaired consciousness.

rhabdomyosarcoma Extremely malignant neoplasm that originates in skeletal muscle.

RICE *Rest, ice, compression, and elevation; used to treat soft tissue injury.

rickets A disease of the bones, caused by lack of calcium or vitamin D.

ritual In psychiatry, a series of repetitive acts performed compulsively to relieve anxiety, as in obsessive-compulsive neurosis.

rooting reflex The infant turns the head toward anything that touches the cheek, as a means of reaching food.

roseola Self-limited infection manifested by high fever followed by maculopapular rash. The child appears well otherwise and usually remains active.

rubella German measles.

rubeola Measles.

S

scoliosis Lateral curvature of the spine.

scurvy A disease caused by the lack of vitamin C in the diet and characterized by joint pains, bleeding gums, loose teeth, and lack of energy.

sebum A fatty secretion of the sebaceous glands of the skin.

self-image How a person views himself or herself.

shunt A bypass.

sibling rivalry Emotional conflict between siblings (brothers and sisters) that arises from a competition for the love, attention, and approval of one or both parents.

sickle cell anemia A disease associated with an inherited defect in the synthesis of hemoglobin, producing sickled cells.

SIDS (sudden infant death syndrome) The sudden and unexpected death of an apparently healthy infant, typically occurring between the ages of 3 weeks and 5 months and not explained by careful postmortem studies; also called *crib death* or *cot death.*

Snellen alphabet chart A device used to measure near and far vision; a variation is the Snellen E chart.

spina bifida A congenital defect in which there is an imperfect closure of the spinal canal.

Standard Precautions Guidelines recommended by the Centers for Disease Control and Prevention (CDC) to reduce the risk for transmission of blood-borne and other pathogens in the hospital.

syndrome of inappropriate antidiuretic hormone (SIADH) Increased ADH activity in spite of reduced plasma osmolarity. First recognized by a relative hyponatremia; most commonly associated with CNS disorders, various tumors, and drugs.

T

talipes equinovarus *See* Clubfoot.

tantrum A violent display of temper.

Tay-Sachs disease A degenerative, fatal brain disease caused by a lack of hexosaminidase A in all body tissues. Seen mostly in Eastern European Jews and genetically transmitted.

tenesmus Spasmodic contraction of anal or vesical sphincter with pain and persistent desire to empty the bowel or bladder, with involuntary ineffectual straining efforts.

tetralogy of Fallot A congenital heart defect involving pulmonary stenosis, ventricular septal defect, dextroposition of the aorta, and hypertrophy of the right ventricle.

thalassemia A hereditary blood disorder in which the patient's body cannot produce sufficient hemoglobin.

thelarche The beginning of breast development.

therapeutic holding A secure, comfortable, temporary holding position that provides close physical contact with the parents or caregivers.

thrombosis The formation, development, or existence of a blood clot, or thrombus within the vascular system.

thrush An infection of the mucous membranes of the mouth or throat caused by the fungus *Candida.*

tinea A contagious fungus infection; ringworm.

TORCH Acronym used to describe a group of infections that represent potentially severe fetal problems if infection occurs during pregnancy. *TO,* Toxoplasmosis; *R,* rubella; *C,* cytomegalovirus; and *H,* herpesvirus.

torticollis A condition in which the head inclines to one side because of a shortening of either sternocleidomastoid muscle. Also called *wryneck.*

total parenteral nutrition (TPN) Providing for all nutritional needs by administration of liquids into the blood; used in life-threatening conditions. Also called *hyperalimentation.*

toxin A poison; frequently used to refer specifically to a protein produced by some higher plants, certain animals, and pathogenic bacteria, which is highly toxic for other living organisms.

tracheoesophageal fistula The esophagus, instead of being an open tube from the throat to the stomach, is closed at some point. A fistula between the trachea and the esophagus is common.

transfusion The introduction of whole blood or blood components directly into the bloodstream.

transillumination Inspection of a cavity or organ by passing a light through its walls. When pus or lesion is present, the transmission of light is diminished or absent.

transitional object A child's favorite possession brought from home to ease the transition into the hospital and promote the child's sense of control.

transport team A team or group of health care professionals that move a patient from one place to another.

triage The sorting out and classification of casualties to determine priority of need and proper place of treatment.

tripod position Posturing that a child uses when in respiratory distress; the child sits upright, leaning forward, with the chin up and mouth open while leaning on the arms.

truncus arteriosus A single arterial trunk leaves the ventricular portion of the heart and supplies the pulmonary, coronary, and systemic circulations.

tuberculosis A disease caused by the tubercle bacillus and characterized by inflammatory infiltration, formation of tubercles, caseation, necrosis, abscesses, fibrosis, and calcification. Commonly affects the respiratory system but can affect other body parts.

turgor Elasticity of the skin.

tympanography Process of recording the relative compliance and impedance of the tympanic membrane and ossicles (small bones) of the middle ear.

tympanometry Measurement of mobility of the tympanic membrane of the ear and estimation of middle ear pressure.

U

uncover test Test in which the eye is covered and the child looks at a light source. When the eye is quickly uncovered, it should not move; this indicates alignment. Used to detect strabismus.

V

varicella Chickenpox.

variola Smallpox.

ventriculography Radiographic examination of the ventricles of the brain after the injection of air into the ventricles.

vernix caseosa A cheeselike substance that covers the skin of a newborn infant.

viral agent One of a group of minute infectious agents (with certain exceptions, such as poxviruses) not resolved in the light microscope; characterized by a lack of independent metabolism and by the ability to replicate only within living host cells.

volvulus A twisting of the loops of the small intestine, causing obstruction.

W

weaning Discontinuation of breastfeeding of an infant, with substitution of other feeding habits.

wheal Large, slightly raised red or blistered area of skin; may itch.

White House Conference on Children and Youth Government commission that issued recommendations for children and their well-being.

Wilms tumor A malignant tumor of the kidneys.

Z

zygote A fertilized egg.

Index

A

Abdomen, 32t
Abduction, 285
Absence seizure, 253t
Abuse, child, 170-175, 171f-172f, 174f, 203
Accidents, 188-190, 192, 234, 336
Acetaminophen
  poisoning caused by, 216-217, 217t
  suppositories, 46
Acne vulgaris, 338-340, 339f
Acquired immunodeficiency syndrome,
  86-89, 359t
Acrocyanosis, 52
Activated charcoal, 216
Active listening, 6
Acupuncture, 46
Acute glomerulonephritis, 257-258, 259t
Acute lymphoblastic leukemia, 241, 242t,
  243
Acute myeloid leukemia, 241
Acute otitis media, 142-143, 143b
Acute rheumatic fever, 308, 311-312
Adenoiditis, 247-249
Admission to hospital, 28-29
Adolescence
  chronic illness during, 330-331
  definition of, 324
  growth and development during, 327t
Adolescent
  biological development of, 324-325
  career plans for, 328-329
  confidentiality concerns, 332-333
  dating by, 330
  death as perceived by, 402t
  dental care by, 335
  developmentally disabled, 331
  diabetes mellitus in, 302t
  dying, 402
  emancipated minor doctrine, 333
  emotional needs of, 329-330
  gastrointestinal disorders in, 342-345
  genitourinary disorders in, 352-362
  growth and development of, 324-331
  health examination of, 332-333
  health promotion and maintenance for,
    331-337
  hematologic disorders in, 340
  heterosexual relationships, 330
  hospitalization reactions by, 27
  hygiene by, 335
  independence by, 324, 326
  Internet solicitation of, 337
  lymphatic system disorders in, 340-342
  medication administration to, 383t
  musculoskeletal disorders in, 345-352
  nutrition for, 334-335
  oxygen therapy for, 398t
  parents/parenting of, 327t, 331-332
  peer influences, 328
  preventive health care recommendations
    for, 413-414
  responsibility by, 329
  safety concerns, 335
  self-concept concerns, 324, 326
  sexuality of, 333-334

Page numbers followed by f indicate figures;
t, tables; b, boxes

Adolescent—cont'd
  skin disorders in, 338-340
  sleep requirements for, 335
Adolescent pregnancy, 362-363
Aerosol therapy, for cystic fibrosis, 154
African-Americans, 7t
Aganglionic megacolon. See Hirschsprung's
  disease
Airway
  in newborn, 48-49
  tracheostomy. See Tracheostomy
Albuterol, 305t
Alcohol, 366t
Allergens, 136
Aloneness, 403
Alopecia, 245
Alpha-fetoprotein, 15
Amblyopia, 240-241
American Academy of Pediatrics, 2, 42
American Pain Society, 42
Amniocentesis, 15, 15f
Amyl nitrite, 370t
Anabolic steroids, 335, 370t
Anastomosis, 95
Anemia, iron-deficiency, 144-145
Animal bites, 192
Animism, 25, 220, 222t
Anorexia nervosa
  description of, 343-344
  medication-induced, 322
  nursing care for, 344-345
  physiological, 183
  signs and symptoms of, 344
  treatment of, 344
Anthelmintics, 202
Anthrax, 5-6, 263t
Anticipatory grieving, 405-406
Anticipatory guidance, 6, 280
Anticonvulsants, 254, 255t
Antigliadin antibody test, 250
Antihistamines, 137
Anti-IgE antibodies, 305t
Antiinflammatory drugs, 311
Antiretroviral medications, 86b
Anuria, 57
Apgar score, 50, 50t, 56
Apnea, 75-76
  infantile, 169
Appendectomy, 313
Appendicitis, 312-314
Art therapy, 233
Arthritis. See Juvenile rheumatoid arthritis
Arthroscopy, 350
Artificialism, 222, 222t
Asepsis, medical, 38-39
Aspartame, 300
Aspirin toxicity, 217
Asthma
  classification of, 304b
  description of, 303
  exacerbations of, 307
  management skills for, 307-308
  nursing care plan for, 309b-310b
  self-care skills for, 307-308
  signs and symptoms of, 304

Asthma—cont'd
  treatment of
    gas exchange, 307
    hydration, 307
    medications, 304-307, 305t
    metered-dose inhaler, 304, 306f
Astrocytoma, 319t
Ataxia, 209
Atelectasis, 73
Athetoid cerebral palsy, 209
Atomoxetine, 322t
Atopic dermatitis, 136-140
Atraumatic care, 372
Atrial septal defect, 94, 95f
Attachment, 68
Attention deficit/hyperactivity disorder,
  321-323
Audiometry/audiometer, 196
Auditory brainstem response, 56
Aura, 253
Auscultation, of blood pressure, 33
Autism, 131, 215, 260, 262
Automatisms, 254
Autonomy, 178, 401t
Autosomes, 12
Autosyringe, 388
Axillary temperature measurements, 34, 78
Azotemia, 391

B

Baby. See Infant; Newborn
Baby bottle tooth decay, 134, 181
Back, 32t
Baclofen, 210
Bacterial infections, 113
Bacterial meningitis, 165-167
Bad language, 226-227
Bathing, 67-68, 137, 373-374
Battered child syndrome, 170
Beclomethasone dipropionate, 305t
Behavioral disorders, 320-323
Benevolence, 401t
Bereavement, 406
Bicycle safety, 286, 286f
Biofeedback, 403b
Birth defects, 85-86
Biting, 179t
Black cohosh, 9t
Bladder training, 186
Bleeding. See also Hemorrhage
  in hemophilia patients, 247
  in leukemia patients, 244-245
Blood glucose monitoring, 296b, 298-299
Blood pressure
  definition of, 32
  measurement of, 32-34
  of newborn, 52
Blood pressure cuffs, 33f, 40
Blood specimens, 376, 378, 378f
Body mass index, 17, 17b, 342
Body piercings, 334
Body proportions, 16
Body spica cast, 108
Body surface area, 380
Body temperature
  in head-injured patients, 213
  measurement of, 34, 51-52
  newborn assessments, 51-52

Body temperature—cont'd
  normal ranges for, 34t
  postnatal changes in, 51
  in preterm infant, 78
Body weight composition, 390f
Bonding, 68, 82f, 174
Bone growth, 17
Bone marrow transplantation, 243
Bottle feeding, 65-66
Bowel training, 186
Bracing, for scoliosis, 345, 347f
Brain tumors, 318-320
Brazelton Neonatal Behavioral Assessment
    Scale, 61
Breast engorgement, 64
Breast milk, 63-64, 132
Breast self-examination, 325
Breastfeeding
  advantages of, 62-63
  contraindications, 63
  problems with, 64
  technique of, 63, 64b
  weaning from, 134
Breathing. *See* Respirations
Bronchiolitis, 149-151
Bronchitis, 199
Bronchodilators, 304
Bronchopulmonary dysplasia, 75, 151-152
Brown fat, 50
Bryant traction, 203-204
Buck extension traction, 205f
Budesonide, 305t
Bulb syringe, 67, 373, 373f, 375
Bulimia, 345
Bullying, 280, 281b
Burn(s)
  depth of, 236, 238t
  description of, 236
  emotional issues, 240
  fluid resuscitation for, 239
  full-thickness, 236-237, 238t, 239f
  nutritional management, 240
  pain control, 240
  partial-thickness, 236-237, 238t
  preschool child, 234, 236-240
  prevention of, 190
  scald, 192
  scarring from, 239-240
  signs and symptoms of, 236-237, 237f-238f
  total body surface area calculations, 237f
  treatment of, 237, 239
  wound management, 239-240
Burn shock, 239
Burning, 7
Butyl nitrite, 370t

C

Calcium, 182, 335
Calcium disodium edetate, 218
Camp nurses, 10-11
Capsules, 381-382
Caput succedaneum, 52, 53f
Car seat, 189, 192, 234
Carbamazepine, 255t
Carbohydrates, 300, 335
Cardiovascular disorders
  acute rheumatic fever, 308, 311-312
  congenital heart disease. *See* Congenital
      heart disease
  newborn, 92-101
  in school-age child, 308, 311-312
  treatment of, 99-101
Career plans, 328-329
Case manager, 10
Cast
  body spica, 108
  clubfoot treatment with, 106

Cast—cont'd
  developmental dysplasia of the hip treated
      with, 108-109
  fractures treated with, 202, 203f
Catheterization, for urine specimen
    collection, 375
Catheters, 388
Catholic, 8t
Celiac sprue, 249-250
Cellulitis, 140
Centering, 222
Centers for Disease Control and Prevention,
    39
Cephalhematoma, 52, 53f
Cephalocaudal development, 16
Cerebellar astrocytoma, 319t
Cerebral palsy
  athetoid, 209
  causative factors, 204, 206
  definition of, 204
  dyskinetic, 209
  infant weight and, 206
  mental health needs, 211
  nursing care for, 210-211
  signs and symptoms of, 206, 209-210
  spastic, 209
  treatment of, 210
Cerebrospinal fluid, 110
Cervical traction, 205f-206f
Chancre, 360
Chelating agents, for lead poisoning, 218
Chemotherapy
  in adolescent, 341t
  brain tumors treated with, 320
  leukemia treated with, 243
  nausea and vomiting caused by, 245
Chest
  assessment of, 32t
  circumference of, 178
Chest tubes, 100
Chickenpox, 263t, 270b, 270f
Child. *See* Adolescent; Infant; Newborn;
    Preschool child; School-age child; Toddler
Child abduction, 285
Child abuse and neglect, 170-175, 171f-172f,
    174f, 203
Child Coma Scale, 213, 214t
Child health
  cultural considerations, 6-8
  government programs, 2, 3t
  history of, 1
  preventive health care recommendations,
      412-414
  religious considerations, 6-8
Child predators, 337
Child Protective Services, 172
Childhood mortality, 3
Children's Bureau, 2
Chinese-Americans, 7t
Chiropractors, 46
Chlamydia, 353, 354t
Chlamydial ophthalmia, 62
Chlorthiazide, 100
Choking, 183, 190-193, 193f
Chordee, 168
Chorea, 312
Chorionic villi sampling, 15
Choroid plexus, 111
Christian Scientist, 8t
Chromosomes, 12-14
Chronic illness, 330-331
Circulatory system, 56-57
Circumcision, 57, 58f
Clean-catch urine specimen, 373, 375
Cleft lip, 101-102, 103f
Cleft palate, 102-104
Clonazepam, 255t

Clubbing, 93f, 95
Clubfoot, 106, 106f
Cluster suicide, 363
Coarctation of the aorta, 94-95, 97f
Cocaine, 368t
Cognition, 19
Cognitive development, 19-20
Cognitive intellect, 19
Coining, 7, 174f
Colic, 122b
Colostomy, 393
Colostrum, 63
Coma, 213, 214t
Comedo, 338
Comminuted fracture, 203f
Common cold, 148-149
Communicable diseases, 260, 263t-269t
Communication
  with adolescent, 329
  methods of, 401
  with toddler, 180-181
Compartment syndrome, 202
Complementary and alternative medicine,
    8-9, 46
Compound fracture, 202
Compulsive overeating, 342
Concussion, 212t, 350b
Conditioned responses, 61
Conduction, 51t
Conductive hearing loss, 195-196
Confidentiality, 332-333, 401t
Congenital heart disease
  atrial septal defect, 94, 95f
  classification of, 92-93
  coarctation of the aorta, 94-95, 97f
  description of, 92
  hypoplastic left heart syndrome, 96, 99f
  patent ductus arteriosus, 93-94
  signs and symptoms of, 92b, 93
  tetralogy of Fallot, 95-97, 98f
  transposition of the great arteries, 96, 98f
  ventricular septal defect, 94, 96f
Congestive heart failure, 96-97
Constipation, 60
Contractures, 210
Contusion, 212t
Convection, 51t
Convulsive seizures, 253
Cor pulmonale, 153
Cord. *See* Umbilical cord
Corneal light reflex, 241
Corrosives, 216
Corticosteroids, 305t
Cow's milk, 132
Crack, 368t
Cradle cap, 53
Cradle position, 38f
Credé's method, 114
Critical thinking, 29-30
Cromolyn sodium, 305t
Croup, 197-199, 198f
Cryotherapy, 77
Cryptorchidism, 167
Culture (family), 6-8
Culture (specimen)
  nasopharyngeal, 378-379
  throat, 378, 379b
Cushing triad, 213
Cuts, 191
Cyanosis, 97
Cystic fibrosis
  complications of, 153-154
  description of, 152
  emotional support for, 155-156
  hygiene considerations, 154-155
  long-term care for, 155
  nursing care plan for, 157-159

Cystic fibrosis—cont'd
  pancreatic involvement in, 152-153
  signs and symptoms of, 152-153
  treatment of, 154

D

Dactylitis, 145, 147f, 147t
Dancing reflex, 56
Dantrolene, 210
Date rape, 330
Dating, 330
Daycare, 188
Daydreams, 330
Deafness, 195-197
Death and dying. *See also* End-of-life care
  of adolescent, 336, 402
  anxiety about, 402
  care after, 406
  child's reaction and awareness of, 402-403
  cultural issues, 404
  ethical issues, 400-401, 401t
  family considerations, 403-404, 406
  fears associated with, 403
  hospice care, 404-405
  legal issues, 400-401
  palliative care, 401-402
  preparations for, 405-406
  preschool child's awareness of, 225
  reflection on, 406-407
  self-exploration before, 400
  sibling reactions to, 404
  signs and symptoms of, 405-406, 406b
  stages of, 404
Decerebrate posturing, 211, 213f
Deciduous teeth, 134, 135f
Decorticate posturing, 211, 213f
Dehydration, 90b, 100, 163-165, 389
Deltoid, injections in, 384, 386f
Dental health
  for adolescent, 336
  for toddler, 181-182
Denver II Developmental Screening Test, 128, 169, 180
Depakene. *See* Valproic acid
Department of Health and Human Services, 6
Dependence, 365
Depression, 363-365
Dermabrasion, 339
Desferrioxamine, 147
Desmopressin acetate, 228, 247
Desquamation, 59
Development. *See* Growth and development
Developmental disability
  in adolescent, 331
  autism, 131, 215, 260, 262
  definition of, 260
  IQ scores, 270
  mental retardation, 262, 270-271
  nursing care for, 271-272
  parental considerations, 272
  signs and symptoms of, 270-271
  treatment of, 271-272
Developmental dysplasia of the hip, 107-109
Dextroamphetamine (Dexedrine), 322t
Diabetes mellitus
  acidosis in, 295f
  in adolescent, 302t
  alcohol intake, 303
  blood glucose monitoring, 296b, 298-299
  classification of, 293, 294t
  definition of, 292
  description of, 292-293
  exercise for, 300
  family effects, 301
  foot care in, 300
  glucose-insulin imbalances in, 301

Diabetes mellitus—cont'd
  hypoglycemia management, 298, 299b
  incidence of, 293-294
  in infant, 302t
  insulin for, 296t, 296-298, 297t
  insulin-dependent, 292-293
  maternal, 83
  nurse's role, 303
  nutritional management of, 299-300, 303
  in preschool child, 302t
  psychosocial considerations, 301
  signs and symptoms of, 294-295
  skin care considerations, 300
  stress associated with, 302b
  in toddler, 302t
  travel considerations, 301
  treatment of, 295-301
  urine checks, 300-301
Diabetic ketoacidosis, 294-295, 301
Diagnosis-related groups, 4
Diarrhea, 89-91
Diet. *See* Feeding; Foods; Nutrition
Digestion, 59-60
Digoxin, 99-100
Dilantin. *See* Phenytoin
Diphtheria
  characteristics of, 264t
  diphtheria-tetanus-pertussis vaccine for, 130, 130t, 408-409
Discharge planning, 30-31
Discharge teaching, 69
Discipline
  consistency in, 226
  for preschool child, 225-226
  for toddler, 179-180
Dislocations, 204
Distraction, 403b
Diuretics, 100
Divorce, 285
DNA, 18
Documentation, 30
Dominant gene, 12
Dominant inheritance, 13f
Dorsogluteal injection site, 384, 387f
Down syndrome, 12-13, 109-110, 111t
Dramatic play, 26
Drawings, 26-27
Dressing up, 222, 222f
Drooling, 134
Drowning, 191, 234
Drug reactions, 380
Duchenne muscular dystrophy, 250-251, 251f
Ductus arteriosus, 93
Dunlop traction, 205f-206f
Dying. *See* Death and dying
Dysarthria, 209
Dyskinetic cerebral palsy, 209
Dysmenorrhea, 352-353

E

Ear(s)
  assessment of, 32t
  disorders of
    in infant, 141-144
    otitis media, 141-144
    in toddler, 195-197
Eardrops, 384
Early Language Milestone Scale, 128
Eating disorders
  anorexia nervosa. *See* Anorexia nervosa
  bulimia, 345
Echinacea, 9t
Ectasy. *See* 3, 4-Methylenedioxymethamphetamine
Eczema, infantile, 136-140

Edema
  in congenital heart disease, 99
  periorbital, 258
  treatment of, 258
Egocentrism, 220, 222t
8-year-old child, 275t-276t, 277
Elbow dislocation, 204
Elbow restraint, 39f, 39t
Elective surgery, 10
Electrical shock, 192
Electroencephalography, 318
Electromyogram, 250
Emancipated minor, 333
Emergency preparedness, 4-6
EMLA, 46, 385
Emotional disorders, 320-323
En face position, 68, 68f, 115
Encephalitis, 251-252
Endocrine disorders, 292-303
End-of-life care. *See also* Death and dying
  palliative care, 401-402
  psychosocial issues in, 401b
Enema, 391-393, 393t
Enterobius vermicularis, 201. *See also* Pinworms
Enuresis, 228
Ependymoma, 319t
Epicanthal folds, 241
Epiglottitis, 199, 200f
Epilepsy, 252-256
Epinephrine, racemic, 198-199
Epispadias, 167-168, 168f
Epstein-Barr virus, 340
Equinovarus, 106
Erikson, Erik, 19, 21t, 24, 178, 274, 326
Erythema infectiosum, 264t
Erythema marginatum, 311f
Erythroblastosis fetalis, 115-116
Esophageal atresia, 104-106
Esotropia, 241, 241f
Ethical decision making, 6
Ethics, 400-401, 401t
Eustachian tube, 142
Evaporation, 51t
Evidence-based practice, 6
Exanthema subitum, 265t
Exercise
  by adolescent, 335
  diabetes mellitus managed with, 300
  intolerance of, in congenital heart disease, 99
Exercise-induced bronchospasm, 304
Exotropia, 241
Extremely low-birth weight, 71
Extremities, 32t
Extrusion reflex, 131
Eye(s). *See also* Vision
  assessment of, 32t
  in school-age child, 273
Eye disorders
  amblyopia, 240-241
  in preschool child, 240-241
  strabismus, 241, 241f
Eyedrops, 384, 385f
Eyewear, 41

F

Factor IX deficiency, 246
Factor VIII deficiency, 246
Failure to thrive, 169-170
Falls, 190
Family. *See also* Parents
  of diabetes mellitus patient, 301
  discharge teaching for, 69
  of dying patient, 403-404, 406
  education of, 41
  hospitalization reactions by, 27-28

Family—cont'd
parenthood transition for, 68
of preterm infant, 82-83
structure of, 19
Fantasy, 25-26
Fast foods, 334
Fat embolism, 203
Fears, 223
Febrile seizures, 252
Feeding. *See also* Nutrition
of cerebral palsy patient, 210
cleft lip and palate patient, 101-103
of infant, 131-134
nasogastric tube, 99
preterm infant, 80-81
spina bifida patient, 115
Female genitalia, 58-59
Femoral traction, 206f
Femur fractures, 203-204
Fetal circulation, 48, 49f, 57
Fetal monitoring, 15
Fever, 35-36, 373, 376b
Fidelity, 401t
Fifth disease. *See* Erythema infectiosum
Firearms, 191, 286, 336
5-year-old child, 221t, 225
FLACC scale, 43, 45t
Fluid balance
for nephrotic syndrome patient, 259
oral fluids, 389-390
parenteral fluids, 390-391
principles of, 389-391
total parenteral nutrition, 391
Fluid resuscitation, 239
Flunisolide, 305t
Fluorinated water, 182
Fluorosis, 182
Fluticasone propionate, 305t
Fontanels, 53-54, 54f, 113
Foods. *See also* Feeding; Nutrition
buying, storing, and serving of, 133-134
for infant, 133
Foot care, in diabetes mellitus patients, 300
Football position, 38f
Foreskin, 57, 58f
Formoterol, 305t
Formula, 65, 132
4-year-old child, 221t, 224-225
Fractures, 202-204, 203f, 212t
Freud, Sigmund, 19, 21t, 178, 223, 274, 328
Friendships, 278, 279f
Fruit juice, 182
Full-thickness burns, 236-237, 238t, 239f
Functional diarrhea, 89

G

Galactosemia, 62
Gamma hydroxybutyrate, 369t
Gangs, 336
Gastric lavage, 216
Gastrointestinal system
digestion, 59-60
disorders of
in adolescent, 342-345
appendicitis, 312-314
celiac sprue, 249-250
cleft lip, 101-102, 103f
cleft palate, 102-104
esophageal atresia, 104-106
fluid imbalance, 163-165
gastroschisis, 104, 104f
Hirschsprung's disease, 162-163
infant, 156-165
inguinal hernia, 156
intussusception, 160-162
newborn, 101-106
obesity, 342-343

Gastrointestinal system—cont'd
omphalocele, 104, 104f
pinworms, 201-202
in preschool child, 249-250
pyloric stenosis, 156, 159-160, 160f
in school-age child, 312-314
in toddler, 201-202
tracheoesophageal atresia, 104-106
umbilical hernia, 156, 159f
vomiting, 163
newborn assessments, 59-60
Gastroschisis, 104, 104f
Gastrostomy, 391, 392b
Gastrostomy button feeding, 391, 393f
Gender
prepuberty, 279
pubertal differences in, 324
school performance and, 280
10-year-old child differences, 278
Gene mapping, 12
Generalized seizures, 253t
Genetic counseling, 14
Genitourinary system
assessment of, 32t
disorders of
acute glomerulonephritis, 257-258, 259t
in adolescent, 352-362
dysmenorrhea, 352-353
epispadias, 167-168, 168f
hydrocele, 167
hypospadias, 167-168, 168f
in infant, 167-168
nephrotic syndrome, 258-262, 259t
in preschool child, 256-260
sexually transmitted diseases. *See* Sexually transmitted diseases
in toddler, 214-215
urinary tract infection, 256-257
Wilms tumor, 214-215
female, 58-59
male, 57-58
newborn assessments, 57-59
Genotype, 12
German measles, 266t-267t
Gestational age, 71
Ginkgo, 9t
Glasgow Coma Scale, 213, 214t
Glioma, 319t
Glomerulonephritis, acute, 257-258, 259t
Gloves, 40
Glucagon, 298
Glucocorticoids, 243
Glucose-electrolyte solutions, 90
Glucosuria, 294
Gluten, 249
Gluten-sensitive enteropathy. *See* Celiac sprue
Gomco clamp, 58, 58f
Gonococcal ophthalmia, 62
Gonorrhea, 353, 354t, 360
Government programs, 2, 3t
Gower sign, 251f
Gowns, 40-41
Grasp reflex, 56f, 119
Greenstick fracture, 203f
Grief, 404-406
Group A ß-hemolytic streptococci, 269t, 308, 312
Group therapy, 11
Growth and development
of adolescent, 324-331
bone growth, 17
characteristics of, 16-17
definition of, 15-16
factors that affect, 18-19
of infant, 119-120

Growth and development—cont'd
nursing implications of, 20-21
of preschool child, 220-223
of school-age child, 273-279
standards of, 17-18
theories of, 19-20, 21t
of toddler, 176-179
Guarding, 313
Guided imagery, 403b

H

Haemophilus influenzae type B
epiglottitis caused by, 199
immunizations, 130, 130t, 142, 196, 408-409
Halo cast/vest, 206f
Hand-eye coordination, 278
Handwashing, 40, 67
Head
assessment of, 32t
fontanels, 53-54, 54f
of newborn, 52-54, 53f
sutures of, 54f
Head circumference
measurement of, 36-37, 51, 52f
in toddler, 178
Head injuries, 211-214
Healing touch, 46
Health care delivery settings, 9-11
Health examination
of adolescent, 332-333
of school-age child, 286, 288, 289f
Health history, 31
Health maintenance organizations, 4
Health promotion, 4
Healthy People 2010, 4, 5b
Healthy Youth 2010, 332
Hearing assessments, 56
Hearing loss, 195-196. *See also* Deafness
Heart
anatomy of, 94f
assessment of, 32t
Heart murmurs, 57
Heart rate, 52
Heat loss, 50, 51t
Heel puncture, 378, 378f
Height
measurement of, 36
of newborn, 16-17
of preschool child, 220
Heimlich maneuver, 193f
Hemarthrosis, 244-246
Hematemesis, 244
Hematologic disorders
in adolescent, 340
hemophilia, 245-247
in infant, 144-148
infectious mononucleosis, 340
iron-deficiency anemia, 144-145
leukemia. *See* Leukemia
in preschool child, 241-247
sickle cell disease, 145-148
Hematoma, 52, 212t
Hemodynamics, 93
Hemoglobin A, 145
Hemoglobin F, 148
Hemoglobin S, 145
Hemoglobinopathies, 62
Hemolytic disease of the newborn, 115-116
Hemophilia, 245-247
Hemorrhage. *See also* Bleeding
intracranial, 116-117
leukemia-related, 244-245
Hemorrhagic cystitis, 244
Hemorrhagic disease, 77
Heparin lock, 388

Hepatitis A
  characteristics of, 265t
  vaccine against, 130t, 131, 408-409
Hepatitis B
  characteristics of, 265t-266t, 358t
  vaccine against, 62, 129, 130t, 408-409
Herbs, 8, 9t
Hernia
  inguinal, 156, 156f, 167
  umbilical, 156, 159f
Herniorrhaphy, 156
Heroin, 368t
Herpes simplex virus, 356t, 360-361
Heterosexual relationships, 330
Hiccups, 60, 122b
High-risk infant, 71, 83. *See also* Postterm
  infant; Preterm infant
Hindu, 8t
Hip dysplasia. *See* Developmental dysplasia
  of the hip
HIPAA (Health Insurance Portability and
  Accountability Act), 2
Hirschsprung's disease, 162-163
H5N1, 200
Hodgkin's disease, 340-342
Home care, 10
Home phototherapy, 69
Homicide, 336
Homosexuality, 333-334
Hospice, 10, 404-405
Hospitalization
  admission, 28-29
  of adolescents, 27
  for cardiovascular disorders, 100
  child's reactions to, 24-27
  critical thinking, 29-30
  data collection, 31-37
  discharge planning, 30-31
  documentation, 30
  family and, 27-28, 41
  head circumference measurements,
    36-37
  height measurements, 36
  of infant, 24-25
  infection transmission prevention, 39-41
  measurements, 34, 36-37
  of preschoolers, 25-26
  safety during, 37-41
  of school-age children, 26-27
  settings of, 23-24
  stressors of, 25b
  of toddler, 24-25
  vital signs. *See* Vital signs
  weight measurements, 34, 36
Human Genome Project, 14
Human immunodeficiency virus, 86, 359t
Human papillomavirus, 355t, 409
Hyaline membrane disease. *See* Respiratory
  distress syndrome
Hydration, 307
Hydrocele, 167
Hydrocephalus, 110-113
Hydrotherapy, 239
Hydroxyurea, 148
Hyperbilirubinemia, 116
Hyperglycemia, 294, 299b
Hyperlipidemia, 259
Hyperpnea, 217
Hyperpyrexia, 373
Hypertonic dehydration, 164t
Hypnosis, 46
Hypocalcemia, 77
Hypoglycemia, 77, 298, 299b
Hypoplastic left heart syndrome, 96, 99f
Hypoproteinemia, 259
Hypospadias, 57-58, 167-168, 168f
Hypostatic pneumonia, 112

Hypothyroidism, 62
Hypotonic dehydration, 164t

I

Ibuprofen poisoning, 217
Icterus neonatorum, 59
Identification, 61, 381
Ileostomy, 393
Immunizations
  contraindications, 129
  diphtheria-tetanus-pertussis, 130, 130t
  Haemophilus influenzae type B, 130, 130t,
    142, 196, 408-409
  hepatitis A, 130t, 131, 408-409
  hepatitis B, 129, 130t, 408-409
  influenza, 130t, 131, 408-409
  mechanism of action, 128-129
  meningococcal, 130t, 131, 408-409
  mumps measles, and rubella, 130, 130t,
    408-409
  pneumococcal, 130t, 131, 408-409
  poliovaccine, 130, 130t, 408-409
  precautions for, 129-131
  respiratory syncytial virus, 150
  rotavirus, 130t, 131, 408-409
  schedule for, 129, 408-409
  side effects of, 129-131
  varicella, 130t, 130-131, 408-409
Immunotherapy, 243
Impetigo, 138, 140, 141f
Inborn errors of metabolism, 14
Indwelling catheters, 388
Infant
  bathing of, 373-374
  death as perceived by, 402t
  diabetes mellitus in, 302t
  ear disorders in, 141-144
  gastrointestinal disorders in, 156-165
  gender differences, 18
  genitourinary disorders in, 167-168
  growth and development of, 119-120
  health promotion and maintenance of,
    120-128
  hematologic disorders in, 144-148
  hospitalization reactions by, 24-25
  month-by-month milestones for, 121b-128b
  mortality rate for, 2-3
  nervous system disorders in, 165-167
  nutrition for, 131-134
  oral medication administration to, 382,
    382f, 383t
  oxygen therapy for, 398t
  physical development of, 121b-128b
  preterm. *See* Preterm infant
  preventive health care recommendations
    for, 412, 414
  respiratory disorders in, 148-152
  skin disorders in, 136-141
  social behavior of, 121b-128b
  teething in, 134
  weighing of, 34, 36
Infantile apnea, 169
Infection
  bacterial, 113
  handwashing protection against, 66
  in newborn, 66-67
  signs and symptoms of, 66
Infection prevention
  description of, 66-67
  in leukemia patients, 243-244
  for nephrotic syndrome patient, 260
  transmission, 39-41
Infectious diarrhea, 89-91
Infectious mononucleosis, 340
Influenza
  characteristics of, 264t
  vaccine against, 130t, 131, 408-409

Influenza A, 200
Inguinal hernia, 156, 156f, 167
Inhalants, 370t
Inheritance patterns, 13f
Injections
  intradermal, 387
  intramuscular, 384-385, 385f
  intravenous, 387-388, 388f
  sites for, 385f-386f
  subcutaneous, 387
Injury prevention
  epidemiological framework for, 193-194
  for preschool child, 234
  safety measures for, 189f
  for school-age child, 287b-288b
  for toddler, 188-193
In-line skating, 285
Insulin, 296t, 296-298, 297f
Insulin pumps, 296
Insulin shock, 298
Insurance, 4
Integumentary system. *See also* Skin
  assessment of, 32t
  newborn assessments, 59
Intention tremor, 209
Internet solicitation, 337
Interpreter, 6
Intracranial hemorrhage, 116-117
Intracranial pressure, increased, 211, 212b
Intradermal injections, 387
Intramuscular injections, 384-385, 385f
Intranasal administration, 46
Intravenous infusions, 390-391
Intravenous injections, 387-388, 388f
Intussusception, 160-162
Ipecac syrup, 215-216
Ipratropium bromide, 305t
Iridocyclitis, 315
Iron, 335
Iron-deficiency anemia, 144-145
Isolation, 41b
Isoniazid, 91
Isotonic dehydration, 164t

J

Jacket restraint, 39f, 39t
Jacobi, Abraham, 1
Jaundice
  description of, 78
  pathological, 116
  physiological, 59, 69
  true breast milk, 63
Jealousy, 227
Jehovah's Witness, 8t
Jewish, 8t
Justice, 401t
Juvenile rheumatoid arthritis
  description of, 314-315
  signs and symptoms of, 315, 317
  treatment of, 317
  types of, 315, 316t

K

Kangaroo care, 81, 82f
Karyogram, 12
Karyotype, 12-14
Kava, 9t
Kernicterus, 116
Ketoacidosis. *See* Diabetic ketoacidosis
Ketogenic diet, 255
Kohlberg, Lawrence, 20, 21t, 178, 222, 274, 328
Korotkoff sounds, 33
Kussmaul breathing, 295

L

Laminar flow patient isolation rooms, 244
Landau-Kleffner syndrome, 253t

Language
development of, 180
impairments in, 228-229
in school-age child, 274
Lanugo, 59, 59f
Laryngotracheobronchitis. See Croup
Latchkey child, 284
Lead poisoning, 217-219
Lecithin/sphingomyelin ratio, 75
Legg-Calvé-Perthes disease, 314
Length, 17
Let-down reflex, 63
Leukemia
bleeding management, 244-245
bone marrow transplantation for, 243
chemotherapy for, 243
description of, 241-242
extramedullary, 242
hair care in, 245
immunotherapy for, 243
incidence of, 242
infection prevention, 243-244
nutrition in, 245
signs and symptoms of, 242
transfusions for, 245
treatment of, 242-245
Leukotriene modifiers, 305t, 306
Levalbuterol, 305t
Level of maturation, 71
Lice. See Pediculosis
Lichenification, 136
Lindane, 292
Lip, cleft, 101-102, 103f
Lipoatrophy, 297
Lipohypertrophy, 297
Liquid ventilation, 75
Logan bow, 102
Log-roll, 347, 347f
Long-term care facilities, 11
Long-term venous access, 388
Low-birth weight
description of, 2, 71
factors associated with, 73b
Lumbar puncture, 379-380
Lungs, 32t
Lyme disease, 266t
Lymphatic system disorders, 340-342
Lysergic acid diethylamide, 367t

M

Macrosomia, 83
Male genitalia, 57-58, 58f
Mantoux test, 91
Marijuana, 369t
Masks, 40
Maslow's hierarchy of needs, 19, 20f
Massage therapy, 46
Masturbation
by preschool child, 227-228
by school-age child, 283
Maternal diabetes mellitus, 83
Maternal-infant bonding, 174
Maturation, 16
Mature minor doctrine, 333
McBurney's point, 313
Measles, 266t-267t
Measurements
head circumference, 36-37, 51
height. See Height
of newborn, 51
weight. See Weight
Mebendazole, 202
Meconium, 60
Meconium aspiration syndrome, 73
Meconium ileus, 152-153
Medical asepsis, 38-39

Medication administration
dosage calculations, 380-381
eardrops, 384
eyedrops, 384, 385f
factors that affect, 381f
intradermal, 387
intramuscular injections, 384-385, 385f
intravenous, 387-388, 388f
long-term venous access, 388
in newborn, 61-62
nosedrops, 383-384, 384f
oral medications, 381-382, 383t
rectal, 388-389
routes for, 46
subcutaneous, 387
Medulloblastoma, 319t
Meiosis, 13
Menarche, 324
Meninges, 111, 165
Meningitis, bacterial, 165-167
Meningocele, 113, 114f
Meningococcal vaccine, 130t, 131, 408-409
Meningomyelocele, 113, 114f
Mental retardation, 262, 270-271
Meperidine, 46
Mesentery, 160
Metabolic rate, 16-17
Metered-dose inhaler, 304, 306f
Methamphetamine, 366t
Methicillin-resistant *Staphylococcus aureus*, 140
3,4-Methylenedioxymethamphetamine, 367t
Methylphenidate, 322t
Methylprednisolone, 305t
Mexican-Americans, 7t
Midazolam, 248
Milwaukee brace, 345-346
Mittelschmerz, 352
Modeling, 226
Molding, 52, 52f
Mongolian spots, 59, 59f
Monilial vaginitis, 89
Mononucleosis, infectious, 340
Montelukast, 305t
Moral development, 20
Morbidity, 3
Moro reflex, 54, 55f
Morphine, 44, 46
Mortality rates, 2-3
Motor vehicle accidents, 188-190, 192, 234, 336
Mouth, 32t
Mummy restraint, 39t
Mumps
description of, 267t
immunization for, 130, 130t, 408-409
Munchausen syndrome by proxy, 173
Murmurs, 57
Musculoskeletal disorders
in adolescent, 345-352
clubfoot, 106, 106f
developmental dysplasia of the hip, 107-109
dislocations, 204
Duchenne muscular dystrophy, 250-251, 251f
fractures, 202-204, 203f
juvenile rheumatoid arthritis. See Juvenile rheumatoid arthritis
Legg-Calvé-Perthes disease, 314
newborn, 106-109
in preschool child, 250-251, 251f
in school-age child, 314-317
scoliosis. See Scoliosis
in toddler, 202-204
Music, 233
Muslim, 8t

Mutations, 14
Mycobacterium tuberculosis, 91
Myelinization, 273
Myelodysplasia, 113-115
Myoclonic seizure, 253t
MyPyramid, 183, 184f-185f, 289, 334
Myringotomy, 144
Mysoline. See Primidone

N

N-acetylcysteine, 217
NANDA diagnoses, 29, 410-411
Nasogastric tube
feedings through, 99
medication administration through, 382
Nasopharyngeal culture, 378-379
Nasopharyngitis, 148-149
Nausea, chemotherapy-induced, 245
Navajos, 7t
Neck, 32t
Necrotizing enterocolitis, 76-77
Nedocromil, 305t
Needles, 39
Neglect, child, 170-175, 171f-172f, 174f
Neisseria gonorrhoeae, 353. See also Gonorrhea
Neonatal tetany, 77
Neonate. See Newborn
Nephroblastoma. See Wilms tumor
Nephrotic syndrome, 258-262, 259t
Nervous system
disorders of
bacterial meningitis, 165-167
brain tumors, 318-320
cerebral palsy. See Cerebral palsy
Down syndrome, 109-110, 111t
encephalitis, 251-252
head injuries, 211-214
hydrocephalus, 110-113
in infant, 165-167
myelodysplasia, 113-115
in newborn, 109-115
in preschool child, 251-256
Reye's syndrome, 318, 318t
in school-age child, 318-320
seizures. See Seizures
spina bifida, 113-115, 114f
in toddler, 204, 206, 209-214
function of, 54
newborn assessments, 54-56, 55f
Newborn
adaptations of, 48
bathing of, 67-68
behavioral states of, 61, 61t
bottle feeding of, 65-66
breastfeeding of, 62-64
cardiovascular system disorders in, 92-101
examination of
airway, 48-49
Apgar score, 50, 50t, 56
blood pressure, 52
circulatory system, 56-57
gastrointestinal system, 59-60
genitourinary system, 57-59
heart rate, 52
integumentary system, 59
measurements, 51
musculoskeletal system, 57
nervous system, 54-56, 55f
reflexes, 54-56, 55f
respirations, 52
respiratory system, 56
sensory system, 56, 56f
skin, 59
umbilical cord, 49-50
vital signs, 51-52
family of, 68-69
gastrointestinal disorders of, 101-106

Newborn—cont'd
handling of, 38f
head of, 52-54, 53f
heat loss in, 50, 51t
height of, 16
identification of, 61, 381
infection prevention in, 66-67
maturity of, 52
movements of, 57
musculoskeletal disorders of, 106-109
nervous system disorders of, 109-115
nutrition for, 63-66
oxygen therapy for, 398t
physical development of, 121b
positioning of, 38
postterm, 71, 83
preterm. *See* Preterm infant
reactivity of, 60
restraining of, 38, 39f
screening tests in, 62
sleep by, 60
transporting of, 38
warmth for, 50
weight of, 16
Nicotine, 366t
Nifedipine, 258
Nightmares, 179t
9-year-old child, 275t-276t, 278
Nipple soreness, 64
Nitric oxide, 75
Nomogram, 380, 382f
Nonmaleficence, 401t
Nonopioid analgesics, 43
Nonshivering thermogenesis, 50
Nonsteroidal anti-inflammatory drugs, 317
Nose, 32t
Nosedrops, 383-384, 384f
Nursing Interventions Classification, 29-30
Nursing Outcomes Classification, 29-30
Nursing process, 29-30
Nutrition. *See also* Feeding; Foods
adolescent, 334-335
burn patients, 240
cleft palate newborn, 103
cystic fibrosis patient, 154
diabetes mellitus, 299-300, 303
infant, 131-134
leukemia patients, 245
preschool child, 229
preterm infant, 80-81
school-age child, 289-290
toddler, 182-183
total parenteral, 391

O

Obesity, 342-343
Oblique fracture, 203f
Omalizumab, 305t
Omphalocele, 104, 104f
Opioids, 43-44, 46
Oral candidiasis. *See* Thrush
Oral fluids, 389-390
Oral hygiene, 134
Oral medications, 381-382, 383t
Oral rehydration therapy, 90
Oral temperature measurements, 34
Orchiopexy, 167
Ordinal position, 18
Ortolani's sign, 107
Ossification, 17
Osteochondroses, 314
Osteomyelitis, 204
Osteopenia, 315
Osteoporosis, 153-154, 335
Ostomy, 393, 394f
Otitis media, 141-144
Otoscope, 197

Oucher Scale, 42
Overeating, 334, 342
Overhydration, 165
Oxygen tents, 397
Oxygen therapy
administration methods for, 397-398
considerations for, 398b
for pneumonia, 201
safety considerations for, 396-397

P

Pacifier, 122b
Pain
burn-related, 240
challenges associated with, 41-42
complementary and alternative medicine
for, 46
complementary methods for, 403, 403b
in dying patients, 403
evaluation of, 42-43
interventions for, 43-44, 46
nonopioid analgesics for, 43
nursing care plan for, 45
otitis media, 143
pharmacologic therapy for, 43-44, 46
rating scales for, 42-43, 44f, 45t
Palate, cleft, 102-104
Palliative care, 401-402
Palpation, 33-34
Pancreatic lipase, 60
Papilledema, 319
Parachute reflex, 119
Parallel play, 187
Paralysis, 210
Parenteral feedings, 80-81
Parenteral fluids, 390-391
Parents. *See also* Family
of adolescent, 327t, 331-332
of cardiovascular disorder patient, 100
of developmental disabled child, 272
discharge teaching for, 69
during hospitalization, 28-29
hospitalization reactions by, 27-28
of preterm infant, 82-83
Parish nursing, 10
Parkland formula, 239
Partial seizures, 253t
Partial thromboplastin time, 246
Partial-thickness burns, 236-237, 238t
Patent ductus arteriosus, 93-94
Patient-controlled analgesia, 46
Pavlik harness, 107-108, 108f
Peak expiratory flow rate, 304, 307, 307b
Pediatric nurse practitioner, 9
Pediatric surgery
postoperative care, 43t
preparations for, 41, 42t
Pediatrics, defined, 1
Pediculosis, 291-292
Peers, 282, 328, 331
Penis
circumcision of, 57, 58f
pubertal growth of, 326
Penrose drains, 314
Percutaneous umbilical blood sampling, 15
Periorbital edema, 258
Peripherally inserted central catheters, 388
Pertussis, 267t, 408-409
Petechiae, 242
Phencyclidine, 367t
Phenobarbital, 255t
Phenylketonuria, 62
Phenytoin, 255t
Phototherapy, 69, 78, 79b-80b, 116
Physical, 350, 352
Physiological anorexia, 183
Physiological jaundice, 59, 69

Piaget, Jean, 20, 21t, 274, 326
Pica, 218
Pilocarpine iontophoresis, 153
Pincer grasp, 120f
Pinworms, 201-202
Plastibell, 58, 58f
Play
hospitalization adjustments through, 26
nurse's role in, 231-232
parallel, 187
by preschool child, 224, 229-234
by school-age child, 288
by 7-year-old child, 277
therapeutic, 233
by toddler, 181, 182f, 187-188
toys for, 232b, 233
Plumbism. *See* Lead poisoning
Pneumococcal vaccine, 130t, 131, 408-409
Pneumocystis carinii pneumonia, 244
Pneumonia, 199-201, 244
Poisoning
acetaminophen, 216-217, 217t
aspirin, 217
corrosives, 216
emergency care for, 216
ibuprofen, 217
lead, 217-219
by preschool child, 234
prevention of, 191-192, 215-216
salicylate, 217
by toddler, 216-217, 217t
Poliovirus
characteristics of, 268t
vaccine against, 130, 130t, 408-409
Polydipsia, 294
Polyphagia, 294
Polyuria, 294
Postoperative care, 43t
Poststreptococcal glomerulonephritis,
257-258, 259t
Postterm infant, 71, 83
Potty chair, 186
Prednisolone, 305t
Prednisone, 243, 305t
Preferred provider organizations, 4
Pregnancy, adolescent, 362-363
Prehension, 119
Prematurity, 71-72
Premenstrual syndrome, 352-353
Preoperational thinking, 220
Prepuberty, 278-279
Preschool, 230
Preschool child
bad language by, 226-227
burns. *See* Burn(s)
daily care of, 229-230
death as perceived by, 402t
diabetes mellitus in, 302t
disciplining of, 225-226
enuresis in, 228
eye disorders in, 240-241
5-year-old, 221t, 225
4-year-old, 221t, 224-225
gastrointestinal system disorders in,
249-250
genitourinary system disorders in, 256-260
growth and development of, 220-223
health promotion and maintenance,
229-234
hematologic disorders in, 241-247
hospitalization reactions by, 25-26
injury prevention for, 234
jealousy by, 227
language impairment in, 228-229
leukemia in. *See* Leukemia
masturbation, 227-228
medication administration to, 383t

Preschool child—cont'd
  motor development of, 221t
  musculoskeletal disorders in, 250-251, 251f
  nervous system disorders in, 251-256
  nutrition for, 229
  oxygen therapy for, 398t
  play by, 229-234
  preventive health care recommendations for, 413-414
  respiratory system disorders in, 247-249
  seizures in. *See* Seizures
  sibling rivalry, 227
  skin disorders, 236-240
  sleep by, 230
  speech impairment in, 228-229, 229t
  3-year-old, 221t, 223
  thumb sucking, 227
Pressure sores, 112
Preterm infant. *See also* Infant
  body temperature control of, 78
  causes of, 71
  description of, 71
  family reaction to, 82-83
  feeding of, 80-81
  full-term infant vs., 52
  needs and care of, 78, 80-82
  nutrition for, 80-81
  observation of, 81
  positioning of, 81
  REM sleep by, 60
  risks for, 72
  skin care in, 82
  transportation of, 83
Primidone, 255t
Procedures
  lumbar puncture, 379-380
  preparations for, 372
  specimens. *See* Specimens
  sponge bathing, 373, 376b
Protein, 182
Proximodistal development, 16
Psychiatrist, 320
Psychosocial development, 19
Psychosomatic, 320
Puberty, 324-325
Pulse
  congenital heart disease and, 97
  measurement of, 31, 32f
Pulse oximetry, 201, 396, 397f
Punishment, 225-226
Pyloric stenosis, 156, 159-160, 160f
Pyloromyotomy, 159
Pyrazinamide, 91

Q

Quadriplegia, 210

R

Radiation, heat loss through, 51t
Radiation therapy, for brain tumors, 319-320
Reactive airway disease. *See* Asthma
Reactivity periods, 60
Recessive gene, 12
Recessive inheritance, 13f
Recombinant factor VIII concentrates, 246
Rectum
  assessment of, 32t
  body temperature measurements, 34
  medication administration, 388-389
Reed-Sternberg cell, 340
Reflexes, 54-56, 55f
Relaxation, 403b
Religion, 6-8, 8t
REM sleep, 60
Research centers, 9-10

Respirations
  assessment of, 32, 32t
  in newborn, 52, 97
Respiratory distress syndrome, 74f, 75
Respiratory syncytial virus, 149, 200
Respiratory system
  disorders of
    adenoiditis, 247-249
    asthma. *See* Asthma
    bronchiolitis, 149-151
    bronchitis, 199
    bronchopulmonary dysplasia, 151-152
    croup, 197-199, 198f
    cystic fibrosis. *See* Cystic fibrosis
    epiglottitis, 199, 200f
    in infant, 148-152
    nasopharyngitis, 148-149
    in newborn, 91-92
    pneumonia, 199-201
    in preschool child, 247-249
    in school-age child, 303-308
    in toddler, 197-201
    tonsillitis, 247-249
  inadequate functioning of, 73
  newborn assessments, 56
Restraints, 38, 39f, 103-104
Retinoic acid derivatives, 339
Retinopathy of prematurity, 77
Reye's syndrome, 217, 318, 318t, 373
Rh antigens, 116f
Rheumatic fever, acute, 308, 311-312
Rheumatoid arthritis. *See* Juvenile rheumatoid arthritis
RhoGAM, 115
RICE, 350, 352f
Ricin, 6
Rickets, 63
Ringer's lactate solution, 239
Ritalin. *See* Methylphenidate
Rituals, 179, 183
Rivotril. *see* Clonazepam
Rocky Mountain spotted fever, 268t
Rohypnol, 330, 369t
Rooting reflex, 54, 55f, 131
Rotavirus
  description of, 89
  vaccine for, 130t, 131, 408-409
Rubella, 266t-267t
Rubeola, 266t
Rule of nines, 236
Russell traction, 205f

S

Safety
  adolescent, 335
  bicycle, 286, 286f
  hearing-impaired toddler, 197
  during hospitalization, 37-41
  injury prevention through, 189f
  Internet, 337b
  oxygen therapy, 396-397
  for school-age child, 285-286
Salicylate poisoning, 217
Salmeterol, 305t
SARS. *See* Severe acute respiratory syndrome
Scald burns, 192
Scalded skin syndrome, 141t
Scalp injuries, 212t
Scarring, from burns, 239-240
School, 279-280
School nurses, 9
School-age child
  abduction of, 285
  anticipatory guidance of, 280
  behavioral disorders in, 320-323
  biopsychosocial development of, 274-279
  bullying effects, 280, 281b

School-age child—cont'd
  cardiovascular disorders in, 308, 311-312
  daily care of, 288
  death as perceived by, 402t
  diabetes mellitus in. *See* Diabetes mellitus
  8-year-old, 275t-276t, 277
  11- to 12-year-old, 276t, 278
  emotional disorders in, 320-323
  endocrine disorders in, 292-303
  environmental influences on, 279-282
  friendships, 278, 279f
  gastrointestinal disorders in, 312-314
  growth and development of, 273-279
  guidance for, 282-286
  health examination of, 286, 288, 289f
  health promotion and maintenance for, 286-290
  hospitalization reactions by, 26-27
  injury prevention in, 287b-288b
  language in, 274
  latchkey child, 284
  medication administration to, 383t
  musculoskeletal disorders in, 314-317
  nervous system disorders in, 318-320
  9-year-old, 275t-276t, 278
  nutrition for, 289-290
  oxygen therapy for, 398t
  peer influences, 282
  play by, 288
  preventive health care recommendations for, 413-414
  respiratory disorders in, 303-308
  safety of, 285-286
  school influences on, 279-280
  7-year-old, 275t, 276-277
  sex education of, 283-284
  6-year-old, 274-276, 275t
  skin disorders in, 291-292
  television influences on, 280-281, 282b
  10-year-old, 276t, 278
  video game influences on, 281-282, 282b
  vital signs of, 274
Scoliosis
  bracing for, 345, 347f
  definition of, 345
  nursing care plan for, 348-349
  screening for, 347, 349, 351f
  signs and symptoms of, 345, 346f
  surgery for, 346-347
  treatment of, 345-347
Screenings
  description of, 62
  scoliosis, 347, 349, 351f
Sebum, 338
Secretions, 100, 373, 394, 395b
Security, 61
Seizures
  absence, 253t
  anticonvulsants for, 254, 255t
  convulsive, 253
  epileptic, 252-256
  febrile, 252
  generalized, 253t
  myoclonic, 253t
  partial, 253t
  signs and symptoms of, 253-254
  tonic-clonic, 253t
  treatment of, 254-256, 255t
Self-acceptance, 282
Self-concept, 324, 326
Sensorineural hearing loss, 195
Sensory system, 56, 56f
Separation anxiety, 24-26
Sepsis, 67b, 76
"Setting sun" sign, 111, 112f
7-year-old child, 275t, 276-277
Severe acute respiratory syndrome, 200

Sex chromosomes, 13
Sex education
    of adolescent, 333
    of school-age child, 283-284
Sexual abuse, 173
Sexuality, 333-334
Sexually transmitted diseases
    acquired immunodeficiency syndrome,
        359t
    chlamydia, 353, 354t
    description of, 353
    genital warts, 355t
    gonorrhea, 353, 354t, 360
    hepatitis B, 358t. *See also* Hepatitis B
    herpes simplex virus, 356t, 360-361
    human immunodeficiency virus, 359t
    reporting of, 362
    signs and symptoms of, 353, 360-361
    syphilis, 357t, 360
    treatment of, 361t, 361-362
Shaken baby syndrome, 173
Shin splints, 350b
Shunt, 112-113
Sibling(s)
    of dying child, 404
    fighting with, 179t
    hospitalization reactions by, 28
    preparations for newborn, 68-69
Sibling rivalry, 227, 273
Sick-child care centers, 188
Sickle cell disease, 145-148
Sickle cell trait, 145
Side-arm traction, 205f-206f
SIDS. *See* Sudden infant death syndrome
Silvadene, 239
Simian crease, 110, 110f
Simple fracture, 202
6-year-old child, 274-276, 275t
Skating, 285
Skeletal muscle relaxants, 210
Skeletal traction, 206f
Skin
    anatomy of, 238t
    newborn assessments, 59
    of postterm infant, 83
    preterm infant, 82
Skin disorders
    in adolescent, 338-340
    atopic dermatitis, 136-140
    burns. *See* Burn(s)
    eczema, 136-138
    impetigo, 138, 140, 141f
    in infant, 136-141
    pediculosis, 291-292
    in school-age child, 291-292
    Staphylococcus aureus infection, 140-141,
        141f
Skin grafts, 239-240
Skin traction, 205f
Skull injuries, 212t
Sleep
    adolescent requirements, 335
    newborn requirements, 60
    by preschool child, 230
    school-age child requirements, 288
    toddler requirements, 181
Sleeping sickness, 251
Smallpox, 268t-269t, 270b, 270f
Smoke detectors, 192
Socialization, 279
Spanking, 226
Spasmodic croup, 199
Spastic cerebral palsy, 209
Specimens
    blood, 376, 378, 378f
    nasopharyngeal culture, 378-379
    stool, 376, 377b

Specimens—cont'd
    throat culture, 378, 379b
    urine, 373, 375-376, 377b
Speculum, 197
Speech impairments, 228-229, 229t
Spina bifida, 113-115, 114f
Spiral fracture, 203f
Spiritual care, 69
Splenectomy, 148, 341
Splenic sequestration, 147t
Split Russell traction, 205f
Sponge bathing, 373, 376b
Sports
    injuries caused by, 349-350, 352
    nutritional considerations, 335
    preparticipation physical, 350, 352
Sprain, 350b
St. John's wort, 9t
Standard precautions, 40-41
Staphylococcus spp.
    S. aureus infection, 140-141, 141f
    scarlet fever caused by, 141t, 142f
State Children's Health Insurance Program, 4
Status asthmaticus, 303-304
Status epilepticus, 253
Stealing, 277
Stem cell transplantation, 148
Sternal retractions, 56
Steroids, anabolic, 335, 370t
"Stinger," 350b
Stoma, tracheal, 395-396, 396f
Stomach capacity, 60
Stools
    in breastfed infants, 60
    specimen collection, 376, 377b
Strabismus, 241, 241f
Strain, 350b
Strangers, 234
Strangulated hernia, 156
Strattera. *See* Atomoxetine
Streptococcal infection, 269t
Streptococcus pneumoniae, 142
Stress, 11
Stress fracture, 350b
Stridor, 197
Subacute bacterial endocarditis, 312
Subcutaneous administration, 46
Subcutaneous medications, 387
Substance abuse, 365, 366t-370t
Sucking reflex, 56f
Suctioning
    of secretions, 56f, 67, 373, 375
    of tracheostomy, 394, 395b
Sudden infant death syndrome, 60, 168-169
Suffocation, 190-191
Suicide, 336, 363-365
Sulfamethoxazole/trimethoprim, 257
Sulfamylon, 239
Sullivan, 19, 21t
Sunscreen, 181
Surfactant replacement therapy, 75
Sutures, of head, 54f
Swearing, 226-227
Sweat test, 153
Syndrome of inappropriate antidiuretic
    hormone, 165-167
Syphilis, 357t, 360
Syrup of ipecac, 215-216
Systems review, 31, 32t
Systems theorists, 19

T

Tachycardia, 97
Talipes, 106
Tattoos, 334
Teenage pregnancy. *See* Adolescent
    pregnancy

Teeth
    deciduous, 134, 135f, 181
    loss of, 274
    of toddler, 181-182
Teething, 134
Tegretol. *See* Carbamazepine
Television, 280-281, 282b
Temper tantrums, 179t
Temperature. *See* Body temperature
Tenesmus, 90
TENS. *See* Transcutaneous electrical nerve
    stimulation
Teratogens, 14-15
Terbutaline, 305t
Terrorism, 5
Testes
    self-examination of, 326
    undescended, 167
Tetanus. *See* Diphtheria-tetanus-pertussis
    vaccine
Tetralogy of Fallot, 95-97, 98f
Theophylline, 305t
Therapeutic holding, 38
Therapeutic play, 233
Thermoregulation
    in newborn, 50, 51t
    by toddler, 178
Thimerosal, 131
13-*cis*-retinoic acid, 339
Thomas ring, 206f
Thoracolumbosacral orthosis, 346
3-year-old child, 221t, 223
Throat culture, 378, 379b
Thrombosis, 391
Thrush, 89
Thumb sucking, 227
Time outs, 179-180, 226
Tissue turgor, 59
Tobacco, 366t
Toddler
    behavior problems in, 179t
    choking risks in, 183
    communicating with, 180-181
    daily care of, 181
    daycare for, 188
    death as perceived by, 402t
    definition of, 176
    dental health for, 181-182
    diabetes mellitus in, 302t
    ear disorders in, 195-197
    gastrointestinal disorders in, 201-202
    genitourinary disorders in, 214-215
    growth and development of, 176-179
    guidance and discipline for, 179-180
    health promotion and maintenance for,
        181-194
    hospitalization reactions by, 24-25
    injury prevention for, 188-193
    language development by, 180
    medication administration to, 383t
    musculoskeletal disorders in, 202-204
    nervous system disorders in, 204, 206,
        209-214
    nutrition for, 182-183
    oxygen therapy for, 398t
    play by, 181, 182f, 187-188
    respiratory disorders in, 197-201
    thermoregulation by, 178
    toilet training of, 183, 186-187
Toilet training, 183, 186-187
Tolerance, 365
Tonic neck reflex, 54, 55f
Tonic-clonic seizure, 253t
Tonsillitis, 247-249
Toothbrushing, 182, 229
TORCH infections, 111
Total parenteral nutrition, 80, 391

Toxic shock syndrome, 141t, 142f
Toys, 232b, 233
Tracheoesophageal atresia, 104-106
Tracheostomy
 definition of, 393
 patency of, 394
 stoma, 395-396, 396f
 suctioning of, 394, 395b
Traction
 Bryant, 203-204
 fractures treated with, 203-204
 nursing care plan for, 207-209
 skeletal, 206f
 skin, 205f
Trampoline injuries, 234
Transcutaneous electrical nerve stimulation, 46
Transfusions, 242, 245
Transillumination, 111
Transitional stools, 60
Translocation, 14
Transmission-based precautions, 40-41
Transposition of the great arteries, 96, 98f
Transverse fracture, 203f
Treponema pallidum, 360. *See also* Syphilis
Triage, 9
Triamcinolone acetonide, 305t
Trimethoprim-sulfamethoxazole, 86, 88
Trisomy 21. *See* Down syndrome
True breast milk jaundice, 63
Tube feedings
 gastrostomy, 391, 392b
 nasogastric, 99
Tuberculosis, 91-92
24-hour urine specimen, 375-376
Tympanic temperature measurements, 34
Tympanography, 196
Tympanostomy tubes, 144

U

Umbilical cord
 assessment of, 49-50
 blood from, 50
 care of, 68

Umbilical hernia, 156, 159f
Undescended testes, 167
Upright position, 38f
Urinary system. *See* Genitourinary system
Urinary tract infection, 256-257
Urine checks, in diabetes mellitus patients, 300-301
Urine specimen, 373, 375-376, 377b
Urostomy, 393

V

Vaccinations. *See* Immunizations
Valproic acid, 255t
Vancomycin-resistant *Staphylococcus aureus*, 140
Varicella vaccine, 130t, 130-131, 408-409
Varicella zoster immune globulin, 244
Variola. *See* Smallpox
Vasoocclusive crisis, 147t
Vastus lateralis, 384, 386f
Venipuncture, 378, 378f
Venous access, long-term, 388
Ventricles, 111
Ventricular septal defect, 94, 96f
Ventrogluteal injection site, 384, 385f
Veracity, 401t
Vermox. *See* Mebendazole
Vernix caseosa, 59
Very low-birth weight, 71
Vesicoureteral reflux, 256-257
Video games, 281-282, 282b
Vietnamese-Americans, 7t
Vision. *See also* Eye(s)
 description of, 56
 in school-age child, 273
Visual acuity testing, 240
Vital signs
 blood pressure, 32-34, 52
 body temperature. *See* Body temperature
 newborn, 51-52
 pulse, 31, 32f, 97
 respirations, 32, 32t
 of school-age child, 274

Vitamin C, 144
Vitamin D, 63, 182
Vitamin K, 61-62, 217
Voiding cystourethrography, 257
Vomiting
 chemotherapy-induced, 245
 description of, 163
 inducement of, 215-216
Vulva, 58-59

W

Weaning, from breastfeeding, 134
Weight
 of adolescent, 325
 of infant, 34, 36
 measurement of, 34, 36
 of newborn, 16, 51
 of preschool child, 220
 of toddler, 178
Whooping cough, 267t
Wilms tumor, 214-215
Women, Infants, and Children, 2
Wong-Baker FACES Pain Rating Scale, 42, 44f
Wound, burn, 239-240

X

X chromosome, 13
X-linked inheritance, 13f

Y

Y chromosome, 13

Z

Zafirlukast, 305t
Zinc, 335

Student Name _____

Date _____

CHILD HEALTH EVOLUTION

Matching Questions

1. ___ evidence-based practice
2. ___ Children's Bureau
3. ___ pediatrics
4. ___ DRGs
5. ___ morbidity
6. ___ WIC
7. ___ Mexican-American
8. ___ *Healthy People 2010*
9. ___ hospice
10. ___ anticipatory guidance

a. food program that provides nutritious food and nutrition education to low-income women and children
b. illness, chronic disease, and disability
c. health promotion and disease prevention objectives for the future

d. examines research literature and focuses on important evidence for quality of care
e. providing families with information on normal growth and development and nurturing child-rearing practices before the child enters that stage of development
f. seeks a *curandero* for treatment remedies and spiritual healing
g. a program that provides palliative and supportive care for terminally ill patients and their families, either directly or on a consulting basis
h. national activity focused on the problems of infant and maternal mortality
i. branch of medicine that deals with children and their development and care
j. structure for prospective health insurance payments for hospital stay

Multiple Choice

1. Childhood became a separate stage in child development when:
   1. the Child Labor Act was passed
   2. middle-class leisure time increased
   3. child development specialists identified it
   4. youths were freed to attend school
2. The infant mortality rate in the United States is decreasing. Which of the following describes the infant mortality rate?
   1. the number of infant deaths per 1000 live births
   2. the number of infant deaths per 10,000 live births
   3. the annual number of infant deaths
   4. the number of infants with fatal illnesses
3. In the United States, the leading cause of death in children less than 1 year of age is:
   1. congenital anomalies
   2. respiratory illness
   3. accidents
   4. suicide
4. Which of the following is a major contributor to infant mortality in developed countries?
   1. low birth weight
   2. communicable diseases
   3. contaminated water supply
   4. underimmunization
5. Children are at greater risk than adults for the effects of bioterrorism because they:
   1. breathe at a slower rate
   2. have less fluid reserve than adults

   3. can outrun danger
   4. have thicker skin
6. A 26-year-old single mother with one child, age 7 years, meets the guidelines for low-income families. Which of the following programs could this mother access for her child to ensure adequate nutrition?
   1. Social Security
   2. Children and Youth Project
   3. National School Lunch Program
   4. Head Start
7. Which of the following provides screening, diagnosis, and treatment for low-income children?
   1. Medicaid EPSDT
   2. WIC
   3. SCHIP
   4. UNICEF
8. Home care nursing is important because it:
   1. includes assessment of the total needs of children and their families
   2. supplies appliances and equipment
   3. provides nursing care
   4. allows time for the parents to go to the grocery store or run other errands
9. One of the fastest growing areas for primary health care for children and adolescents is the:
   1. home
   2. children's camp

3. outpatient surgery center
4. school-based health center
10. The herb used today for anxiety, insomnia, and menopausal symptoms is:

1. kava
2. St. John's wort
3. gingko
4. echinacea

Community Search

1. Attend a Pediatric Nurse Society meeting in your area and discuss the role of this organization. (Reference section: Current Practice)

2. Investigate a local WIC center. Observe various aspects of the programs and determine its major objectives. (Reference section: Government Programs)

3. Visit a school-based health center in your area. Explore the role of the nurse in that setting.(Reference section: Health Care Delivery Settings—Clinics and Offices)

Case Studies with Critical Thinking Questions

An 18-month-old toddler is seen by the nurse practitioners at a local community clinic. Her diagnosis is failure to thrive, and she is behind on her immunizations. Her mother is a single parent who earns minimum wage at a grocery store.

1. What criteria does the family have that make them eligible for assistance?

2. Which programs would be available for this family?

A 3-year-old is brought to the pediatrician's office. During the history, the mother discusses the use of herbs when her child is ill.

1. What questions should be asked of the mother?

2. Discuss the pros and cons of CAM.

Internet Activity

Investigate the Maternal and Child Health Bureau (MCHB), part of the U.S. Dept of Health and Human Services (www.hrsa.gov) to find out what programs are available.

Student Name _____

Date _____

GROWING CHILDREN AND THEIR FAMILIES

Matching Questions

1. ____ growth
2. ____ development
3. ____ maturation
4. ____ amniocentesis
5. ____ CVS (chorionic villi sampling)
6. ____ BMI (body mass index for age)
7. ____ PUBS (percutaneous umbilical blood sample)

a. fetal blood sample that provides genetic information
b. an increase in physical size, measured in pounds or kilograms
c. type of prenatal sampling that can be done early in pregnancy for detection of possible defects
d. the total way in which a person grows and develops, as dictated by inheritance
e. procedure done after 16 weeks of gestation
f. calculated with height and weight measurements
g. a progressive increase in the function of the body (e.g., a baby's ability to digest solids as he or she matures)

Multiple Choice

1. A normal karyotype is made up of:
   1. 23 pairs of chromosomes
   2. 47 chromosomes
   3. 22 pairs of sex chromosomes
   4. 49 individual chromosomes
2. An example of a sex-linked genetic disorder is:
   1. phenylketonuria
   2. hemophilia
   3. cystic fibrosis
   4. Down syndrome
3. Amniocentesis for genetic counseling is performed at:
   1. 4 weeks of gestation
   2. 12 weeks of gestation
   3. 16 weeks of gestation
   4. 36 weeks of gestation
4. Growth occurs in all of the following ways *except:*
   1. cephalocaudal
   2. proximodistal
   3. general to specific
   4. posterior to anterior
5. Birth weight usually triples by age:
   1. 1 year
   2. 2 years
   3. 3 years
   4. 6 months

6. In comparing a child's growth with the standards, the nurse can recognize that further investigation is needed if the deviation is _____ or more percentiles from the median.
   1. 20
   2. 10
   3. 5
   4. 2
7. Knowledge of developmental theories is useful for the nurse because it:
   1. allows the nurse to know exactly what to do
   2. provides a framework to guide the nurse in caring for the patient
   3. is a set of facts that each child follows in a prescribed method
   4. is predictable and aids in controlling the child's development
8. BMI is used in children to:
   1. estimate the child's height when fully grown
   2. identify underweight, at risk for overweight, and overweight
   3. identify children who will have a heart attack
   4. evaluate need to change formula calories

Study Questions

1. Identify the different tests that are available for genetic testing and compare the results and risks of each procedure. (Reference section: Advances in Perinatology)

Community Search

1. Research what specific natal testing in done in your state.

Case Study with Critical Thinking Questions

A pregnant couple is seen in the Genetic Clinic because they have family history of sickle cell disease. They are scheduled to have a genetic amniocentesis.

1. Knowing this amniocentesis is being done for genetic studies, how advanced is this woman's pregnancy?

2. How is the sickle cell trait carried?

3. If both parents have the trait, what is the possible risk for their fetus to have the disease?

Internet Activity

With a search engine such as Google (www.google.com), search for any of the following topics:

- Genetics
- Moral development
- Erikson developmental theory
- Maslow's hierarchy of needs

Visit the CDC website (http://www.cdc.gov/nccdph/dnpa/growthcharts/) and explore the 2000 CDC Growth Chart Training Modules and Resources.

Student Name _____

Date _____

CARE OF THE HOSPITALIZED CHILD

Matching Questions

1. ___ discharge
2. ___ play room
3. ___ rectal temperature
4. ___ hospital unit
5. ___ apical pulse
6. ___ blood pressure
7. ___ cross contamination
8. ___ patient's room
9. ___ disposable mask
10. ___ handwashing

a. considered a "safe place" for the child
b. pediatric setting differs from adult setting
c. variety of toys available for play
d. begins on admission
e. protects from respiratory droplets
f. counted for 1 full minute
g. pressure of the blood on the walls of the arteries
h. contraindicated in newborns
i. most important barrier against transmission of disease
j. the spread of germs from one child to another

Multiple Choice

1. Safety is important; it reduces unnecessary accidents and:
   1. sets a good example for parents
   2. keeps the play room in order
   3. ensures that accidents will never happen
   4. guarantees that errors will never be made
2. All invasive procedures should be performed in the:
   1. patient's bed
   2. treatment room
   3. morning
   4. evening
3. A 2-year-old with pyelonephritis is admitted to your hospital unit. Her mother needs to go home this evening to be with her other children. Which of the following reactions do you anticipate when her mother leaves?
   1. laughter
   2. silence
   3. crying and screaming
   4. quiet conversation with her doll from home
4. A 4-year-old preschooler is screaming for a Band-Aid after you obtain a capillary blood sample. You know he is upset because one of the major fears of preschool children is that:
   1. their hearts will stop beating
   2. their insides will leak out
   3. they were responsible for their illness
   4. the injury will be permanent
5. A preschooler that received an injection specifically requested a Band-Aid with the picture of a popular fictional hero. Use of fantasy by preschool children:
   1. helps them avoid reality
   2. diminishes guilt
   3. decreases nightmares
   4. helps them cope with their environment

6. A major fear of school-age children is:
   1. that their parents will abandon them
   2. bodily harm
   3. loss of sexual function
   4. not being able to play
7. Normal respiratory rate (per minute) for a 1-year-old to a 3-year-old is:
   1. 10-20
   2. 20-30
   3. 30-40
   4. 40-50
8. When the nurse chooses a blood pressure cuff:
   1. it should cover one third of the upper arm
   2. it should be long enough to encircle the extremity
   3. it should cover the entire upper arm
   4. it should encircle half the extremity
9. Hospital-acquired infections are called
   1. nosocomial
   2. disinfection
   3. medical asepsis
   4. contamination
10. The most appropriate restraint to use when a 5-year-old child receives venipuncture for laboratory work is
    1. therapeutic holding
    2. jacket restraint
    3. mummy restraint
    4. elbow restraints

Study Questions

1. Compile a list of safety measures that would be effective on the children's unit of your hospital. (Reference section: Safety)

2. Describe how and why measurement of blood pressure differs when patient is a child. (Reference section: Data Collection-Vital Signs)

3. The charge nurse has just told you to prepare Room 101 for a new admission who is suspected of having meningitis. The patient is 6 years old. How would you do this? (Reference section: Safety)

4. Discuss how you would evaluate a 4-year-old child for pain. (Reference section: The Child in Pain)

Case Study with Critical Thinking Questions

A 7-year-old boy is admitted to the outpatient surgery section of the hospital where you work.

1. How will you discuss his surgery with him?

2. What will you need to do before surgery?

3. What are normal vital signs for this age?

4. What are the types of things to consider after surgery with a 7-year-old?

Internet Activity

Visit http://www.kidshealth.org and click on Parents. Under "What's New for Parents," review the section on "Preparing Your Child for Anesthesia." If the article is not in the featured list, type in a key word or two (e.g., Anesthesia) in the Search box. Make a list of all the helpful suggestions you can offer parents.

Student Name _____

Date _____

THE NEWBORN INFANT

Matching Questions

1. ___ Moro reflex
2. ___ tonic neck reflex
3. ___ anterior fontanel
4. ___ posterior fontanel
5. ___ acrocyanosis
6. ___ icterus neonatorum
7. ___ desquamation
8. ___ meconium
9. ___ let-down reflex
10. ___ cold stress

a. can cause metabolic and physiological problems
b. closes by 2 months of age
c. closes by 12 to 18 months of age
d. may be seen when infant's crib is bumped
e. peeling of the skin
f. physiological jaundice
g. release of milk in the breast
h. the first stool
i. the "fencing" position
j. bluish discoloration of the hands and feet

Multiple Choice

1. The Apgar score is used to determine:
    1. the gestational age of the newborn
    2. major body systems' responses at birth
    3. the future intelligence of the newborn
    4. the level of parent and newborn interaction
2. The umbilical cord will most likely be off by:
    1. 2 days of age
    2. 3 to 5 days of age
    3. 10 to 14 days of age
    4. 24 hours of age
3. Because of the neonate's sterile intestinal flora at birth, the newborn receives an injection of:
    1. AquaMephyton
    2. erythromycin
    3. vitamin C
    4. tetracycline
4. In fetal circulation, the structure located between the pulmonary artery and the aorta is the:
    1. ductus venosus
    2. foreman ovale
    3. ductus arteriosus
    4. truncus arteriosus
5. The most effective prevention of infection in the newborn is:
    1. administration of antibiotics on time
    2. use of disposable items
    3. keeping others away
    4. proper handwashing by staff and family
6. Of the following, the description of the most likely sign of infection in the newborn is:
    1. temperature of 96.6° F, vomiting, and lethargy
    2. temperature of 97.8° F, alert, and fussy about every 4 hours

3. temperature of 98° F, central cyanosis, and fatigue with feedings
4. temperature of 98.4° F, ruddy pink coloring, and active with stimulation
7. Which of the following responses most indicate bonding is occurring?
    1. The mother speaks to her newborn while holding and stroking him.
    2. The mother allows her newborn to cry for a minimum of 10 minutes before checking on him.
    3. The mother is reluctant to hold her newborn and describes her role of mother as burdensome.
    4. The mother desires others to always care for the newborn.
8. All newborns are screened for:
    1. phenylketonuria and hypothyroidism
    2. hemoglobin, hematocrit, and blood sugar
    3. blood group, RH type, and direct Coombs test
    4. sickle cell disease and HIV status
9. In identifying the newborn, which of the following is most important? Identification is done:
    1. at the earliest convenient time
    2. before the mother and newborn are separated
    3. at least by 30 minutes of age
    4. by footprinting the newborn
10. The second period of reactivity occurs:
    1. during the first 30 minutes of life
    2. at 1 to 2 hours of age
    3. at 2 to 6 hours of age
    4. after 10 hours of age

Community Search

1. Visit a parenting class at a local hospital and be able to discuss content covered. (Reference section: Care of the Newborn)

2. Visit a breastfeeding class at a local hospital and be able to discuss tips and techniques given to parents planning to breastfeed. (Reference section: Nutrition)

Study Questions

1. What differences occur in caring for the circumcision done with the Gomco clamp versus the Plastibell? (Reference section: Genitourinary System)

2. Discuss behavioral states in the newborn and their importance. (Reference section: Activity and Table 4-4)

Case Study with Critical Thinking Questions

A young, expectant mother has attended a breastfeeding class but was unable to attend a parenting class. She is in labor and is asking what happens to the baby after birth.

1. What procedures are done immediately after birth?

2. What procedures are done prior to discharge?

After the birth, she has additional questions about providing cord care and about bathing the baby.

3. How will she provide cord care?

4. What advice needs to be given regarding bathing the baby?

Internet Activity

Explore reliable Internet resources related to care of the newborn.

Student Name _____

Date _____

THE HIGH-RISK NEONATE

Matching Questions

1. ___ grunting
2. ___ cyanosis
3. ___ retracting
4. ___ atelectasis
5. ___ lanugo
6. ___ liquid ventilation
7. ___ gestational age
8. ___ level of maturation
9. ___ nitric oxide

a. a bluish discoloration of the trunk
b. unexpanded lung tissue
c. audible sound heard with respirations
d. fine, downy hair
e. pulling in of tissue above, between, or below the ribs with each respiratory effort
f. how well the baby is developed at birth
g. gas that improves oxygenation
h. actual time from conception to birth
i. fluid ventilation for the infant

Multiple Choice

1. A low-birth weight infant is one who is:
   1. less than 2500 g
   2. less than 2000 g
   3. less than 1500 g
   4. less than 1000 g
2. The goal for treatment of the high-risk newborn is:
   1. delay conception until maternal age is greater than 34 years
   2. education of parents before conception
   3. a NICU in every hospital
   4. prevention or early detection
3. Which of the following situations is least likely to result in a premature birth?
   1. teen pregnancy
   2. multiple births
   3. maternal illness
   4. maternal consumption of 2500 calories per day
4. The reason for the development of respiratory distress syndrome in the preterm infant is:
   1. lack of surfactant
   2. too much surfactant
   3. lack of vitamin K
   4. unknown at present
5. Neonatal apnea may be treated with which of the following medications?
   1. AquaMephyton
   2. ampicillin
   3. caffeine
   4. Lanoxin

6. Necrotizing enterocolitis can be a complication of:
   1. breastfeeding
   2. elevated oxygen levels
   3. hypoglycemia
   4. prematurity
7. The best nursing action in response to an alarming apnea monitor would be to:
   1. suction the nose
   2. begin the treatment for cardiac arrest
   3. silence the alarm
   4. assess for respiratory distress and color.
8. If the fluid needs of a preterm infant are 100 mL/kg/24 hr and the weight of the newborn is 1200 g (1.2 kg), what will the infant's hourly intravenous rate be?
   1. 0.5 mL/hr
   2. 5 mL/hr
   3. 50 mL/hr
   4. 120 mL/hr
9. In the NICU, discharge planning begins:
   1. at birth
   2. on admission to the transitional area
   3. 2 days before discharge
   4. when the parents are completely comfortable
10. The infant of a mother with diabetes is most likely to:
    1. be small for gestational age
    2. be appropriate for gestational age
    3. be large for gestational age
    4. have intrauterine growth retardation

Study Questions

1. List the risks related to preterm births. (Reference section: The Preterm Infant)

2. How does the nursing care of the premature baby differ from that of the full-term neonate? (Reference section: The Preterm Infant)

3. Close observation is extremely important in the care of the premature infant. List several significant changes that should be reported to the nurse in charge. (Reference section: Table 5-1)

4. What problems do the parents of a premature infant face? In what ways might the nurse facilitate maternal-infant bonding? (Reference section: Family Reaction to the Preterm Infant)

Community Search

1. Visit the CDC website and select your state statistics for infant mortality. Identify the top causes and discuss what community projects can assist in decreasing the risks.

Case Study with Critical Thinking Questions

A 32-week gestation female is born to a mother who had preterm labor for 2 weeks. The mother received Celestone. The baby at birth weighed 1.54 kg.

1. With the Ballard maturational assessment (Appendix F), determine this newborn's classification for gestational age.

2. What care will be needed for this preterm infant?

3. The infant has developed a distended abdomen and bloody diarrhea. What is the possible problem that has presented? Why is this patient at risk for this? What will the nursing care involve with this problem?

4. An intravenous line is needed, and the order is for 80 mL/kg/24 hr. What will be the amount for 24 hours? What will be the amount for each hour?

Internet Activity

With a web browser or search engine, find sources of information for parents or health care providers related to the premature infant. Using the Internet, visit the KidsHealth for Parents website (http://www.kidshealth.org/parent/) and review the topics discussed in this chapter.

Student Name _____

Date _____

DISORDERS OF THE NEWBORN

Matching Questions

1. ___ birth defect
2. ___ hydrocephalus
3. ___ spina bifida
4. ___ meningocele
5. ___ meningomyelocele
6. ___ ventricular septal defect
7. ___ coarctation of the aorta
8. ___ tetralogy of Fallot
9. ___ transposition of the great vessels
10. ___ thrush
11. ___ functional diarrhea
12. ___ infectious diarrhea
13. ___ TB

a. an example of a congenital heart defect resulting in increased pulmonary blood flow
b. involve the membranes and cerebrospinal fluid
c. an example of a congenital heart defect resulting in mixed blood flow
d. an abnormality of structure, function, or metabolism that the child has at birth
e. an example of a congenital heart defect resulting in obstructive blood flow
f. diarrhea caused by an infection
g. increase of cerebrospinal fluid in the ventricles of the brain
h. causative organism is *Candida*
i. diarrhea from an organic disease
j. embryonic neural tube defect
k. causative organism is the mycobacterium
l. involves the membranes, the spinal cord, and cerebrospinal fluid
m. an example of a congenital heart defect resulting in decreased pulmonary blood flow

Multiple Choice

1. According to the March of Dimes classification of birth defects, an example of a metabolic defect would be:
   1. Rh disease
   2. Down syndrome
   3. Sickle cell anemia
   4. PKU
2. A nurse would suspect a TEF in a newborn with:
   1. excessive flatus
   2. blue extremities that are cold to touch
   3. coughing, choking, and cyanosis
   4. weak sucking
3. The most severe form of spina bifida is:
   1. meningomyelocele
   2. meningocele
   3. spina bifida occulta
   4. lipoma
4. The most common cardiac condition is:
   1. patent ductus arteriosus (PDA)
   2. pulmonary stenosis
   3. tetralogy of Fallot
   4. truncus arteriosus
5. Of the following congenital heart defects, the one least likely to present initially with cyanosis is:
   1. tetralogy of Fallout
   2. truncus arteriosus
   3. transposition of the great vessels
   4. ventricular septal defect (VSD)

6. Talipes equinovarus is the most common form of a:
   1. cleft palate
   2. clubfoot
   3. cleft lip
   4. defect of the hand
7. The infant born with an omphalocele is at risk for:
   1. hypercalcemia and hypokalemia
   2. polycythemia
   3. blood loss
   4. infection and hypothermia
8. RhoGam has significantly decreased the incidence of:
   1. ABO incompatibility
   2. Rh incompatibility
   3. genetic disease
   4. pathologic defects
9. In children, the most common transmission of HIV is through:
   1. perinatal exposure
   2. close family contact after birth
   3. blood transfusions
   4. unknown sources
10. Transmission of TB is by:
    1. direct contact of the organism on the skin
    2. handling of feces or urine
    3. ingestion of the organism
    4. inhalation of an infected droplet

Study Questions

1. List the symptoms of increased intracranial pressure. (Reference section: Nervous System)

2. Discuss the nursing goals in caring for a child with a heart defect. Also include the care for the family. (Reference section: Nursing Goals and Treatment in Congenital Heart Disease)

3. Discuss the multidisciplinary team approach needed in the treatment of a newborn who has a gastroschisis. (Reference section: Gastroschisis/Omphalocele)

4. Review cast care and anticipate potential problems associated with a pediatric patient who has a cast. (Reference section: Cast care)

5. Discuss the special needs of a family who has a child with Down syndrome. (Reference section: Down Syndrome)

6. Discuss the method for treatment of a child who has TB. Include the family support that will also be needed with this child. (Reference section: Tuberculosis)

Case Study with Critical Thinking Questions

A male child who is term (40 weeks' gestation) is delivered to first-time parents. He has a cleft lip and cleft palate. The parents are distraught.

1. What will be the first concern for this newborn?

2. What resources are available for his parents?

3. What can the nurse do to help with the bonding process for this family?

4. What method of feeding will most likely be recommended for this newborn?

Internet Activity

Go to the March of Dimes website (www.modimes.com) and find statistics and information regarding birth defects.

Student Name _____

Date _____

THE INFANT

Matching Questions

1. ___ baby teeth
2. ___ grasp reflex
3. ___ Moro reflex
4. ___ pincer reflex
5. ___ prehension reflex

a. flexion of the fingers or toes in response to pressure
b. intentional grasping of objects between thumb and all the fingers
c. coordination of index finger and thumb
d. generalized response to noise or loss of balance
e. deciduous

Multiple Choice

1. If the needs of the infant are met in a consistent manner, the infant will develop:
   1. independence
   2. responsibility
   3. trust
   4. love
2. The first year of life involves a great deal of growth and development. Parents need to anticipate what their child will be doing next, not only to enjoy their child's accomplishments but also for the child's:
   1. love
   2. freedom
   3. dependence
   4. safety
3. The ability to hold the head erect in midposition occurs during the _____ month of life.
   1. first
   2. second
   3. fourth
   4. sixth
4. The polio vaccine, diphtheria-tetanus-pertussis, and *Haemophilus influenzae* type b immunizations are begun at _____ months of age.
   1. 1
   2. 2
   3. 3
   4. 4
5. Sleeping all night (8 to 10 hours) may not occur until the infant is:
   1. 2 weeks old
   2. 2 months old
   3. 4 months old
   4. 8 months old
6. Speech begins with cooing. This behavior is typical at:
   1. 2 months of age
   2. 4 months of age
   3. 6 months of age
   4. 8 months of age

7. Crawling has usually been developed by the time the infant is:
   1. 4 months old
   2. 6 months old
   3. 8 months old
   4. 12 months old
8. Walking around objects for support can be observed in the infant who is:
   1. 4 months old
   2. 6 months old
   3. 8 months old
   4. 10 months old
9. By 12 months of age, the infant has _____ its birth weight.
   1. doubled
   2. tripled
   3. quadrupled
10. The first solid food item to be introduced into an infant's diet is:
    1. vegetables
    2. meat
    3. fruit
    4. cereal
11. The infant's first tooth is usually anticipated around the _____ month of age.
    1. second
    2. fourth
    3. sixth
    4. twelfth
12. The initial MMR (mumps, measles, rubella) vaccination is recommended at:
    1. 12 to 15 months of age
    2. 6 months of age
    3. 6 weeks of age
    4. 9 months of age

Study Questions

1. Why must the pediatric nurse be able to recognize the various stages of growth and development in the infant? (Reference section: General Characteristics and Development)

2. Discuss the needs of the newborn infant. How do these needs change during the first year? (Reference section: Physical Development, Social Behavior, Care, and Guidance)

3. What is the value of attending to the needs of an infant promptly and cheerfully during the first year? (Reference section: General Characteristics and Development)

4. A mother has been bringing her 4-month-old daughter, to the well-child clinic since she was 1 month old. What services are provided by a well-child clinic? (Reference section: Health Promotion and Maintenance)

5. How does the infant's environment affect physical growth and development? Mental health? (Reference section: General Characteristics and Development)

Case Study with Critical Thinking Questions

A 4-month-old infant is brought to the well-child clinic. He weighs 15 pounds 11 ounces and is 25 inches long. He is being breastfed and eats every 4 to 6 hours. At 2 months of age, he received the second Hep B and the first dose of the DTaP, HIB, IPV, Rotavirus, and PCV.

1. Using a growth chart in Appendix F, what is this infant's percentile for weight and length?

2. What immunizations will he need to receive at this visit?

3. What instructions need to be given to the mother related to the reactions the infant may have regarding the immunizations?

4. What type of information does the mother need for anticipatory guidance?

Internet Activity

Explore the Immunization Action Coalition website (http://www.immunize.org) and review the parent/patient information sheets (vaccine information statements) on various immunizations. Be prepared to discuss how you would explain various immunizations to parents.

Student Name _____

Date _____

DISORDERS OF THE INFANT

Matching Questions

1. ___ acetaminophen
2. ___ anemia
3. ___ child abuse
4. ___ cryptorchidism
5. ___ cystic fibrosis
6. ___ eczema
7. ___ failure to thrive
8. ___ impetigo
9. ___ inguinal hernia
10. ___ meningitis
11. ___ myringotomy
12. ___ otitis media
13. ___ RSV
14. ___ sickle cell anemia
15. ___ SIDS

a. middle ear infection
b. a small incision into the eardrum
c. used to reduce fever
d. respiratory syncytial virus
e. inherited disease involving the red blood cells
f. hemoglobin less than 10 g/dL
g. more common in boys than girls
h. inherited disease involving the exocrine glands
i. spinal tap used as a diagnostic procedure
j. undescended testicles
k. atopic dermatitis
l. caused by staphylococci
m. also known as crib death
n. below the 5th percentile in growth
o. prevention and early intervention is the best approach

Multiple Choice

1. When a child has otitis media and begins therapy with an antibiotic, this medication should be taken:
   1. until the symptoms go away
   2. until the entire prescription is gone
   3. only when the child has symptoms
   4. as long as fever persists
2. To increase the absorption of iron, _____ is/are added to the diet.
   1. B complex vitamins
   2. vitamin C
   3. vitamin A
   4. vitamin D
3. A sickle cell crisis can be precipitated by an episode of:
   1. anemia
   2. hyponatremia
   3. hypoxia
   4. hypercarbia
4. Dehydration is of concern in the pediatric population because the child has a:
   1. higher percentage of fluid to body weight
   2. lower metabolic rate
   3. smaller amount of surface area to body weight
   4. more stable heat-regulating system
5. When an oral pancreatic extract is given, which of the following should be considered?
   1. give with meals or snacks
   2. give even if the child is ill or not eating

3. the enteric-coated tablets may be crushed or chewed
   4. the medication is given between meals
6. When failure to thrive is the result of an environmental cause, which of the following is correct?
   1. A sense of trust is missing in the child.
   2. The growth of the child is above the 50th percentile.
   3. The mother cannot be helped.
   4. The mother has the ability to tolerate high levels of stress.
7. Infants and young children can become dehydrated from a respiratory infection because of:
   1. loss of fluids through increased temperature and respirations
   2. decreased intake resulting from anorexia
   3. vomiting
   4. all of the above
8. The most common surgical condition of the digestive tract in infancy is:
   1. pyloric stenosis
   2. umbilical hernia
   3. intussusception
   4. meconium ileus
9. Infantile eczema is seen:
   1. after 2 years of age
   2. as an allergic response to a substance
   3. frequently in breastfed infants
   4. more frequently in the summer

10. Bacterial meningitis:
1. may be preceded by cold or upper respiratory tract infection
2. has declined as a result of the *H. influenzae* type b vaccine
3. causes the patient to be overly sensitive to stimuli
4. all of the above

11. A symptom of Hirschsprung's disease is:
1. reflux
2. hyperactive bowel sounds
3. constipation
4. diarrhea

Study Questions

1. An infant, age 11 months, is admitted to the hospital with the diagnosis of meningitis. List the symptoms of meningeal irritation. (Reference section: Bacterial Meningitis)

2. List the symptoms of pyloric stenosis. Why must infants with pyloric stenosis be fed so carefully? (Reference section: Pyloric Stenosis)

3. Discuss the pathophysiological process of cystic fibrosis as it relates to the following structures: respiratory system, sweat glands, pancreas. (Reference section: Cystic Fibrosis)

4. Prepare a day's menu for an 11-month-old baby with anemia. (Reference section: Iron Deficiency Anemia)

Case Study with Critical Thinking Questions

A 10-month-old African-American child is admitted to the hospital with a severe infection. The physician suspects that she may also be experiencing a sickle cell crisis. Intravenous fluids are started, and she is medicated for the infection and pain. She was diagnosed with sickle cell disease at birth by the newborn screen. Her parents have some knowledge about the disease.

1. Develop a care plan for this child that includes her immediate needs for tissue perfusion, fluids, pain, infection, and knowledge deficit related to sickle cell crisis.

2 After being hospitalized for a week, the child's parents are preparing for her discharge in the morning. What information regarding home care is necessary to discuss with them?

Internet Activity

Explore the Internet and find sites that provide information regarding sickle cell disease.

Student Name _____

Date _____

THE TODDLER

Matching Questions

1. ___ ritualism
2. ___ right and wrong
3. ___ egocentric thinking
4. ___ anal phase
5. ___ autonomy versus shame or doubt
6. ___ negativism
7. ___ autonomy
8. ___ ambivalence

a. Freud's stage of personality development
b. Erikson's developmental task
c. Kohlberg's moral development
d. self-confidence
e. fluctuation of emotions
f. increases a toddler's sense of security
g. opposition to suggestion or advice
h. difficulty seeing anyone else's point of view

Multiple Choice

1. A child at which of the following ages runs clumsily, throws a ball overhand without falling, and builds a tower of three to four cubes?
   1. 15 months
   2. 18 months
   3. 24 months
   4. 30 months
2. The toddler gains about how many pounds per year?
   1. 2
   2. 5
   3. 8
   4. 10
3. Which is the appropriate description of a 2-year-old's sentence?
   1. five-word complex sentences
   2. two-word noun-verb simple sentences
   3. use of adjectives and adverbs when describing nouns and verbs
   4. cannot speak in sentences
4. When a 2-year-old needs to be disciplined:
   1. spanking works best because it is the most effective
   2. a 5-minute time out is most effective
   3. a 2-minute time out is most effective
   4. no method is effective, so the parent need not bother
5. Physiological anorexia is a phenomenon of toddlerhood that occurs because of:
   1. decreased appetite and increased nutritional need
   2. increased appetite and lack of food preferences
   3. increased appetite and strong food preferences
   4. decreased appetite and decreased nutritional need

6. One indication that the toddler is ready to toilet-train is:
   1. the ability to climb onto the toilet
   2. the ability to stay dry for 1 hour
   3. the ability to communicate being wet or needing to urinate or defecate
   4. the willingness to sit on the potty for 2 to 3 minutes
7. Which type of play do toddlers exhibit?
   1. associative
   2. team
   3. solitary
   4. parallel
8. Toys that parents should buy for toddlers include:
   1. toys with small, removable parts
   2. wind-up toys
   3. toys that can be pushed or pulled
   4. balloons because they often come in bright colors
9. The leading cause of death in childhood is:
   1. accidents
   2. child abuse
   3. burns
   4. drowning
10. The most common type of burn injury in children is from:
   1. chemicals
   2. radiation
   3. electricity
   4. scalds

Study Questions

1. Prepare a day's menu for a toddler. Include between-meal snacks. (Reference section: Nutrition Counseling)

2. Define parallel play. Of what value is play to the child? (Reference section: Play)

3. Review your newspaper for 1 week. Bring to class accounts of various accidents that occurred to children during that week. Be prepared to discuss how they might have been prevented. (Reference section: Injury Prevention)

Case Study with Critical Thinking Questions

You are the nurse in a community clinic. A 2-year-old boy comes in for a routine physical. The mother states he is very healthy and "all boy." On examination, the physician states he is "doing well" physically. Routine immunizations are ordered. After you administer them, the mom asks you why her child is such a "picky eater" and when he will be ready to "potty train?"

1. What is the anticipatory guidance that needs to be provided to this child's mother in regard to nutrition and toileting?

2. What other anticipatory guidance is needed for a child of this age?

Internet Activity

Explore the Internet and find sites that provide information on concepts of growth and development related to the toddler, including safety, nutrition, and daycare.

Student Name _____

Date _____

DISORDERS OF THE TODDLER

Matching Questions

1. ___ plumbism
2. ___ stridor
3. ___ dysarthria
4. ___ tympanography
5. ___ dyskinetic
6. ___ decerebrate
7. ___ Mucomyst
8. ___ epiphyseal plate
9. ___ *Haemophilus influenzae*
10. ___ idiopathic

a. posturing indicating injury to the midbrain
b. involuntary, purposeless movements
c. antidote for acetaminophen poisoning
d. found at the end of long bones
e. problems with coordination of muscles needed for speech
f. no known cause
g. most common cause of epiglottitis
h. graphic picture of eardrum motion
i. high-pitched sounds on inspiration
j. lead poisoning

Multiple Choice

1. Parents would suspect hearing loss if their child did not:
   1. babble at 2 months
   2. startle with sudden loud noises
   3. talk at 6 months
   4. turn toward a sound immediately after birth
2. When collecting data about a child with suspected epiglottitis, the nurse keeps in mind that, unlike croup, epiglottitis:
   1. has a brassy cough
   2. develops rapidly
   3. occurs in infants
   4. is worse at night
3. One of the major goals when caring for children with cerebral palsy is to:
   1. prevent further brain damage
   2. maximize their physical and intellectual potential
   3. recommend they be placed in special classes
   4. keep them from taking undue physical risks
4. One of the *first* signs of increasing intracranial pressure in a nonverbal toddler is:
   1. decreasing blood pressure
   2. behavior changes
   3. seizures
   4. sudden vomiting episodes
5. When a family is treated for pinworm infestation, the nurse recommends which of the following additional actions?
   1. washing all kitchen utensils in the dishwasher
   2. washing underwear and bed linens in very hot water
   3. airing out blankets and pillows
   4. throwing away all "dress-up" clothes
6. A child with a head injury exhibits a rise in systolic blood pressure, a decrease in pulse, and an uneven respiratory pattern. The nurse's *first* action is to:
   1. notify the charge nurse or physician
   2. lower the head of the bed
   3. measure the child's head circumference
   4. take the child's temperature
7. Wilms tumor is a tumor that affects the:
   1. kidney
   2. brain
   3. cartilage
   4. blood
8. A young child with a lower extremity cast has swelling of the toes. The toes are bluish in color, and capillary refill is slow. The child is crying. The parents are worried. The nurse *first*:
   1. calls to have the cast removed
   2. reassures the child's parents that this is normal
   3. notifies the charge nurse or physician
   4. takes measures to stop the child's crying
9. A serious complication for children with fractures is:
   1. discoloration of the skin
   2. injury to the epiphyseal plate
   3. a greenstick fracture
   4. swelling over the fracture
10. Treatment for Wilms tumor can involve the following:
    1. chemotherapy
    2. surgery
    3. radiation
    4. all of the above

Study Questions

1. An 18-month-old has been seen in the office by the family pediatrician. He has been diagnosed with croup. List the home care instructions for caring for this child. (Reference section: Croup)

2. List the symptoms for epiglottitis. Why do these symptoms occur with this disease? (Reference section: Epiglottitis)

3. A young child is hospitalized with Wilms tumor. A sign is posted above his bed that reads "Do Not Palpate Abdomen." Explain to the mother why this sign has been posted. (Reference section: Wilms Tumor)

4. A 2-year-old in traction needs diversional activities. What toys/activities are appropriate for this age of a child? (Reference section: Care of the Child in Traction; also see Chapter 9, section on play.

Case Study with Critical Thinking Questions

A 2-year-old child is admitted with pneumonia.

1. List the problems that would be expected for a child with this diagnosis.

2. What nursing interventions are appropriate?

3. What discharge instructions would be expected with this child?

Internet Activity

Explore the Internet and locate sites that have information that would be beneficial for caretakers of children with cerebral palsy. Start with the United Cerebral Palsy website (www.ucp.org).

Student Name _____

Date _____

THE PRESCHOOL CHILD

Matching Questions

1. ____ preoperational phase
2. ____ artificialism
3. ____ speech
4. ____ sense of initiative
5. ____ phallic phase
6. ____ 3-year-old
7. ____ 4-year-old
8. ____ 5-year-old
9. ____ stuttering
10. ____ centering

a. posturing repetition of sounds
b. a stage in Erikson's development theory
c. reflected in child beginning to make friends outside of the family
d. a stage in Freud's theory of the psyche
e. more responsible, have more patience
f. boisterous, stormy age
g. a stage in Piaget's development theory
h. the world and everything in it are created by human beings
i. tendency to concentrate on a single characteristic of an object while excluding its other features
j. utterance of vocal sounds conveying ideas

Multiple Choice

1. Thumb sucking is considered:
   1. normal in the preschool child
   2. detrimental to the preschool child
   3. normal until age 8 years
   4. dangerous and must not be allowed
2. Masturbation in the preschool child is viewed as:
   1. disruptive to the family
   2. embarrassing to the parents
   3. normal behavior that can best be dealt with by ignoring the behavior and providing distraction
   4. abnormal behavior that needs to be dealt with immediately
3. The most effective management of children with enuresis is:
   1. an aggressive, overzealous approach
   2. encouraging the use of punishment so that children will gain control more quickly
   3. making children feel guilty so that they will get over the problem quickly
   4. providing reassurance, teaching, and support for the parents
4. An important aspect of the preconceptual stage is:
   1. the increasing development of language and symbolic functioning
   2. the development of moral thinking
   3. the development of spiritual thinking
   4. the development of socialization of the individual
5. Three-year-olds will:
   1. play cooperatively for long periods of time
   2. play well with new friends
   3. revert to parallel play if placed in a strange situation with children they do not know
   4. share toys eagerly when others want them
6. The presence of an imaginary friend generally occurs around age:
   1. 3 years
   2. 4 years
   3. 5 years
7. The play activity best suited to a 4-year-old is:
   1. pretending
   2. any game with numbers or letters
   3. riding a two-wheeler
   4. hopscotch
8. An effective means of establishing rapport with the hospitalized preschooler is through:
   1. lengthy discussion
   2. explanation with drawings and models
   3. play
   4. silence
9. A sexually abused child may be able to express feelings best through:
   1. therapeutic play
   2. play therapy such as dramatic play
   3. talking quietly with the nurse
   4. drawing a picture
10. A preschooler pretending to do the dishes is an example of:
    1. centering
    2. artificialism
    3. magical thinking
    4. domestic mimicry

Study Questions

1. How do you think the preschool child would react to hospitalization? Give reasons for your answer. (Reference section: Theories of Development)

2. A 4-year-old's father dies unexpectedly. What special problems will this present to the preschool child? (Reference section: The 4-Year-Old Child)

3. Visit a preschool. Evaluate a child based on observations listed in Box 11-1. (Reference section: Preschool)

Case Study with Critical Thinking Questions

You are the nurse in a preschool clinic, working with a nurse practitioner. A 4-year-old girl comes in for a well checkup. The parents state she is "doing great." Their only concerns are occasional "bad language" and that she still sucks her thumb.

1. What advice needs to be given?

2. What other anticipatory guidance is needed for a child of this age?

Internet Activity

Explore the Internet and find sites that provide information on the concepts of growth and development related to the preschooler, including safety, play, and preschool advice.

Self-Assessment—Chapter 12

Student Name _____

Date _____

DISORDERS OF THE PRESCHOOL CHILD

Matching Questions

1. ___ smallpox
2. ___ rubeola
3. ___ partial thromboplastin time
4. ___ prodrome
5. ___ amblyopia
6. ___ simple partial motor seizure
7. ___ autograft
8. ___ Gower maneuver
9. ___ PL 94-142
10. ___ morphology

a. vision loss caused by confusing retinal images
b. structure of cells
c. characteristic movement of children with muscular dystrophy
d. time immediately before the onset of a communicable disease
e. potential bioterrorism agent
f. Education for All Handicapped Children Act
g. helps determine the blood factor VIII level
h. measles
i. area of undamaged skin used to cover a burn wound
j. muscle movements involving face, neck, and extremities

Multiple Choice

1. Patching the unaffected eye is a method of treatment for amblyopia because it:
   1. forces the weaker eye to function
   2. automatically enlarges the pupil of the opposite eye
   3. decreases abnormal eye muscle movement
   4. decreases sensory input to the brain
2. When the nurse is planning care for the child who has had surgery to remove the tonsils and adenoids, a major goal is to:
   1. prevent hemorrhage
   2. decrease dehydration
   3. prevent pneumonia
   4. control activity
3. First-aid measures during a tonic-clonic seizure are based on the understanding that the child:
   1. is aware of what is happening
   2. might injure others
   3. is unconscious
   4. has control over muscle action
4. Nursing care for a child with encephalitis includes which of the following?
   1. monitoring intravenous fluids
   2. providing a quiet environment
   3. providing seizure precautions
   4. all of the above
5. When teaching the parents about home management of the child with nephrotic syndrome, the nurse emphasizes:
   1. daily blood pressure measurements
   2. strict activity restrictions
   3. very low-sodium diet
   4. accurate testing for urine protein
6. Which of the following symptoms might indicate urinary tract infection in an infant?
   1. frequency, urgency
   2. poor feeding, unexplained fever
   3. flank pain, chills
   4. incontinence, foul-smelling urine
7. A mother calls to report that her 8-year-old has chickenpox. Her children have not been immunized. She wants to know about how long it will be before his 5-year-old sister gets them. You tell her:
   1. 7 to 10 days
   2. 2 to 6 days
   3. 14 to 48 days
   4. 10 to 21 days
8. An important intervention for infants who have developmental disabilities is to:
   1. have them institutionalized as soon as possible
   2. help the parents realize that their child will never develop further
   3. stress the importance of early infant stimulation programs
   4. have children reevaluated at 2 years to confirm the diagnosis
9. Whooping cough (pertussis) consists of what symptoms?
   1. brassy cough, worse at night
   2. loose, wet productive cough that patient recovers from easily
   3. paroxysms of several sharp coughs in one expiration followed by a whoop
   4. coughing that responds to nebulizer treatment

10. The common symptoms for acute poststreptococcal glomerulonephritis are:
    1. increased urine output with marked periorbital edema
    2. urine may be clear but child has painful urination
    3. diarrhea, nausea, and vomiting accompanied with a high fever
    4. bloody or smoky urine that is decreased in output

11. Duchenne muscular dystrophy:
    1. is a random occurrence
    2. is sex-linked, with the mother as the carrier
    3. only occurs in girls
    4. can be contagious

12. Which statement about smallpox is true?
    1. Lesions appear on the palms and soles.
    2. Lesions first appear on the face or trunk.
    3. Lesions are superficial vesicles.
    4. There is no fever before the rash.

Study Questions

1. Discuss the preoperative teaching and postoperative care for the child who is undergoing tonsillectomy and adenoidectomy. (Reference section: Tonsillitis and Adenoiditis)

2. Discuss clinical signs and symptoms of the child with leukemia (reference section: Leukemia)

3. Compare the symptoms and rash characteristics of the following communicable diseases: chickenpox, measles, German measles, roseola, and fifth disease. (Reference section: Communicable Diseases and Table 12-7)

4. Discuss several nursing measures to help a toddler with nephrotic syndrome eat. (Reference section: Nephrotic Syndrome)

Case Study with Critical Thinking Questions

A 5-year-old has full-thickness burns on his legs after mimicking his older brother by stomping out a camp fire. He weighs 24 kg.

1. Discuss the initial ABCs of this child's care. Include the IV fluid volume calculation for the first 24 hours of care based on his weight.

2. Devise a nursing care plan for his initial care, including wound management, nutrition, and pain control.

Internet Activity

Explore sites for children with cancer. Include reliable resources/sites for parental use.

Student Name _____

Date _____

THE SCHOOL-AGE CHILD

Matching Questions

1. ___ 6 years
2. ___ 7 years
3. ___ 8 years
4. ___ 9 years
5. ___ 10 years
6. ___ 11 to 12 years
7. ___ sibling rivalry
8. ___ self-image

a. emotional conflict between brothers and sisters
b. period of complete disorganization
c. can be bossy, rude, sensitive to criticism
d. beginning of preadolescence
e. easiest age to teach
f. group fads begin, hero worship is evident
g. how a person perceives himself or herself
h. worries, compulsions, and nervous habits may be common

Multiple Choice

1. Erikson believes that the school-age child is in the stage of:
   1. self-esteem versus shame and doubt
   2. identity versus identity confusion
   3. industry versus inferiority
   4. autonomy versus inferiority

2. According to Piaget (cognitive development), the school-age child:
   1. thinks and reasons in concrete terms
   2. thinks and reasons in abstract terms
   3. thinks and reasons in philosophical terms
   4. thinks and reasons in preoperational terms

3. The best guidelines to use when answering children's questions related to sex include:
   1. answering questions simply and at the child's level of understanding
   2. answering questions with complex terms because the school-age child is old enough to understand
   3. answering questions in a matter-of-fact way so that the child does not become embarrassed
   4. deferring questions back to the child's teachers because they are better at answering these types of questions

4. The American Academy of Pediatrics suggests how much television viewing per day by school-age children?
   1. none
   2. 1 to 2 hours
   3. 2 to 3 hours
   4. 3 to 4 hours

5. An advantage of playing video games includes:
   1. dominating leisure time
   2. promotion of eye-hand coordination
   3. teaching acceptance of violence
   4. promotion of competition among friends

6. A 7-year-old girl is caught stealing. Which course of recommended action should her mother take?
   1. tell her how wrong she was and what a bad child she is
   2. tell her what she did wrong and that she must return the item to the store with an apology
   3. tell her it is okay to steal only when she really needs something and cannot afford it
   4. tell her in front of the store manager that she has done a terrible thing and certainly was not brought up this way

7. A 9-year-old boy has been repeatedly biting his fingernails at school. His mother wants advice on how to handle this problem. The best advice is to tell her:
   1. this is a normal nervous habit that will disappear when tension disappears
   2. this is a dangerous habit and should discuss the problem with her physician
   3. she should ignore the problem because "all kids do it"
   4. this is not normal for a child this age and he must be having emotional problems

8. A 10-year-old child whose parents are going through a divorce will likely demonstrate:
   1. open grieving
   2. uncontrollable crying in the classroom
   3. hatred toward the teacher
   4. school performance problems

9. Children in which of the following age groups begin to use the clock for practical purposes and to use cursive writing?
   1. 6 years
   2. 7 years
   3. 8 to 9 years
   4. 10 to 12 years

10. Children in which of the following age groups can think about social problems and see others' points of view?
  1. 6 years
  2. 7 years
  3. 8 to 9 years
  4. 10 to 12 years

Study Questions

1. Discuss activities enjoyed by the child of 8 years. What diversion would you suggest for the long-term patient of this age? (Reference section: Eight Years)

2. Plan a day's menu for the school-age child. What foods should be included? (Reference section: Nutrition)

3. Investigate after-school programs in your community. What types of guidance/activities are provided? What is the cost involved? (Reference section: Latchkey Children)

Case Study with Critical Thinking Questions

You are the elementary school nurse.

1. How will you determine whether health needs are being met for children in your school? What resources are available if needs are not being met?

2. Develop a teaching plan for a parent who wants to introduce measures to prevent child abduction for a specific age group.

3. What signs might a child demonstrate when being bullied? What are some of the interventions that the school nurse could initiate?

Internet Activity

Using the Internet, investigate drug abuse prevention in your community.

Student Name _____

Date _____

DISORDERS OF THE SCHOOL-AGE CHILD

Matching Questions

1. ___ hyperglycemia
2. ___ peak expiratory flow rate
3. ___ nystagmus
4. ___ avascular necrosis
5. ___ McBurney's point
6. ___ pediculosis
7. ___ hemoprophylaxis
8. ___ "gel" phenomenon
9. ___ polydipsia
10. ___ psychosomatic
11. ___ glargine

a. midway between the umbilicus and the right iliac crest
b. bone tissue death from inadequate blood supply
c. thirst
d. preventing disease with medications
e. low blood sugar
f. force of expiration from maximum lung inflation
g. dysfunctions with an organic and emotional component
h. constant jerky motion of the eyeball
i. stiffness after a period of inactivity
j. head lice
k. long-acting insulin that cannot be mixed with other insulins

Multiple Choice

1. A 6-year-old is admitted to the hospital with wheezing. He was well until a few days ago, when he developed a cold. Which of the following signs and symptoms suggest that he has respiratory distress?
   1. cough, fever, sore throat
   2. flushed, skin, thirst, increased breathing
   3. decreased pulse, restlessness, clammy skin
   4. retractions, increased respirations, pallor

2. A child is diagnosed with asthma. The nurse needs to administer albuterol via nebulizer every 20 minutes. Albuterol is:
   1. a bronchodilator
   2. an antiinflammatory
   3. a cough suppressant
   4. an antiallergenic agent

3. Which of the following is a long-term nursing goal for a child with asthma?
   1. maintaining hydration
   2. appropriate home monitoring of respiratory status
   3. decreasing exercise
   4. oxygen saturation of 92%

4. Which of the following are major manifestations of acute rheumatic fever, according to the Jones criteria?
   1. fever, evidence of a previous streptococcal infection
   2. carditis, subcutaneous nodules
   3. elevated ESR and ASO
   4. arthralgia, ECG changes

5. An 8-year-old boy is receiving radiation therapy for treatment of a brain tumor. Which of the following would be an appropriate intervention to address his major body image concerns?
   1. encourage increased protein in his diet
   2. administer antinausea medications before treatment
   3. erase the pen marks on his head
   4. allow him to wear his favorite baseball hat

6. A 12-year-old girl has juvenile rheumatoid arthritis, polyarticular type. Which of the following is the best advice to give to help her cope successfully with the school day? Tell her to:
   1. not go to school when she does not feel well
   2. allow a lot of extra time in the morning to get ready for school
   3. get up and walk around the classroom if she feel stiff
   4. take a warm shower after gym

7. The major pathophysiological difference between type 1 and type 2 diabetes is that:
   1. children with type 2 never need insulin
   2. children with type 1 can take insulin orally
   3. type 1 results from pancreatic islet cell destruction
   4. affected children with type 1 are obese

8. When the nurse reviews nutritional management with a school-age child with type 1 diabetes, which of the following would be an expected outcome?
   1. strict adherence to the prescribed diet
   2. complete avoidance of sweets
   3. appropriate choices of a wide variety of foods
   4. no episodes of hypoglycemia

9. The three hallmarks of attention deficit with hyperactivity disorder are:
   1. organization, intelligence, and distractibility
   2. impulsivity, excess energy, and inattention
   3. poor school performance, dyslexia, and poor gross motor skills
   4. learning disability, below-average IQ, and difficulty communicating

10. Head lice can be transmitted by:
  1. sitting next to a child with lice
  2. wearing the headphones of a child with lice
  3. spraying hairspray used by child with lice
  4. using the shampoo used by child with lice

Study Questions

1. Describe what factors could precipitate an attack of asthma. (Reference section: Asthma)

2. Demonstrate how to measure the PEFR and explain what the results may mean. (Reference section: Asthma)

3. What factors would you consider when determining whether a 9-year-old is ready to administer her own insulin? How would you best teach her this skill? (Reference section: Insulin-Dependent Mellitus)

4. A young girl has joined the school softball team, which practices twice a week after school. How will this affect her diabetes? What factors would you consider when providing anticipatory guidance to her and her parents regarding this new activity? (Reference section: Insulin-Dependent Mellitus)

5. A 7-year-old has a brain tumor. He wishes to go to summer camp for children with cancer. How would you help the family prepare him for camp? Discuss both the physical and psychological considerations. (Reference section: Brain Tumors)

Case Study with Critical Thinking Questions

A 9-year-old girl has been recently admitted to the hospital for juvenile rheumatoid arthritis. Her parents are very concerned with the drugs she is receiving. They have heard over the years that children are not to take aspirin, but their daughter is receiving this medication.

1. What information can you tell the parents to relive their anxiety?

2. The parents also express concern about how they are going to take care of their daughter when she is discharged. Develop a home care plan for this child, including activities.

Internet Activity

Use the Internet to find information about juvenile arthritis. Visit www.arthritis.org and select the section on juvenile arthritis. What information did you find? Is there information that would be helpful to parents?

Student Name _____

Date _____

THE ADOLESCENT

Matching Questions

1. ___ asynchrony
2. ___ adolescence
3. ___ sense of identity
4. ___ preadolescence
5. ___ puberty
6. ___ menarche
7. ___ androgens
8. ___ estrogens

a. developmental stage in Erikson's theory
b. male hormones
c. onset of menstruation
d. different body parts mature at different rates
e. to "grow up"
f. female hormones
g. marked by rapid changes in the structure and function of various parts of the body
h. reproductive organs become functional

Multiple Choice

1. The years of greatest turmoil for most families include those of:
   1. preadolescence
   2. early adolescence
   3. middle adolescence
   4. late adolescence
2. Which of the following statements is *true* regarding puberty?
   1. Puberty begins around age 15 years in both boys and girls.
   2. Puberty occurs about 2 years earlier in girls than in boys.
   3. Puberty occurs about 2 years earlier in boys than in girls.
   4. Puberty begins around age 14 years in boys.
3. The first sign of puberty in boys is usually:
   1. enlargement of the testes
   2. the beginning of nocturnal emissions
   3. production of sperm
   4. changes in the voice
4. Which of the following statements best describes how parents should act with regard to limit setting during adolescence?
   1. Limit setting is not necessary because teens are very responsible individuals.
   2. Limit setting is essential because teens still need guidance.
   3. Limit setting is a waste of time because most teens will do what they want anyway.
   4. Limit setting is necessary only in certain situations.
5. When adolescents can see a situation from many points of view and can imagine or organize unseen or unexperienced possibilities, they are said to be in the stage of:
   1. concrete operations
   2. postconventional thinking
   3. identity versus role confusion
   4. formal operations
6. Iron is an essential element in a teenager's diet. Which of the following are good sources of iron?
   1. oysters and nuts
   2. milk and cheese
   3. hamburgers and french fries
   4. fish and dried beans
7. A healthy lunch that meets mineral needs and avoids high fat intake for a teenager would include:
   1. skim milk, tuna on wheat bread, and salad
   2. chocolate milkshake, hamburger on a bun, and french fries
   3. cola drink, roast beef sandwich, and chips
   4. whole milk, hamburger on a bun, and salad
8. Confidentiality cannot be maintained by the physician if:
   1. the adolescent has questions about birth control
   2. the adolescent has questions regarding nocturnal emissions
   3. the adolescent is so angry that he or she is considering running away
   4. the adolescent has questions regarding HIV
9. A 15-year-old girl is taller than everyone in her class. During a health examination, she tells the nurse that she feels everyone is always staring at her and she does not want to go to school anymore. The nurse's best response would be to say:
   1. "That is okay. It will not be that way forever."
   2. "Everyone feels that way at some point during adolescence."
   3. "Just ignore everyone. That will make you feel better."
   4. "Tell me more about your feelings."

10. Which of the following age groups often participate in activities that center around teen nightclubs and rock concerts?
    1. early adolescence
    2. middle adolescence
    3. late adolescence
    4. early adulthood

Study Questions

1. A boy and a girl are each beginning to establish a sense of identity. What does this mean? How may this development be reflected in their behavior? (Reference section: Development Theories)

2. Investigate a babysitting course in your area and discuss what information is presented to adolescents regarding babysitting skills. (Reference section: Responsibility)

3. Plan a day's menu for a 15-year-old girl and a 17-year-old boy. What are the nutritional requirements in terms of calories, protein, calcium, and iron? (Reference section: Nutrition)

Case Study with Critical Thinking Questions

You are the high school nurse.

1. What are the needs of the teenagers in your school?

2. What resources do you have to help meet their needs?

Internet Activity

Explore the Internet and find sites that provide information on anticipatory guidance with the adolescent.

Student Name _____

Date _____

DISORDERS OF THE ADOLESCENT

Matching Questions

1. ___ arthroscopy
2. ___ bulimia
3. ___ Reed-Sternberg cell
4. ___ sebum
5. ___ polypharmacy
6. ___ amenorrhea
7. ___ Harrington rods
8. ___ RICE
9. ___ Epstein-Barr virus
10. ___ Accutane

a. double-nucleated cell that is diagnostic for Hodgkin's disease
b. cause of infectious mononucleosis
c. surgical procedure designed to assess joint damage
d. absence of menses
e. initial treatment of soft tissue injury
f. systemic treatment for severe acne
g. use of several drugs together
h. binge eating
i. instrumentation used to repair scoliosis
j. fatty substance secreted by the sebaceous follicles

Multiple Choice

1. An important nursing goal for the adolescent required to be in a shell brace for the treatment of scoliosis is:
   1. restoring normal spine curvature
   2. maintaining normal activity levels
   3. decreasing pain
   4. ensuring compliance
2. When screening for scoliosis, the nurse looks at the child from front and back to determine:
   1. symmetry
   2. degree of curve
   3. flexibility
   4. muscle spasm
3. An important clue that might tell the nurse there is a problem with a particular sports activity is:
   1. the coach demands that all team members sit on the ground when an athlete has been injured
   2. boys and girls are playing on the same team
   3. a limping player is removed from the game for the day
   4. 10-year-old and 14-year-old boys are playing on the same team
4. A major difference in the clinical manifestations of adolescents with anorexia nervosa and those with bulimia is:
   1. binge eating
   2. body image distortion
   3. purging
   4. decreased self-esteem
5. Which of the following is the most frequently seen sexually transmitted disease in the United States?
   1. syphilis
   2. gonorrhea
   3. *Chlamydia*
   4. genital herpes

6. When reviewing the prevention of STDs with sexually active adolescent girls, it is important to tell them that:
   1. all STDs can be prevented through condom use
   2. if their sexual partner is not symptomatic, disease is unlikely
   3. having sex with only one partner usually is safe
   4. they should request routine *Chlamydia* and *Gonorrhea* cultures
7. An adolescent who is a model is being treated with chemotherapy for cancer. She is particularly concerned about what the medications will do to her appearance. An important nursing intervention for her would be to:
   1. help her pick out a wig, eyebrow pencil, and false eyelashes before treatment begins
   2. reassure her that she will be beautiful even without hair
   3. tell her that the chemotherapy probably will not affect her appearance
   4. advise her that her hair will probably grow back in curly
8. A teacher in a school where you are the school nurse shows you a poem written as a class assignment by a student. In the poem, the student has expressed a desire to "end it all." Your first action should be to:
   1. ignore it because it is just poetry
   2. ask the student, "Are you planning to kill yourself?"
   3. alert the student's parents
   4. ask the teacher whether the student is really suicidal

Study Questions

1. A young male wants to join the high school swimming team. What health factors need to be considered in investigating this possibility? (Reference section: Sports Injuries)

2. You are working with a very obese 13-year-old. His favorite foods are french fries and Coca-Cola. What nutritional principles would you discuss with him? How does "being fat" alter his psychosocial development? (Reference section: Obesity)

3. An 18-year-old girl has anorexia nervosa. Define this condition and its causes. What approach would you take when meeting with her for the first time? Discuss the reasons for your approach. (Reference section: Anorexia Nervosa)

4. A 17-year-old star basketball player has seemed unusually tired. His mother says he has had a sore throat for several weeks. After examination by a physician, a diagnosis of infectious mononucleosis is made. What laboratory test would support this diagnosis? Outline the nursing management for this condition. (Reference section: Infectious Mononucleosis)

Case Study with Critical Thinking Questions

A 13-year-old who has been diagnosed with scoliosis is being admitted to the hospital. Admission information indicates that she was identified with this problem at the age of 10 years and that she has been wearing a brace for the past 3 years. She has indicated that she does not like to wear the brace because it makes her "look funny," and her mother has indicated that compliance with wearing the brace has been a problem. Her orthopedic physician has decided to perform a surgical procedure (TSRH) on the patient because of the progressive curvature. She is scheduled for the surgical procedure in 2 days. You are to develop a preoperative teaching plan.

1. What issues—preoperative, intraoperative, and postoperative—should be covered during this part of the teaching?

2. After her surgical procedure, what issues should be addressed in preparing the child for discharge?

Internet Activity

1. Explore the National Institute on Drug Abuse website (www.nida.nih.gov) for information related to substance abuse. What are the current statistics for marijuana use with preadolescents and adolescents? What are some of the common street names for this drug? From this site, explore other links to related topics.
2. What sites are available to parents and adolescents regarding eating disorders? To start, visit the website for the behavioral health department of the St. Francis Health System (www.laureate.com/behaviorhealth). In addition, visit www.edap.org, the website for Eating Disorder Awareness and Prevention, Inc.

Student Name _____

Date _____

PEDIATRIC PROCEDURES

Matching Questions

1. ___ metabolic rate
2. ___ nomogram
3. ___ tepid baths
4. ___ gastrostomy feeding
5. ___ heel warmer
6. ___ nasopharyngeal culture
7. ___ fever
8. ___ 1 mL
9. ___ enema
10. ___ half-strength hydrogen peroxide

a. should take 20 to 25 minutes to complete
b. temperature should not exceed 42° C
c. rules out pertussis
d. maximum volume administered to one site via IM route
e. used for temperature over 104° F
f. body temperature above 38° C
g. increases 10% for every 1° C
h. calculates body surface area
i. used to clean tracheal stoma
j. should be administered over 10 to 15 minutes

Multiple Choice

1. The age group that benefits most from explanations through drawings, pictures, and contact with equipment is the:
   1. toddler group
   2. preschool group
   3. school-age group
   4. adolescent group
2. The rule of thumb for urine output is:
   1. 0.5-2 mL/kg/hr
   2. 3-4 mL/kg/hr
   3. 5-6 mL/kg/hr
   4. 10-12 mL/kg/hr
3. For which of the following must children be monitored after a spinal tap?
   1. fever, CSF leakage, and headache
   2. use of playtime, headache, and urine output
   3. urine output, fever, and headache
   4. naptime, headache, and decrease in appetite
4. Subcutaneous medication is administered using a
   1. 21-gauge, 1-inch needle
   2. 23-gauge, $^5/_8$-inch needle
   3. 25-gauge, $^1/_2$-inch needle
   4. 27-gauge, 1-inch needle
5. The best procedure to follow if an infant clenches the eyes shut when you are administering eyedrops is to:
   1. call the doctor
   2. apply the drops in the nasal corner where the lids meet
   3. try to open the eyelids and administer
   4. notify the charge nurse

6. The recommended injection site for children less than 2 years of age is the:
   1. dorsogluteal site
   2. ventrogluteal site
   3. vastus lateralis site
   4. deltoid site
7. Thrombosis, hyperglycemia, and contamination are all potential complications of which therapy?
   1. TPN
   2. intravenous infusion
   3. gastrostomy feedings
   4. IM medications
8. During a spinal tap procedure, the nurse should be constantly assessing the child's:
   1. spine alignment
   2. respiratory status
   3. crying
   4. temperature
9. When the nurse is suctioning a tracheostomy, suction should be held no longer than:
   1. 5 seconds
   2. 15 seconds
   3. 25 seconds
   4. 35 seconds
10. Signs of inadequate oxygenation include:
    1. increased restlessness, decreased pulse oximetry, and increased respiratory rate
    2. decreased restlessness, increased pulse oximetry, and increased respiratory rate
    3. increased restlessness, increased pulse oximetry, and increased respiratory rate
    4. increased restlessness, decreased pulse oximetry, and decreased respiratory rate

Study Questions

1. What special precaution must be taken when giving medications to children? Explore a drug circular and the information provided for administering this drug to a child. Is the information adequate for your purposes? Discuss how and where medications are charted in your hospital. Are there differences between documentation of a medication to a child and an adult? (Reference section: Administrating Medications)

2. A 6-month-old has an order for obtaining a sterile urine culture. The mother is extremely anxious and tearful. This is her first child and the child's first hospitalization. Discuss what you will need to explain to the mother regarding the procedure. How can you reduce the mother's anxiety? Outline the steps for obtaining a culture from this infant.

Case Study with Critical Thinking Questions

A 12-month-old girl is scheduled for a lumbar puncture (spinal tap). The child is extremely fearful of any health care providers. She screams and kicks and bites. The mother is very anxious and tearful.

1. What approach is needed for the child?

2. What approach is needed for the mother?

3. What steps are necessary during this procedure?

Student Name _____

Date _____

END-OF-LIFE CARE FOR CHILDREN AND THEIR FAMILIES

Matching Questions

1. ___ palliative care
2. ___ anticipatory grief
3. ___ anxiolytics
4. ___ grief
5. ___ pain

a. whatever the person experiencing it says it is and existing whenever he or she says it does
b. a functional category of drugs used in the treatment of anxiety that do not cause excessive sedation
c. occurs before the loss
d. subjective and unique to the individual
e. care and comfort at the end of life

Multiple Choice

1. Which of the following children would realize death is permanent?
   1. a 2-year-old who sees a dead puppy
   2. a 4-year-old whose grandmother dies
   3. a child in kindergarten who hears his friend's grandfather has died
   4. a 10-year-old whose classmate dies of complications from a medical condition
2. Which age group sees death as a person (personification of death)?
   1. toddler
   2. preschool
   3. school-age
   4. adolescent
3. In dealing with death, which of the following would be the most positive way for a nurse to cope?
   1. becoming secluded from family and friends
   2. isolating herself from her peers
   3. discussing the event with her supervisor
   4. relating the story to several of her friends
4. The death of a child will change the dynamics of the family because:
   1. death is final
   2. the parents disagree
   3. siblings will resent the attention given to the dying child
   4. death is an event when new mechanisms for coping need to be established
5. Anticipatory grief begins:
   1. at the time of death
   2. during the dying process
   3. during the funeral
   4. after the loss

6. Shortness of breath and dyspnea can lead to the feeling of "air hunger." Which medication can help with this discomfort?
   1. Tylenol
   2. morphine
   3. glycerin suppository
   4. Phenergan
7. Nursing care for a 4-year-old who is dying will be based on the knowledge that:
   1. he has no understanding of death
   2. the nurse should provide all the care
   3. his primary fear is separation from his parents
   4. he is too young to sense his parents' anxiety
8. As a dying child's condition deteriorates, the mother angrily shouts at the nurse, "This isn't fair. Why can't you do something?" The most appropriate response by the nurse would be:
   1. "I will not discuss this until you can calm down."
   2. "Please calm down. You are upsetting your daughter."
   3. "You are right. This is not fair. What would you like me to do?"
   4. "Being angry is not going to help anyone. Now what can I help you with?"
9. A dying child's desire is to be at home, and a referral is made to hospice. The goal of hospice is to:
   1. provide for the physical needs of the child
   2. teach the family how to care for the child
   3. enhance the quality of life that remains
   4. provide all the care so the family can rest
10. As death is approaching, the child's respirations become labored and noisy. Nursing care at this time would be to:
    1. do deep suctioning
    2. let the family know this is expected
    3. give the child something to drink
    4. call the physician

Study Questions

1. How will the child and family express their psychological and social needs? (Reference section: Table 18-2)

2. In discussing a 4-year-old child's knowledge of death, what can you tell the parents regarding the child's understanding of death? (Reference section: Table 18-3)

3. What is a cause of the cool hands and feet that the dying child will have? (Reference section: Box 18-3)

Case Study with Critical Thinking Questions

An 8-year-old boy has a diagnosis of advanced lymphoma. A bone marrow transplant has been unsuccessful. There is no longer a hope for a cure, and the disease is advancing at a rapid rate. The parents are undecided about what and when to tell their child.

1. How can you help the parents?

2. How can you help the child?

3. What reaction would you expect from the child when he is told that he is dying?

4. When is the most appropriate time to discuss death with the patient?

5. When would you recommend the referral be made to hospice?

Internet Activity

Explore hospice organizations online such as HospiceNet (www.hospicenet.org) or Hospice International (www.chionline.org). Explore websites of support groups such as The Compassionate Friends (www.compassionatefriends.org).